D0894409

AIDS: Plague or Panic?

AIDS: Plague or Panic?

AN EDITORIALS ON FILE BOOK

EDITOR: Oliver Trager

Facts On File Publications
New York, New York • Oxford, England

AIDS: Plague or Panic?

Published by Facts On File, Inc.
460 Park Ave. South, New York, N.Y. 10016
© Copyright 1988 by Facts On File, Inc.

Library of Congress Cataloging-in-Publication Data

Main entry under title:

AIDS: plague or panic/ editor, Oliver Trager.

p. cm -- (An Editorials on file book)
Includes Index
Summary: A collection of editorials on the AIDS crisis and its implications for the nation.

ISBN: 0-8160-1938-X
1. AIDS, (Disease)--United States. 2. American newspapers-
- Sections, columns, etc.--Editorials. [1. AIDS (Disease)]
I. Trager, Oliver   II. Series   88-6889
RC607.A26A3487 1988   CIP
362.1'9697'92009--dc 19   AC

Printed In The United States of America

9 8 7 6 5 4 3 2 1

14307

CONTENTS

Preface 1

Part I:
AIDS Research and the Public Health Response 2

Research '83, Blood Transfusions, French Research, Research '84, Africa, Research '85, AZT '86, Infection Projections, New England Journal of Medicine Report, AZT '87, Health Workers Infected

Part II:
AIDS and the Reagan Administration Response 44

AIDS Funds, Koop Responds to the Crisis, Justice Department Sets Guidelines, Reagan Addresses the AIDS Issue, 3rd AIDS Parley Held, Reagan Names AIDS Panel, Leaders Quit AIDS Panel

Part III:
AIDS, Education and Schools 94

Schoolchildren With AIDS Becomes an Issue, AIDS Education, Ryan White Returns to School, AIDS Rocks Arcadia, Florida

Part IV:
AIDS and the Law 124

AIDS in the Prisons, AIDS Testing in the Military Ordered, AIDS Testing 1985-1987, Immigrant AIDS Testing Considered, Insurance Companies React to Crisis, Supreme Court Rules on Georgia Sodomy Law, Supreme Court Rules on Contagious Diseases, House Backs Catastriphic Health Plan

Part V:
AIDS and American Lifestyles 172

AMA Sets Guidelines, Bathhouses Ordered Shut, Concern Sweeps Nation, Rock Hudson Dies, AIDS and Narcotics Addicts, Condom Ads Broadcast

Index 213

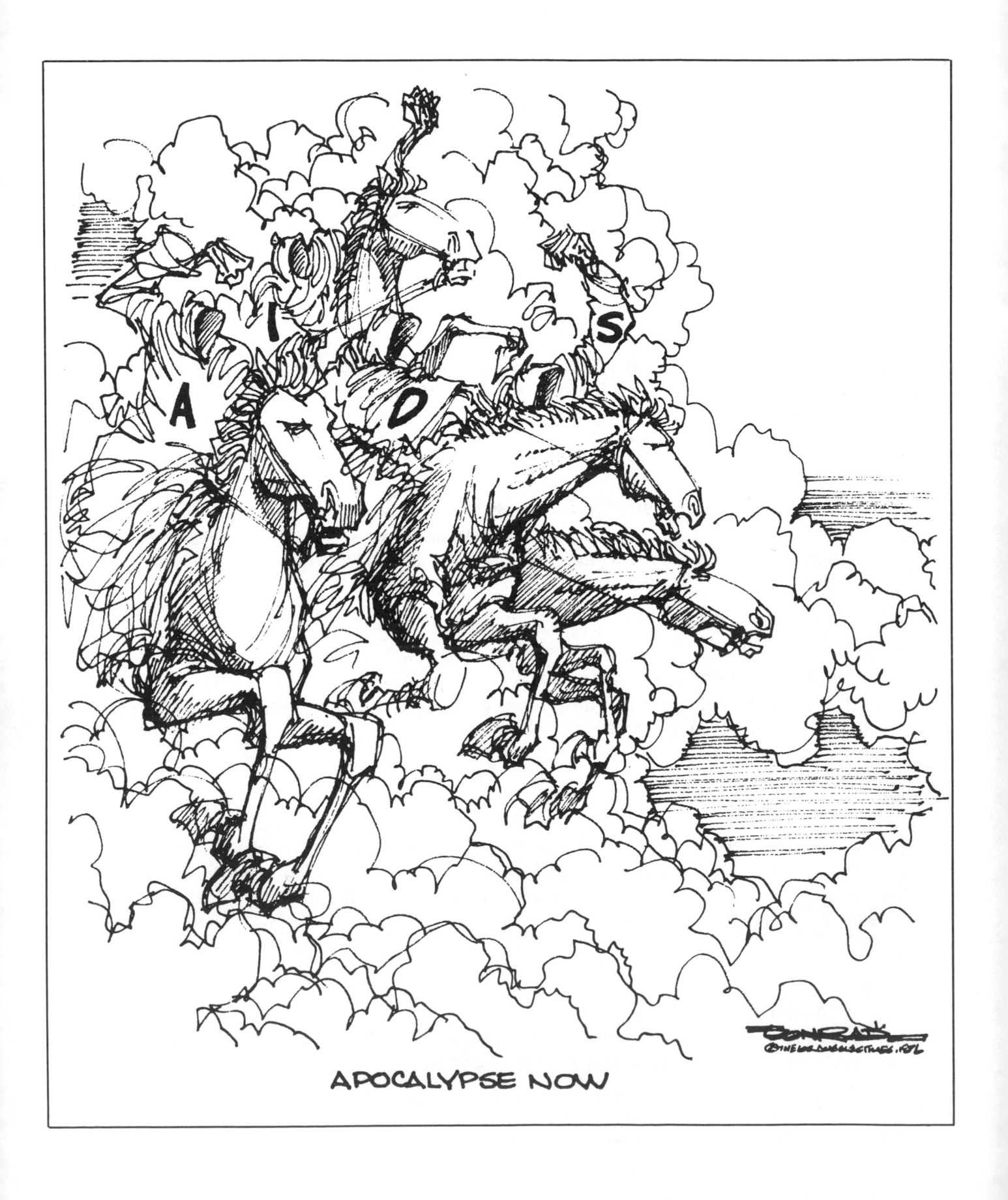

APOCALYPSE NOW

Preface

In September 1987, the Centers for Disease Control in Atlanta announced that 25,000 lives had been claimed by Acquired Immune Deficiency Syndrome, or AIDS, in the United States since the first cases were detected in 1981. In addition, officials estimated that as many as 1.5 million Americans had been infected by the virus that causes AIDS. Contradicting the initial public perception of AIDS as a male homosexual disease, 7% of all reported cases were women, 2% were recipients of blood transfusions and 10,000 people had contracted AIDS through the intravenous use of illicit drugs.

The controversy surrounding the tragic emergence of AIDS has shaded virtually every aspect of American public and private life. The educational and legal systems, health care departments, insurance companies, broadcasting companies, hospitals, the medical establishment and even the federal government are all faced with questions that are new, confusing and frightening. For instance, should AIDS testing be mandatory and what are the implications for society as a whole if it is? Should schoolchildren infected with the AIDS virus be allowed to attend school? How do recent Supreme Court decisions affect the rights of AIDS victims or members of high-risk groups? Should condom advertising be allowed to run on television? Have the sexual habits of the American public changed since awareness of AIDS has become widespread? What of the ethics of doctors and other health care workers who refuse to treat AIDS patients for fear of becoming infected themselves? Has the Reagan administration's concentration on sexual abstinence as the primary way to avoid infection helped slow the spread of AIDS? What of the new drugs that have shown promise and the problem of making them available to AIDS sufferers? Should awareness of AIDS be incorporated into our schools' sex education curriculums?

AIDS is one of the most serious epidemics to confront modern medicine and is now a commonly encountered clinical problem, especially in the cities. As the incidence of the disease has grown, so has its coverage in the media. Although the enormous amount of information conveyed is often incomplete, taken out of context, tainted by social prejudice or premature in its optimism, the information has helped physicians, researchers, politicians and others in battling this major health dilemma.

As the national preoccupation with the AIDS question reaches a peak, *AIDS: Plague or Panic?* takes a look at the AIDS crisis and its implications for the nation.

April, 1988   Oliver Trager

Part I: AIDS Research and the Public Health Response

Since its initial description in 1981, Acquired Immune Deficiency Syndrome, or AIDS, has become a major public health problem in the United States. Although other epidemics in recorded history have killed many more people, AIDS presents a unique challenge to the public health and medical community, political leaders and the general public.

AIDS is a unique condition marked by a collapse of the body's immune system and a consequent vulnerability to infections that healthy people are usually able to fight off. A person who is sick with AIDS is in the final stages of a series of health problems caused by the AIDS. The virus can be passed from one person to another chiefly during sexual contact or through contact with infected blood, as in the sharing of intravenous drug needles and syringes used for injecting drugs. Scientists have named the AIDS virus HIV, HTLV-III or LAV. These abbreviations denote a virus that attacks white blood cells (T-lymphocytes) in the human blood. The AIDS virus attacks a person's immune system and damages its ability to fight off other disease. Without a functioning immune system, the victim is vulnerable to infection by bacteria, other viruses and other microorganisms that may cause life-threatening illness, such as pneumonia and cancer. There is presently no cure for AIDS and no vaccine to prevent it.

It is necessary to understand how the normal immune system works if one is to understand the malfunction of an immune system damaged by AIDS. When the AIDS virus enters the blood-stream, it begins to attack certain white blood cells, the T-lymphocytes. Substances called antibodies are produced by the body in response to invasions by alien substances. The antibodies produced in response to the AIDS virus can be detected by a simple blood test, usually two weeks to two months after infection. But even before the antibody test is positive, the victim can pass the virus to others during sexual contact or through the sharing of intravenous drug paraphernalia. But, for reasons not yet understood, the antibodies in the blood of carriers of the AIDS virus fail to check the damage caused by the virus, which is by then present in large numbers in the body. Researchers still do not know why the AIDS virus is not destroyed by the body's immune system.

Once an individual is infected, there are several possibilities. Some people remain well, but even so they are able to infect others. Others develop a disease less serious than AIDS referred to as AIDS Related Complex or ARC. In some people the protective immune system may be destroyed by the AIDS virus and then other germs and microorganisms that ordinarily would never get a foothold cause "opportunistic diseases"—using the *opportunity* of lowered resistence to infect and destroy. Some of the most common opportunistic diseases are *Pneumocystis carinii* pneumonia and tuberculosis. Individuals infected with the AIDS virus may also develop certain types of cancers such as Kaposi's sarcoma. Evidence shows that the AIDS virus may also attack the nervous system, causing damage to the brain.

In September 1986, health officials cautiously announced a new drug, azidothymidine (AZT), which showed promise in the treatment of some types of AIDS infection. Although by no means a cure for AIDS, AZT was widely publicized as a possible breakthrough in the fight against AIDS.

In all but a few notable exceptions, the story of the battle against AIDS is also the story of international cooperation at its best as efforts to develop viral inhibitors and therapies for the specific symptoms and infections progress. Until an effective prevention or treatment is made available, transmission of the AIDS virus can be reduced only by avoidance of certain risk-taking behaviors, such as intravenous drug abuse and promiscuous sexual behavior, both heterosexual and homosexual. Another factor that has contributed to preventing the spread of the disease is the screening of blood and blood products, organs for transplant and other biological materials.

Although AIDS is still a mysterious disease in many ways, scientists have learned a great deal about it. In the five years that it has been seriously researched scientists have come to know more about it than they do about many diseases that have been studied even longer. Presumably, research will ultimately reveal answers to the question of AIDS prevention and treatment. As is often the case in the aftermath of disasters, the lessons learned in dealing with a crisis will provide benefits to both sufferers and society in general. The knowledge gained in immunology, virology and other branches of science will assist research on cancer and on neurologic and rheumatic diseases, thus benefiting all mankind.

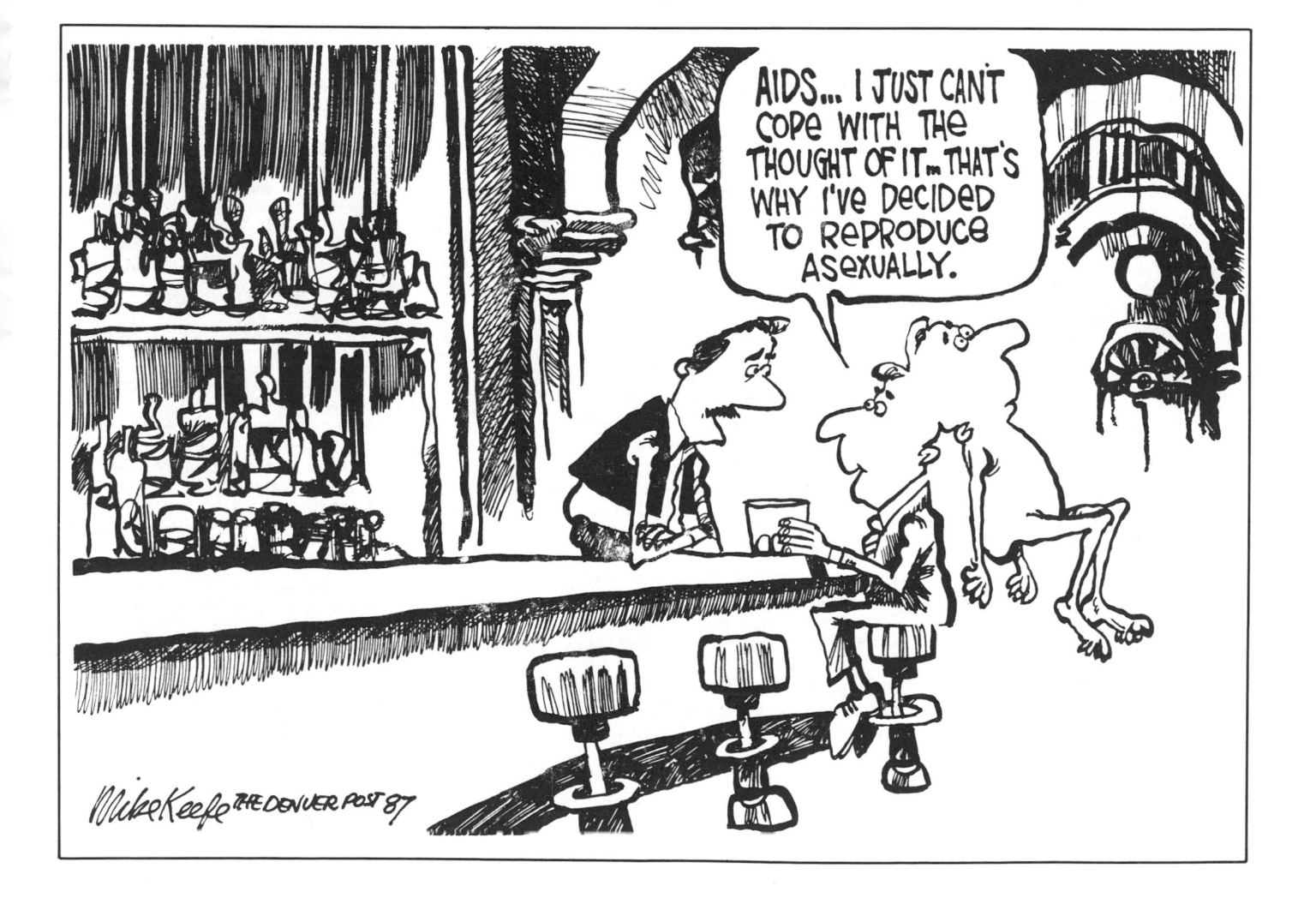

Leukemia Virus Linked to AIDS; New Findings Reported

Research reports published in the May 20, 1983 issue of *Science* linked AIDS with a virus known to cause a kind of cancer, the human T-cell leukemia virus (HTLV). AIDS had come to public attention in 1981, and since then more than 1,350 cases had been reported in the U.S. So far about 40% of those who had contracted AIDS had died, and doctors feared that the mortality rate might eventually rise to 70% or higher, making the epidemic one of the deadliest to hit the U.S.

Research had suggested that an infectious agent, probably a virus, was a cause of AIDS, but efforts to identify that agent had run into difficulties. The studies published in *Science* showed that 25% to 35% of AIDS victims had been infected by HTLV, a fairly rare virus. Although the studies demonstrated a link between the virus and AIDS, scientists carefully refrained from saying that HTLV had been shown to be a cause of AIDS. It was possible that the virus was a consequence of the breakdown initiated by AIDS, rather than a cause of the disease. Nevertheless, the studies were seen as affording a significant step in the attempt to understand the disease.

In a related development, use of interferon, an infection-fighting protein, appeared helpful in fighting a rare form of cancer, Kaposi's sarcoma, that often developed in victims of AIDS, according to preliminary research results reported in the *New England Journal of Medicine* May 4, 1983.

A letter to the British medical journal *Lancet*, described in the press April 29, 1983 had suggested that a swine virus found in Africa and Haiti might be a cause of AIDS. The letter, written by Harvard scientist Jane Teas, noted that the virus produced an AIDS-like virus in animals, and the viral infection could conceivably be acquired by a human who ate raw or insufficiently cooked pork. Haitians were one of the groups at risk in connection with AIDS. "The similarities in geography, symptoms and timing between AFSV [African swine fever] and AIDS are striking and deserve further investigation," Teas wrote.

The Hartford Courant

Hartford, CT, August 4, 1983

If the number of acquired immune deficiency syndrome, or AIDS, victims multiplies at the present rate of reported cases, some 3 million Americans will have been stricken by the mysterious disease by the end of 1988.

A mortality rate of at least 60 percent applied against the number of potential victims yields the ghastly specter of nearly 2 million deaths. That is a public health threat of staggering proportions.

Yet, the nation's "quests for cause and cure represent little more than mere shooting in the dark with scientific scatter guns," according to a former president of the American Public Health Association. Government agencies are "underfunded, understaffed and overworked," and are operating without an organized plan to guide them, he noted in testimony at a House subcommittee hearing.

The government's response to the AIDS menace lacks focus and a sense of urgency, critics claim, because the disease primarily attacks homosexual and bisexual men.

The response to AIDS probably does suffer from quiet discrimination and cruel political opportunism of the sort that can arise whenever unpopular minorities are in need of government intervention. It is also undoubtedly hampered by an institutional lethargy that has nothing to do with bias.

The anti-AIDS effort must gather momentum if the cause of the disease is to be found, a cure developed, and lives saved. It isn't enough for Health and Human Services Secretary Margaret M. Heckler to simply declare AIDS her department's number one health priority. It isn't enough to claim, as one congressman has, that the government has put more money into AIDS research than it sank into research on legionnaire's disease and toxic shock syndrome combined.

More obviously needs to be done. The disease has spread apparently unabated since it was identified in the late 1970s.

Rep. Theodore S. Weiss, chairman of the House Government Operations subcommittee which held the hearing, has introduced legislation to create a federal fund of $60 million with which states and communities could respond more quickly to such emergencies.

Dr. Marcus Conant of the University of California Medical Center told the subcommittee that the government should provide more money and aggressively promote research, create a high-level task force to coordinate action and speed up the process of approving studies that will help explain the disease.

The government has the resources to undertake a program within those broad outlines. What's missing is a sense of urgency.

Rocky Mountain News

Denver, CO, June 14, 1983

WHEN the Center for Disease Control identifies AIDS as America's No. 1 health concern, action to fight it should be immediate. But acquired immune deficiency syndrome carries a lot of baggage that could work against dealing with the problem.

Part of that baggage involves the fact that the majority of its victims, so far, have been homosexual males. Some 1,500 cases have been confirmed nationwide, and about half the victims have died. In Colorado, 14 confirmed cases of AIDS include 12 in Denver.

The mysterious illness, which breaks down the body's ability to produce antibodies that fend off usually harmless germs, is believed to be transmitted through blood transfers and sex. It is considered to be on the verge of becoming epidemic.

Like many unknown and threatening illnesses, AIDS also damages by triggering fear. And fear is an accomplice of hostility. In the matter of AIDS, fear is a monster with two heads.

Many people fear homosexuals as a threat to traditional values and would treat their sexual orientation as a crime. They would deny homosexuals access to jobs and housing if the law permitted. AIDS has caused some cities to propose banning homosexual meeting places and certain sexual activities.

This long-held hostility may explain the slowness of a full-scale fight against the disease.

It may also explain the delay of some homosexuals in seeking treatment. Many of them have lived for years in fear that they will be discovered and stigmatized. Many still are unwilling to publicly identify themselves.

But all of them are right to fear AIDS, which apparently can be transmitted to sexual partners before the victim experiences any symptoms.

In addition, homosexuals also fear the loss of their hard-fought but still tenuous acceptance in society. With that could come new, restrictive legislation against sexual activities among consenting adults.

So for homosexuals, AIDS is not just a physical threat — it's a social one as well.

It is important that Congress vote the funds needed to research the causes and find a prevention or cure for this grim disease. And it is equally important that we refrain from attaching moral judgment to it.

EVENING EXPRESS
Portland, ME, August 11, 1983

The federal government has authorized $1.7 million for two major New York City medical research centers to develop a blood test that will identify carriers of AIDS, acquired immune deficiency syndrome, a virulent and frequently fatal disease.

Good. Development of the test will enable blood collection agencies to screen the blood, not only the responses, of donors. And that's important if AIDS can be transmitted, however infrequently, through blood transfusions.

Primarily, of course, AIDS is transmitted by sexual contact among homosexual men. As of last month, 1,922 people had contracted the disease and 743 have died. In addition, many AIDS victims have been subjected to hate-mongering and mindless fear generated either by ignorance or by those who would use the disease to further their own interests.

While an effective blood test would protect society in general, the U.S. Public Health Service should not relax its efforts to establish the cause and discover a cure for AIDS.

Earlier this year, the Public Health Service made AIDS its top priority. More than that, it has backed that priority with money, spending $5.5 million last year and allocating $14.5 million for 1983.

But money to develop blood tests or eventually to find the cause and cure for the disease can do little immediately for the five to seven new AIDS victim who report to the federal Centers for Disease Control each day.

They deserve understanding and compassion, not hatred and ignorance.

The Charlotte Observer
Charlotte, NC, May 20, 1983

When a deadly new disease called Acquired Immune Deficiency Syndrome (AIDS) first surfaced in this country two years ago among homosexual men, health officials were baffled.

Since then the so-called "Gay Plague" has spread to intravenous drug users, Haitian immigrants, hemophiliacs, recipients of blood transfusions and a growing number of people who fit in none of these high-risk categories. More than 1,300 cases of AIDS have been reported so far, and more than 500 deaths.

Yet the frightening fact is that health officials are *still* baffled — about where the disease came from, how it is transmitted, what is the period of communicability, how it can be treated.

Throwing money at AIDS isn't likely to produce a miracle cure overnight, of course. Yet declining government support for the research-oriented National Institutes of Health (NIH) and the lack of any federal emergency fund for medical crises have hampered investigation of the AIDS epidemic even as the mortality rate soars.

Clearly, federal budget-makers cannot foresee such emergencies or plan for them in making annual health appropriations. That's why the legislation introduced by Rep. Henry Waxman, D-Calif., to allocate $40 million for a standby fund for research into public-health emergencies, makes sense.

Though Rep. Waxman's bill has so far been opposed by the Reagan administration, it should gain momentum as AIDS continues to invade the general population. Every six months since the first case was diagnosed in June 1981, its incidence has doubled; today three to five new cases are reported daily. The disease — which ravages the body's natural immune system and leaves victims easy prey for a rare form of cancer and a host of infections — already has claimed more lives than the highly publicized Legionnaire's Disease and Toxic Shock Syndrome combined.

As long as AIDS seemed confined to one or two distinctive groups, existing research funds may have been adequate. But as it spreads, researchers have had to beg, borrow and steal resources from other deserving projects. And new studies are beginning to cast doubt upon early theories that AIDS — which researchers believe is a virus — is spread only through blood and other body fluids, requiring either intimate contact or exposure to blood to be transmitted from one person to another.

The Journal of the American Medical Association recently noted that AIDS now appears to be striking some children, apparently through routine contact with other family members. If such routine contact can indeed spread the disease, wrote Dr. Anthony Fauci of the NIH, "then AIDS takes on an entirely new dimension . . . (and) the scope of the syndrome may be enormous."

Yet we simply don't know — and until we are willing to put adequate resources into research about this terrifying new disease, we may not find out. Prompt congressional approval of Rep. Waxman's bill would be a step in the right direction.

Minneapolis Star and Tribune
Minneapolis, MN, August 14, 1983

AIDS could be the most serious public health emergency since polio. But that does not mean the public should react with panic. The more appropriate response is research — a concerted effort to uncover the cause and cure for the disease.

AIDS (Acquired Immune Deficiency Syndrome) attacks the body's natural immune systems, leaving the victim defenseless against even a summer cold. No one knows exactly what causes it, but most doctors now agree that AIDS can be transmitted only through intimate sexual contact, a shared hypodermic needle, or, in rare cases, through blood transfusions.

The disease primarily afflicts male homosexuals with multiple sex partners, intravenous drug users and hemophiliacs. (Haitian immigrants are often cited as another risk group, but the justification for that classification has recently been challenged.) As of the first of this month, 1,972 AIDS victims had been diagnosed; the number of cases doubles every six months. At least 743 AIDS victims have died, three in Minnesota; no one has been cured.

The medical consequences of AIDS are reflected in the death statistics. But the stigma of the disease is painful as well: First stricken by a deadly illness, then shunned by those who fear that they will somehow catch it, many AIDS victims live out their lives in isolation. And the disease may yet cause other tragedies: It has led some people to defend discrimination against homosexuals on public-health grounds; others have welcomed AIDS as the "proper punishment" for homosexuality. Unfounded fear of contracting AIDS also appears responsible for a dangerous drop in blood donations.

Much of the fear and prejudice would dissolve if more people listened to the facts learned so far about AIDS. Doctors agree that the disease isn't highly contagious. It can't be contracted from giving blood, from walking down a city street, from shaking hands — or even from working or living with an AIDS victim. Neither can the illness be blamed on any particular group: Although homosexuals appear to be the main carriers, they are no more responsible for AIDS than polio victims were for polio epidemics.

Paranoia will not help solve this health disaster; only research will. After a slow start, the federal government is working vigorously to unravel the AIDS mystery. The Department of Health and Human Services will spend some $37 million to study and combat AIDS through 1984, more than was spent in eight years on both Legionnaire's disease and toxic shock syndrome.

When Congress reconvenes in September, it will consider adding even more research money. Such acts are prudent. Federal research is the best way to learn how to fight a frightening illness.

AIDS Linked to Blood Transfusions; Donor Screening Begins

The Centers for Disease Control (CDC) in Atlanta January 11, 1984 reported evidence linking the possible transmission of AIDS through blood transfusions. The first transfusion-associated AIDS case had been reported to the centers in 1982. Since then, a total of 40 such cases had been diagnosed. Twenty additional cases of the disease had developed among hemophiliacs since that time. The 60 cases associated with blood or blood products represented approximately 2% of the total AIDS cases reported. A study published in the Jan. 12 issue of the *New England Journal of Medicine* reported that 18 of the transfusion-associated AIDS cases had no known risk factors for AIDS other than that they had received blood 15 to 57 months prior to the start of their illness. Health workers at the CDC had identified eight donors who were in one of the high-risk categories of AIDS, but reported that no donor was known to have had the disease. CDC officials cautioned that the risk of getting AIDS from a blood transfusion remained small.

A $23.9 million study had been launched by researchers in Los Angeles and five other cities to evaluate the effectiveness of ongoing tests to detect the AIDS virus in humans, it was reported October 17, 1984. The study would check the usefulness of screening blood donors for signs that they might carry the virus. The test was the first breakthrough in AIDS research to result from the discovery of the virus in April 1984. Its main drawback was said to be its potential for alarming people unnecessarily; a positive test result would indicate that a person had been exposed to the virus, but not whether that person would subsequently develop the disease.

The U.S. Department of Health and Human Services January 10, 1985 announced that the new test to detect the AIDS virus would soon be commercially available. The new test was expected to indicate with a high level of accuracy whether an individual had been infected with the virus but would not indicate whether the individual was likely to develop AIDS. It was hoped that the new test would reduce the incidence of AIDS transmitted through donated blood. However, the department's figures continued to indicate that only about 2% of known AIDS cases—162 of 7,788 AIDS cases nationwide as of Jan. 7—were related to blood transfusions.

It was "essential" that blood banks adopt improved tests for AIDS, a panel of health experts said July 9, 1986 in Washington, D.C. Panel members said the chance of catching AIDS through a transfusion was "substantially less than one in 10,000" and that the U.S. blood supply was "much safer than it was two to four years ago." But they estimated that each year current screening tests were unable to block 120 of the 12,000 whole blood units that were believed to be infected with AIDS viruses. Current tests detected antibodies to the viruses themselves. The panel said more sensitive tests were required. The panel recommended that blood banks allow patients facing surgery to set aside some of their own blood for any necessary transfusions. Commercial blood-freezing centers for long-term individual storage had opened in eight cities, an August 17, 1986 news account said. The panel did not recommend the growing practice of asking friends or relatives for donations. It said the blood would probably be no safer than the general supply, a view some medical experts disputed. The group had been called together by the National Institutes of Health, the federal Centers for Disease Control, the Food and Drug Administration and the National Institute of Mental Health.

The CDC March 19, 1987 said that physicians should consider recommending the blood test for AIDS virus infection for some people who received transfusions of blood and blood products from 1978 to the spring of 1985. An earlier version of the federal recommendation, leaked March 19, had generated considerable alarm as well as widespread criticism of the CDC. Some officials had interpreted the earlier draft to imply that all recipients of transfusions of blood and blood products from 1978 to early 1985 be urged to undergo AIDS testing. Immediately following the leak, telephone lines at blood centers and American Red Cross chapters had been flooded by panicky transfusion recipients, and top public health officials from New York State, New York City and New Jersey had issued a statement questioning the wisdom of the CDC proposal. Health officials estimated that from 1978 to April 1985 only one in every 2,500 units of blood was contaminated. Mandatory testing of donated blood had reduced that risk by a factor of 100.

THE DENVER POST
Denver, CO, May 26, 1983

ACQUIRED Immune Deficiency Syndrome (AIDS) isn't something to snicker about just because it's been linked to homosexuals. As Marjie Lundstrom reported in The Post's Contemporary magazine last Sunday, this mysterious, incurable disease has reached Colorado. At least 14 cases have been confirmed, 11 in the Denver area, and three of the victims died.

AIDS was recognized about two years ago by epidemiologists at the federal Center for Disease Control in Atlanta. More than 1,400 cases have been identified nationally. The incidence has been doubling every six months. Within two years of diagnosis, 80 percent of the victims have died.

Equally alarming, it is believed the disease may not become noticeable until 6 to 30 months after exposure. "The long induction period," says epidemiologist James W. Curran, "means it's not going to explode across the country. But it also means the implication won't be fully known for several years."

About half the cases have been discovered in New York City. San Francisco and Los Angeles also have a high incidence. A large percentage of the victims are male homosexuals, drug abusers who have used contaminated needles, people who received blood transfusions, and Haitian immigrants.

Since it is not known what causes AIDS, there is no diagnostic test and no known cure. It is detected by what it does — it breaks down the body's ability to resist diseases. Many victims have contracted and died of lethal forms of cancer and pneumonia.

One recent study has indicated that the disease also may be sexually transmitted between heterosexual men and women, which makes the possibility of its spread through the general population a much greater risk. Some scientists consider AIDS already a national epidemic.

About all that can be done so far is to urge precautions. Blood donors need to be screened more carefully. And people must be warned about activities that have been linked to AIDS. But if there is indeed the danger of a national epidemic, more of the nation's resources must be devoted to the task of conquering it. New grants for research announced this week are a good first step. AIDS is no laughing matter.

Detroit Free Press

Detroit, MI, June 19, 1983

FEAR — worse, baseless fear — is preventing the Red Cross from obtaining the blood it needs to service the people of Southeastern Michigan. Too many would-be blood donors, misled by publicity about the malady known as AIDS, have been needlessly frightened about the possibility of contracting the disease.

Although some hemophiliac AIDS victims are reported to have acquired the disease from receiving contaminated blood, there is no record of anyone acquiring AIDS by *giving* blood. From what is known of the transmission of the disease, there is virtually no possibility of blood donors doing so. The disposable equipment used by the Red Cross for blood donations bars any known health risk. The donor collection bag has a self-contained sterile needle that is used once, then discarded.

The majority of known victims of AIDS, an acronym for acquired immune deficiency syndrome, are male homosexuals who contracted the disease through sexual contact. Other groups, notably Haitians, drug addicts using intravenous needles, and women and children living in households with AIDS sufferers have also contracted the malady, presumably through injection or constant, intimate contact.

Much remains unknown about AIDS. What is noteworthy, however, is that no medical technician, doctor or nurse working with AIDS patients in New York City, which has the largest number of victims, is known to have come down with the disease. Apparently, it takes more than daily handling of AIDS sufferers to become one.

Summer is traditionally a bad time for blood donations. Many institutions that lend themselves easily to large blood drives, such as schools, are closed. Businesses that are short-staffed for the summer discourage their remaining employes from taking time off. Other plants, hard-hit by the economy, are shut down or functioning at reduced levels. Numerous individuals who regularly give blood during the colder months leave town for vacations.

What has made the difference this summer, however, between a normally slow season and a dangerous dip in blood donations is the unnecessary fear of AIDS. But the need remains. Call the Red Cross at 833-4440, any time night or day, for more information on where you can help by giving blood.

The Orlando Sentinel

Orlando, FL, August 14, 1983

Yes, the people in the blood supply business should have let Richard Studer of St. Cloud give his own blood to his hospitalized, infant son last week.

But this is a particularly unfortunate flap for the blood banks because they are right when they argue that the concern over getting some disease from a blood transfusion is way out of proportion to the problem. Those fears don't justify turning the blood bank program upside down even though common sense says that surely parents should be able to give blood to their own flesh and blood.

The pressure on both sides comes from AIDS, an incurable, often-fatal disease whose victims typically are homosexual, drug-addicted, hemophiliac or Haitian. Families want to eliminate the risk of getting AIDS from a stranger's blood. Those refusing them want to avoid a disruptive panic based on misinformation.

The chances of getting AIDS from a transfusion are remote indeed — perhaps one in a million. Researchers are investigating about two dozen AIDS cases that may be linked to tranfusions. Also, the nation's three major blood bank groups have tightened their own defenses. Since March, all donors are asked if they're in a high-risk group. They are asked about any of the AIDS symptoms: night sweats, unexplained fever, unexplained weight loss, swollen lymph glands, pink or purple blotches on their skin.

One of the concerns of the blood banks is that someone who is asked to donate blood specifically for one person may be more likely than the routine volunteer donors to lie about risk factors. More important, they worry that such "directed" donations would reduce the supply of blood.

Their concern is more valid than their conclusions. They're guessing that permitting any directed donations would lessen the supply of blood. The banks say current donors might hold off in case they are asked to give for someone later. They show too little faith in the real foundation of the blood business — millions of people who care enough to share their blood with others.

The banks also speculate that *any* directed option would make people afraid that, contrary to the evidence, the normal supply of blood is unsafe. That's a communications challenge that they should be able to handle.

The experts also claim it would be a nightmare to administer — and that more mistakes would be made. But currently, someone who expects surgery can give blood for his own use. In fact, the strict rule against other directed donations was agreed to nationally only in June.

The nation's system of blood supplies is working well overall, and blood banks don't want to disrupt it. But all the blue-ribbon reasoning just doesn't justify last week's hard line. This time, a little give by the blood banks could go a long way.

Newsday

Long Island, NY, July 16, 1983

The Greater New York Blood Program, which serves Long Island, New York City, northern New Jersey and the lower Hudson River valley, has reported an alarming decline in its blood supply.

Donations at the New York Blood Center and Long Island Blood Services, for example, were down 25 per cent in the first half of July compared with the same period last year. And similar declines are being reported nationally. The supply has dwindled so low that some elective surgery has been postponed until more blood is available.

While some of the falloff is attributable to normal seasonal fluctuations, much of it is being blamed on fear by prospective donors that they might contract the disease known as AIDS by donating their blood.

The cause of AIDS — acquired immune deficiency syndrome — remains a medical mystery. But experts say that one thing about it is certain: It can't be contracted by donating blood.

AIDS typically hits members of a few specifically vulnerable groups: homosexuals, who apparently contract it during sexual contacts; hemophiliacs, who need frequent transfusions of blood, some of which apparently carries the agent that transmits AIDS, intravenous drug abusers, and Haitians.

As medical experts have noted repeatedly, the method used to draw blood from donors protects them from any possibility of contracting the disease. The needle inserted into the vein of a donor is used only to take that donor's blood and no one else's. Then it is thrown away.

So, according to all the experts, there's no reason whatever to worry about contracting AIDS by donating blood. It remains a safe and easy way to contribute to the health and well-being of the community.

The Seattle Times

Seattle, WA, July 26, 1983

A FEDERAL study committee has faced an extremely ticklish task in advising the Food and Drug Administration regarding blood donations and transfusions in relation to the mysterious disease called acquired immune deficiency syndrome, or AIDS.

The committee recommended that the government not have an "automatic policy" of destroying a large reserve of blood just because one donor is suspected of having AIDS.

We're not sure how helpful that recommendation will be to the FDA. Not having an "automatic policy" could mean anything from destroying 99 percent of suspect blood reserves to destroying none.

But the committee did base its recommendation on three seemingly sound factors. First, although a few people have contracted AIDS after receiving blood transfusions, it is unclear what the cause-and-effect relationship is.

Second, any contaminated blood from a potential AIDS victim would be diluted in a large pool. And in addition, widespread destruction of blood pools could put people who suffer bleeding diseases at a "great risk."

The problem, of course, is that so little is known about AIDS other than that homosexuals and drug abusers are among the high-risk groups.

Two other advisory-committee recommendations to the FDA are of unquestioned validity. The committee called for a public-education campaign and the screening of blood donors who are in the high-risk categories.

The latter point can scarcely be overemphasized. The government should take every possible step to ensure that the screening is thorough and that it is so perceived by a concerned public.

Seattle, WA, September 6, 1983

WHEN AIDS has been conquered by medical science, the irrational fear it engendered may be looked back upon with wonder one day. But this disease, which has infected only 2,000 people in a society of 226.5 million, is the source of widespread panic and threatens to disrupt an important institution.

News that AIDS can be transmitted through blood transfusions has shaken the foundation of the voluntary donor program. It has raised needless controversy over a vital community service.

Until AIDS became a focal point, few people worried about keeping blood donations in the family. Now policies against intrafamily donations have been raised as an issue reflecting distrust of blood-donor programs. Family members should have the right to donate blood to one another, but the question has everything to do with individual rights and little to do with AIDS.

(Sponsors of blood-donor programs including the Puget Sound Blood Bank argue that if intrafamily donations were allowed routinely, the voluntary programs might collapse, leaving thousands of people who need transfusions without blood.)

Mistrust and fear are spread further by some hospitals' statements that patients may have their own blood, lost during surgery, recycled or stored for future need.

Obviously, since so little is known about AIDS and because it is contagious, certain precautions are wise. Close screening of blood donors is common sense (not only to protect against AIDS but to limit the spread of other diseases such as hepatitis). And the government properly has invested heavily in research to find the causes and cure for the disease.

But turning AIDS victims into the lepers of the 1980s or looking for AIDS in every drink of water, in every needle, in every breath of shared air, seems unreasonable and counterproductive.

The Houston Post

Houston, TX, August 24, 1983

The trouble with jumping to conclusions is that most jumpers fail to notice either take-off point or landing point, much less the trajectory between the two. Jumping to conclusions is often a flight of fancy rather than a process of thought. Take public reaction to AIDS.

Because of the national and international publicity given to the acquired immunity deficiency syndrome, blood banks across the country have experienced a sharp and distressing decline in the number of voluntary blood donors. This is, of course, nonsensical. The acquired immunity deficiency may presumably be acquired from receiving blood. But it is hard to argue that you can catch it from *giving* blood. You would think that an experienced blood donor would figure that out unaided.

THE ANN ARBOR NEWS

Ann Arbor, MI, July 13, 1983

AIDS, or Acquired Immune Deficiency Syndrome, is near to fostering hysteria in some parts of the country, according to Health Secretary Margaret Heckler.

It shouldn't. Research shows AIDS is not spread through casual relationships, such as between children and parents or friends. Contact with the same bus seats or restaurant utensils does not spread the disease.

If you're not a member of one of the risk groups, the chances of contracting and dying of AIDS are remote. And blood donations under reliable auspices of a blood bank or hospital are completely safe and sterile.

Nevertheless, Red Cross officials say the AIDS scare caused blood donations to drop 16.4 percent nationwide during one week last month.

Donations are down in Washtenaw County, too. In June of 1982, collections totalled 2,278 units of blood in the county; in June of '83, collections dropped to 1,535.

NEWS ILLUSTRATION•CATHY GENDRON

County Red Cross people say that blood collections always decline at the onset of summer. Students, a big donor group, are gone, and long periods of heat discourage giving. The big decline from last year, however, is attributable in large measure to the scare over AIDS, according to a Red Cross spokeswoman.

The medical tragedy of AIDS is that we really don't know much about the nature of the enemy. There is no cure; there isn't even a test for the suspected virus. Early diagnosis helps, but AIDS may take more than one form.

AIDS attacks the immuno-suppressive system and increases the body's vulnerability to infections. AIDS victims have developed a particularly virulent form of pneumonia and Kaposi's sarcoma — two rare, potentially deadly diseases.

The social tragedy is already apparent. The unknown nature of AIDS feeds a public concern bordering on panic. High risk groups — sexually active male homosexuals, Haitian immigrants, intravenous drug users and hemophiliacs — are stigmatized. A leper class in society is created.

Meanwhile, it's vitally important that local blood supplies be maintained at comfortable levels and that potential donors be encouraged to give. When the facts on AIDS are more generally known and taken to heart, available supplies of blood should rise accordingly. The need is still there.

The Hartford Courant

Hartford, CT, September 3, 1983

The facts are these: Only about 24 blood transfusions out of 10 million given nationally since 1980 have had even tentative links to the disease AIDS.

The chance of being infected with AIDS (acquired immune deficiency syndrome) from a blood transfusion is negligible.

Yet the American Association of Blood Banks claims there has been a "dramatic increase" in the number of people who want to recruit their own blood donors, since the public alarm over AIDS began to grow last spring. The Connecticut Red Cross has also received many similar requests.

Blood donation agencies should not feel compelled to change their longstanding practices because some people are needlessly panicked. A system of so-called directed donations would invite an "administrative, scientific and medical nightmare," according to a state Red Cross official.

The selflessness of the present blood donation system is one of its beauties as well as one of its administrative strengths. No grand acknowledgment comes with this most personal donation, and there is no promise of individual reward.

People give blood for the satisfaction of contributing to the common good.

The present system is also safe. Blood donation groups have responded to concerns about AIDS by asking more questions of potential donors.

People have little reason to fear that they will become infected with AIDS as a result of donating blood or receiving transfusions. There is something to worry about, though, if people become too afraid to help each other.

The Evening Gazette

Worcester, MA, June 30, 1983

There was a dark edge to the weekend celebrations by homosexuals in New York, San Francisco, Chicago and other cities. The dread disease known as AIDS (acquired immune deficiency syndrome) kept unnumbered thousands away and spread new fears in communities with concentrations of homosexuals.

AIDS seems to afflict only certain kinds of people. Promiscuous male homosexuals are most at risk. Of the 1,641 known cases and 644 known deaths from the disease, 70 percent involve male homosexuals. But fear of AIDS is spreading rapidly. Some hospital workers have refused to treat AIDS victims. Some television crews have refused to get near enough to them to allow them to be interviewed. Private blood banks are being set up in some places, to avoid the risk of AIDS blood contamination. One AIDS victim in San Francisco carried a pathetic sign: "I have AIDS, not leprosy." AIDS victims most likely will be treated as lepers until more is known about the mysterious disease that so far is untreatable.

What is needed is a definitive, authoritative statement on AIDS. So far, the federal government and the medical societies have said that the public's fears may be exaggerated. There is no evidence that there will be a plague of AIDS or even that AIDS will spread into the general population. But the medical people are the first to say that they don't have much information to go on.

In the meantime, the blood supply must be protected. Homosexuals who give blood should be willing to give the facts to the authorities so that their blood can be segregated for special purposes, if that is deemed wise. This is not a matter of anti-homosexual bigotry but plain common sense.

The Kansas City Times

Kansas City, MO, August 20, 1983

Possibly because so much is unknown about acquired immune deficiency syndrome, people are paying attention poorly, if at all, to what is known. Excessive anxiety is one result.

It's ironic that institutions such as community blood centers, which are singularly successful in this country, should be caught in a backlash of ignorance and smoldering rumor. In fact, it's quite contradictory.

Since AIDS was identified in 1979, about 15 million people have received blood tranfusions. In the same four years, there has been one case where a patient contracted AIDS after receiving blood apparently supplied by an individual who later developed the condition. Even that linkage is being questioned. About 10 other cases are under investigation.

Yet public discussions routinely include blood transfusion recipients among those threatened by AIDS. That is a factual error.

Last year, 25,000 people died in alcohol-related car accidents. On any Friday or Saturday night, one in every 10 drivers on the road is driving under the influence of alcohol. Saturday night driving is a high-risk pastime. That is a statistical fact.

Concern about AIDS, and precautions against it, are understandable and sensible. But health officials are confounded when off-the-top-of-the-head notions are repeated often enough to sound authentic though they lend nothing to prevention and can cause disruptions in other crucial areas of health care. The suggestion that a drop in donations is a result of volunteer questions about getting AIDS by giving blood — a groundless idea — is an example. It has always been much more difficult to get blood donors in the summer. The weather, vacations and other competing activities are obvious factors. Blaming an old phenomenon on a new problem is ridiculous.

Working together, millions of volunteers and community blood center staffs have provided a safe and reliable supply of blood here and around the country. The facts simply do not warrant fiddling with that system.

The TENNESSEAN

Nashville, TN, July 15, 1983

THE Red Cross here is running low on blood because many prospective donors are afraid of contracting AIDS (acquired immune deficiency syndrome).

Medical authorities have given assurance that there is no danger of contracting AIDS by giving blood. Some doctors suspect that AIDS is transmitted through blood — but that is blood received not blood donated.

AIDS is generally thought to be confined to homosexual and bisexual men, hemophiliacs, intravenous drug abusers and Haitians. The medical profession in general regrets that the danger posed to the general population is greatly exaggerated.

It is most regrettable that the unfounded fear of AIDS may keep blood from reaching those who need it for their survival. If anybody gets AIDS from the blood transference, it will be the recipient and not the donor — and some critically ill recipients probably would be glad to take the chance.

The Red Cross supplies blood to all local hospitals and 108 hospitals in Middle Tennessee and southern Kentucky. Its reserve supplies at times recently have been dangerously low.

The mistaken attitude that giving blood might transmit AIDS could cause some people to die for lack of blood. It is hoped that doesn't happen.

DESERET NEWS

Salt Lake City, UT

July 22, 1984

Should blood banks screen donors more rigorously to prevent those with acquired immune deficiency syndrome (AIDS) from donating?

That's the path that may become necessary if a cure for AIDS doesn't materialize and the disease continues to grow. According to a Los Angeles Times writer, at least 70 deaths have been linked in recent years to blood transfusions when no other factors were present. Only 24 of those cases were hemophiliacs — a high-risk group because they so frequently need transfusions.

Other high-risk groups that demand large supplies of blood are patients who undergo open-heart, hip-replacement, or other surgeries in which loss of blood is high. Also vulnerable are newborn babies who require transfusions.

Risks of blood-passed AIDS disease, however, may be significantly higher in some East or West Coast areas than it is in Utah. For one thing, AIDS disease is almost non-existent in Utah. The State Health Department reports that in 1983, two residents and two non-residents contracted the disease. Three of those were homosexuals and one an intravenous drug abuser. Of those four, one resident and one non-resident died. So far in 1984, only one person has contracted AIDS.

The State Health Department last September took steps to require blood banks to screen donors more carefully and to keep track of any donated blood suspected of contamination. A folder given to each prospective donor now cautions about AIDS symptoms and the risks of passing the disease on in donated blood. Nurses, too, are more cautious in approving donors.

If patients are still uneasy about accepting blood bank donations, they can designate their own donors.

There are, of course, additional precautions that could be taken to assure wholesome blood supplies: Making up registries of pre-selected repeat donors in good health, for example; or adding additional screening measures in the present process. But for now, those steps seem superfluous. Utahns can have considerable confidence in the integrity of the present system.

The Courier-Journal

Louisville, KY, March 4, 1984

THE LOUISVILLE chapter of the American Red Cross has been both helped and hindered by the reduced blood needs being experienced in its three-state, 62-hospital region. The demand may have fallen, but the need for a steady supply of donors hasn't.

Possible reasons for lower blood needs are many, and experts can't pin down the exact causes of the present slump. For instance, fewer patients are being hospitalized nationwide, but in Kentucky the number seems to be rising. The recession seems to have reduced elective surgery. Federal cost-containment programs may have shortened hospital stays and lowered treatment costs for some Americans.

But the blood needs in some area hospitals either have remained the same or have fluctuated unpredictably. And despite the lowered demand, the Red Cross has been chronically short of blood in recent years. The AIDS scare last summer caused some donors to stay away for fear of contracting the disease, though only blood recipients, not donors, might have anything to worry about. And collections from industrial Bloodmobile sites have declined because of plant closings, layoffs and other recession-related factors.

The Red Cross has cut back its budget and laid off employees; those actions, coupled with the publicized decrease in demand for blood, might tend to give potential donors the impression that there is sufficient supply. If donors are discouraged, it will be a disservice to the entire region.

Blood is perishable. The Red Cross must balance its limited, short-lived supply against the changing needs of 62 hospitals in widely varying locales. Without a steady supply of donors, the task becomes difficult. Regular donors shouldn't become complacent; new donors shouldn't hesitate or feel their contribution isn't needed.

Blood, as the Red Cross often emphasizes, is the gift of life. Better to have too much of it than not enough.

Richmond Times-Dispatch

Richmond, VA, February 5, 1984

That mysterious killer-disease, acquired immune deficiency syndrome (AIDS), has thrown a fright into many Americans who face the prospect of receiving or giving blood. As a result, the potential exists for serious disruptions of the blood supply system upon which public health depends. According to the American Council on Science and Health (ACSH), a nonprofit organization composed of prominent scientists and physicians, fears have been exaggerated so far beyond any actual danger that the consequences of those fears could be more of a threat to health than AIDS itself.

Since first being identified in 1981, AIDS has stricken fewer than 3,000 Americans. Most at risk are homosexual and bisexual men who are promiscuous; also at increased risk are intravenous drug users and recent Haitian immigrants. What spread the alarm about the blood supply was the finding (as of last Nov. 1) that seven persons not fitting those profiles had contracted AIDS after receiving blood transfusions from AIDS carriers. But consider these perspective-restoring facts supplied by ACHS specialists:

● In the past three years, 10 million Americans have received 30 million units of blood. With only a handful of AIDS cases firmly linked to those transfusions, the risk of getting AIDS from a blood transfusion can be calculated at approximately one in a million.

● You would incur this same one-in-a-million risk of death if you rode a bicycle for 10 minutes, a car for 300 miles, or a jet plane for 1,000 miles.

● Actually, one-in-a-million overstates the risk for most blood recipients. Because most blood is used in the region where it is collected, the risk for persons outside the large metropolitan areas reporting most of the AIDS cases is undoubtedly smaller. Also, since last spring, the voluntary blood banking organizations have taken steps to exclude members of high-risk groups from donating blood.

● Despite all the care that is exercised in collecting, testing and processing blood, a blood transfusion is not, and never has been, risk-free. (No medical procedure is.) The chance of death as a result of being given the wrong unit of blood is one in 500,000. And there is a 7 in 100 risk of acquiring a hepatitis infection from transfused blood. But the great majority of blood recipients benefit from a transfusion.

And what is the risk of acquiring AIDS as a result of donating blood? *Zero*, states ACHS emphatically. Underline that: There is absolutely no chance of contracting AIDS or any other infection from donating blood because the blood collection centers use sanitary disposable needles — use them once, and then throw them away.

Besides unduly scaring off some blood donors, the AIDS spectre also has prompted some people to seek or make "directed donations" of blood for family or friends. But blood banking organizations point out that segregating blood donations according to kith and kin isn't necessarily safer, and could actually increase the danger of fatal errors as a result of the extra clerical work needed to separate supplies. And the blood supply could be disrupted to the extent that even emergency rooms might fall short.

AIDS is a horrible disease that has been mostly confined to the homosexual communities of a few large cities. That does not justify indifference toward efforts to eradicate this scourge. But neither does it call for hysteria on the part of households more likely to be felled by a meteorite than by AIDS.

The Birmingham News

Birmingham, AL, July 11, 1983

Thinking about giving blood? Worried about contracting AIDS if you do? You needn't. Giving blood is about as safe as can be insofar as contracting AIDS or any other disease for that matter.

To give weight to that assessment, Health and Human Services Secretary Margaret M. Heckler last week donated a pint of her own blood at a Red Cross facility in Washington.

"This year, because of the fear of AIDS, the donation level has seriously been undermined," Mrs. Heckler said. "I want to assure the American people that donating blood is 100 percent safe."

Those who have given blood in the past know that blood banks are sterile and that the Red Cross uses only disposable sterile needles and equipment in extracting blood from donors. None of this equipment is used a second time.

According to the Red Cross blood donations for the week of June 13 were down 16.4 percent nationally. In some urban areas, spot shortages have been as high as 30 percent below last year's levels. One hopes the news gets around. Adequate supplies of whole blood have been one of the keys to saving lives following accidents and surgery. We can't afford to let unfounded fear turn back the clock.

AKRON BEACON JOURNAL

Akron, OH, August 19, 1983

BLOOD donations are lower than normal this summer, because fear surrounding AIDs has accompanied the usual vacation slump.

That means potential blood shortages across the country after Labor Day, when doctors and patients end their summer hiatuses and hospital operating rooms are back in full swing. As a result, blood banks are furiously trying to increase their collections. The Red Cross in Washington, D.C., has chosen a novel approach: It is showing free movies.

A donor can relax with his feet up, give a pint of blood, and weep over Ingrid Bergman's farewell to Humphrey Bogart in *Casablanca*. The more adventurous may watch *Goldfinger* or *Close Encounters of the Third Kind* on video terminals that are used for medical instruction films when donors aren't around.

The sales scheme is working, even without popcorn. Washington's August blood drive is a success and hospitals will benefit. This could become great summertime entertainment, as long as Bela Lugosi isn't the featured attraction.

The Miami Herald

Miami, FL, February 7, 1984

IT WOULD be hard to imagine anything that hurts the cause it intends to help any more than does state legislator Tom Woodruff's proposal to ban "high risk" blood donors. Representative Woodruff's suggestion is poorly conceived and needless. It potentially could provoke reactions that curtail donations to blood banks.

The legislator from St. Petersburg says that persons designated as risk-prone to Acquired Immune Deficiency Syndrome (AIDS) should be jailed if they donate blood — even if they don't have AIDS. Moreover, Mr. Woodruff says, persons in the risk groups should be required to sign oaths swearing that they don't have the disease.

The "risk groups" include homosexual and bisexual males, intravenous-drug users, hemophiliacs, and Haitians.

There's plenty wrong with the legislator's suggested bill. Foremost is that it is entirely unnecessary. Blood centers nationwide adhere to rigorous screening procedures before, during, and after accepting blood. At most blood banks in Florida, standards are even tighter.

At the South Florida Blood Service in Miami, for example, each donor is individually examined and questioned. Donated blood is further tested for AIDS, venereal diseases, and other potential contaminants. Certain categories of people — any recent immigrant from a country with malaria, such as Haiti, for example — automatically are rejected as potential donors.

Representative Woodruff says that "the number of cases is increasing among people who are getting [AIDS] through transfusions." No evidence supports that conclusion.

In the past five years, the Government's Centers for Disease Control (CDC) have found 39 persons with AIDS who also have had blood transfusions. No information suggests that these victims contracted AIDS through transfusions. In fact, the CDC found no blood donors who were AIDS victims among 50 million blood donations.

If Representative Woodruff's suggested bill somehow managed to become law, it would have an adverse effect on some blood banks. Gay-male donors are the primary source for producing hepatitis-B vaccine. Mr. Woodruff's proposal would seriously jeopardize production of the vaccine by eliminating its main plasma source — gay men.

Moreover, suggestions that transfusions are causing AIDS are likely to frighten potential donors and recipients. No good reason argues in favor of the legislator's suggestion to ban risk donors.

The Legislature ought to reject the idea outright.

Rocky Mountain News

Denver, CO, July 6, 1983

NOT all dangers are created equal. People will go out of their way to take risks skiing, mountain climbing or driving their cars, yet devise elaborate precautions to avoid the more than one in a million shot of contracting a disease like AIDS.

And that's exactly what some Denver-area patients are doing, doctors say.

Not that anyone really objects. No one minds, for example, if people insist that only their own blood be used during surgery — anymore than people mind if those same patients, upon recovery, decide to spend every summer day facing the far greater risk of white-water rafting.

What would be unfortunate, however, is if the exaggerated fears of a few people came to infect everyone else and alter attitudes on a host of issues involving AIDS. Acquired Immune Deficiency Syndrome is not a pretty disease — and it is almost always fatal. It somehow destroys the body's immune system, thus opening the way for rare forms of cancer and pneumonia. And no cure is known.

Yet in the two years since AIDS was discovered, it has affected only about 1,600 people, primarily sexually promiscuous homosexual men and drug-users.

In short, it is still extremely rare, and it simply should not generate panic.

There is some evidence, however, that it has. Firemen in San Francisco have refused to give mouth-to-mouth resuscitation to suspected victims of AIDS. In San Antonio, paramedics have been issued protective clothing because of their fear.

Other instances exist of unrealistic concern, but the most alarming and potentially harmful manifestation is the sudden decline in blood donations.

Chicago and New York City report decreases of 10 and 12 percent. In Detroit, Red Cross officials say that fear of AIDS has resulted in a 33 percent drop in blood donations and brought the city's supplies to a critical low.

According to Margaret Heckler, secretary of Health and Human Services, not a single doctor, nurse or other health provider has contracted AIDS while treating a victim, and the probability of contracting it from blood transfusions or other routine medical treatment is minimal.

"One epidemic is enough to combat," she says, noting that HHS will spend more on AIDS research this year than it has spent on Legionnaires' disease and toxic shock syndrome over the past eight years. "We do not need an epidemic of unreasoned fear as well."

She is right. In other words, while the decision to accept someone else's blood is the individual patient's business, it is everyone's business to see that unnatural fear of AIDS does not get in the way of facts.

The Courier-Journal

March 17, 1985
Louisville, KY

THE BLOOD testing now underway at the Red Cross and other collection centers in some cities is, in a sense, an insurance policy to protect the country's blood supplies against the virus suspected of causing AIDS. It's not a 100 percent safeguard, but an important tool to keep the disease from spreading through transfusions.

So far, of nearly 8,500 diagnosed cases of AIDS, the disease that destroys the body's ability to fight off diseases, 113 have been linked to transfusions of blood or plasma. More than 4,000 have died from the Acquired Immune Deficiency Syndrome. But until now, the only way to safeguard the blood banks was asking those most likely to contract the disease — homosexual men, intravenous drug users and hemophiliacs — to refrain from donating blood.

There are critics of the test. Some argue that the number of AIDS cases among blood recipients is too small to warrant the cost and inconvenience of testing everyone. Others fear that a donor may be misdiagnosed, since the test is not foolproof, and that the resulting worries will be compounded by public embarrassment. They aren't entirely consoled by pledges of confidentiality and bids to be retested free.

These critics also fret that mentioning AIDS to donors will scare some of them off. They recall that blood supplies dropped sharply in some areas two years ago, when AIDS seemed to be an epidemic, because many people erroneously believed they could get the disease by merely donating blood.

Others worry that offering the tests might, paradoxically, encourage people in high-risk groups to donate blood just to obtain free, periodic testing. But there's a simple alternative. Indiana's health department is among those planning to make tests available to anyone who asks, without having to donate blood. The same option probably will be offered in Louisville when testing begins soon.

But all of these concerns pale beside the need to safeguard blood supplies. Red Cross officials say the fear of receiving transfusions tainted by AIDS has prompted some families to contemplate "directed" donations, an agreement among relatives to donate blood to each other. Such private agreements could dangerously undermine the system of assembling stockpiles of blood for instant benefit to anyone in need.

Admittedly, the blood test isn't perfect. It measures antibodies, which the body produces to fight off the AIDS virus, not the virus itself. The problem is that some people with the disease don't produce the antibodies, so their blood wouldn't be screened out. And there's the opposite flaw: Of 100 people testing positively for the antibody, federal officials say about 17 won't have the illness or even develop it later.

But the main goal must be to make the blood supply as safe as possible. Despite its shortcomings, the test still identifies blood likely to be contaminated and, according to federal officials, that should prevent 50 to 150 cases of AIDS a year. For a disease that so often is fatal, the benefit of safeguarding the nation's blood supply and preventing AIDS from spreading further is clearly paramount.

Rockford Register Star

Rockford, IL, October 22, 1985

Acquired Immune Deficiency Syndrome is a disease that kills people. The recent death of movie star Rock Hudson has brought that fact home to any Americans who were still unaware of AIDS' deadliness.

Now, the medical community and blood bank officials here and everywhere must try to match that almost total awareness of the threat with the knowledge that *donating* blood will not transmit AIDS to the donor.

Ironically, the tragedy of AIDS now threatens to spread tragedy to many others who cannot survive without the life-saving flow of new blood.

Closely following reports of national concern that AIDS fear had reduced blood donations is a similar report from the Northern Illinois Blood Bank. An official says he believes the bank is losing an average of one donor a week from its active list because of fear of AIDS.

This illogical change in public attitude about blood donations comes at a critical time, too. In September, the local blood bank recorded the second highest need for blood in its history.

In the last six years, more than 100,000 blood transfusions were provided by local donors. That's a proud record of community concern for others.

Since April the blood bank has been testing for AIDS antibodies in blood donated. That's understandable since the blood bank wants to be sure no contaminated blood is given to others.

But the sterile process of giving blood cannot transmit AIDS — or any other disease — to the donor

AIDS is spread only through: contaminated needles shared by intravenous drug abusers, *receiving* transfusions of infected blood, or sexual contact.

These limits on exposure must be made as well known to the public as the threat of AIDS. Our vital reservoir of donated blood must not be lost to ignorance.

DESERET NEWS

Salt Lake City, UT, October 21-22, 1985

How safe is America's blood supply from AIDS, the acquired immune deficiency syndrome?

That's a question increasingly raised by recipients of blood transfusions as the deadly disease grows in the number of victims and jumps from the homosexual to the heterosexual population. Even children have acquired AIDS from blood transfusions.

The whole question of blood safety is being discussed during the current annual meeting of the American Association of Blood Banks in Miami Beach. As one official put it, AIDS is one of the most delicate problems to arise in the 38 years of the AABB's blood-banking experience.

Misleading information has been rife. Some people have been unwilling to donate blood, for instance, because they're afraid they could catch AIDS merely from the giving. That's nonsense.

Others have put off elective surgery because they fear tainted blood supplies. Since blood banks have initiated the AIDS test and started turning away donors with even a possibility of being an AIDS carrier, supplies are "measurably safer," say officials of the National Institutes of Health, the Food and Drug Administration, and the Centers for Disease Control. The Red Cross agrees.

Still, there's lingering controversy over that issue. Just recently Dr. Myron Essex, chairman of the department of cancer biology at the Harvard School of Public Health, told an AIDS meeting in Boston that screening tests had failed to detect some infected individuals. Dr. John Ward of the Centers for Disease Control — which has monitored the spread of AIDS since 1981 — says only 6 percent of those individuals who test positive will be AIDS carriers. And those will be screened out, he adds.

What it comes down to is percentages: what's the chance of getting tainted blood? As Eugene Jeffers of the American Red Cross puts it: "There is only a 1/1000th chance of getting AIDS from a transfusion."

Detroit Free Press

Detroit, MI, November 19, 1985

THE BLOOD bank, one of this nation's best egalitarian institutions, is on the skids. Fear of contracting Acquired Immune Deficiency Syndrome (AIDS) through blood transfusions has caused thousands of Americans to ask not what they can do for the good of the order but what they can do for themselves. In several cities, people are donating blood, not to a community reserve, but solely for themselves against the day of surgery or serious illness — this despite assurances that any accredited hospital these days uses techniques to screen out AIDS-contaminated blood, if only to avoid being sued for malpractice.

Americans are a people who have generally banded together to battle common enemies, because there is not only strength in numbers but community as well. While acknowledging the private property rights of one's own blood, we think that the social order will be far better served by our continuing to donate to a common cause rather than a singular one — especially in such a life-and-death matter as life-saving blood.

DAYTON DAILY NEWS

Dayton, OH, October 21, 1985

The Community Blood Bank is sticking with a bad decision and ought to reverse it. Promptly.

The blood bank wants to have a private-sector support team in place before it tells three blood donors that antibodies of the acquired immune deficiency syndrome virus have been found in their blood serums.

At least 33,000 people have given blood at the blood bank since AIDS testing began there in April. That's a great number of apprehensive people forced to wait until the blood center has its support team in place so it can notify the three who need to know. There also is the possibility that the three have AIDS and could be exposing other people to the disease because they don't know they have it.

There is another, quicker way than waiting for the development of a private sector team: use the Montgomery County Health District. As one of eight alternative AIDS testing sites in Ohio, the health district already has a support team of counselors and private-sector physicians in place.

The Community Blood Bank, however, has chosen to set up a private-sector network because the blood donors were volunteers and should have some support system available to them other than a public health one.

This reasoning implies that for a donor to be seen at a public health center is as terrible as being told he or she has AIDS antibodies.

The other implication is that somehow the people tested at the health district, mostly homosexuals and intravenous drug users, are different from the volunteer blood donors who have no reason to believe they've been exposed to the AIDS virus and therefore the two should be kept apart.

That's nonsense. AIDS is a disease that doesn't distinguish between those whose life styles "ask for it" and those who happened to be exposed to the virus. The medical tests and support for every potential AIDS victim is the same, and that local help, already available, ought to be taken advantage of promptly.

THE ATLANTA CONSTITUTION

Atlanta, GA, August 12, 1985

1) No medical test is foolproof, but one with a reported 99.8 percent accuracy rate is almost as reliable as humankind can make it.

2) Donated blood customarily is used within a month's time of being drawn.

Putting 1) and 2) together, America's public-health establishment has come to the immensely reassuring conclusion that the nation's blood supply is safe from contamination from the dreaded AIDS virus.

The test, which spots not the virus itself but the presence of AIDS antibodies, was licensed last spring. Since that time, it has been used to screen hundreds of thousands of units of blood. Researchers who don't think 99.8-percent detection is good enough, bless 'em, are working to narrow the margin for error still further.

The news lifts a heavy weight of fear from candidates for surgery, accident victims and hemophiliacs. No longer need they put off elective procedures or worry themselves sick that their life-sustaining treatment might possibly be life-threatening.

All told, more than 200 Americans are known to have contracted AIDS through blood transfusions. Because the virus can incubate for indefinite periods before the disease symptoms are manifest, that number is sure to rise. Bear in mind, though, these will be almost exclusively cases of persons infected prior to the testing.

When one considers AIDS was all but unknown five years ago, the speed with which medical detectives isolated the virus and developed this screening test is extraordinary. The Centers for Disease Control here in Atlanta are playing an important part in this continuing and daunting battle against AIDS and deserve the nation's — make that the world's — thanks.

One more thing: Blood-bank operators are concerned there's a fear abroad that giving blood exposes the donor to AIDS. Not so. Needles used for the procedure are always discarded and never reused. The risk isn't even .2 percent; it's nil, nothing, *nada*. You can give to your heart's content.

The Miami Herald

Miami, FL, August 27, 1985

THE UNFORTUNATE death in Saudi Arabia of a man who received AIDS-tainted blood from a Miami blood bank in 1981 brings to light something that healthy people can do to fight back against AIDS (acquired immune deficiency syndrome). They can donate blood to voluntary blood banks, boosting supplies of infection-free blood available for the entire community. Now is a good time, too: Blood supplies are low in August, and accidents that accompany the Labor Day weekend typically increase demand.

Many eligible donors are reluctant because they fear they can contract AIDS by giving blood. That is impossible because only sterile, disposable needles are used. And now, because of testing, the risk of getting AIDS through transfusions has decreased to "essentially zero," says Dr. Peter Tomasulo, president of the South Florida Blood Service. That reduction in risk from transfusions is one of the few victories medical science can claim at this stage of the battle against AIDS.

The Saudi received blood from a commercial blood bank four years ago, *before* blood banks could screen donors for the AIDS virus or antibodies. Few specialists knew then that AIDS kills. Now potential donors are asked if they belong to high-risk groups, and tests have been in use for five months to screen donors scientifically.

Dr. Tomasulo says that studies show that the safest blood is from a donor "who just wants to help a patient he or she doesn't know." An incentive of any kind, particularly a monetary incentive, he adds, could induce a donor to lie about his medical history. Nationwide, more than 98 percent of the whole blood and blood components used in transfusions comes from volunteers; in Florida all of it does.

Because of the incubation period for AIDS — the Saudi didn't develop it until two years later — cases of transfusion-transmitted AIDS may still crop up, Dr. Tomasulo explains. Still, there's little risk from blood donated today.

The South Florida Blood Service is a nonprofit agency that distributes blood to those who need it on a medical-priority basis in about 60 health-care centers in Dade, Broward, and Monroe counties. The more healthy people who give blood, the healthier and more abundant the community's blood supply. It's just that simple.

The Pittsburgh PRESS

Pittsburgh, PA, January 11, 1986

At first, the situation looked dismal. A Pittsburgh transplant recipient had been given a liver that tested positive for AIDS antibodies.

In addition, another recipient in another city was given the same donor's heart.

In the week since the operations took place, with the threat of possible AIDS infection, though, the outlook has swung from dismal to optimistic.

The chance that the recipient of the liver had been given a dread disease along with his life-saving replacement part was charted as just about nil by Dr. Thomas Starzl, director of organ transplantation at Presbyterian-University Hospital. It's unclear how many of those who test positively will develop AIDS, and the donor was determined to have a low level of the antibodies present.

Even more welcome is the news from the state of Indiana, where the organs were taken from a 19-year-old man who was brain dead after being injured in an auto accident. A more definitive test yesterday showed no infection.

Indiana Gov. Robert D. Orr, reacting to initial reports on the transplantation of the organs, had ordered the formation in his state of an organ transplant task force to make certain the scenario is never repeated.

The AIDS-detecting tests on the donor last week were not started until so late that the recipients of his heart and liver already were on the operating tables when the possible contamination results became known. Because of that, the task force will push for legislation that would require that all prospective organ and tissue donors be tested for AIDS or its antibody.

With all the moral and ethical problems already dogging transplant surgery in Pittsburgh and the nation, there is absolutely no room for deadly chance that a terminal disease will be transferred along with an organ.

Transplant hospitals by now should have instituted immutable and unpliable policies that would require that AIDS testing be done and the results determined before operations begin.

Since they haven't, Pennsylvania should follow Indiana's lead and make it mandatory.

DESERET NEWS

Salt Lake City, UT, January 10, 1986

Sometimes it's amazing how a wrong idea can become embedded in the public consciousness — and stay there despite common sense.

A poll taken by national blood bank officials showed this week that one in every three Americans believes it is possible to get AIDS by donating blood.

That is utterly untrue, but such misunderstanding about how AIDS is spread is causing the worst January blood shortage in history, according to the American Association of Blood Banks. Shortfalls of up to 13 percent are common nationally. Many hospitals are postponing non-emergency surgery.

In answer to another question in the blood bank poll, more than half of the people said they believed a person was "likely" to get AIDS by receiving a blood transfusion — although the facts indicate otherwise.

In the early stages of the AIDS story, before awareness of the disease had really blossomed, a few people were infected by receiving tainted blood transfusions. However, since all donated blood is now screened for evidence of AIDS virus, scientists say the risk from transfusions is very remote.

At least the concern over transfusions — even if wildly exaggerated — had some basis in fact. But it's hard to understand how people jumped to the conclusion that donating blood could cause AIDS.

Apparently some things need to be repeated over and over again. For the record, it is NOT possible to catch AIDS simply by giving blood. So go sign up at the nearest hospital or Red Cross blood bank and give a pint. They need it badly.

Pittsburgh Post-Gazette

Pittsburgh, PA, January 13, 1986

Acquired immune deficiency syndrome — AIDS — is a serious health problem. So, in time, may be the epidemic of unreasoning fear that has accompanied the AIDS outbreak.

According to the American Association of Blood Banks, widespread ignorance about how AIDS is transmitted has produced the worst January shortage of blood in history. Although the shortage has yet to result in loss of life, many hospitals are postponing emergency surgery. (Fortunately for Pittsburgh, local blood bank officials report that donation levels remain high.)

What is most depressing about the decline in blood donations is that it is based on a demonstrably absurd premise: that *giving* blood can expose someone to the risk of contracting AIDS. Amazingly, a recent telephone survey conducted for the blood banks showed that 34 percent of Americans believe

AIDS can be contracted by donating blood.

That bizarre misapprehension presumably can be traced to the fact that, before blood supplies were screened for the AIDS virus, a few people did contract the disease by *receiving* tainted blood. (Dr. Eugene Berkman, the president of the blood banks association, notes that the risk of contracting AIDS from donated blood is now "exceedingly small.")

"The linkage of the words AIDS and blood is causing a great deal of fear," a spokesman for the blood banks observed. Obviously, but Americans owe it to themselves — literally, in the sense that everyone is a potential recipient of a blood transfusion — to get the facts straight. AIDS is a deadly enough disease without the avoidable side effects of hysteria-induced blood shortages.

THE TENNESSEAN

Nashville, TN, February 17, 1986

NASHVILLE'S chapter of the American Red Cross believes that healing is an emotional as well as a physical process.

The chapter recently decided to allow surgical patients to receive direct donation of blood from friends or family members. Several patients had made such requests in the past few months because of the fear of contracting AIDS from a transfusion.

Previously, direct donations were only allowed when a physician could cite a medical cause. Now the attending physician will only have to request the direct donation.

The Red Cross's decision should not, however, be interpreted as a shift of its position concerning AIDS. The Red Cross has repeatedly assured the public that there is absolutely no danger of contracting AIDS by either donating blood, or being transfused with blood from a Red Cross source.

All blood products handled by all chapters of the American Red Cross are now carefully screened for the AIDS virus. According to Dr. Kenneth Fawcett, director of the Nashville chapter, 90,000 units of blood have been tested in Nashville since last April, and only nine have been confirmed as carrying the AIDS virus.

The best medical evidence indicates that AIDS may be contracted from a blood transfusion, but only when the blood supply or the needle used for the transfusion has been contaminated with the virus. Neither is the case with blood received from the American Red Cross.

Nevertheless, the Red Cross's decision is welcome. Anyone who has ever been seriously ill, has needed an operation, or has gone through those medical traumas with a family member knows that peace of mind can be potent medicine.

People who are facing surgery have enough anxiety. If knowing whose blood they will receive eases their anxiety, they should have that opportunity. ∎

Chicago Defender

Chicago, IL, September 10, 1986

Acquired Immune Deficiency Syndrome (AIDS) has hit society so hard that many people are afraid to accept blood from anyone except family members or other loved ones. Some are hesitant to give blood for fear of catching the dreaded disease. Others still are having units of their own blood frozen (directed donations) to be used when and if they ever have to undergo surgery.

These new fears and changes in donor activity have not made blood program administrators happy because, reportedly, the blood supply has been reduced. And since there is no known cure for AIDS, it is understandable that terrifying questions about the disease abound in the minds of many people.

Fear, ignorance, and wrong information have contributed to a generally low-key but injurious feeling of terror in many people about the ways in which AIDS can be caught. Such feelings, whether overt or partially concealed, can spread harmfully through individuals like fire through a forest.

The fear is understandable. AIDS is a killer. It has also made various people question whether the country's blood supply is, as it has been reported, safer than ever. Some persons are so confused by the epidemic that they believe a person can get the deadly disease by donating blood (which is not possible under the methods of hygiene used in current donation programs). This feeling has forced many people to stop giving blood.

We want to emphasize that a person *cannot* catch AIDS by donating blood since the instruments used are sterilized and are never exposed to the virus or syndrome of the disease. Therefore, we encourage healthy individuals to give blood. It's needed now as much as ever.

We also agree with the concept of directed donations programs although·they create problems by having to be logged and stored separately from other blood supplies. But they should be allowed to exist, not because they insure safety (they don't), but because they contribute to the public's peace of mind.

To a limited extent, the programs also: benefit hospitals and the medical profession by reducing the number of potential lawsuits which might otherwise be filed; and assure that patients don't become physically and emotionally traumatized before surgery out of an overactive fear of catching AIDS through a tranfusion.

Again, we understand that directed donation programs are not a guarantee against AIDS because some of the people making such donations might have an AIDS virus in their blood which is undetectable at the time the donation is made. And also, as Dr Bruce Newman, medical director of the University of Chicago's blood bank said, in emergencies, such "insurance" is not practical since frozen blood requires hours of preparation before use.

In the final analysis, however, this is an instance where the public's perception and requests should be respected until a vaccination is created or a cure is found.

During the interim, individuals should make liberal blood donations to save the lives of others.

The Morning News

Wilmington, DE, January 11, 1986

EVERY WINTER blood banks send out alarm signals. Their supply of blood is low, they say, and they may not be able to meet normal demands, let alone any sizable emergency. This winter, the warning bell rings a bit louder.

For most blood banks, 1985 was a lean year and the effect lingers. What made 1985 so difficult was the link between AIDS (acquired immune deficiency syndrome) and being the recipient of a blood transfusion. A few hemophiliacs as well as some individuals who in the past had received blood for other life-saving reasons have since come down with the dreaded AIDS disease.

These unfortunate sufferers, however, received their transfusions before much was known about AIDS and, more importantly, before a test had been developed to check blood for the AIDS virus. That test is now used by all blood banks and should eliminate the hazard of contracting AIDS from blood transfusions.

There is, however, still some reluctance to donate blood, and that reluctance is based on a false premise. Mistakenly, people confuse blood giving with blood receiving. For blood donors, blood banks use only disposable equipment — the needle inserted in the donor, the bag for collecting the blood, even the thermometer used for checking the donor's health — they are packed in sterile condition and discarded after one use. This means that contamination of blood bank equipment is as impossible as humans can make it.

There should, therefore, be no fear of giving blood.

Fortunately, Delaware has not been beset by the blood shortages afflicting some other areas. This is not necessarily because Delawareans are smarter and understand the absence of a link between donation and AIDS, but because the blood bank in the state is run on a membership-insurance basis. Persons join the Blood Bank of Delaware; they pay a small annual membership fee and agree to donate blood periodically (every two or three years) or make an equivalent money contribution if they or members of their family are unable to give blood.

This organized system of blood donation assures a steady supply. Most other blood banks have no memberships and do not insure donors for blood; the other blood banks depend on volunteers. And folks shrink from volunteering when there is talk about AIDS, however mistaken that talk may be.

It's too bad that so few blood banks have adopted the membership-insurance system. We would be spared the annual alarm ringing if they had.

Chicago Tribune

Chicago, IL, April 14, 1987

It was one of the nightmares about AIDS come true, this one from the records of the U.S. Centers for Disease Control. A toddler, born in 1980, gradually developed what doctors call "failure to thrive." Six years later he died of the form of pneumonia characteristic of AIDS. Blood tests of his mother, father and older brother showed all of them infected with the AIDS virus. The mother had acquired it from blood transfusions during her first pregnancy in 1978, years before AIDS was recognized as a disease, and had passed it on to her husband and both sons.

How many other people were unknowingly infected with AIDS virus by blood transfusions before tests were developed to screen donated blood in the spring of 1985? No one knows. Blood banks have been able to trace and notify some individuals at risk because they received blood from donors who again gave blood after April, 1985, and were then identified through screening tests as infected at that time.

Now, efforts are underway to extend this Operation Look-Back to find other individuals who might have been infected with the AIDS virus via transfusion before April, 1985, and to urge them to be tested. It's a commendable effort. But it has emotional and practical pitfalls.

Hospitals and blood banks are concerned lest their attempts to find a few individuals who need testing scare many other people unnecessarily. They don't want to frighten patients who now need transfusions away from accepting them or discourage potential donors from giving life-saving blood. No one gets AIDS from donating blood, they stress. A patient who needs a transfusion runs enormously greater risks by refusing it than by consenting; screening tests make the current American blood supply virtually free from the AIDS virus.

The Centers for Disease Control estimates that of about 30 million people who received at least one blood transfusion between 1978 and April, 1985, about 12,000 may have been infected with the AIDS virus. Risks are higher in areas where the epidemic is most widespread (New York, California, Florida, Texas, Washington, D.C.). The more transfusions received and the closer to April, 1985, the greater the risk.

Despite the encouraging odds, hospitals and blood banks do recommend testing for individuals who got multiple blood transfusions between 1978 and April, 1985, and especially if they are about to make changes in their lives that would increase chances of spreading the virus should they be infected. For example, testing is urged for blood transfusion recipients who now plan to marry, begin a relationship with a new sex partner or become pregnant.

It costs about $25 to be tested. Every effort is made to keep the testing and its results confidential. And it is one small, commendable step toward getting control over the spread of this terrible new epidemic.

The Cincinnati Post

Cincinnati, OH, May 12, 1987

Congressman Stewart B. McKinney may not have intended it, but the statements about his AIDS-related death have maligned this country's systems for collecting and supplying blood.

The fact is, blood collection centers such as Hoxworth in Cincinnati are taking greater pains than ever to ensure their blood supply is safe.

Upon McKinney's death last week, his physician said he had contracted AIDS from blood transfusions during heart bypass surgery in 1979. Since then, however, friends and associates have acknowledged the Connecticut Republican's homosexual activities.

Of course, we'll never know exactly how the congressman was infected. We do know that only about 2 percent of AIDS-related diseases are caused by transfusions, while the percentage caused by sexual contact is much higher.

We also know there is little reason these days for hysteria about the nation's blood supply. For the past two years, blood centers such as Hoxworth have screened all blood for AIDS antibodies. Out of 180,000 units of blood collected in that time, only 18 have tested positive and have been discarded. Their donors are barred from giving blood again.

And to date, not one AIDS case in Greater Cincinnati has been traced to a blood transfusion.

For those who remain worried about AIDS—and about the more troublesome problem of hepatitis—Hoxworth has long had a program in which those who are having scheduled surgery can stockpile blood for themselves.

In the past few weeks, Hoxworth also has allowed directed donations, in which family members may give blood for a relative due to have surgery. It is doing so despite the extra paper work and with the knowledge its blood is as safe as is scientifically possible.

Despite these precautions, Hoxworth is running 1.6 percent below last year's donations, which were already inadequate to meet demand.

Much of that drop can be traced to AIDS paranoia. Even though Rep. McKinney said he wanted his death to underscore the need for an AIDS cure, it may have the unintended result of simply compounding AIDS myths.

Blood is a vital medical need, and Hoxworth Blood Center is doing everything possible to meet that need—even opening a downtown donation center this week at 417 Vine St. More than ever, Hoxworth deserves widespread support. Phone 569-1100 to find out how you can help.

Omaha World-Herald

Omaha, NE, March 20, 1987

The American Red Cross has recommended that people who had blood transfusions between 1978 and 1985 take a blood test for the AIDS virus. Red Cross officials in Omaha said Midlands residents who had transfusions during that time span and who are concerned should ask a doctor whether a test would be advisable. The recommendations are sensible.

Nationwide, a person who received a transfusion between 1978 and 1985 has only a one in 10,000 chance of being infected. The odds of being exposed to the virus are believed to be less in the Midlands, where the disease has been less common.

Still, anyone who has been exposed deserves to know it — for the safety of others.

The number of Americans infected with the AIDS virus is estimated at more than 1 million. Many of them don't know they are infected and consequently may be passing the virus to everyone with whom they have sexual relations.

A voluntary testing program, such as that proposed by the Red Cross, is a sensible precaution. The 1978-1985 period covers the years between the appearance of AIDS in this country and the point at which blood tests were taken to protect the nation's blood supply from AIDS contamination.

The Red Cross testing recommendation was made by Dr. S. Gerald Sandler, associate vice president of the organization's medical operations. "As long as we have a relatively inexpensive, highly reliable test, let's use it," Sandler said. "Let's find out where that virus is."

One of the odd aspects of the AIDS epidemic is the apparent reluctance of some people, including some health officials, to take the threat as seriously as it warrants. In calling for voluntary tests for people with even a slight chance of exposure to the virus, the national Red Cross organization has taken a responsible position.

The Times-Picayune
The States-Item

New Orleans, LA, March 20, 1987

Since testing donated blood for the AIDS virus began in 1985, the threat of receiving AIDS-contaminated blood in transfusions has been virtually eliminated. The problem of previous contamination is being dealt with now by urging people who received transfusions in the period 1978-1985 to have their blood tested for the antibody to the AIDS virus.

The AIDS virus began to appear in 1978.

The figures suggest that residents of our metropolitan area have a relatively low chance of having received blood contaminated with the virus. Medical statisticians say that about 230 of the 84,000 persons in our area who received transfusions during that period may have been infected with the virus and that about half of them could actually develop the disease. The odds are lower for those who did not get many transfusions and lived in areas with low case counts. During 1978-85, New Orleans was such an area.

Though having the virus in one's blood does not necessarily mean one will contract the disease, the chances of doing so are 1 in 2. One can also transmit the virus to others, increasing the overall public exposure.

State and federal health records show that there have been 393 AIDS cases and 255 deaths in Louisiana. Fifteen of the reported cases have been related to transfusions.

The local Blood Center, which furnishes blood to about four dozen hospitals in 14 parishes, began screening donated blood for the AIDS virus two years ago. Since then, it reports that only 70 of the 200,000 pints it has tested have come up positive. They were discarded.

The local response to the urging that transfusion receivers have their blood tested has been immense. Doctors and the free clinics that offer the service with anonymity report being swamped by telephone calls and visits.

The necessity is particularly poignant because contaminated transfusions can put at risk people whose lifestyles did not place them in the high-risk category. AIDS is contracted and transmitted through sexual activity — primarily male homosexual activity — and from hypodermic needles shared by intravenous drug users.

Infected women can also transmit the disease to their unborn children. This is a significant — and heartbreaking — risk group and, like the transfusion recipients, a group of utter innocents.

We would like to point out again, however, that the risk related to blood transfusions is not related to blood donations. While it was possible, during the period 1978-85, for one to get AIDS or the AIDS virus from receiving contaminated blood, one could never have gotten them by giving blood.

The early, relatively unfocused AIDS scare led to a dangerous drop in blood donations in some areas, though not ours.

We urge the public not to be frightened of giving blood, but to continue to give it and to begin to do so if it has not been one's practice. Giving one's own life's blood to others who need it is perhaps the best and easiest human service an individual can render. The procedure is painless and short, and it is done by able, appreciative medical technicians. And it can be the difference between someone else's life and death.

The Kansas City Times

Kansas City, MO, March 19, 1987

Precautionary checks for the AIDS virus are being recommended by the American Red Cross and other national authorities. People urged to consider them are those who have had a transfusion between 1978 and April, 1985, when centers began routinely testing all donated blood for evidence of exposure.

This is preventive community health care in the best sense of the words. Individuals who received transfusions ought to listen to the good advice of the experts this time. The test is reliable and not expensive. At the very minimum it would provide peace of mind to the former patient and the family.

Beyond that, in the small number of instances where the virus is found to be present, habits could be changed so that it would not be passed on to unsuspecting spouses, children or other members of society. The devastating nature of AIDS is enough to strike terror into a victim's soul. Rightly so. Responsible individual efforts to block its spread should be consistent with that level of danger and concern. Every possible method

of learning facts to spare loved ones should be made. If it's too late to do anything else, that's the least a conscientious person can do.

Suggestions that assorted groups of Americans be made to take tests for AIDS have been flying about as more people get sick. Serious consideration of the tests is increasingly replacing a credulous reaction that society could dismiss personal rights so easily. This Red Cross suggestion that transfusion recipients seek out their own tests voluntarily is a good way to avoid another set of demands for mandatory examinations.

The Centers for Disease Control says that of the 32,825 cases of AIDS reported, only 683 have resulted from blood transfusions. All but two happened before 1985. Moreover, it's expected that probably as few as 1/100th of 1 percent of those who received transfusions in the pre-screening period are carrying the virus.

But no one would want to risk spreading the disease of AIDS if he or she is in that tiny, innocent group.

Newsday

*Long Island, NY
March 19, 1987*

The American Red Cross is urging everyone who received a blood transfusion between 1978 and April of 1985 to do what President Ronald Reagan has already done — get tested for the AIDS antibody.

That recommendation may panic 25 to 30 million people who received transfusions before blood donors were routinely screened for evidence of the AIDS virus. It shouldn't.

As the Centers for Disease Control make clear in their weekly health bulletin released today, the risk of infection is slight, and routine testing for every transfusion patient is *not* recommended. How much blood you received, where and when you received it and where it came from all affect the odds of getting the AIDS virus from a transfusion. Someone who got a single unit of blood in South Dakota in 1978 would be at much less risk than someone in the New York metropolitan area who underwent major heart surgery in early 1985 — when the incidence of AIDS was higher and comprehensive screening was not yet done.

Yet even in this area, risk of infection from a transfusion is small. New York City Health Commissioner Stephen Joseph estimates that out of 2.1 million transfusions in that time period, only about 420 people received contaminated blood units.

Besides, many who were exposed to the virus through a blood transfusion will be discovered through "look-back" programs, where health workers track down those who might have received bad blood.

So before rushing off to the nearest testing center, those who received a transfusion during the blood bank's 7½-year window of vulnerability should first consult with their doctor or the hospital where they had the transfusion.

Voluntary testing — done with a patient's informed consent, with guarantees of confidentiality and in conjunction with counseling — can provide useful diagnostic information and reduce spread of the deadly disease. Now more than ever, these testing guidelines should be foremost in the minds of public health officials — particularly when they're talking about a testing alert that could affect millions of people.

French, U.S. Researchers Report Finding Probable AIDS Virus

The U.S. Centers for Disease Control in Atlanta had recorded 3,775 cases in the U.S. of AIDS through mid-March of 1984, of which 1,624 had been fatal. Of the U.S. cases reported through December 1983, 71% were among homosexual and bisexual men, 17% among intravenous drug abusers and 5% among U.S. residents born in Haiti. Hemophiliacs, recipients of blood transfusions and people having heterosexual contact with members of risk groups made up an additional 1% each of the reported cases. Since AIDS was labeled the "No. 1 priority" of the U.S. Public Health Service in May 1983, new research grants connected with the effort to find the cause of AIDS were announced, and an effort was made to quell the public panic over a feared spread of the disease to the general population.

The CDC April 21, 1984 confirmed news reports that French researchers had isolated a virus thought to be the cause of AIDS. Only two days later, Health and Human Services Secretary Margaret Heckler announced a parallel discovery by a U.S. National Cancer Institute team of a virus believed to be the cause of the disease. Though neither set of findings had yet been published in the scientific literature, and many details remained in doubt, Heckler said at her news conference that she thought the two viruses ultimately "will prove to be the same." Identification of the virus was regarded as the first necessary step toward developing a cure for the disease. Both viruses were retroviruses that attacked the same white blood cells attacked by AIDS. In neither case, however, had it yet been possible to establish positively a causal relationship between the virus and AIDS. Because of the alarm the disease had caused, research efforts had been unusually intense, and it was expected to be some time before the significance of the discoveries and the competing claims of priority could be firmly established.

The Seattle Times
Seattle, WA, April 30, 1984

NO ONE yet is declaring an unequivocal victory over AIDS (for Acquired Immune Deficiency Syndrome), but the speed with which researchers have accomplished a breakthrough is a tribute to the ever-astonishing skills of medical science.

Last week, scientists in both the U.S. and France announced that they think they've identified a virus that causes the untreatable, often deadly disease that strikes down the body's defenses against cancer and other disorders. Identification of the virus opens the door to devising a blood test to identify carriers of AIDS and, eventually, to a preventive vaccine.

Because AIDS has been identified principally with homosexuals, it has produced a good deal of tasteless gallows humor. But the menace it poses to overall health care is serious business. Because AIDS can be transmitted through blood transfusions, blood donations have shown an alarming decline in many parts of the country.

Although incontrovertible proof of the discovery awaits further laboratory work, the breakthrough is utterly remarkable both for its medical significance and its pace. The announcement came less than three years after AIDS first was identified.

Richmond Times-Dispatch
Richmond, VA, April 30, 1984

Secretary Margaret Heckler spoke modestly of adding "another miracle to the long honor roll of American science and medicine." Why did her Department of Health and Human Services boast so confidently last week of scoring a breakthrough against the mystery disease AIDS? Consider that:

• The government's scientists have discovered a virus that *probably* causes acquired immune deficiency syndrome, the killer disease that has terrorized (primarily) homosexual communities in major cities. But French scientists a week earlier had identified a virus of a different name that *probably* is guilty. Mrs. Heckler says the two viruses *probably* will prove to be one and the same.

• If tests prove this viral strain actually triggers AIDS, scientists *probably* can produce a test within six months to identify carriers and screen blood donors. (That should help end the hysteria concerning blood transfusions, but the actual present danger of contracting AIDS from donated blood is extremely small. The American Council on Science and Health has calculated that Americans run less than a one-in-a-million chance of getting AIDS from a transfusion; by contrast, they incur a 7 in 100 risk of acquiring a hepatitis infection.)

• If research proceeds according to a best-case scenario, HHS says a vaccine for AIDS *probably* will be available in two years. However, some non-government researchers temper that optimism by noting that a vaccine for hepatitis B, also a viral disease, took 10 years.

Any progress against an incurable disease that has killed nearly 2,000 persons since it was first identified in 1981 is worth cheering. But since HHS dealt in probabilities, some of which more accurately appear to be possibilities, why the big blast of the publicity trumpets?

Explained The New York Times, editorially: "... what you are hearing is not yet a public benefit but a private competition — for fame, prizes, new research funds." From Paris to Cambridge, Mass., from the Centers for Disease Control in Atlanta to HHS' National Institutes of Health near Washington, the race is on not only to discover the cause of a deadly disease but also to be credited with being first.

The Times, for once, is probably right. And wouldn't it be great if a similar frenetic competition developed to discover the cause of such veteran scourges as, say, cancer of the pancreas and of the liver, which still kill more than 95 percent of their victims within five years?

The Hartford Courant
Hartford, CT, April 27, 1984

The headlines are hopeful, but the reality is this: Acquired immune deficiency syndrome, or AIDS, can neither be cured nor prevented at the present time, and it could be years before the medical mystery is completely solved.

French and American scientists, working independently but sharing their findings, think they have discovered the virus that causes the disease. American researchers call their find HTLV-3; the French have isolated a virus they call LAV. The two viruses may prove to be the same, because it is believed that a single micro-organism causes AIDS.

Discovery of the cause would mean that scientists are on the right track to finding sure means to detect, cure and prevent the disease. The American researchers predict that a test to detect AIDS in victims even before symptoms develop will be widely available within six months. The test can be used to screen donated blood, which is considered a transmitting agent. The test could help restrain the spread of AIDS through transfusions and will offer peace of mind to users of donated blood. That's the most important short-term benefit of the work on the viruses.

But discovery of the viruses, while significant, should not be blown out of proportion. A medical problem of enormous dimensions still exists.

The progress in research thus far presents no immediate hope to those now suffering from the disease and those in whom the virus is incubating. Since AIDS was recognized in 1981, it has been detected in some 4,000 Americans and more than 1,700 have died. If the incidence of the disease advances at the present rate and no preventive is developed, there is no telling how many thousands, or millions, more could be afflicted.

Scientists, while rejoicing at the apparent successes announced in the last few days, don't agree on how soon the real victories will come. Some say a vaccine to prevent AIDS can be developed in two to three years; others say five years or longer.

So no one should be lulled into thinking the disease has been conquered. The further commitment of public and private resources to research must be generous. Providers have to anticipate even greater demands on treatment and counseling services for victims and those in the high risk categories — mainly homosexual and bisexual males, intravenous drug users and regular users of donated blood. Efforts must continue to educate the public about the disease so that ignorance and fear — and thus discrimination — are minimized.

And caution and recognition of the costs are still the watchwords for those whose sexual behavior and other habits put them at risk.

Science has taken great strides in understanding AIDS, but nothing much can yet be done about it.

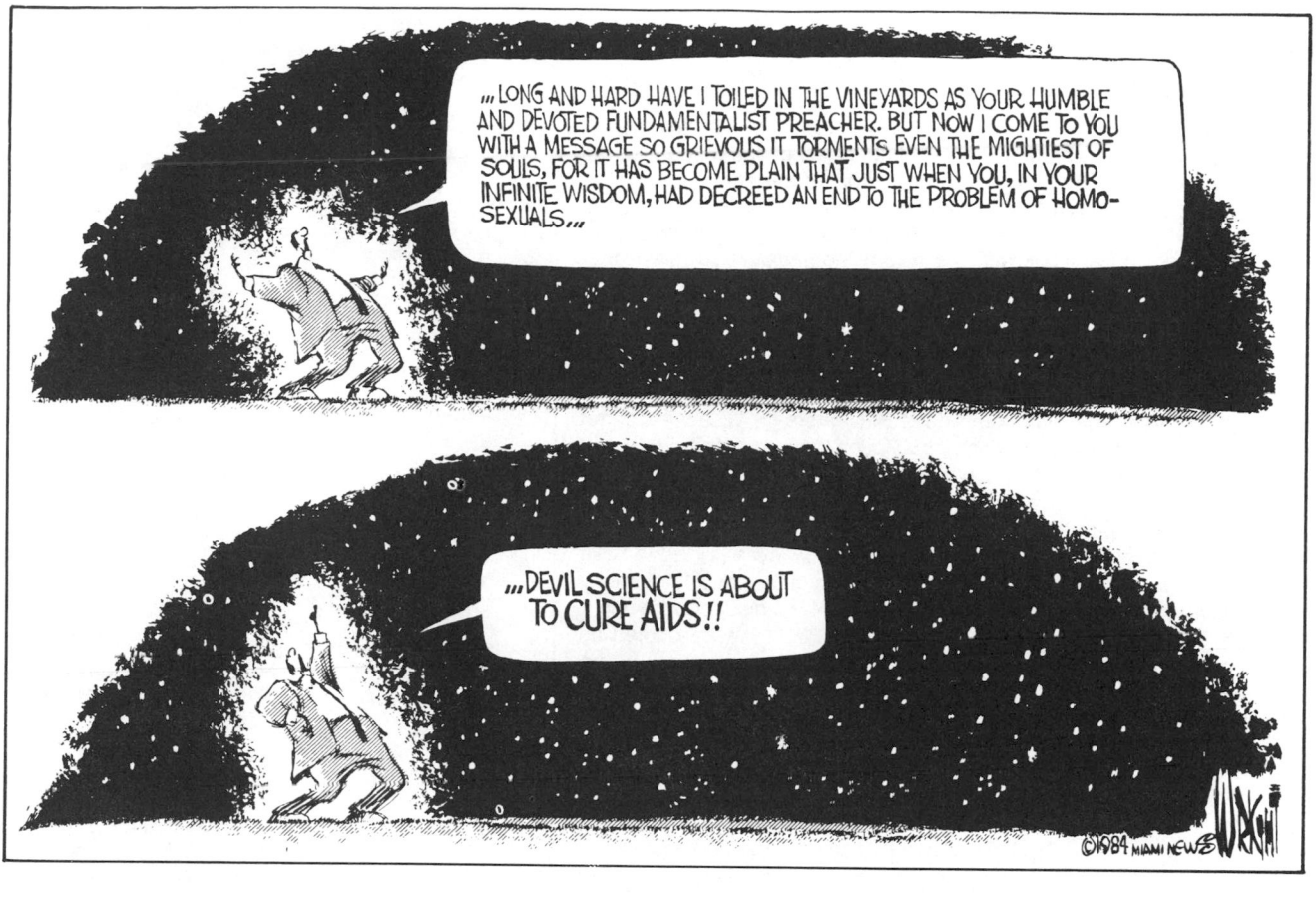

Pittsburgh Post-Gazette
Pittsburgh, PA, April 25, 1984

In the annals of medical research, the fight against the insidious killer called Acquired Immune Deficiency Syndrome will occupy a celebrated chapter one of these days. And, while it is too early to celebrate, that day has now come a little closer.

Federal researchers have announced that they have discovered the virus that appears to cause AIDS. Although a cure is still not assured, there is hope of a vaccine being developed. Moreover, within six months a test should be widely available to identify the virus, which among other things will enable blood banks to ensure that prospective donors are not infected. (This, as with everything else about AIDS, has been the subject of exaggerated public fears).

The American announcement comes hard on the heels of a similar one from France, and hints at the prestige at stake in this great scientific endeavor. It is not clear who first cleared the initial obstacle, or indeed if it is the same one; more pertinent is the intensity of the chase. By throwing light on the unknown, this international effort should do much to defuse the hysterical public reaction to the AIDS outbreak.

It may also have a soothing effect on hysterical overreaction by some at the fringes. When AIDS first struck about three years ago, certain fire-and-brimstone types could not resist seeing it as a divine judgment against homosexuals, who are the group most affected. This un-Christian salivating, devoid as it was of any charity, in turn seemed to prompt some in the gay community to assume an official lack of interest on the part of a moralizing Reagan administration.

Both views were outrageously wrong.

AIDS is clearly an urgent public health problem and one with implications for the whole country. This compelling public interest, as well as the natural drive of scientific curiosity, should ensure that the heartening breakthrough announced this week is not the last.

Los Angeles Times
Los Angeles, CA, April 25, 1984

It has been a little less than three years since the first cases of a mysterious disease known as acquired immune deficiency syndrome (AIDS) were reported in the United States. Since then, nearly 4,100 people have been identified as victims of the disease that impairs the body's natural system for fighting infections, and at least 1,758 of them have died. Now medical researchers believe that they have found a virus that probably leads to the onset of AIDS. If they prove to be right, the way could be open to devise a method for the early detection of AIDS and to develop a vaccine to prevent it.

The proof is not yet at hand. Laboratory test animals have been inoculated with the suspect virus, but insufficient time has passed to determine whether AIDS has developed in them. AIDS most commonly occurs among male homosexuals as a result of intimate sexual contact. It has also been found among intravenous drug users, recent immigrants from Haiti, and hemophiliacs. Because AIDS can be transmitted by blood transfusion, persons known to have received blood from donors who subsequently developed AIDS are also being closely monitored. This latter study could rather grimly provide definitive human tests on unwitting potential victims of the disease.

Dr. Robert C. Gallo of the National Cancer Institute, who headed the main American AIDS research team, hopes that a vaccine to prevent AIDS can be developed in as little as two years, using recombinant DNA techniques. Before then, though, there seems to be a good chance that an accurate test for AIDS will be devised. Margaret Heckler, secretary of Health and Human Services, thinks that such a test could be widely available within six months. For the population at large, the great promise of such a test would be to insure that blood for transfusions is free from the virus that is thought to trigger AIDS.

Simultaneously with the claimed successes by American researchers has come word that a French medical team believes that it has found an AIDS-causing virus. Whether this is the same virus as that identified by the American team ought to be known in the next few weeks. Whether one or the other or both are responsible for the onset of AIDS will almost certainly take longer to determine. Only after that determination is made will it be possible for a vaccine to be created.

What can be said for now is that the effort to find a cause for AIDS and in so doing devise measures that could prevent its spread appears to have made remarkable progress in a relatively brief time. If the answer has not yet been found it has, at a minimum, been brought measurably closer.

AIDS Virus Evidence Mounts; Exposures Feared Wider

Accumulating evidence linked AIDS to a class of viruses called retroviruses. Retroviruses had been identified as the cause of the disease by French and American research teams in April 1984. The leader of the American effort, National Cancer Institute researcher Dr. Robert Gallo, June 13, 1984 said he and his French counterpart, Dr. Luc Montagnier, had recently compared notes. Gallo said that he and Montagnier had agreed that the virus called LAV by the French and the virus called HTLV-3 by the Americans were "close relatives." The identification was already widely accepted in the medical community but the question of which team could claim credit for the potentially momentous discovery was still in dispute.

New evidence for viral transmission of the disease was cited in the July 6, 1984 issue of the journal *Science*. The U.S. Centers for Disease Control (CDC) in Atlanta cited a case in which it had found the suspected virus in the blood of a blood donor and of a patient who had received the donor's blood. The donor had not shown symptoms of AIDS, but both donor and recipient subsequently developed the disease.

Separate CDC research teams October 7, 1984 were reported to have found active forms of the AIDS virus in semen and saliva of healthy individuals, suggesting that there were "carriers" of the disease who might unwittingly infect others. Two of the researchers Oct. 9 were quoted as emphasizing, however, that there was no evidence that discovery of the virus in saliva posed any greater risk to the public at large. Contact with contaminated saliva alone, one argued, "cannot be important in spreading AIDS or the disease would be more widespread than it is."

A federal health official feared that exposure of Americans to the virus believed to cause AIDS was much higher than had been previously suspected, it was reported November 5, 1984. Dr. James Curran, head of the AIDS task force at the CDC, estimated that at least 300,000 people had already been unknowingly exposed to the virus. He said that preliminary research indicated that perhaps 10% of that group—most of them homosexual men—would come down with the severe form of the deadly disorder over the following five years. "There's a tendency for all of us to underestimate the problem because we don't want to believe it's true," Curran said.

THE BLADE
Toledo, OH, May 8, 1984

IN the annals of medical research, the fight against Acquired Immune Deficiency Syndrome will occupy an important chapter one of these days. And, while it is too early to celebrate, that day is now a little closer.

Federal researchers have announced that they have discovered the virus that appears to cause AIDS. Although a cure is still not assured, there is hope of a vaccine being developed. Moreover, within six months a test should be widely available to identify the virus, which among other things will enable blood banks to insure that prospective donors are not infected.

The American announcement comes hard on the heels of a similar one from France, and hints at the prestige at stake in this medical-research endeavor. It is not clear who first cleared the initial obstacle, or indeed if it is the same one; more pertinent is the intensity of the chase. By throwing light on the unknown, this effort should do much to defuse the panicky public reaction to the AIDS outbreak.

It also may have a soothing effect on hysterical overreaction by some at the fringes. When AIDS first struck about three years ago, certain fire-and-brimstone types could not resist seeing it as a divine judgment against homosexuals, who are the group most affected. This un-Christian salivating, devoid as it was of any charity, in turn prompted some in the gay community to assume an official lack of interest on the part of a moralizing Reagan administration.

Both views were outrageously wrong. AIDS is clearly an urgent public health problem and one with implications for the whole country. This compelling public interest, as well as the natural drive of scientific curiosity, should be assurance enough that this heartening breakthrough is not the last.

The Evening Gazette
Worcester, MA, April 27, 1984

It's heartening that government medical researchers may have discovered the cause of the deadly disease AIDS — Acquired Immune Deficiency Syndrome — that already has killed 1,758 people in the United States alone. The source is probably a cancer virus that American and French scientists successfully have isolated. Finding the cause is an important achievement and a first step to developing a cure.

Unfortunately, the latest breakthrough won't immediately help those stricken with this virus, which breaks down the body's immune system, leaving victims defenseless against infection. In the past, effective antiviral vaccines have proved difficult to create, and it may be six months to two years before an AIDS vaccine can be produced and tested.

But discovery of the AIDS virus has immediate benefits: Scientists now can develop a blood test to identify AIDS victims, and keep AIDS-infected blood out of the nation's transfusion supply — causes of much concern since the outbreak of the disease. As one scientist said, the breakthrough "just begins a whole series of miracles that can occur."

Government and medical authorities — and the majority of the public — should be given much credit for taking a calm, responsible approach to the AIDS outbreak. Because a large number of the victims have been homosexuals, a homophobic hysteria has surfaced in some quarters, threatening to add a scourge of prejudice to what is essentially a public health problem. Clearly, what researchers are fighting is one more loathsome disease, not divine retribution, and the latest hopeful developments show that the battle, although far from over, can be won.

The Birmingham News

Birmingham, AL, November 19, 1984

Most of the news about AIDS — Acquired Immune Deficiency Syndrome — has been bad news. A recent study continues in that vein.

According to Dr. Jeffrey Laurence of the New York Hospital-Cornell Medical Center and other researchers, persons who show no symptoms of the virus and are otherwise healthy can be carriers of the disease. That conclusion was reached after researchers studied cases in which drug-using mothers passed AIDS on to their babies, despite themselves having no symptoms of the disease.

The mothers, researchers said, proved to have the AIDS antibodies, but the antibodies failed to prevent them from "carrying" the disease or otherwise do the mothers any good.

The findings suggest that current research on AIDS antibodies to produce a vaccine which will protect human beings from the disease may have to be revised, and research be broadened to include other possibilities.

Meanwhile in Australia, the Queensland state legislature approved legislation that would make donating blood by one knowing he had AIDS a criminal offense. The legislation was prompted by the deaths from AIDS of three babies who had received blood donated by a male homosexual. A fourth baby is near death.

The disease is likely to be passed on only by intimate contact with a person with AIDS or with a carrier, not by normal contact or by using sterile needles. Even so, one hopes the findings of the study increase the determination of the medical research community to find a defense against the disease.

The Dispatch

Columbus, OH, May 13, 1984

The discovery of the probable cause of acquired immune deficiency syndrome (AIDS) is exciting news, offering the first real chance of combating the mysterious and often fatal ailment.

Almost as exciting is the comparative speed with which medical science, with its sophisticated new accesses to the most minute particles of tissue, was able to pinpoint the probable virus culprit.

AIDS, a collapse of the body's immune systems which leaves its victims prey to certain cancer types, pneumonia or other infections, was not identified until 1981. Believed to be transmitted through contact with body fluids, it strikes mainly promiscuous homosexual males, intravenous drug abusers, Haitian immigrants and hemophiliacs who are treated with blood products.

Some initial confusion resulted from the almost-simultaneous disclosure of a suspected causal virus by a Pasteur Institute team in France and an American team at the National Institutes of Health.

However, Dr. Robert Gallo of the National Cancer Institute, leader of the U.S. team, said he believes with many scientists that the two finds, although labeled differently, may be the same virus, a member of the human T-cell leukemia virus family.

Since its discovery, AIDS has struck more than 4,000 U.S. victims and caused more than 1,700 deaths.

The scientists' ultimate task now, development and testing of a safe and effective vaccine from a virus believed capable of causing cancer, is at least several years away — offering no immediate hope to present AIDS sufferers and those at high risk of getting it.

However, Gallo outlined possible intermediate steps toward a vaccine cure that could check the rising incidence of AIDS cases.

A blood screening test being developed at NIH, which could be available in six months, would permit identification of AIDS victims and help ensure that donated blood and blood products used for transfusions and other treatments are free of the virus.

Doctors at NIH said the blood test would also help define the disease course at earlier stages and possibly allow for more effective treatment. They also saw possibilities, short of a vaccine, for developing super antibodies to help victims fight AIDS infection and for tailoring a portion of the virus, by genetic research techniques, to stimulate immunity without causing the disease.

Although U.S. scientists are collaborating with the French scientists, there is an element of national pride involved in work which is already being labeled of Nobel Prize stature and in which the U.S. team believes it has a developmental edge.

The work itself is the important achievement, against an awful disease. If it is a contest, too, it is the kind of international competition to which we can be most proud and happy to see U.S. talent and resources devoted.

THE TENNESSEAN
*Nashville, TN,
April 28, 1984*

GOVERMENT scientists have announced discovery of a virus which causes the killer disease known as AIDS — acquired immune deficiency syndrome.

The discovery also includes the technique for growing the virus routinely and a blood test which can identify the carriers of AIDS in virtually all cases.

AIDS has struck more than 4,000 people and caused more than 1,700 deaths in the United States since 1981. But since it is an incurable disease and an almost certain killer, it has filled countless others with fear. The prospect that the virus can be identified and the disease prevented by vaccine should be a comfort to many.

AIDS is contracted mainly by male homosexuals, intravenous drug users, hemophiliacs who are treated with blood products, and others who receive blood transfusions.

A vaccine for the disease could be developed within three years, according to the scientists. Unfortunately, this will not help those who already have AIDS. But identifying the virus that causes it should be of tremendous benefit in preventing the spread of the disease by detecting it in the blood of victims before it is passed on to others.

"We should be able to assure that blood for transfusion is free from AIDS," said Secretary Margaret M. Heckler of the Health and Human Services Department. "With the blood test, we can now identify AIDS victims with essentially 100% certainty."

Scientists at the National Institutes of Health, especially Dr. Robert Gallo of the National Cancer Institute, are credited with isolating the virus and devising the system to detect and grow it.

French scientists reported a similar discovery a week earlier. The French and the Americans have been cooperating in the research. But because of some "miscommunications and misunderstandings," it was not determined if the discovery reported by the French was exactly the same as that of the Americans.

But regardless of who gets the final credit, the identification of the cause of AIDS is a major medical breakthrough which should bring cheer to all nations.

WHO Gives Alert on AIDS in Africa

AIDS was spreading in central Africa, and people there appeared to be getting it through heterosexual contact, according to a study the *New England Journal of Medicine* published February 23, 1984. No African countries reported AIDS cases in 1985, although doctors there had found hundreds, if not thousands of the virus' victims, according to the United Nations World Health Organization (WHO). The *New York Times* reported the situation November 8, 1985. In central Africa the disease had been found to strike women and men in roughly equal numbers and to be spread largely by heterosexual contact. Six nations—Zaire, Zambia, Tanzania, Kenya, Uganda and Rwanda—had all been hit.

WHO said that since 1980 at least 50,000 Africans had probably contracted AIDS, according to a June 6, 1986 news account. The figure, the highest and most definite WHO had yet offered on the subject, appeared in a report that the group had not officially released. The report estimated that at least one million to two million Africans had been infected with the disease. It said that by "the most conservative rate of annual progression," a "minimum of 10,000 AIDS cases annually may be occurring in Africa." The group based its estimate of 50,000 on this figure. The number was double that for the U.S., where AIDS had been thought to be most widespread. Health workers in Africa had reported a mounting AIDS toll, but nations there had acknowledged only a handful of cases. Their motive for secrecy was said to be fear of jeopardizing tourism and development aid. The WHO report said the continent's total of 378 officially reported cases had been supplied by just nine countries.

Five top AIDS experts, including Dr. James W. Curran, director of the AIDS program at the Centers for Disease Control, and Dr. Jonathan Mann, director of the WHO program to fight AIDS, in a report described in news accounts October 27, 1986 and November 14, 1986, warned that the disease had become "a major health threat to all Africans." The report asserted that "eductional programs and blood bank screening must become an immediate public health priority." The meager funds of the African nations meant that "an international concerted effort" would be needed to contain the spread of the disease on the continent, the report said.

LOS ANGELES Herald Examiner

Los Angeles, CA, December 1, 1985

The AIDS epidemic has crossed both the U.S. and Western Europe like a winter storm, leaving in its wake scattered deaths and widespread fear. But, in some parts of Africa, the disease's impact can best be described as a ravaging cyclone. A recent study by a National Cancer Institute researcher shows that the AIDS virus has affected from 10 to 50 percent of the population in some central and east African countries.

It is in that part of Africa where, some scientists say, the AIDS virus may have begun its spread more than 20 years ago. This hypothesis has led researchers to search for possible clues to a cure in such countries as Zaire, Rwanda and Uganda. Recent reports that some Senegalese may have a natural immunity to AIDS have also raised hopes that links to a cure may be found there.

African leaders are understandably loathe to accept both the theory that AIDS originated in their lands and the basis of the theory. An international game of hot-potato can hardly be productive, however; quarrels over place-of-origin must not impede valuable research, particularly on the continent where the disease's ravaging impact is felt so powerfully. In capitals like Kinshasa, Zaire, the epidemic's victims have filled up half the city's hospital beds. During a recent visit to one such hospital, whispers of *"l'horreur"* drifted between the narrow aisles in a ward packed with beds and infested with malarial mosquitoes.

Because AIDS in Africa is transmitted primarily by heterosexuals, and because unsanitary conditions there often encourage the spread of disease, hopes of containing the epidemic are dim. In fact, as AIDS works its way across the globe, there is a rising fear among epidemiologists that it will become a scourge in most Third World countries. The cost in lives and already limited services could be devastating.

AIDS is now a world crisis that calls for international solutions. It will not be in anyone's best interest to confuse politics with science while solutions are sought. Finding a cure is a major concern for everyone — and for no one more than the people of central and east Africa.

ST. LOUIS POST-DISPATCH

St. Louis, MO
November 23, 1985

Who, or what, is to blame for the deadly disease Acquired Immune Deficiency Syndrome? And where did AIDS originate? Those are the questions being tackled by scientists around the world as they search for ways to halt the growing epidemic and to successfully treat current AIDS victims, who now face an almost certain death sentence.

But the search has run into roadblocks in some countries, particularly in Africa, that are defensive about the notion that the disease might have originated within their borders. *The New York Times* reports that the result has been the suppression, and in some cases destruction, of research and information. Some are denying the existence of the disease within their borders at the same time doctors are reporting epidemics. Such actions do nothing to help stem the disease.

Africa offers some of the most fascinating clues because the disease appears to have been detected there 20 years ago and it is spreading by conventional heterosexual practices. In addition — unlike elsewhere, where the victims are primarily male — it is striking both sexes equally in Africa and a greater number of children. Scientists are particularly interested in certain species of African monkeys that appear to naturally carry viruses similar to AIDS.

It's unfortunate that politicians are treating AIDS, like its victims, as an untouchable subject. Finding the place of origin is crucial to AIDS research because it could explain how the disease took hold in humans and could offer the best clues on how to stop it. Where AIDS began is an act or accident of nature, not the fault of any government. But while man may not be blamed for initiating the disease, he can be held responsible for impeding a cure.

THE ATLANTA CONSTITUTION
Atlanta, GA, December 27, 1985

Up until a week ago, Acquired Immune Deficiency Syndrome didn't exist in Kenya and Zaire — that is, officially. Oh, Kenyans and Zaireans were becoming infected with AIDS, all right. But some government officials were loathe to scare off prospective tourists or to admit their countrymen might have been touched by a disease associated with taboo practices. In Kenya, censors went so far as to confiscate copies of the International Herald Tribune documenting cases of AIDS there.

Now, in a major turnabout hailed by the World Health Organization, Kenya has become the the first black African government to report verified cases of AIDS to WHO's Geneva headquarters; and in Zaire physicians, with government approval, have begun passing out AIDS informational pamphlets, a tacit admission the disease is a problem there, too.

The WHO is appealing to developed countries for a $30 million fund to build a global reporting network to trace and check the spread of AIDS. Additionally, it hopes to start a public health informational campaign to combat the disease, with a special emphasis on reaching the huge transistor-radio audience in the Third World.

But vast areas where AIDS is already prevalent may not be drawn into the WHO campaign simply out of some leaders' irrational feelings of shame. Kenya and, to a lesser extent, Zaire have set examples that may crack that reticence, and they should be commended. The idea, after all, should be: It's OK to tell.

The Boston Globe
Boston, MA, November 14, 1985

The worst news is yet to come about AIDS. Even as the American public takes some reassurance from the limited transmission of the disease here, reports emerging from some African countries are ominous.

Coupled with a newer understanding of the AIDS virus as an insidious infection of the brain as well as the body, the reports make the disease even more calamitous.

What had been suspected in central and east Africa now is confirmed: AIDS is rampant. One-tenth of the residents are infected by the virus; in time, at least half will become sick.

They number more than 10 million people, five times as many as are infected in the far more populous United States. There is less reason to think the spread of AIDS can be slowed in Africa, although it may be in the United States.

Last summer, two American medical scientists Drs. Bruce Johnson and Charles Oster of the Kenya National Research Institute, expressed anxiety over the heavy seeding-in of the AIDS virus.

Blood donations indicated that 10-15 percent of Kenya's population carried the virus. A blood screening of 90 Nairobi prostitutes showed that half were infected and that three out of four had symptoms. A sampling of the 250,000-member Turkana tribe showed that two out of three were AIDS-positive.

Although Kenya lists only three official cases of AIDS, the doctors had heard through colleagues that a lethal new sickness was widespread in neighboring Rwanda and Uganda. They fear that it is only a matter of time until it moves into Kenya and other countries. It is known as "slim disease" because its victims waste away and die. The doctors suspected it was a new form of AIDS.

They were right.

Now, reports in the British medical journal The Lancet show that slim disease is an African version of AIDS. Its spread into Uganda — both to rural villages and the capital, Kampala — is linked to traveling traders and troops from Tanzania, which borders on the south. The prostitutes tested in Nairobi were migrants from Tanzania, where nothing is known about the status of AIDS.

The AIDS outbreak is no less dismal in Rwanda and Zaire. As early as 1983, a higher rate of acute AIDS cases was detected in Zaire's capital city, Kinshasa, than in New York or San Francisco, the American cities with the highest incidence of AIDS. In Rwanda, AIDS cases in children are 15 times higher than in the United States.

Up to half the hospital beds in Kinshasa are reported to be occupied by AIDS-infected patients. Twenty percent of the pediatric beds in Kigali hold children with slim disease. Since the AIDS virus can be passed from mother to child during pregnancy and breast-feeding, the high birthrate in Africa compounds the AIDS problem.

In Africa, as in Haiti, AIDS occurs almost equally in men and women. The disease seems to be spread in the same ways that it is in the US — sexually and through contaminated blood.

Opportunities for transmitting the AIDS virus in Africa are believed to be enhanced, however, by certain practices. Injections are commonly given by folk-medicine practitioners who reuse unsterile needles. Cutting the skin is another folk-medicine practice, and the blade is reused. Tribal circumcision rites, piercing of the ear, nose and lip, and ritual scarring are often performed under unsanitary conditions.

Beyond that, the miserable overcrowdedness "in which the bulk of the people live, combined with a high frequency of infections, injuries and sores which break the skin, make blood contact among family members practically inevitable, with the transmission of the virus likely," says Dr. John Seale, an AIDS specialist and researcher in London.

In an editorial in the Journal of the Royal Society of Medicine, Seale emphasizes the singularly dangerous threat posed by the AIDS virus over the next decade, as a "slow, irreversible and cumulative" brain infection. Because the virus persists for life, "it would produce a self-sustaining epidemic.

"Indeed," wrote Seale, "it would produce a lethal pandemic throughout the crowded cities and villages of the Third World of a magnitude unparalleled in human history. That is what the AIDS virus is now doing."

The specter of an AIDS catastrophe looms over Africa, driving home the desperate need to find an effective treatment and making urgent the call for a US research effort on the scale of the Manhattan Project. Not a moment can be lost.

THE KANSAS CITY STAR
Kansas City, MO
November 11, 1985

Conflicts brew in East and Central African countries about coping with acquired immune deficiency syndrome. They illustrate clearly the pitfall of treating this fatal disease as a political question instead of the major public health problem it is.

Information is being collected, and sluggishly disseminated, that AIDS patients in African countries are primarily heterosexual or infants. The normal route of transmission of the virus is by conventional sexual behavior and pregnancy. Unlike in the United States and other Western countries where most victims are homosexual or bisexual men, it apparently is almost as common there among women as male heterosexuals. A study discussed recently in the *Journal of the American Medical Association* documented findings of the AIDS antibody in male and female African patients in Rwanda in Central Africa and in Brussels. Prostitutes should be considered a new high risk group, the researchers believe.

"These studies suggest that human T-cell lymphotropic virus type III (AIDS) has already spread extensively into the general African population and that female prostitutes could be an important human reservoir of AIDS virus in the heterosexual population," the scientists advised. Other medical analyses have drawn similar conclusions, offering no explanation why the disease has taken a different course in Africa. One risk similarity in both countries seems to be the large number of sexual contacts of victims — homosexuals, prostitutes, their liaisons.

On top of the terrible urgency to find the cause and cure of this disease on both continents, it is complicated by African political leaders' unwillingness to release information about its course there. Some even refuse to acknowledge its existence. Independent physicians' reports show the disease exists in 20 African countries, but none has reported cases to the World Health Organization.

Leaders fear attacks blaming Africans, or criticism of health care there, for the disease. It's understandable. The ignorant and bigoted prefer such outbursts to a problem over deliberate work toward a solution. But data from Africa are greatly needed for the implications they contain on the course of the disease here and in other countries.

U.S. Tests of French AIDS Drug OK'd

An official of the U.S. Food and Drug Administration (FDA) September 18, 1985 announced that the agency had approved human tests in the U.S. of HPA-23, a French drug that appeared to be scoring successes in the treatment of AIDS. The drug was developed at the Institut Pasteur in Paris, where the AIDS virus had been isolated in 1983. Institute scientist Jean Claude Chermann February 8, 1985 told a U.S. symposium that the new drug, HPA-23, had appeared for the first time to have inhibited the replication of the virus believed to cause AIDS. Tests had been completed in only four patients, he said, but in all four the virus seemed to have disappeared, at least temporarily. Chermann stressed, however, that the treatment should not be regarded as a cure. The drug was believed to have severe side-effects. Discovery of the treatment spread hope among AIDS sufferers and put pressure on the FDA to approve use of the drug in the U.S. on at least an experimental basis.

Other drugs currently being evaluated experimentally included Suramin, a 50-year-old antiparasitic drug that appeared to inhibit the multiplication of the AIDS virus; alpha-interferon, an antiviral agent; and phosphoformate, a drug originally developed to combat the Herpes virus infection.

Forming a backdrop to the ongoing AIDS research was a continuing controversy over the discovery of the virus. Not only scientific prestige but also money was involved, because of potential revenues from both tests and treatments for the disease. The U.S. test kit market alone was estimated at $80 million. Patent rights for the tests depended in part on who had actually first isolated the virus.

Scientists July 10, 1985 reported that they had identified the crucial defect in the immune system caused by the AIDS virus. Writing in the July 10 issue of the *New England Journal of Medicine*, a team led by Anthony S. Fauci reported finding that the AIDS virus selectively destroyed members of a key set of blood cells. It had been known that AIDS victims showed a sharp decrease in the number of T4 helper cells. The new discovery established that while some T4 helper cells survived, such as those that produced against infecting organisms, a particular subset of the T4 helpers that was responsible for detecting invading infections was either missing or inactive.

St. Petersburg Times

St. Petersburg, FL, August 1, 1985

The speed with which the Food and Drug Administration (FDA) approves the experimental use of new drugs to combat disease should correlate with the severity of the disease being fought. If that standard is applied by the FDA, HPA-23 — the drug has shown some promise in France in treating patients with acquired immune deficiency syndrome, or AIDS — should be available for testing in this country in a matter of weeks.

Many of the normal tests of drug safety and effectiveness can be bypassed with HPA-23 and other experimental drugs to be tried on AIDS patients. Those afflicted with the disease have little need to worry about the side effects of potential medication: They are already under a death warrant. In the past five years, almost 12,000 Americans have been diagnosed with AIDS. Half of those are already dead, and the rest are almost certain to die soon unless some new treatment is discovered.

FRENCH PHYSICIANS who have used HPA-23 on many patients — including about 100 Americans — in recent months, stress that the drug is no panacea. It seems to inhibit the advance of the disease in some patients, but it offers no cure. A vaccine against the virus that causes AIDS is the only long-term answer, and researchers apparently aren't close to developing one.

Why has it taken the world — especially the United States — so long to make a concerted fight against such a deadly and devastating disease? The answer is obvious: Almost three-fourths of all AIDS victims are homosexual men. Many of the others are intravenous drug users. The stigma of the disease has caused many victims to hide the true nature of their illness; it also seems to have delayed proper financing and research in this country.

Actor Rock Hudson's bravery in openly fighting AIDS seems to have helped to erase whatever remained of that stigma. His story has the effect of turning the public image of all AIDS victims into flesh and blood instead of stereotype.

UNFORTUNATELY, as the disease spreads to other segments of the population, the stigma of AIDS will disappear long before the disease itself. The FDA at least seems to be cutting through much of the normal red tape involved in approving the use of HPA-23, as well as a half-dozen other experimental drugs used on AIDS patients.

Those drugs which bypass normal approval procedures are limited to "compassionate use" on patients already diagnosed as terminally ill. But that definition currently applies to all AIDS victims. Approval of HPA-23 may at least give AIDS patients new hope that finding a cure for their disease is now the priority that it should have been long before now.

DESERET NEWS

Salt Lake City, UT
September 29, 1985

National concern about the disease acquired immune deficiency syndrome, better known as AIDS, is mounting as reports come in about its spread beyond the realm of male homosexuals and drug abusers to other sectors of the population.

Parents are keeping their children out of schools in which infected children have been enrolled. Show business people have become hesitant about stage kissing. Medical personnel are becoming cautious as they hear of a nurse and laboratory technician becoming accidentally infected by contaminated needles.

Though the concern is understandable, compassion should not be allowed to overwhelm good judgment in dealing with this problem. This observation is prompted by the comment that Gov. Richard D. Lamm of Colorado made the other day in one of the brutally frank statements for which he is becoming nationally famous.

In answer to a question from a physician about what level of care should be given AIDS patients, Gov. Lamm stated his opposition to spending unlimited amounts of money on victims who have no chance of recovery. Do what is necessary to alleviate pain and suffering but skip the expensive, heroic measures to treat terminal cases. Rather, use the money to find a cure for AIDS, the governor recommended. At present, no cure is known and the disease is fatal.

While Lamm's remarks may be stark and jarring, they reflect considerable common sense. But then it's the same kind of common sense being used by the Denver hospital where Colorado's AIDS surveillance is located, and, no doubt, by numerous other health care facilities throughout the country.

An encouraging development in keeping with this approach is the proposed merger of two organizations dealing with AIDS research, the National AIDS Research Foundation in Los Angeles, and the AIDS Medical Foundation in New York. The two will form a single national organization to raise money and provide research grants for AIDS research.

The federal government also is moving toward augmenting its funding of programs to combat AIDS. Former Utahn James O. Mason, assistant secretary for health in the Department of Health and Human Services, said the disease is the department's number one public health priority.

Certainly, the proposed $200 million government appropriation to combat AIDS — or whatever the final amount may be — will, coupled with the resources of the proposed new foundations, give strong impetus to the AIDS combat effort. Care should be taken to make sure the bulk of the money goes for research rather than for needlessly elaborate patient treatment.

THE TENNESSEAN
Nashville, TN, July 27, 1985

ACQUIRED Immune Deficiency Syndrome, an often fatal disease which destroys the body's immune system and leaves it vulnerable to numerous other diseases, is a national health threat and should be combated on an urgent basis.

As of July 15, the national Centers for Disease Control had recorded 11,737 cases of AIDS, including 5,812 deaths. The disease, which attacks people at all socio-economic levels, is believed to be triggered by a virus that spreads through sexual contact, use of contaminated needles and blood or blood products.

AIDS was originally thought to be a threat only to homosexuals, people receiving blood transfusions and drug addicts. But more recent evidence indicates that in some cases it has been spread by heterosexual contact.

The CDC said the number of AIDS cases initially seemed to double every six months, but more recently appear to be doubling every 12 months. This could indicate preventive steps and changes in lifestyles by those in the vulnerable groups. But AIDS remains a very dangerous disease and calls for a crash program to find a cure or preventive vaccine. This will require a considerable investment.

The Reagan administration, which previously had not seemed to recognize the seriousness of the threat, has now asked that its original request for $86 million in AIDS research money be increased by $40.7 million for next year. The money would go for epidemiological studies, research on prevention and control and community health education.

This is an encouraging step. Unfortunately, however, the increased request does not call for a hike in the national health budget but would be skimmed from other important programs such as the National Health Service Corps and the Indian Health Service. Also, the administration's initial request was a $10 million cut from the previous year's spending for aids, so that the new request does not represent such a large increase. It can hardly be called a deep commitment to public health.

In any case, health officials have told Congress that the administration's additional request is inadequate and would hardly begin to halt the advance of AIDS.

AIDS is a killer much in the same class as smallpox, polio and other communicable diseases that are no longer serious threats to the nation's health. It will require the same kind of national commitment that led to the elimination of those diseases. Congress should see that medical researchers have the tools they need to put an end to AIDS.

The Boston Globe
Boston, MA, November 30, 1985

It is time to rename and redefine the disease called AIDS – acquired immune deficiency syndrome. Until a broader designation is adopted, many cases will go undetected, the pattern of the disease's spread will not be clear, and its full impact will not be known.

The term "AIDS" no longer encompasses the growing list of illnesses that can be brought on by the disease's virus. Nor does it convey a true picture of how the virus can do harm.

The original definition of AIDS fails to elicit an accurate reporting of the numbers of people being stricken by the virus. Significant underreporting may be occurring, because doctors are noting only those cases that fit the narrow definition. Many are unaware of the multiple disorders now linked to the virus.

At a conference on AIDS in Africa, Dr. Robert Gallo of the National Cancer Institute emphasized that "this virus causes much more than AIDS, and most of it goes unreported."

In the beginning, AIDS was defined by the federal Centers for Disease Control as a disease characterized by acquired (not inborn) defects in a person's immune system – the system that normally protects against infection. As a consequence, patients develop an unusually deadly form of cancer known as Kaposi's Sarcoma, or an unusually deadly pneumonia, Pneumocystis carinii, or both. The definition has since been broadened to include a few other cancers and rare infections and, in cases of AIDS in children, another kind of pneumonia.

For good disease-detection reasons, the original definition was deliberately narrow. Otherwise, similar but unrelated cases might have confused the early attempts to track the disease. Now, however, the virus has been identified – designated HTLV-III by Gallo's American team, which isolated it, and LAV by the French team that first identified it. Now, when unusual cancers or infections are diagnosed, it is possible to find out whether they result from infection with HTLV-III/LAV.

Moreover, many illnesses have now been linked to the virus. They include a chronic glandular illness, peculiar bleeding disorders, the resurgence of latent diseases such as malaria and tuberculosis, new syndromes such as "slim disease" in Africa, and most of all, dire brain and nervous-system disorders.

"Most important is that this virus is causing primary brain disease with no other abnormalities detected in some people," Gallo said. "This is likely to be the future, most serious problem from this virus, in America anyway."

"We need a name for the whole spectrum of disease that this virus causes," he said, recommending the term "HTLV-III Related Disorders" or "HRD," coined by Dr. William Haseltine of the Dana-Farber Cancer Institute in Boston. Since studies by Gallo's team and others are beginning to show that the virus can directly infect the brain – possibly without first infecting immune cells – there no longer is any justification for the name "acquired immune deficiency syndrome."

The disease is too important, its threat too far-reaching, to continue a designation that signifies only the propensity of the virus to attack the immune system. That designation ignores the virus' effect on the brain and undermines detection of the actual spread of the disease. It should be dropped and a better name assigned.

WORCESTER TELEGRAM
Worcester, MA October 31, 1985

The televised announcement from Paris that three French doctors have found an effective treatment for AIDS was one of the more remarkable medical publicity events of recent history. In this case it was the medical profession, not the media, that jumped the gun.

On the basis of treating two patients for less than a week, the doctors asserted that a drug known as Cyclosporine-A saved one of the patients from certain death and enabled him to start walking around again.

Doctors and AIDS researchers around the world are upset, even furious, and understandably so. They will be deluged with demands for treatment with Cyclosporine-A before they have a chance to assess its effectiveness and risks. AIDS victims who have been wasting away from the debilitating disease will see no reason why they shouldn't be given this one last chance of life. But there's no reason to raise unsupported hopes, as has been done so often with quack remedies for cancer, for example.

The French doctors are not quacks, nor is the medication something to be dismissed outright. Cyclosporine-A is used to weaken the body's natural immune system so that foreign objects, such as transplanted hearts, will not be rejected. Some specialists think it at least possible that the drug may work in reverse to help the body's immune system rebuild itself after AIDS attacks.

Everyone hopes that the French announcement proves true, and that there is a treatment for AIDS. At the same time, the experts fear that unwarranted hopes have been built up for thousands of people, who will be devastated if those hopes are dashed.

The French doctors will be proved either heroes, or false and dangerous prophets. How soon the facts will be known cannot be said with any certainty.

Newsday

Long Island, NY
November 17, 1985

Late last month, three French scientists called a full-dress news conference to announce important progress in the treatment of acquired immune deficiency syndrome, the dreaded disease better known as AIDS.

The French researchers said that by administering the drug cyclosporine A — which is normally used to prevent the rejec- on of transplanted organs — they had re-.uced the ravages of AIDS on the body's immune system.

Scientists in the United States and elsewhere were extremely dubious. For one thing, the French doctors were announcing their findings after only *five days* of experimentation. For another, the research sample was small; it consisted of only six patients.

Observers now have even more reason for skepticism. Two patients given cyclosporine A have died since the Oct. 29 news conference. And it turns out that another AIDS victim who was undergoing the treatment had died even before the French doctors announced to the press that in two experimental cases "the growth of the disease was stopped; it is the first time in the world that this has happened."

Despite the negative results, Dr. Philippe Even, a member of the team of Paris doctors from Laennec Hospital who administered cyclosporine A to AIDS victims, said Monday that the treatment of nine other patients looked promising and that he and his team intended to broaden the test to include about 20 patients in five other hospitals.

Dr. Even denied that either he or his colleagues had ever claimed that cyclosporine A was an effective treatment. "We said it was a reasonable hope for a cure," he said.

Even assuming that's all they said, the question still remains: Why say anything at all at a news conference after testing a drug on six patients for five days? Why not simply publish research findings in scientific journals, as scientists normally do, and allow other researchers to examine, test and verify the results?

As a French physician said the other day, commenting on the Laennec Hospital team's approach: "We do not have the right to say things in this manner. We gave hope to people. We must now go back to scientific testing."

The Globe and Mail

Toronto, Ont., January 2, 1985

AIDS is an extraordinarily intelligent, dastardly disease.

It is communicable by intimate contact, usually sexual and apparently involving exchange of bodily fluids. What better means to assure transmission than sex, which is assured of popularity?

AIDS has a long gestation period — from a few months to several years — possibly allowing transmission by apparently healthy people.

It does not attack its victims superficially; rather, AIDS depresses the human immune system, allowing any number of other deadly diseases to do the actual damage. The present fatality rate for AIDS victims is 100 per cent after three years.

This is Acquired Immune Deficiency Syndrome, first noted in the United States in 1981. Last year, there were some 3,000 confirmed cases in the U.S. By Nov. 5 of this year, there were 6,791 cases in the U.S., with 24 new cases reported every day. As of July 15, there were 451 cases in Western Europe, double the number eight months before. In Canada, there have been 51 new male cases in the last four months; 85 had been reported in the previous 29 months. There have been 78 deaths in Canada, 3,164 in the U.S.

AIDS is apparently caused by a variation of the leukemia virus HLTV. The AIDS virus has been found in the blood, semen and saliva of its victims. It seems unlikely that transmission occurs through saliva, though research has not yet determined the actual route.

Although homosexual and bisexual men account for 73 per cent of U.S. cases, intravenous drug users, hemophiliacs (who depend on external blood products) and Haitians in some localities also appear among higher risk groups. However, AIDS is common among heterosexuals in Zaire and, of 221 cases diagnosed in France to mid-October, 63 (more than a quarter) had no apparent link to any of the higher risk groups.

The Centre for Disease Control in Atlanta, Georgia, estimates that as many as 200,000 American men may have been exposed to AIDS. Indications are that only a minority will develop the disease in its complete form, and that 10 times the number who develop full-blown AIDS will suffer from non-fatal AIDS-Related Complex — swollen lymph glands and a depressed immune system. Research on the incidence and variations of AIDS is just getting under way in various locales, including the University of Toronto.

The disease has the potential to be socially as well as medically damaging. Although there is no evidence that AIDS can be transmitted by casual contact, members of higher risk groups have experienced discrimination by people afraid of the disease. Transmission through transfusions of infected blood is causing concern, although the number of cases is low.

While a vaccine for AIDS appears several years away (the virus is reportedly changing to become more infectious), a test may soon be generally available to detect the presence of AIDS antibodies in the blood. While this would not indicate whether a person might develop AIDS, it would allow screening of blood donors to eliminate those exposed to the disease.

AIDS is not a "gay disease," nor is it a moral judgment by some deity against purported wrongs. It is a new virus entering Europe and North America through certain communities, and apparently capable of spreading beyond. It is a common problem requiring a common front.

The first line of defence is information. AIDS must become a topic for polite society, because AIDS is anything but polite.

The Evening Gazette

Worcester, MA, July 11, 1985

Government researchers may have made a key discovery in the fight against AIDS.

Scientists at the National Institute of Allergy and Infectious Diseases have discovered the AIDS virus wrecks the immune system by "blinding" sentry cells in the blood so they cannot recognize protein labels that ordinarily give away germs' presence in the body. The so-called "helper T cells" orchestrate the immune system, and among their important jobs is spotting hostile invaders and sounding an alarm.

The new study shows that long before these helper cells are wiped out, they lose the internal radar that enables them to recognize germs. Since the body can't detect them, it doesn't destroy them.

The researchers established the body's inability to recognize disease as the key cause of the eventual breakdown in the body's immune system that accompanies AIDS. Up until now scientists have been unable to determine which of AIDS' many effects on the immune system are most important and what causes them.

The discovery may not quickly lead to any cure for the wasting disease. But it does suggest that the best treatment is the current approach of developing drugs to inactivate the AIDS virus in combination with boosting the immune system.

A cure to AIDS may still be a long way off. But the researchers may have taken the first critical step.

THE WALL STREET JOURNAL

New York, NY, October 31, 1985

Once again, a large class of seriously ill people is being yanked around between reports of a promising drug therapy and the American research community's injunction that no one shall be cured of any disease without permission from the appropriate bureaucrats.

Yesterday morning's news was filled with stories about the unorthodox manner in which a team of French physicians had announced the results of its work on AIDS with a drug called cyclosporine, which up to now has been famous for making organ transplants more successful. Two out of six patients with AIDS showed "spectacular" improvements within two days of receiving the drug. One patient had been close to death. If Hippocrates were alive today and learned this, we're sure his first instinct would be to share the drug with AIDS sufferers everywhere.

We're sure that Hippocrates would do this even though he recognized that initially promising results might be a blind alley. At their news conference, the French doctors said the drug didn't constitute a cure but that it might keep AIDS patients alive on a maintenance program until a virus-killing drug is actually discovered. This sounds like perfectly good common sense to us, as we suspect it does to many AIDS patients or anyone else terminally ill with an incurable disease. Or for that matter, to non-terminal patients who think that as adults they can be trusted to know the latest possibilities about their disease.

In the modern U.S. health community, however, what quickly developed is another example of the Catch-22 situation terminally ill patients are encountering. News travels fast now of promising therapies for diseases, but dying patients run smack into a united wall of medical officials—led by the Food and Drug Administration—who say, "Despite what you've read, we won't let you use this drug until we've thoroughly checked it out and approved it or unless you can finagle your way into one of our clinical trials. Check back in a year or two, if you're still alive."

Consider the reactions to the French announcement being heard from important parts of the U.S. research community:

Dr. Anthony S. Fauci of the National Institutes of Health: "There's not a scientist I know who'd give something for one week to six patients and make an announcement in the press. If you want to talk about ethics, you want to make sure something works before you announce it."

William Haseltine of Harvard Medical School: "It takes at least several weeks to measure the amount of virus in a patient," and "You might as well say chicken soup works."

Dr. Samuel Broder, director of clinical oncology at the National Cancer Institute: "I think on the basis of the evidence presented thus far in scientific journals, no patient need feel that he is being deprived of a curative therapy" for AIDS.

Consider, then, the traditional route to official acceptance. First, a researcher either presents a paper on his or her work at a professional meeting, or submits it for publication to a professional journal, which in turn will circulate it for preliminary approval among a committee of the researcher's peers. Then, in this country, the drug will enter clinical trials using a limited number of test subjects, under protocols established by the Food and Drug Administration, which may or may not approve it years hence.

Though in many ways admirable for its medical achievements, the system's serious flaws are becoming increasingly evident. It takes up to 10 years to approve a drug, for example, and in that time patients die. Naturally, shortcuts develop. The cyclosporine used in the French tests had been approved by the FDA for other uses already, for example, and thus competent U.S. doctors can legally prescribe it for anyone afflicted with AIDS. But the ethos of the research community is to censor the French doctors.

Let Drs. Fauci and Broder by all means proceed with their time-honored methods for finding a "curative" therapy that "works" according to criteria they and their peers have established. But they need to entertain the possibility that there should be an alternative "parallel track" for making promising therapies more widely available to dying people who wish to assume the risks of using them.

Put it another way: If the child of an American AIDS researcher were dying of AIDS and his wife said—For heaven's sake, can't we at least administer the cyclosporine to see if there's a response—does anyone seriously believe that this researcher would tell his wife they can't do it until the FDA approves the drug for marketing in the U.S.?

The Miami Herald

Miami, FL, August 15, 1985

CONCERNED by an alarming and inexplicable incidence of AIDS in rural Belle Glade, state health officials rightly plan to test residents to determine how many may have been exposed to the fatal disease. The pilot project could lead to the much-needed Federally funded study of environmental links to AIDS sought by pioneer researchers Caroline MacLeod and Mark Whiteside.

Drs. MacLeod and Whiteside repeatedly have urged such a study to explain why the small, rural community of Belle Glade has an incidence of AIDS (acquired immune-deficiency syndrome) that is four times greater than the incidence in New York or San Francisco. Half of the 43 victims in Belle Glade fall outside the national profile of persons at risk: They are not homosexuals, drug abusers, hemophiliacs, or heterosexual partners of infected persons.

Drs. MacLeod and Whiteside have drawn national attention to Belle Glade's anomalies. Regrettably, that attention also has spurred a new round of hysteria, victimizing healthy area residents who predictably resent the spotlight on problems beyond their control.

Yet without outside attention and assistance there is little hope that Belle Glade can cure its clearly evident health problems. AIDS may be the community's newest threat, but the familiar maladies of malnutrition, tuberculosis, high-risk pregnancy, and venereal disease are — for most residents — the more-serious risks. Those diseases thrive in an area where income and education levels are far below the state and county averages, housing is inadequate and overcrowded, and sanitation is woeful. The link between an impoverished environment and poor health has not yet been made for the spread of AIDS, but it has for those other health threats.

Financing the prescribed treatment is beyond the means of the community alone. That prescription includes a renewed effort to clean up slums, including state and Federal assistance for the new and promising housing programs already under way; the extension of specialized health services to the Glades; instruction for slum residents on hygiene, sanitation, and nutrition; the hiring of more interpreters to assist doctors in treating Haitian and Hispanic patients; a formal system for transferring uninsured Glades residents to coastal hospitals for treatment unavailable at local tax-supported hospitals; and a residential center for the mentally ill of the Glades area.

Research on the cause and treatment of AIDS is needed and must continue. Belle Glade is a good "laboratory" for a specific aspect of that research. But when AIDS is placed in perspective, it also is clear that the area suffers more-immediate and wholly curable health problems.

Only a broad-based attack can hope to cure the Glades's ills. Such an attack is welcome — even if it rides piggyback on a fearsome, unpopular disease.

Anti-AIDS Drug, AZT, Found Successful

Federal health officials September 19, 1986 announced at a Washington, D.C. news conference that testing had found significant success for the drug azidothymidine as a palliative for some cases of AIDS. The drug, often referred to as AZT, was the "first therapeutic agent which seems to hold promise for some AIDS patients," said Dr. Robert E. Windom, assistant secretary of health and human services. But he stressed that the drug was not a cure and that much remained uncertain about its effects. Windom said he had asked the federal Food and Drug Administration (FDA) to approve the drug swiftly for commercial sale. Until the drug could be sold, the National Institutes of Health (NIH) would distribute it for treatment of some AIDS victims. Burroughs Wellcome Co., maker of the drug, would supply it to the NIH free of charge.

The latest AZT test had begun in February 1986. The drug had been given to 145 AIDS victims, while 137 others had been given placebos. Researchers found that there had been 16 deaths among placebo recipients but only one among those taking AZT. The number of "serious medical events"—which included not only death but also such phenomena as the appearance of a life-threatening infection—was 59 among placebo recipients and 36 among subjects taking AZT. The test also found that patients taking AZT gained weight on the average, that the drug halted deterioration in some patients' immune systems, and in some cases even allowed the systems to regain some strength.

Another benefit of AZT was that it appeared able to move from the recipient's blood system into the brain, an organ often invaded by the AIDS virus. Side effects of the drug seemed to be limited to nausea, mild headaches and a few instances of anemia. AZT operated by stopping the virus from taking over the cell's genetic material. Upon entering the cell, the genetic material of the AIDS virus, in the form of RNA, took over the cell's machinery to produce viral DNA, which in turn directed the synthesis of new viruses. The new viruses eventually budded off and infected healthy cells. AZT stopped the process by blocking the viral enzyme that transcribed the virus's RNA code into DNA.

WORCESTER TELEGRAM
Worcester, MA
October 7, 1986

Azidothymidine, or AZT, an experimental drug, is being distributed on a limited basis to help prolong the lives of patients with some forms of aquired immune deficiency syndrome. It's on the market lacking the normal testing period because there is certain death for those with AIDS. In this case, the decision to make it available is appropriate.

There is no history and little data on side effects from AZT, but the drug has been around for 25 years. The compound, made first from herring and salmon sperm, was considered as a treatment for tumors because it seemed to halt the multiplication of cells. It failed, but the emergence of AIDS brought AZT back into the laboratory in hopes it would stop the spread of the virus that causes AIDS.

Initial indications are encouraging. AZT has stopped the spread of the virus in some test cases, although it provided no cure. When that was discovered, the AIDS patients who had been given placebos as controls in testing AZT were immediately given the drug.

It usually takes eight to 10 years of testing before the Food and Drug Administration clears a drug for general use; AIDS patients don't have that kind of time.

Burroughs Wellcome Co. has been successfully synthesizing AZT. The drug company will provide AZT to doctors for AIDS patients, if the physicians agree to supply research data.

AIDS victims who have contracted pneumonia associated with the disease will receive the drug first. Burroughs Wellcome will supply AZT free to as many patients meeting the criteria as possible until a license is granted, probably in January. Children and pregnant or nursing women will not be given AZT.

Other types of drugs are in test phases. They will be distributed for general use as soon as possible. Ribavirin is being studied to find if it is effective against the AIDS virus; Interferon and Interleuken-2 may combat certain cancers; and a group of natural substances that might induce bone-marrow cells to boost white-blood cells' effectiveness against AIDS is under study.

The fight against AIDS has just begun. The question of whether untested, experimental drugs ought to be given to terminally ill patients is not peculiar to AIDS victims. At this stage of treatment, however, there seems to be no other option available in treating those who suffer from this deadly disease.

Los Angeles Times
Los Angeles, CA, September 23, 1986

For the first time, a drug exists that has been shown to help AIDS patients in controlled studies. The final test results are not in, and there are no definitive conclusions about possible long-term effects, but the government has wisely decided to allow the drug—azidothymidine, or AZT—to be made available to the thousands more people who are suffering from the deadly disease. In doing so, the National Institutes of Health is striking the proper balance between protecting the public and providing effective medication to people who need it.

The six months of tests so far involved 282 patients with *Pneumocystis carinii* pneumonia, an opportunistic infection that commonly attacks people whose immune systems have been crippled by AIDS. Only one of the 145 people who received AZT died, while 16 of the 137 people who were given a sugar pill—a placebo—died. The odds against these results occurring by chance are just five in 10,000, according to researchers. In addition, the patients who received AZT had fewer serious medical problems than the others.

This is most encouraging news, so encouraging that the National Institutes of Health and the drug's manufacturer, Burroughs Wellcome Co., have decided to cut short the first round of tests and to give AZT immediately to those patients who had been receiving the placebo. In addition, Burroughs Wellcome will make the drug available free of charge on a "compassionate-plea basis" to others with AIDS-related pneumonia. As many as 6,000 people in the country may be eligible to get this drug. So far, AIDS has struck about 25,000 Americans, of whom 14,000 have died.

When to approve the use of a promising but unproven drug is a continuing dilemma for health authorities. AZT is not a cure for AIDS, and no one knows how long its beneficial effects will last or whether it will present a dangerous side effect, as yet unknown, that would be as bad as the disease—or worse. The U.S. government has traditionally been extremely cautious in approving the use of new drugs, judging that the doctor's oath to "do no harm" means that drugs that have not been proved safe and effective should not be dispensed.

But that attitude has been changing. Increasingly, "do no harm" is interpreted to mean that drugs that show promise, such as AZT, should not be withheld. Although it involves greater risk, this seems to be a better policy, especially when the disease being treated is fatal. Still, health authorities must continue to insist that drugs show some degree of effectiveness before being made widely available.

If all goes well, AZT will be tried on AIDS patients with other infections, including Kaposi's sarcoma, and the Food and Drug Administration may approve it for general commercial use by January. In the long fight against this terrible disease, this is the first real ray of hope.

THE COMMERCIAL APPEAL

Memphis, TN, April 26, 1986

BANNED in the U.S.A.

That's the status of some of the most promising drugs in the fight against AIDS.

The antiviral agent Ribavirin is legal in more than two dozen countries. But not here.

HPA-23, administered to Rock Hudson in Paris, still isn't approved for widescale use here. The same goes for Isoprinosine.

That last example is especially baffling. Isoprinosine has been around for 18 years and has been described in more than 170 medical-journal articles worldwide. Nobody has found any evidence that it is toxic.

But there is evidence that it boosts the immune system. It helps in treatment of hepatitis B and rheumatoid arthritis. It has proved valuable in cancer therapy. And it has aided sufferers of AIDS-related complex (ARC), the set of symptoms that sometimes leads to the full-blown disease.

Eighty-nine countries allow Isoprinosine treatment for at least some illnesses. The United States isn't one of them, though the Food and Drug Administration acknowledges it does no harm.

Some observers say the agency won't approve any AIDS-related medication unless it actually kills the virus. Isoprinosine can't do that. But it could give some AIDS victims more time, and perhaps the chance to see more solid breakthroughs.

Bureaucratic inertia is nothing new at the FDA. But the AIDS crisis is giving it added attention. We hope the result is change at the agency.

The FDA has an important mission — protecting Americans from clearly dangerous drugs. But they don't need shielding from helpful ones.

Such inhumane "protection" is an abuse. The agency's molasses-like review process needs reforming. If change isn't forthcoming from within, then Congress should force it from without. AIDS victims, and all sick people running low on hope, deserve nothing less.

The Salt Lake Tribune

Salt Lake City, UT, September 23, 1986

Maybe this society is not as excessively super-cautious and mercenary as it sometimes appears. Take the rather unusual case of approving a new anti-AIDS drug before it has been fully tested.

According to a news account out of Washington, D.C., the federal Food and Drug Administration has been authorized to accelerate availability of the drug azidothymidine (AZT) for some 6,000 AIDS victims on an experimental basis. Even while this action remains to a certain extent a sort of qualified accommodation, it is also extraordinary. Understandably and acceptably so.

Although, evidently, tests found AZT unpromising for its original purpose, treating cancer patients, a particular fatal version of AIDS is responsive. If this can be confirmed, it would be a breakthrough of definitely welcome proportions.

AIDS victims, their families and friends, the doctors, nurses and other medical professionals directly involved with this especially pernicious disease are currently condemned to experience only futility and despair. Once active, the virus is so relentless in attacking the human immune system that death becomes inevitable. While fatal illnesses are by no means uncommon, for most of them some sort of hope-giving therapy has been developed, at least when early detection occurs. Not yet, however, for Acquired Immune Deficiency Syndrome.

But now comes AZT. Since some medical authorities wonder if enough laboratory and field tests have been conducted to detect every possible fatal side-effect, and realizing how painstakingly thorough federal evaluations of any new drug usually are, reluctance and delay would have seemed the more likely approach.

Moreover, at a time when medical research and practice have become so gun-shy of anything which might prompt even more liability lawsuits, hurrying a new drug into use looks downright impulsive. But for once, better instincts prevailed.

In the first place, AZT is thought destined for only 60 percent of AIDS cases, those involving Pneumocystis carinii pneumonia. And it will still be prescribed on a controlled, experimental basis. Possibilities remain that it damages bone marrow, could have other harmful incidental effects and that it merely prolongs life without actually being a cure.

Nevertheless, if it helps at all, gives some hope to those who now have none, equips medical practitioners with confidence they can do more than simply prepare their patients to die, rushing AZT into use makes sense. With this unprecedented move, a formerly more important precedent of placing humanitarianism above practical materialism seems to have been rediscovered.

Chicago Tribune

Chicago, IL, September 29, 1986

All the news about AIDS has been bad for so long that the first glimmerings of hope offered by the new drug azidothymidine (AZT) is particularly cheering. AZT isn't a cure. It won't protect potential victims against AIDS or keep AIDS patients from dying eventually. But it is the first drug that affects AIDS victims' underlying disease and gives them realistic hope of longer life.

Despite some reported bickering, controversy and apparent jealousies, scientists have acted with unprecedented speed to recognize AIDS as a new disease, classify its symptoms, discover how it is transmitted, recommend ways to guard against becoming infected, find the responsible virus and develop a helpful drug. It has been only five years since the first known cases of AIDS in the United States were reported by the Centers for Disease Control.

Government regulators also deserve credit for acting with uncharacteristic speed to make AZT available to AIDS victims as quickly as possible. The drug was being tested in double-blind, placebo studies in which half of the volunteer patients got AZT while the others received identical-looking dummy pills. Such research is the surest, quickest and easiest way to get objective data about a drug's effects.

But once it became evident that the AIDS test subjects getting AZT were faring better and living longer than those receiving placebos, researchers and regulators decided to end the test and arrange for those getting the placebos to receive the real drug.

Burroughs Wellcome Co., which produces AZT, intends to supply it to physicians and pharmacists as quickly as possible for what are, in effect, greatly expanded drug trials. The company will provide it free until it is approved for sale, probably in December or January. Final criteria for getting the drug now have not yet been made public. The government has set up a telephone hotline to answer questions. And the message is being repeated that the drug is effective only in patients with a kind of pneumonia characteristic of AIDS and that it can cause toxic side effects.

Much more research is essential to develop not only a complete cure for AIDS but also a vaccine to prevent it. The complex nature of the AIDS virus makes this particularly difficult. But AZT is a welcome sign that progress is possible and that when new developments do show promise, the government is willing to cut some red tape to benefit as many victims as possible. Patients with other intractable, incurable illnesses would be fortunate to get the same kind of urgent attention.

Rockford Register Star

Rockford, IL, September 25, 1986

AIDS sufferers, the medical community and society in general must welcome each advance — great or small — in finding a cure and treatment for the deadly disease.

A newly-developed drug that could extend the lives of AIDS victims and reduce their symptoms could be a major breakthrough. The drug is being anxiously awaited by the 12,000 living AIDS patients; it comes too late for a larger number who already have died.

This important development comes none too soon. In Winnebago County, the number of reported AIDS cases has tripled this year. Only two cases were reported here during the past three years, while three cases have been reported within the last six months, said Jim Bailey chief epidemiologist for the county Health Department.

Local health officials, while hailing the new drug, point out that it is designed to treat AIDS symptoms, not cure the disease.

Still, any hope in a heretofore hopeless situation must be taken as a positive sign. Perhaps the new drug is the first step toward a cure.

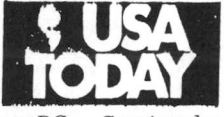

Washington, DC, September 18, 1986

When AIDS was first diagnosed in 1981, medical researchers were thrown into a desperate scramble to find the cause and cure.

While they searched, thousands of AIDS victims lost their deadly race against time. For thousands more, it has been an emotional roller coaster ride as first one hope was raised, then dashed, only to be replaced by another.

Now hopes have been raised once more by the drug azidothymidine, or AZT, being tested by the National Institutes of Health. Sen. Lowell Weicker, who believes AZT can help AIDS patients, has proposed a $47 million increase in AIDS research funds, which would help get the drug to those who need it.

In the tests, 140 patients are being given AZT and 140 patients in a control group are receiving a sugar pill, a placebo. Researchers stress that it's too early to reach conclusions, but results so far indicate that those receiving the drug are gaining weight and living longer, while the condition of those receiving the placebo has continued to deteriorate.

That has raised an ethical dilemma: Should the testing be halted and the drug released, or should the testing continue — which could mean an earlier or more painful death for those in the control group?

And the larger question: Should thousands of AIDS victims not involved in the clinical trials be denied a drug that shows promise of easing their suffering or prolonging their lives? That isn't a casual question — for the victims or the public. So far, AIDS has stricken 24,859 people and killed 13,689. Experts predict the number will increase tenfold by 1991.

What worries those who don't want an early release of the drug? They express a number of concerns:

■ It could cause chaos as victims scramble for a drug the manufacturer might not be able to supply soon enough and in sufficient quantities.

■ It could reduce the pressure to continue the quest for a complete cure. Even AZT's most ardent advocates point out that it only halts action of the AIDS virus. It neither cures nor prevents AIDS.

■ A controlled study is needed to make absolutely sure that the drug doesn't cause unacceptable side effects.

Those are legitimate concerns, but they should not stand in the way of a compassionate solution to this dilemma. AIDS patients whose illness has progressed to the point that side effects are not a consideration should be allowed to get AZT if they want it. It wouldn't be the first time that a promising drug was released before testing was complete.

Testing need not halt; in fact it would be expanded to a larger group. And if the drug isn't released, it's possible that a black market will develop or that victims will be forced to go outside the USA to get the drug.

The reluctance of scientists to raise false hopes is understandable. But when so many lives are on the line, even faint hope is better than no hope at all.

THE WALL STREET JOURNAL

New York, NY, October 15, 1986

After federal officials announced recently that an experimental drug had successfully delayed death and relieved the suffering of AIDS patients, the National Institutes of Health had to set up a telephone hot line to handle calls from sick patients wanting to know how to get it. Calls came in at the rate of 1,000 a day. The Food and Drug Administration hasn't approved the drug for sale yet, but the government's fast-track processing for AIDS drugs may make it available through a doctor's prescription by early next year. In the meantime, the FDA has given Burroughs-Wellcome Co., the developer of azidothymidine (AZT), permission to distribute the drug to certain AIDS patients, so long as it does so for free.

We assume that all those AIDS patients phoning in fully understand that the drug's success is preliminary, that it has toxic side effects, and that other side effects may show up later. Knowing all this they, like people with so many other life-destroying diseases, want to brave the risks and take the drug. Many, however, are told they can't have the drug. The alliance of researchers and regulators says only it will decide who may benefit now from AZT and who may not.

The drug is being offered only to patients who have had a specific kind of AIDS-related pneumonia. About 7,000 people may qualify. The people mainly left out by the FDA's rules have what is known as AIDS-related complex, or ARC, a set of debilitating symptoms similar to AIDS. They number in the tens of thousands.

The decision to forbid ARC patients access to the drug is difficult for them because their malady was included in the clinical trial that precipitated the extraordinary decision to take the control group off placebos and put them on AZT. The test included 282 people with either fully developed AIDS or AIDS-related complex. In the group of 137 patients treated with a placebo (meaning no treatment), 16 died. But of the 145 patients treated with AZT, only one died. With such dramatic results in hand, the company said it couldn't ethically withhold AZT from the placebo patients. It shut down the trial and began distributing the drug free to a restricted class of patients. The formal reason for denying ARC patients access is that the drug's benefits for them were less clearly defined.

Does this make sense? How can the government ethically withhold AZT from one class of AIDS patients while handing it out to another?

The AZT story is an unusually visible example of the arbitrary authority of the research-regulatory alliance in the U.S. Its authority to decide who shall benefit from science and when is too great and deserves challenge. With AZT, another class of gravely ill individuals have found themselves in the unfortunate Catch-22 dilemma of the current drug-approval process. These patients learn of extremely promising therapeutic results with drugs used in research protocols but quickly discover they can't buy the drug or assume its risks until months or even years of additional research make it ready for formal approval by the FDA.

However, AZT raises a particularly volatile issue: What is going to happen when the research-regulatory alliance can't deny that an experimental AIDS drug significantly benefits ARC patients? The costs of distributing that drug "free" will be enormous. The per-patient cost of these free distributions of experimental drugs are substantial and can become prohibitive for a company without the resources of Burroughs-Wellcome.

Current federal regulations effectively prevent companies from recovering distribution costs from patients in large part because of a distaste for "commercializing" a drug prior to its approval for sale. In the event of an ARC breakthrough before the FDA is prepared to release the drug into the tainted world of profit, it's likely that the government would "buy" the unapproved drug from the developer to subsidize distribution.

The government's regulatory apparatus, with its emphasis on "free" or "compassionate" distributions of experimental drugs to restricted patient populations reflects a flawed understanding of the role of capital in bringing benefit to sick people. The deep base of public support for new medical therapies, however, has led to a rediscovery of the fact that research-based companies, large or small, use their income stream to underwrite additional research, whether for AIDS or for other purposes.

The questions before us here are whether the research-regulatory alliance should have such total, unchallenged authority to interpose itself between patients and medicine that promises respite from suffering. And is there a net gain or a net loss to the public's welfare when this alliance holds arbitrary authority to decide at which point a patient's willingness to spend his own money to relieve his suffering is ethical and when it is unethical?

The Hartford Courant

Hartford, CT, October 1, 1986

Sen. Lowell P. Weicker of Connecticut is leading a commendable drive in Congress to provide assistance for AIDS victims to be treated with experimental drugs.

One medication, azidothymidine, or AZT, had been given to 282 people with AIDS in trials at several clinical centers. The drug seemed to have improved the condition of patients in advanced stages of the disease. On Sept. 19 the Department of Health and Human Services approved the distribution of AZT to approximately 60 percent of the estimated 10,000 surviving victims of the fatal disease. Other AIDS victims soon may be made eligible to use the drug.

Mr. Weicker is trying to obtain the money to help pay for the expanded use of AZT and perhaps other experimental drugs. In debate on a major health and human services appropriations bill, he insisted that as many AIDS sufferers as possible should have access to the promising treatments. He sought to add up to $50 million for that purpose to the bill, the money to be administered by the National Institutes for Health.

The widespread distribution of the drugs, Mr. Weicker said, "will accelerate the process" of finding a cure and a vaccine for the disease.

His request for more AIDS money is consistent with Mr. Weicker's praiseworthy record of support for the National Institutes of Health and many of its research programs.

The Senate agreed with Mr. Weicker, and the appropriations measure was sent to a House-Senate conference committee. Funding for AIDS research, prevention and treatment under the Senate bill would total $402 million; the House has approved $336 million.

The higher figure can be readily justified. AIDS is spreading rapidly; thousands have already died because of it. The sensible and humane thing to do is fight it with as many weapons as can be mustered.

ST. LOUIS POST-DISPATCH

St. Louis, MO
December 17, 1986

The search for ways to prevent or treat acquired immune deficiency syndrome is one of the most pressing tasks confounding medical researchers. As difficult as it is, it has been made more so by poor management of the AIDS laboratory at the Centers for Disease Control in Atlanta.

The problems there go beyond the bickering and power struggles that exist in nearly every office. Experiments were sabotaged while others proposed by out-of-favor scientists were handicapped. In interviews with *The Wall Street Journal*, researchers told of grand-standing by Dr. James Curran, who runs the lab. Five of the six senior scientists who started the lab have left, and those who have replaced them are eager to follow suit.

Perhaps worst of all, research showing that a widely available spermicide, nonoxynol-9, killed the AIDS virus under laboratory conditions was kept from the public for months. Two scientists involved in the research attributed the long delay to the sensitivity of Dr. Curran to the Reagan administration's queasiness about AIDS, an attitude that would prefer to stress abstinence or limited sexual contact as the best way of controlling its spread rather than educate a vulnerable population on how to limit exposure without altering lifestyles.

The upshot of this seems to be that the CDC's AIDS laboratory has lost all chance of attracting first-rate scientists. Dr. Curran is accused by his staff of tainting the laboratory's work by imposing his own prejudices on research and publications. Saddest of all, the urgent work that must be done on AIDS has taken a back seat to the pettiest, most niggling disputes.

It might be too late to restore all the lost prestige to the AIDS laboratory at the CDC, but steps should be taken, and at once, to redeem as much of it as possible.

THE ▨ SUN

Baltimore, MD, September 28, 1986

It is a measure of the desperation engendered by the AIDS disease that preliminary results from clinical tests of a new drug have started a near-stampede. Doctors say it's too early to tell whether the experimental drug azidothymidine can actually cure AIDS, but it has at least prolonged the lives of test subjects. That's extremely good news, since almost nothing else has worked.

The drug was developed by a Michigan researcher, Dr. Jerome P. Horwitz, as part of a 1960s cancer project. It didn't show promise then, and was shelved. But in 1984 it was established that AIDS was caused by a "retrovirus," one which used RNA rather than DNA to carry its genetic code. The Burroughs Wellcome Co., a developer of anti-viral drugs, began looking for a retrovirus killer. AZT, which inhibits reproduction of the AIDS virus, was effective in cell-culture tests at the National Cancer Institute in Bethesda. That led to human testing against placebos, pills containing no medication. Only Burroughs-Wellcome knew the distinguishing code, and the company noted which one had been given after a patient's death. Of 137 patients given placebos, 16 died, but only one of 145 treated with AZT died. As a result, placebos were discarded and all patients in the study project were placed in AZT therapy.

As Johns Hopkins specialist Dr. John G. Bartlett noted, AZT may offer only temporary relief, or be required for the rest of a patient's life. It had side effects for some patients, and its full effects are not yet understood. The rush of AIDS patients to get in line for AZT could even hinder the search for more effective treatments if patients spurn other experimental approaches. Moreover, if AZT proves effective over the long term, how could a doctor morally deny it to a person who might die using a drug that turned out to be a dead end?

Thus far, AZT worked best for those who have suffered a rare form of pneumonia. What about the others, and the estimated 150,000 people suffering not from AIDS, but AIDS-related complex? Some ARC patients were included in the study, and AZT seemed to help them as well. But unlike AIDS, ARC is not considered 100-percent fatal, so results were less clear.

It's still too early to cheer, for too much is unknown. Great hopes based on the short-term promise of limited tests could be dashed in the long run. Better to send up a quiet "well done," and keep the lanterns burning for a vaccine that can protect against the infection.

Newsday

Long Island, NY, September 23, 1986

For the first time since Americans learned of AIDS, victims have some reason to hope. A newly developed experimental drug — azidothymidine or AZT — may prolong the lives of some of the afflicted. After only six months of AZT tests, federal health officials have taken the highly unusual step of making the medicine available to thousands of patients.

This landmark decision is undoubtedly a gamble: AZT may prove to be no more than a temporary stay of a certain death sentence. And aside from raising false hopes, it may have dangerously debilitating side effects. But it's a gamble well worth taking; without any treatment, people with AIDS — the acronym for acquired immune deficiency syndrome — will die.

Burroughs-Wellcome Co., which manufactures AZT, will provide it free — under a federal health-policy practice often known as "compassionate use" of experimental drugs. Yet only about 60 percent of the nation's 11,000 AIDS victims have a medical profile that makes them eligible for it. Uncertainty about some of AZT's side effects and the limited availability of the drug itself are other reasons why it's not being given to all AIDS patients.

Logistical as well as financial considerations restrict the supply of experimental drugs. Health officials must, therefore, make agonizing decisions about who will get potentially lifesaving treatment and who won't.

As other promising experimental drugs are developed, this dilemma will become increasingly acute. Officials and doctors must carefully consider every option — from selling experimental anti-AIDS drugs at cost to continuing conventional clinical studies. But at least for the moment, the decision on AZT has struck the right balance among health, head and heart.

Large '91 AIDS Toll Projected in U.S.

The U.S. Public Health Service June 12, 1986 released a report projecting that by 1991 there would be a tenfold increase in U.S. deaths from AIDS and in the country's total number of cases. Government health officials discussed the findings in a Washington, D.C. news conference. Dr. Donald Ian Macdonald, the Health and Human Services Department's acting assistant secretary, said the projections were "staggering." He called for a new commission to map "a national, coordinated response" to the problem. "This is a major problem," he said, "probably bigger than the Public Health Service."

According to the report, 179,000 Americans would die of AIDS by 1991; 54,000 would die in 1991 alone. The total number of AIDS cases, including fatalities, would reach a projected 270,000. During 1991 alone, 74,000 new cases were expected to develop. Most of the victims would already have been infected by the virus at the time of the report. If correct, the projections meant that in 1991 AIDS would claim more lives than had motor accidents during 1982. Medical experts said that figures could place the disease among the country's 10 leading causes of death. The report said its estimates might be as much as 20% too low. In addition, the figures did not include victims of AIDS-related complex (ARC), a disorder resembling AIDS but without its opportunistic infections. Currently, five times as many people suffered from ARC as did from AIDS. The report predicted that the great majority of AIDS cases to be diagnosed over the next five years would still be among intravenous drug users and homosexual and bisexual men. But it acknowledged that some previously unexplained cases, which had probably been brought on by heterosexual transmission, would account for 9% of newly diagnosed cases in 1991, up from 7% in 1986.

Dr. James Curran, director of the AIDS program at the federal Centers for Disease Control, said of the findings: "We recognize now that the disease is transmitted through heterosexual contact as well as homosexual contact...this is a problem that all people have to be concerned about."

BUFFALO EVENING NEWS
Buffalo, NY, June 29, 1986

LAST YEAR, the number of AIDS cases in the nation was doubling every six months. That staggering rate of increase has slowed somewhat, but the disease is still spreading at an epidemic rate.

Federal health officials now estimate conservatively that there will be a cumulative total of 270,000 cases by the end of 1991 — just 5½ years away. There will be 179,000 deaths, 54,000 in 1991 alone.

Federal officials, reporting on a recent conference of physicians and medical researchers, said AIDS — or acquired immune deficiency syndrome — would spread out from New York City and San Francisco, where 41 percent of the cases now occur, and would infect more heterosexual men and women. Such cases will total 7,000 in 1991, or 9 percent of the total new cases.

Dr. James Curran, director of the AIDS program at the Federal Centers for Disease Control, noted the "insidious transmission" of the disease from heterosexual men and women who are intravenous drug abusers. He said "this is not just a problem for gay men."

Another worrisome aspect is that it takes an average of four years to develop the disease after infection. Up to 1.5 million people are believed infected today and are potential AIDS carriers.

In view of the national scope of the problem, the U.S. Public Health Service report urged that a national commission be set up to decide how to cope with the disease. The problem is "bigger than the Public Health Service," one official said. The PHS is spending $234 million on AIDS this year, but the cost of care nationally by 1991 is expected to be from $8 billion to $16 billion a year.

One hopeful note in this gloomy picture is the reduction of the threat of AIDS infection through tainted blood transfusions. "Only a very small number of additional infections are likely to occur through blood and plasma transfusions," the report said.

Intensive efforts are now being made to develop a vaccine to prevent the disease, but this may not come before 1993. Research efforts must be pressed to achieve this goal and also to discover a cure. At present, the disease is 100 percent fatal.

The latest federal report spells out the dread nature of the disease and its rapid spread, but it is no cause for panic. AIDS is caused mostly by sexual contact and contaminated needles of intravenous drug users, not by casual contact. Understanding the disease will help to prevent its spread.

Chicago Tribune
Chicago, IL, July 5, 1986

Deaths from AIDS will increase tenfold in the next five years. Victims will need billions more dollars in health care. And the deadly disease can be expected to spread throughout the country and among heterosexuals as well as homosexuals and intravenous drug users.

That grim new prognosis from public health officials and experts on acquired immune deficiency syndrome is a sharp reminder that AIDS is not simply going to run a limited course in New York City and San Francisco and gradually disappear. According to predictions, 270,000 people will have been diagnosed as having AIDS by 1991; 179,000 of them will have died. Deaths in 1991 alone will total 54,000; many of these victims are already infected with AIDS, although they probably show no symptoms, experts explain.

The scientific fight against AIDS has been progressing with unusual speed and success, compared with battles against dozens of other disabling and fatal ailments. But despite the rapid progress—the virus has been identified, tests for the presence of antibodies have been developed—a vaccine to prevent the infection and drugs to cure it are still unpredictably far in the future.

That leaves prevention as the sole means available now for stopping the spread of AIDS. Unlike with many other serious and deadly disorders, most people who are not now infected can protect themselves from AIDS. It is essential that public health officials step up the clear warnings about the kinds of behavior associated with acquiring AIDS and that high-risk groups look objectively at the facts and help in these educational efforts.

But, as public health officials now say, warnings must no longer be aimed primarily at homosexuals and intravenous drug abusers. The focus should no longer be on high-risk groups, they warn, but on high-risk behavior as evidence grows that AIDS is spreading to heterosexual contacts of infected individuals in this country as it apparently does in Africa. Heterosexuals as well as homosexuals should be wary of sexual contacts with individuals whose backgrounds they do not know well and realize that infected people who do not have active, full-blown AIDS may still be able to spread the disease.

The devastating effects of AIDS, the frightening forecasts about its rapidly increasing incidence and its enormous present and potential strain on health care spending are prompting public health officials to look for more effective ways to use AIDS antibodies tests to help halt the spread of the disease. But there are widespread fears that the tests might be used to deny jobs, insurance or housing or otherwise discriminate against those who have a positive test result and that if names are reported to public health agencies, those at greatest risk of having AIDS will avoid testing.

Six states already have ruled that the names of individuals with positive AIDS tests must be reported. A few states are planning to track down sexual contacts of infected people, warn them to be tested themselves and counsel them on how to avoid spreading the virus even further.

Such measures should not be automatically ruled out because of fears of discrimination. Public health agencies have managed to be discreet and confidential in identifying those who have and could be spreading other venereal diseases, and notifying their sexual contacts. The deadly seriousness of AIDS and the worrisome predictions about its rising incidence should prompt everyone concerned to work out sensible public health measures to protect those not yet infected without infringing on anyone's civil rights.

CHARLESTON EVENING POST

Charleston, SC, June 17, 1986

U.S. Public Health Service predictions on the AIDS toll in only five years are precisely as the service's chief, Dr. Donald I. Macdonald, described them: "staggering." The sheer numbers argue persuasively for the coordinated, national response the PHS has urged.

In 1991, according to the projections, 145,000 people will be stricken with AIDS, or acquired immune deficiency syndrome. In 1991, according to projections, 54,000 will die as a result of AIDS — more than the number of persons killed last year in traffic accidents nationwide. Treatment costs will rise to somewhere between $8 billion and $16 billion during that year.

Computer projections prepared by the federal Centers for Disease Control indicate that the situation will worsen before it improves. The CDC projections say that by the end of 1991, more than 270,000 will have been diagnosed with AIDS, of whom 179,000 will have died. Clearly the disease is reaching crisis proportions.

The PHS has recommended the creation of a national commission, representing public, private and volunteer sectors, and all levels of government, to assess needs and resources and to recommend how all segments of society can handle the AIDs problem. Congress and the president should act accordingly, and as soon as they reasonably can.

Richmond Times-Dispatch

Richmond, VA, June 15, 1986

Cut off one of the Hydra's heads, according to Greek mythology, and two would appear in its place. Acquired immune deficiency syndrome looks distressingly like the 20th century's Hydra. One waits hopefully for solid information that AIDS is slowing down, that predictions of its multiplier effect have been exaggerated. But one waits, so far, in vain.

If anything, it appears that AIDS is causing far more illness in this country than official statistics reveal. Approximately 21,000 Americans, three-fourths of them homosexual men, have been technically classified as AIDS victims, and more than half of them have died. But as data compiled recently by The Wall Street Journal show, another 100,000 to 200,000 persons infected with the AIDS virus are seriously ill with diseases such as hairy leukoplakia, Hodgkin's or dementia, or have alarming symptoms. They are not categorized as AIDS victims primarily because their maladies are not the kinds of infections by which the Centers for Disease Control originally defined AIDS five years ago. They are said to have AIDS-related complex (ARC). An estimated 25 percent of them will contract "full-blown" AIDS.

Additionally, an estimated 1 million to 2 million Americans — again, mostly homosexual men — have been infected with the AIDS virus but as yet have shown no symptoms. A new report by the Public Health Service begins to make clear the huge dimensions of this incipient disease: By 1991, the agency projects that 270,000 persons will be diagnosed as having AIDS and 179,000 of them will have died. Treatment of the sick will cost between $8 billion and $16 billion that year alone.

AIDS-related infections and cancers are multiplying so greatly, according to The Journal's survey, that many physicians are beginning to wonder if the disease has outgrown its narrow definition as an immunity syndrome. Infected persons are now showing up, for examples, with tuberculosis, pneumonia, meningitis, cancer of the mouth, and what one physician describes as "an extraordinarily aggressive glandular cancer that is just ripping through people." Then there are AIDS' neurological afflictions — psychosis, seizure, paralysis — that are so devastating but are not officially linked to AIDS.

Clearly, the nation is facing a public-health problem of staggering proportions. But instead of stopping the spread of the virus through mandatory testing and quarantines, officials of some cities, including the District of Columbia's City Council, seem more concerned about protecting the civil liberties of persons in AIDS high-risk groups, such as homosexual men and intravenous drug users. Moreover, a preliminary paper drafted by Justice Department staffers opines that persons with AIDS should be categorized as "handicapped individuals," with full protection of federal civil rights laws.

Dr. Lewis H. Kuller, a professor of epidemiology at the University of Pittsburgh, disputed such reasoning at a recent scientists' meeting, according to The Chronicle of Higher Education. People who don't have AIDS have rights too, he pointed out.

"AIDS is not a benign skin rash," Dr. Kuller asserted in urging compulsory screenings in high-risk populations. "The individual's right to avoid becoming infected with the HTLV-III virus and dying from AIDS must have the highest priority. This requires a renewed emphasis on basic preventive medicine and infectious-disease control in the community and a strong and responsive public-health system."

Ultimately, Hercules slew the Hydra. It will take a herculean public-health campaign to stop the hydra-headed AIDS monster, but so far the sword's not in sight.

The Boston Globe

Boston, MA, February 17, 1986

Belatedly, President Reagan has called for a "major report" to the American people on AIDS by the surgeon general. At this point, the call is too little, too late. By the time the report can be ready, around the first of June, the horrendous outbreak of AIDS will be five years old.

In many quarters now, the administration's mishandling of the AIDS epidemic looms as a dangerous political issue for the fall congressional elections. Some surmise that it was the political threat posed by AIDS, more than its medical and social consequences, that finally spurred the president's statement. Rep. Henry Waxman (D-Calif.), who has led the fight for federal funds for AIDS research, calls Reagan's sudden directive for a major report "outrageous." He issued it on the same day he submitted a budget that would reduce AIDS research spending.

For 1986, the Reagan administration originally proposed only $85 million for AIDS research. Although Congress raised the AIDS appropriation to $244 million, now the administration wants to rescind $50 million.

That 20-percent cutback would curtail the creation of regional treatment centers for testing experimental drugs — the only immediate ray of hope for AIDS victims.

For fiscal 1987, the administration proposes $214 million for AIDS research and calls it an increase, even though it is far below what Congress voted last year. "It's a shell game," says Waxman. "I can't understand how the president can propose this kind of budget when he talks as if he believes that AIDS is a national emergency. Without the basic research and education work — things we should have been doing for years now — the epidemic will continue to grow."

The president need not wait for the surgeon general's report. He can read the grim statistics on the growth of AIDS cases as they are published weekly by the federal Centers for Disease Control — or their predictions for the months ahead.

By June, at least 21,000 Americans will have been stricken by the most lethal form of the disease, acute AIDS, and 10,000 will be dead. The numbers are easily calculable, as new cases are confirmed at a rate above 200 a week, and are added to the 17,000 already on the books. So far, no one has recovered, and nearly 80 AIDS patients now die every week.

Additionally, 210,000 persons will have a chronic, often debilitating form of the disease, called AIDS Related Complex. This form has still not been officially defined by CDC — many think in an effort to minimize the public's perception of the size of the problem. But doctors diagnose the chronic form of AIDS every day and CDC acknowledges the scope of cases.

An estimated 2.1 million Americans — nearly 1 percent of the population — will carry the infection and be able to transmit it unwittingly to others. Most of the silent carriers do not know they are infected because they seem physically well.

These are the figures that the surgeon general's report should highlight. The president can be sure that congressional candidates will emphasize the even sorrier aspect of AIDS — how those figures grew while the administration ignored them.

AIDS Through Casual Contact Ruled Out

Individuals who lived with victims of AIDS but were not their sexual partners did not become infected with the disease even after months of close personal contact, according to the largest and most thorough study to date. The study, by a team led by Dr. Gerald H. Friedland of Montfiore Medical Center in New York City, was published in the *New England Journal of Medicine* February 6, 1986. The study examined 101 household members who lived with 39 AIDS victims. Those surveyed included the victims' children, siblings, parents and other relatives. All had lived with the AIDS patient for at least three months before the disease was diagnosed, and most had lived with the victims for two years or more. Many of the families were poor and lived in crowded conditions, and hugged or kissed the victims and shared drinking glasses, towels or beds with them. Only one of the 101 subjects, a five-year-old girl whose mother was an AIDS victim, showed signs of infection with the virus. Since the child had suffered related disorders from birth doctors concluded that she had almost certainly been born with the infection. An editorial accompanying the study, which was termed "conclusive," urged that the medical profession "take a more active and influential role in quelling the hysteria over the casual transmission of AIDS."

The Oregonian

Portland, OR
February 10, 1986

The results of a new study reported in the New England Journal of Medicine indicate once again that acquired immune deficiency syndrome cannot be spread by casual contact. Yet that knowledge is likely to make no difference at all in quelling the widespread fear of catching AIDS.

Medical specialists have long asserted that AIDS is transmitted only by intimate contact — by exchange of bodily fluids such as saliva, blood or semen. Of the 101 people observed in the study, all of whom shared homes with diagnosed AIDS patients, only one contracted the disease. That one was a 5-year-old child who is thought to have been born with the disease, which afflicts her mother.

Still, it is a good bet that the results of the study will make not a whit of difference in the thinking of parents who are reluctant to have their children attend classes with an AIDS victim or those who fear they will get the disease from a shared drinking glass or a toilet seat.

Sometimes all the facts in the world cannot make a stand against naked fear.

A safe, inexpensive, easy method of preventing tooth decay has been available to municipalities for decades — yet Portland water is still unfluoridated because a substantial part of the population cannot rid itself of a strong but unfounded fear of the substance used.

AIDS is a far more complex problem than fluoridation — and certainly more deadly. Fears about AIDS and its victims will be allayed only when a foolproof cure for the disease is found.

For fear itself, there is no cure.

The Washington Post

Washington, DC, February 7, 1986

TWO INCIDENTS in the last 10 days illustrate the need for a more intelligent response to AIDS. On Monday, two technicians from the city medical examiner's office refused to remove the body of an AIDS victim from his basement apartment, apparently believing that to do so would jeopardize their own health. A week earlier, at a D.C. council hearing, council member John Ray pressed for action on his bill to prohibit insurers from using AIDS tests in assessing the insurability of persons seeking to buy health or life insurance policies.

Certainly the fear of the technicians is misguided. There is no indication that the AIDS virus can be transmitted by handling a dead body—or even by caring for a live one. Public Health Commissioner Andrew McBride should be commended for traveling to the victim's apartment and personally moving the body, but he should not have to do that again.

The New England Journal of Medicine reported just this week on a study of people sharing households with AIDS patients. Researchers found that friends and relatives who live with and care for these patients do not contract the disease even when they share facilities, eating utensils and toothbrushes. This disease is hard to get. It is transmitted through sexual contact, intravenous

injection and from mothers to unborn babies.

On the other side are those, like Mr. Ray, who seem to shut their eyes to the very real and serious implications of the disease. Certainly people who have insurance and then contract AIDS must be covered, and that is being done. But to suggest that someone who already has AIDS antibodies in his blood should be able to buy a life or health insurance policy on the same terms as a healthy person is ridiculous. Scientists cannot say with certainty how many people with evidence of AIDS antibodies will contract the disease, but estimates are being raised rapidly. Perhaps a third will get it; perhaps they all will. But certainly the risk is great and cannot be ignored.

AIDS is invariably fatal. The majority of its victims are men in their twenties and thirties—just when the actuarial tables indicate they should be healthiest. The government doesn't force companies to sell new health insurance policies at standard rates to people who smoke three packs a day and are 100 pounds overweight, because there is statistical evidence that they run a high risk of heart disease. Why should coverage for AIDS patients be different? Mr. Ray's approach to the disease, though surely well meant, is just as misplaced as others' fears of catching it in a laundromat or on a crowded bus.

San Francisco Chronicle

San Francisco, CA, February 7, 1986

EVIDENCE THAT AIDS is not spread by casual contagion or household contact is reinforced by a detailed, scientific study of 101 New York family members who had prolonged and close contact with AIDS patients in their own homes.

The report in the New England Journal of Medicine should serve as a strong argument to allay the growing public hysteria over fears the disease may spread throughout the population. Researchers found no signs of infection in 100 family members, with the only exception being a 5-year-old daughter of two intravenous drug users who presumably was infected at birth.

A widespread fear of AIDS has led to such unwarranted proposals as mass screening for the AIDS virus, quarantining AIDS patients, excluding pupils with AIDS from classrooms, firing AIDS victims from their jobs and excluding immigrants with AIDS from entering the United States as permanent residents.

IN THE SIMPLEST of terms, all the evidence now indicates that the AIDS virus can only be transmitted by sexual contact with an infected person, or from blood contaminated with the AIDS virus. Emotion and excitability are unjustified reactions to a newly recognized disease that is highly fatal but extremely difficult to acquire.

AKRON BEACON JOURNAL

Akron, OH, February 10, 1986

SOME encouraging news has surfaced in a thorough study of AIDS victims and their families. The study compiled "conclusive" evidence that the fatal disease does not spread through close, personal contact such as that among families.

The study of 101 families, published in the New England Journal of Medicine, said the chance of contracting acquired immune deficiency syndrome from a member of the household is "virtually non-existent" — even though the family members shared drinking glasses, toothbrushes, beds, towels and toilets with AIDS victims, and hugged and kissed them.

The disease is still very deadly, even though it is hard to catch, and the study of these families is continuing, as it should.

But the findings should reassure those who may have come into casual contact with AIDS victims at work or in school. And perhaps such evidence can result in more humane treatment of those with the disease, who are often victims of both the disease and a fearful society.

Pittsburgh Post-Gazette

Pittsburgh, PA, February 12, 1986

It is more in the nature of confirmation than revelation, but a new study on the communicability of AIDS is still good news. Published in the New England Journal of Medicine, the four-year study concludes that close contact with AIDS patients — including the sharing of toothbrushes, bathtubs and toilets — poses virtually no risk of contagion.

The findings are based on the experiences of 101 people who were close relatives of AIDS patients. Of that group, only one — a girl born to an AIDS-infected mother — developed an AIDS-related infection. (Many of the relatives kissed AIDS patients on the lips, a fact that ought to reassure the Pittsburgh police officers who recently refused to simulate mouth-to-mouth resuscitation with a mannequin for fear of contracting AIDS.)

The new study acccords with evidence collected by the Centers for Disease Control. Out of an estimated 12,000 AIDS patients nationally, the centers have reported only one instance in which a family member of an AIDS patient contracted the disease. But in that case the virus was transmitted not through ordinary physical contact but through a mother's extensive exposure to the blood of her AIDS-infected child, who required continual blood transfusions because of an intestinal abnormality.

AIDS remains a deadly disease for members of high-risk groups — male homosexuals and intravenous drug users — and the government should not stint in searching for a cure. But for the vast majority of Americans, including the relatives of AIDS patients, the more dangerous epidemic is the plague of unreasoning fear about catching the disease.

Already, that panic has led to dangerous shortages in blood donations because of the absurd belief that *giving* blood can expose someone to AIDS. It also has needlessly stigmatized schoolchildren and other AIDS patients. Scientific evidence that AIDS is not easily contracted is thus welcome not only for the obvious reason but also because it can serve as a vaccine for that other AIDS epidemic.

Los Angeles Times

Los Angeles, CA, February 10, 1986

Despite repeated assurances from public-health professionals that AIDS is extremely difficult to transmit through casual social contact, many people have urged a policy of "better safe than sorry." As a result, some children with AIDS continue to face opposition to their attending school, and some adult AIDS patients have lost their jobs or homes. Even where the reactions have been less extreme, people with AIDS are frequently treated as modern-day lepers, shunned at the time they most need emotional support.

A report in the New England Journal of Medicine last week provides persuasive evidence that the health professionals have been right and that AIDS is a very, very difficult disease to catch in the absence of sexual contact or direct blood transfer. A study of 101 persons who lived with AIDS patients—including hugging them and sharing dishes and linens, but having no sexual contact—turned up only one person who had caught the AIDS virus. And that person, a 5-year-old girl, almost certainly got it from her mother while in the womb, the study concluded. All of the others not only didn't get AIDS, they showed no sign of infection despite the close and prolonged household contact.

The day after the report appeared, another case seemed to be a counter-example. A mother apparently caught the AIDS virus from her 2-year-old child, who had gotten it through a blood transfusion. But the mother had frequently handled the baby's blood, waste and feed tubes without wearing gloves. "The extent of what she did would be unusual for most parents," Dr. Harold Jaffe of the Centers for Disease Control explained.

So the evidence stands, and it bears repeating. AIDS is transmitted through the exchange of body fluids, principally through sexual contact or through tainted blood. The evidence says there is no danger of infection by being in the same room with an AIDS patient or even by touching. AIDS is not like the common cold or the flu, which can sweep through a classroom or office. No special public-health measures are needed to protect people from casual contact with AIDS patients.

Los Angeles already has an ordinance banning outright discrimination against people with AIDS. The new findings further support the wisdom of that law. But less egregious social discrimination remains. As the number of AIDS cases continues to increase (it passed 17,000 last week), there may be renewed anxiety about the risk to the health of the general public.

These fears are ill-founded. AIDS is a serious epidemic that has killed half of its victims so far while stymieing researchers trying to combat it. But the public need not fear casual infection. In the absence of high-risk activity, AIDS is not a threat.

U.S. FDA Approves Sales of AZT

The federal Food and Drug Administration (FDA) March 20, 1987 gave clearance to Burroughs Wellcome Co., the U.S. unit of the London-based Wellcome PLC, to market azidothymidine, or AZT, in the U.S. The drug had proven to be the first effective palliative for AIDS. The FDA action followed by a little more than two weeks the world's first commercial clearance of AZT—by Great Britain. The drug, which had been given the trade name Retrovir, had also been approved by France. The drug raced through U.S. drug-approval procedures in record time. From the time the first AIDS patient received a test dose until the March 20 commercial approval, only 20 months had elapsed.

In an unprecedented measure to limit distribution, Burroughs Wellcome March 20 said it had set up a registration system whereby doctors would have to apply to a medical board on behalf of their patients. The board would judge which patients fit the criteria for receiving the drug. The limited distribution would continue until the supply met the demand and would then be removed. The drug would initially be distributed to only two categories of patients. These were:

■ Victims of AIDS who had suffered one or more bouts of *Pneumocystis carinii* pneumonia, the opportunistic infection that was the single most frequent cause of death among AIDS victims.

■ Victims of a severe form of the condition known as AIDS-related Complex (ARC). Such patients would have to have a very low white blood cell count to qualify.

Burroughs Wellcome estimated that 15,000 patients in each category would qualify for the drug. The company said a year's supply of AZT would cost an estimated $8,000 to $10,000 per patient. The company attempted to justify the price on the basis of the expense and difficulty of making AZT as well as on the grounds that hospitalization costs would be significantly reduced for those treated with the drug. Nevertheless, the company's announcement generated an immediate outcry among physicians, consumer advocates and AIDS patients around the U.S., who said that the price would force many people to exhaust their savings and go on welfare rolls, relying on programs such as Medicaid to pay for the drug.

ST. LOUIS POST-DISPATCH
St. Louis, MO, March 26, 1987

The Food and Drug Administration's approval of azidothymidine (AZT) for use by AIDS sufferers opens a vast Pandora's box of questions that lie at the heart of public health policy. There's the matter of a private company profiting from a public scourge. The Burroughs Wellcome Co. spent $80 million to develop AZT and has every right to expect a reasonable return. Still, is it conscionable to make AIDS patients or their insurers pay $8,000 to $10,000 a year for the drug? According to industry analysts, that will yield the company a 40 percent profit, more than three times the company's usual rate of return.

There is the further issue of how to distribute the scarce drug until supplies can meet demand. The company's method is not without flaws. While AZT, or Retrovir, to use its brand name, is of most value to people in the earliest stages of AIDS, the system favors victims in the last stages. This might mean that people with the greatest chance of benefiting will be those with the least chance of obtaining the drug. Also, and even more worrisome, the whole decision-making process is put into the hands of a private company, with the government's various health agencies seeming only too happy to stay uninvolved.

Finally, the FDA's review process, speeded up to handle AZT, seems to be moving at its more normal snail's pace for other AIDS treatments. This suggests, at the least, the possibility of favoritism being shown Burroughs Wellcome (a suggestion raised when it became the first company to receive approval for human tests).

In short, approval of AZT has brought with it more than its share of policy questions. How the United States deals with them in the months ahead will do much to determine the quality of life not just for AIDS victims, but for every American.

The San Diego Union
San Diego, CA, March 27, 1987

The AIDS epidemic has been a drain on California's human and financial resources. To date, there have been nearly 6,000 reported cases of AIDS in California and more than 2,800 deaths. Millions of dollars are being spent each year to treat the victims of this terminal disease.

Those outlays are certain to increase now that the state Health Services Department is making the newly approved drug AZT available to eligible patients with AIDS or ARC (AIDS-related complex) through the Medi-Cal program.

AZT, which was approved last week in record time by the U.S. Food and Drug Administration, is not a cure for AIDS. All that it can do is alleviate the symptoms of AIDS and prolong the lives of its victims. Unfortunately, the drug's prohibitive cost, as much as $10,000 per year, places it beyond the reach of many and perhaps most patients. Thus the health department is adding AZT to the list of medications that doctors may prescribe for Medi-Cal recipients.

An estimated 20 percent of the state's AIDS patients could be eligible for AZT at a cost of $290,000 during the current fiscal year that ends June 30. By next year, that amount could exceed $7 million.

The availability of the drug could save the state-run program some money in the short run because patients taking AZT are likely to have fewer life-threatening infections that require hospitalization. Ironically, those savings will almost certainly be negated in the long term as treatment improves, extending the lives of patients. It's only a matter of time, moreover, before the drug's cost erodes the assets of many other AIDS patients who will then qualify for Medi-Cal assistance.

Such grim financial projections notwithstanding, California is obliged, nonetheless, to relieve the suffering of AIDS victims who cannot afford the cost of the new treatment. Meantime, localities must increase the number of testing centers wherein persons can discover whether they are carrying the AIDS virus. Although medical experts estimate that only 20 to 50 percent of these individuals will be afflicted by the disease, every carrier is potentially able to spread AIDS to others.

Increased testing for AIDS and continued medical advances are the surest means of containing and eventually eradicating the first known plague that, thus far, is 100 percent fatal.

THE 🔆 SUN

Baltimore, MD, March 26, 1987

The Federal Drug Administration's decision to allow the first AIDS treatment drug onto the market holds great promise. But AZT isn't a cure; it merely prevents the virus particles from reproducing and growing, arresting the degenerative process. And it has potentially serious side effects, among them bone-marrow suppression and anemia. Yet AZT could buy time while researchers try to uncover a cure. Thus, the risks associated with the drug are worth taking. That said, the more complex question of access comes to the fore.

There are only limited quantities of AZT. The firm that manufactures the drug has enough AZT for about 15,000 people. The cache could double by 1988, but it still does not approach the need.

While AZT certainly should be used to treat AIDS victims, it is most effective in the early stages of the disease, *before* people display severe immune deficiencies. The most recent statistics indicate the number of AIDS cases nationwide was 32,800 in early March. There are 10 times as many cases of Aids Related Complex, a condition in which a patient shows evidence of immune damage, but not enough to be fatal. For them, AZT offers a possibility of keeping the disease from progressing. But the limited quantity of the drug makes wider dissemination impossible. So does

the cost — between $8,200 and $10,000 a year.

FDA approval is pending, after which Maryland Medicaid will be obligated to pick up the cost of AZT for beneficiaries. But only 30 percent to 40 percent of the state's AIDS victims are eligible. The high cost of the drug means AIDS victims will have to "spend down" — sell their houses, cars and deplete their savings on the treatment before they can turn to the state for help. And then, Maryland will be especially vulnerable. Johns Hopkins University is one of only 10 AIDS treatment evaluation units in the country, and as such, a lot of victims come here for help. That, coupled with the escalating number of cases and the high cost of AZT threatens the state with a financial commitment so enormous that it is ludicrous to even image Maryland could underwrite it.

Federal legislation is needed to put AIDS victims in the same category as those who suffer from chronic renal failure and require dialysis, making them eligible for Medicaid benefits by virtue of their medical condition, regardless of their financial status. Sen. Robert Dole, R-Kan., who is one of the GOP presidential front runners in 1988, recently speculated that the country may have little choice but to spend billions of dollars on AIDS treatment and research. Mr. Dole is quite correct.

Despite the FDA's decision on AZT (see above editorial), rising numbers of people are being infected by the AIDS virus, lending new urgency to the search for a vaccine. And despite rapid gains in understanding the human immunodeficiency virus (HIV), researchers say a reliable vaccine is still five to 10 years away.

Here are some of the reasons:

☐ HIV is a complicated beast. Similar viruses that infect humans exist in only a few forms. HIV mutates more rapidly, comes in many strains and has an ability to evade immune system detection until it is thoroughly entrenched.

☐ Humans are the only animal known to contract AIDS. Doctors say chimpanzees can be infected, but they don't develop the disease.

☐ No one knows whether any vaccine can so stimulate the body's defenses it can ward off the virus. Victims produce antibodies now; that's how it's detected. But no one has ever recorded a case of someone successfully fighting off the virus.

The impatience that led a French doctor, Daniel Zagury, to try a U.S.-developed potential vaccine on himself is thus understandable. He is also testing several individuals in Zaire. Early results are encouraging, but doctors expect to learn more about safety than to find a proven preventative. That's true as well for tests planned at Johns Hopkins and the University of Maryland.

Think about it: the way to test a vaccine is to give it to a guinea pig, build up immunities and "challenge" it with the deadly microbe. But humans are the only acceptable guinea pigs, and a "challenge" that succeeded would kill the subject. Researchers will thus be forced to inoculate people thought to be "at risk" and wait to compare disease rates with control groups. Even that is less than satisfying. How do you justify withholding a vaccine that might save lives just to compare death rates? A similar conflict prompted rapid release of AZT, despite still-unsolved problems.

Dr. Zagury must be commended for his courage in injecting himself with parts of AIDS viruses, but let's hope he never gets a real "challenge." Facts known about AIDS are precious few compared with the unknowns. Researchers who can pry loose its secrets are humanity's strongest defense; we need all our Daniel Zagurys, alive and well.

Los Angeles Times

Los Angeles, CA, April 21, 1987

There is reassuring news from Sacramento. The state has decided to seek a waiver from the federal government that will allow the use of Medi-Cal funds to provide care for AIDS patients in homes, hospices or places other than acute-care hospitals.

This follows the earlier decision of the state to extend Medi-Cal coverage for AZT, the medication that can prolong the life of some AIDS patients but that, at an annual cost of about $10,000, is beyond the reach of many.

The waiver for alternative care will be filed by Sept. 1, and funding may be available early next year, according to state officials. It is a welcome step. Our only regret is that it has taken so long.

This will be "budget neutral," according to officials. In fact, there is evidence that there can be significant savings in providing alternatives to in-hospital care while at the same time creating a more amenable and humane situation for patients.

AIDS Project Los Angeles commenced a state-funded study of 131 AIDS patients receiving home

care last May. Preliminary data show a cost of $71.65 per day, compared with an average cost of $963 a day for hospital care. The 131 initially enrolled in the survey ranged in age from 1 to 68, including men and women. Of these, 86 have died, the majority at home. Hospital time has been reduced by at least one-third. Most important, however, is the finding of the researchers of significant benefits for the patient in remaining at home with family and friends. However, under present regulation, Medi-Cal funds are not available for home care. And at least a quarter of all AIDS patients depend on Medi-Cal—a percentage expected to increase in the years ahead.

The waiver will make possible a variety of alternatives to in-hospital care in addition to home care. Among the other alternatives under consideration are hospices, skilled-nursing facilities and day-care centers. State officials are now drafting the program for submission to the federal government, which provides half the Medi-Cal funding.

The Honolulu Advertiser

Honolulu, HI, March 22, 1987

The federal Food and Drug Administration has approved the first drug shown to prolong the lives of AIDS sufferers. It is badly needed.

That drug, AZT, which is derived from herring sperm, now will be available by prescription to those suffering from acquired immune deficiency syndrome. Until now, AZT has only been available to a small group of patients.

The drug's approval reflects a welcome change in policy for the federal agency. Usually, the administration withholds experimental drugs until they have passed a long battery of tests.

In view of the seriousness of the AIDS crisis, the approach is realistic and humanitarian. While AZT is not an AIDS cure, many patients have shown marked improvement after taking the drug. To deny other AIDS patients the drug until testing is complete would have been irresponsible and indefensible.

Approval of AZT comes at a time when AIDS hysteria has been growing, often blocking rational thinking about how to cope with the problem. The danger is that emotional responses will lead governments to promote discriminatory and costly programs that neither protect patients with AIDS or the population at large.

For instance, while it's right to require AIDS screening at blood banks, broad mandatory testing could be counterproductive. Similarly, there's no good reason to quarantine persons who have tested positive for the virus or to ban children with AIDS from schools.

More sensitive and sensible solutions to the problem may include voluntary testing of such groups as drug users and pregnant women. Counseling and sex education also are vital ingredients as ways to instruct the population on ways to avoid AIDS.

By approving AZT as a prescription drug, the federal government is making an important contribution toward prolonging the lives of many AIDS sufferers. Together with other steps, the move offers cautious hope this deadly affliction can soon be conquered.

Newsday

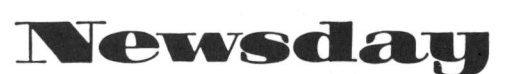

Long Island, NY, March 30, 1987

A controversy surrounding the AIDS drug azidothymidine — better known as AZT — will inevitably replay itself again and again in other contexts. The best approach is to adhere as closely as possible to the principle that everyone, rich or poor, should be able to get quality medical care.

AZT is the first and only drug on the market to show any effect, however modest, against AIDS. Manufactured by Burroughs Wellcome Co. under the brand name Retrovir, it will cost a patient from $7,000 to $10,000 annually — putting this life-prolonging drug out of reach for many AIDS patients.

Gay rights organizations claim that price tag is exorbitant; the company says it's necessary to recoup $80 million in research and development costs before a competitor drug comes out. Yet putting aside that quarrel — which isn't likely to be resolved soon — compassion dictates that needy AIDS patients should get help in paying for drug.

Burroughs Wellcome plans an extremely limited indigent-care program. To subsidize thousands of other AIDS patients desperate for Retrovir, Rep. Henry Waxman (D-Calif.) proposes to earmark many millions in federal assistance for indigent patients who otherwise could not afford approved AIDS drugs.

Is that the right precedent to set? Can the government be expected to pay for every AIDS-related drug that ends up on the market? Will the money spent on such drugs drain resources away from research that could produce a real cure or a vaccine?

What about people suffering from other life-threatening diseases — why not special congressional appropriations for them? And will Waxman's bill have the effect of encouraging pharmaceutical companies to jack up their prices — or motivate more drug developers to join the search for a cure?

Such questions will become increasingly acute as more promising drugs are discovered and resource demands grow. Yet for the moment Retrovir is the sole hope for someone with the deadly disease. To deny patients that hope because they can't afford the drug is a cruel judgment. Compassion may not be the only ingredient of a wise health care policy — but neither is ability to pay.

DESERET NEWS

Salt Lake City, UT, March 16-17, 1987

In proposing to make experimental new drugs more easily available to victims of life-threatening disease, the administration may give dying people a little more hope, but the policy is not likely to save many lives.

New drugs have traditionally been subject to strict controls. The Food and Drug Administration has refused to approve them for experimental use without first showing that they are safe and effective.

But the AIDS epidemic and its lack of any cure is causing great pressure to rush new medication into use — even if it still lacks proof that it will do any good or that it does not have dangerous side effects.

However, dying people are less concerned about safety than the possibility of finding a new miracle drug. If there is only a remote chance or none at all that a new drug might help, they have little to lose in risking the medication.

With this in mind, the administration proposes to take responsibility away from the FDA for deciding who should receive experimental treatments, and put it in the hands of individual physicians. The only way the FDA could refuse a doctor's request would be to have "clear evidence" that the new drug was not safe. That might not be evident early on with a new drug.

There are some concerns about relaxing the rules so drastically. It would make it harder to run tightly controlled experiments if doctors all over the country are giving doses of new drugs to their terminal patients. And it may make it more difficult to identify serious side-effects or potential dangers.

The question of what constitutes a "terminal" illness, and what diseases would be included in the program, are two major loopholes that could open the door to many abuses if every doctor in the nation is allowed to dip into the experimental drug laboratory on behalf of a desperate patient.

The change in rules — to become effective in 90 days — ought to be monitored closely and promptly rescinded if it merely turns patients into human guinea pigs for experimental drugs.

THE LINCOLN STAR

Lincoln, NE, May 26, 1987

The impact of the AIDS virus on America will soon be profound.

Quick vigorous preparation by individuals, institutions and government is imperative. No one will be untouched.

Based on the current estimate of infection — 1.5 million Americans — the Centers for Disease Control expects the number of diagnosed AIDS cases to grow from 35,769 today (20,683 have died) to 324,000 by 1991.

The cost of medical care will grow eightfold, from $1.1 billion last year to $8.5 billion in 1991. In addition, blood-screening, research and education costs will quadruple, to $2.3 billion.

The Office of Technology Assessment reports that by 1991 only cardiac care and car accident casualties will cost more than AIDS care. Those estimates do not include costs for AIDS-related complex, ARC, the initial phase of sickness that can be equally costly, or the lost productivity and wages of working-age people.

AIDS not only kills the infected individuals but frequently reduces them to poverty before they die. In San Francisco, the city with the country's model and most efficient care system, the average AIDS patient's care costs $35,000 a year. From diagnosis to death, an average patient lives two years.

New treatment drugs such as AZT cost as much as $10,000 a year. They prolong and improve life, but do not cure the disease. They may add to the disease cost.

BEYOND THE loss of life and cost of productivity and medical care, the country faces serious challenges to its traditions of individual medical privacy, respect for civil rights and compassion for sick and dying. Fear, divisive stereotypes, misinformation and excessive moralizing threaten to rip our social fabric.

Today's medical opinion overwhelmingly agrees that the AIDS virus is not spread by casual contact. It is contracted in a direct exchange of body fluids, most commonly through sex or use of contaminated needles, from an infected person. Medical experts agree through changes in behavior and use of reasonable precaution it can be personally avoided and its spread in the U.S. can be reduced and controlled without harsh social policies that ostracize, isolate, demean or ignore our fellow humans in need.

YET THERE ARE still many voices using AIDS to abuse others. They see AIDS as retribution for those who have practiced random, anonymous and, in their view, perverse sexual behavior with many partners or have used illicit drugs. Their brand of righteousness reigns over compassion, their fears over reason and understanding.

AIDS is caused by a virus. It does not discriminate between good and evil. It attacks infected human beings — newborn babies, mothers, fathers, sons and daughters alike. To debate morals instead of addressing urgent medical, educational and research needs is itself immoral. Everyone can support action against a common menace without condoning every behavior.

When and if we find a cure and prevention for the disease, we can draw morality lessons until the cows come home. Until then, all humans are at risk. Fraternal squabbles that threaten an essential common effort have no place in a war. They have no place here.

Surgeon General C. Everett Koop has said the traditional American values of personal freedom, mutual assistance and national unity are being tested. He's right.

We must all pay the cost of AIDS by quickly expanding federal research, education and health insurance programs. We must make the disease's control, avoidance and cure a national priority.

Individually, and through our local institutions, we must develop patterns of compassionate care and action. To do otherwise, would be to ignore our collective past and jeopardize our future.

The Providence Journal

Providence, RI, March 26, 1987

Approval of the first drug demonstrated to be effective in treating AIDS raises hopes that eventually a preventive vaccine and a cure will be found. But AZT (azidothymidine) is neither. In some patients it prolongs life by interrupting the reproduction of the AIDS virus in the body. However, it does not eliminate the virus, is highly toxic and can have serious side effects.

Fortunately for those victims who can benefit from AZT (trade named Retrovir) the federal Food and Drug Administration put the drug on a fast track, granting approval less than four months after the manufacturer made its presentation. The 22 months that elapsed from the first human trial to last week's approval for commercial use set a record for this kind of drug, according to Dr. Frank Young, commissioner of the Food and Drug Administration.

Speeding up the approval process was certainly justified, given the nature of this deadly disease. Still, other problems with AZT remain that may not be resolved as easily. Because the drug is still in short supply, it will not be available to all who need it. The supplier, Burroughs Wellcome Co., initially will provide pills only when a physician submits a patient's symptoms. Those considered most suitable for the medication will receive it, others must wait.

The cost for one patient's steady supply for a year is put at between $8,000 and $10,000. Thus, ability to pay is pitted against a desperate medical need. In the case of those who can't afford the cost, who will pay? Health insurance providers? Some, including Blue Cross of Rhode Island, have said they would; for others the jury is still out. Medicaid, the federal-state health program for the poor? Each state must decide.

For someone who has no coverage and doesn't qualify for Medicaid, the prospect is gradually spending down until the patient is impoverished and qualifies for Medicaid, a severe financial penalty for one already fatally stricken. Government undoubtedly would incur less cost if it helped lower-income AIDS victims with expenses before they hit bottom and became totally dependent. California is the first to say it would do this.

Further, other drugs are on the horizon that may warrant FDA's fast track approval because they have been found to be less toxic than AZT and may be more effective. One is ribavirin, which is said to be poised for approval in Britain. Others include Ampligen, Glucan and AL 721, a food product tested at the Weizmann Institute in Israel and found promising. If testing in humans is holding up approval of these drugs, a pool of willing subjects is available among AIDS victims who have nothing to lose.

AZT represents a holding action, a method of buying time for doomed patients who without it would have a life expectancy of perhaps five years at best. "All I know is that I'm still alive," said one patient who started taking AZT experimentally last November. Now he and thousands of others have hope of being alive when more effective drugs are developed or a cure is found.

Hospital Infections Spread Alarm

Three health-care workers had become infected with the AIDS virus after accidentally coming in contact with the blood of infected hospital patients, the federal Centers for Disease Control (CDC) reported May 22, 1987. The report had leaked a few days earlier, causing extensive alarm among health-care workers. In three separate incidents the workers, all women, had been infected with AIDS after their skin was accidentally splashed by blood of infected hospital patients. The three cases caused alarm because they were the first in which health-care workers had become infected with AIDS after a single exposure without being pricked with a needle. But all three women, according to the CDC, had had skin abrasions through which the virus might have entered their bloodstream.

CDC officials sought to put the incidents in perspective, noting that the rate of accidental infection for health-care workers overall was a fraction of a percent. Only nine U.S. workers out of thousands working with AIDS patients had accidentally become infected, and all previous cases had been transmitted by needle. The CDC had documented 103 cases in which health-care workers had accidentally been stuck with contaminated needles and 229 in which health-care workers had splashed infected blood on mucous membranes, usually the mouth—all without any sign of infection in nearly three years of follow-up exams.

"This is an extremely rare situation," CDC official Dr. James Hughes said. "But with more than one million infected people in this country, health-care workers have to take all the necessary precautions."

In a related development, a New York City dentist who rarely wore protective gloves had been infected with AIDS, it was reported June 4, 1987. But the dentist, who was still believed to be practicing, was the only one of 1,231 dentists and dental technicians in a nationwide survey found to have AIDS. Medical authorities said they knew of no legal requirement for the dentist to stop practicing, and they said no effort was being made to contact the dentist.

The Philadelphia Inquirer

Philadelphia, PA
May 22, 1987

Three hospital workers whose skin was exposed briefly to AIDS-contaminated blood are now infected with the AIDS virus as a result, according to federal health officials.

While this latest report does appear to confirm that AIDS may be transmitted via infected blood more easily than previously had been documented, it is not cause for public alarm. These three cases must be weighed in context; so far the government has recorded 35,769 AIDS cases. These patients were attended by tens of thousands of health-care workers who haven't been infected.

It is not news that AIDS-infected blood can transmit the virus. In late 1982, the U.S. Centers for Disease Control warned of the danger. Six previous cases of health workers infected by contaminated blood had been documented. Four of them were pricked accidentally by contaminated needles, and two were infected after prolonged exposure to contaminated blood and bodily fluids.

Moreover, the three new cases don't prove that AIDS can be transmitted through intact skin. In each case, the exposed skin was less than intact, and thus possibly more easily penetrated by the virus. One victim's hands were chapped. Blood splattered onto the acne-inflamed face, and possibly into the mouth, of another. The ungloved hands of the third may have conveyed the virus to a rash on her ears. Moreover, these three cases are the only ones known in which infection has been spread when contaminated blood has come in contact with broken skin — a very low incidence.

Nevertheless, however rare, it is now clear that it can happen. This underscores the imperative for everyone — not just health professionals, but anyone handling blood or other bodily fluids — to take precautions against possible infection, in accordance with federal guidelines. Protective gloves are the first line of defense. When more extensive contact is involved, protective clothing and masks or goggles may be necessary.

As Robert G. Sharrar, director of the Philadelphia Health Department's office of health promotion and disease control, puts it, this report shouldn't make people any more concerned about AIDS than they were before — but it should make them more careful.

Bangor Daily News

Bangor, ME, May 23-24, 1987

The recent discovery that three hospital workers may have contracted AIDS after their skin came into contact with AIDS-infected blood should intensify public concern about the disease and also should make the public more skeptical of official reassurances that the disease is confined to tight, easily identified groups with specific medical and social profiles.

From the beginning, the official response to the potential threat posed by the spread of AIDS has been to downplay and even ridicule the suggestion that it can be innocently transmitted. These new cases, reported from hospitals in different parts of the country, make one wonder if these public health officials have been premature in making absolutist statements about the nature and communicability of this disease.

In one instance, a laboratory worker was splattered with the blood of an AIDS patient. Officials at the Communicable Disease Center are not sure whether the worker contracted the virus through mucus membranes in her mouth or through facial acne. They just don't know. Although the average person does not handle test tubes containing AIDS-infected blood, this and other similar cases raise legitimate questions about the risks of close physical contact between young school children, and among older students who are involved in athletics and other activities.

Unfortunately, for political reasons, public health officials are reluctant to state what is becoming increasingly obvious: They don't have a secure handle on this disease.

AIDS is a relatively recent phenomenon, yet already it has hit 35,769 Americans. More than 20,000 of them have died. By 1991, some experts believe the number of AIDS cases in the United States will reach 270,000, resulting in 179,000 deaths. In other parts of the world, AIDS and other newly discovered related viruses are being compared, in their total potential impact, with the Black Death.

Before this epidemic runs its course, one likely casualty will be the credibility of public health officials who have allowed what should be strictly a medical problem to become hopelessly politicized. Too many of these officials, in Maine and elsewhere, have allowed their states to fall into the trap of dealing with AIDS as a human rights issue. This approach is dishonest, unfair to the public, and potentially deadly.

The Providence Journal

Providence, RI, May 22, 1987

The first three documented cases of AIDS infection in health workers caused by something other than the direct injection of blood, or prolonged exposure to body fluids, have been reported by the federal Centers for Disease Control in Atlanta. Three women tested positive after their skin came in contact with the blood of AIDS patients.

The report, issued this past week, has generated widespread concern. Does this mean that casual contact no longer can be ruled out as a means of spreading AIDS? Not really. Health officials report no evidence that the virus passes directly through skin

that is intact. This does mean, however, that more must be learned about the three cases before any new conclusions about AIDS can be reached.

Two of the women were not wearing gloves. The third was wearing gloves, but was spattered with blood in the face and mouth. According to Dr. James Curran, head of the CDC's AIDS branch, all three had skin problems — dermatitis, chapped hands, or breaks in the skin — through which the virus might have passed. None of the women belongs to a high-risk group considered most likely to contract the disease.

While these developments are likely to stir new concern — particularly among those who provide health care, or others who may come in contact with AIDS patients — it should be noted that the CDC has warned for some time that health workers should wear protective clothing.

Infection through skin breaks has long been considered a possibility. The guidelines say gloves should be worn if there is a chance of contact with blood, and when there is a chance of "more extensive contact with blood or potentially infective body fluids," gowns, masks, goggles or safety glasses may be necessary.

These warnings assume much greater importance now that three cases of infection, probably through skin contact, have developed. Until more is known about these particular cases, extra caution should certainly be exercised. But all facets of the health care delivery system — as well as people who provide emergency care, such as police and firefighters — should insist that the CDC AIDS guidelines are followed to the letter.

The Record

Hackensack, NJ, May 27, 1987

There appears to be a new risk group for AIDS infection: health-care workers.

Federal officials reported last week that three workers contracted the fatal acquired immune deficiency syndrome after blood from infected patients spilled on them. These are the first documented cases in which the AIDS virus has spread to health-care workers in a way not involving accidental injection of tainted blood or prolonged exposure to infected body fluids.

This news is certainly frightening to anyone who works closely with the blood and fluids of AIDS patients. But it's critically important that healthy concern not give way to panic. If these three rare cases of transmission trigger a widespread refusal to treat AIDS patients among health-care workers, that will needlessly escalate this tragedy.

Already, there is a growing ethical debate over whether doctors can refuse to treat AIDS patients. Last week, the New Jersey Board of Medical Examiners formed a committee to address the issue after reports that some physicians at one hospital in the state said they didn't

want to treat AIDS patients. There is nothing in the licensing law that would require doctors to do so.

If this becomes the prevailing attitude, however, New Jersey will soon have a crisis on its hands. Some 2,113 people have been diagnosed as having AIDS in New Jersey, which has the fifth-highest number of cases in the country. In four years, state health officials predict the number could be as high as 10,000. Many more doctors and health-care workers will be needed to treat this population.

It's important to note that two of the three infected health-care workers were not wearing gloves, as recommended by the federal Centers for Disease Control. The guidelines say that workers should wear gloves whenever they expect to be exposed to blood, even if the patient is not known to have AIDS. In some cases, workers should wear gowns, masks, goggles, or safety glasses, according to the guidelines. The latest cases should provoke not alarm among health-care workers but determination to adhere to the guidelines designed to protect them.

THE PLAIN DEALER

Cleveland, OH, May 24, 1987

Should a doctor who is diagnosed to have AIDS be allowed to treat patients? Officials at Cook County Hospital in Chicago have said no. Twice. The Cook County Hospital Board last week and again this week decided that a staff physician with acquired immune deficiency syndrome could perform only diagnostic and research duties. That decision is a step in the wrong direction in terms of allaying public fears about the disease.

It is understandable that the public has misconceptions and fears about the disease, which is projected to have some 270,000 victims by 1991. There is still much to learn about what causes AIDS and how to cure it. But health officials are fairly certain about how it is transmitted: through intimate sexual contact, use of a contaminated hypodermic needle, transfusion of blood containing the virus, or mothers passing the AIDS virus to their babies while in the womb or through breast-feeding. The center says 1,200 health-care workers have AIDS, but that none of them has infected a patient.

The Centers for Disease Control's guidelines say hospitals need not dismiss or change a physician's assignment, as long as doctors take recommended precautions that include wearing gloves, masks and gowns if they have open lesions and contact with a

patient's blood or mucous membranes. It is not recommended that they perform "invasive" procedures such as surgery.

The Cook County doctor has up to 10 days to appeal the board's decision. He currently is working with full staff privileges until the appeal process is completed.

If the public is encouraged to get as much education as it can about the virus and not discriminate ignorantly against its victims, then the public in Chicago is getting mixed signals from the health field—which should be in the forefront in setting a tone to reduce inflammatory panic.

The public has been sensitized over the most recent past about the pervasive impact of the disease. Children with AIDS, for example, were thrown out of classrooms only to be readmitted after people became more informed and less reactionary. The public response should not be a collective gasp and retreat, but a deliberate, progressive search for education, treatment and cures. But it needs consistent and rational direction from the health-care field.

Many things need to be done to ensure that AIDS is understood by the public. Telling a skilled doctor to stop treating patients isn't one of them.

AKRON BEACON JOURNAL
Akron, OH, May 24, 1987

THERE WAS discouraging news last week about the fight against AIDS. Federal officials reported three cases in which health-care workers became infected with the deadly virus after their skin was briefly exposed to blood from infected patients. It was the first documented evidence of AIDS spreading to health workers that did not involve direct injection of the infected blood into the body or prolonged exposure to body fluids.

However, troubling as the news is, unreasonable fears about the spread of AIDS should be resisted.

Federal guidelines recommend that health workers who expect to be exposed to AIDS-infected blood should wear gloves, and in periods of more extensive contact, gowns, masks or goggles may be required. In each of the three cases, the workers were not wearing gloves; nor had other precautions been taken. The infected blood, it is said, probably passed through cracks in the skin caused by chapping or acne. In one instance, the virus may have been transmitted when blood splattered into the mouth of a worker.

Without question, health workers face risks when caring for AIDS patients. But even in extraordinary cases, such as the three reported incidents, precautions can be taken to minimize risks dramatically. And health officials insist there's simply no evidence that the AIDS virus passes directly through intact skin.

Nor, according to the Centers for Disease Control, is there evidence that the AIDS virus can be transmitted through casual contact — shaking hands, working together, sharing the same bathroom. AIDS is a blood-borne disease, most easily transmitted through sexual contact or the sharing of intravenous needles. Thus, the high-risk groups are intravenous drug users and those having frequent sexual contact with multiple partners, especially male homosexuals.

All of us, however, should be concerned about the spread of AIDS. The costs of the disease by any measure — social, economic or individual — are enormous. Clearly, the most effective tool in combating the disease is education. Abstinence from sexual relations is an obvious method of prevention, but it's largely unrealistic. That's why parents, schools and other institutions must do their part to see that society copes intelligently with AIDS.

The news last week was tragic for three health workers. But there was another message in the story: Preventive measures exist, and they must be practiced.

The Kansas City Times
Kansas City, MO, May 21, 1987

An official pronouncement that three health care workers acquired AIDS on the job is alarming. Indeed, like almost all the periodic stories about the fatal disease, this is just one more piece of bad news; worse, if possible, than the one before.

The number of victims is increasing. The number of women and heterosexual victims is increasing. The number of dead is increasing. The cost of treating the ill and dying is increasing. And there is neither prevention nor cure in sight.

In the six years since AIDS has become an official plague and an American household word, there's been no documented case of a nurse, doctor or other professional taking care of someone with AIDS "catching" it from them. But the three publicized cases are not a sign that the disease is acting differently or there's a more virulent strain, or that health workers are generally at risk. These cases are a warning to take federal safety precautions seriously.

What happened to the three health care workers doesn't change the medical position that people cannot acquire AIDS through casual contact. They did not have "casual" contact.

First, they came into direct contact with the blood of AIDS patients, through their own wounds or mouth. Two of the cases involved accidents during special tasks, not routine health care. Finally, the three were not following federal guidelines for working with the AIDS virus. Specifically, none was wearing gloves. Nor were they protected with goggles, gowns, masks or safety glasses as is recommended when there's reason to expect the worker will be involved extensively or intensely with a patient's blood.

The legions of compassionate nurses and other professionals who have spent so much time with AIDS patients have proved panic is not necessary. But as ones now living under the shadow of the AIDS virus testify loudly, in special circumstances special precautions should be taken.

Pittsburgh Post-Gazette
Pittsburgh, PA, May 26, 1987

Reports of three health-care workers being infected with the AIDS virus by being spattered with the blood of infected patients could stir up the senseless early fears that had some funeral directors refusing even to bury AIDS victims. That will not happen, however, if the circumstances of the cases are examined closely.

The real lesson of last week's disclosure is that health-care workers who might be exposed to bleeding should observe scrupulously the safeguards long recommended by the federal Centers for Disease Control. Those precautions include the wearing of surgical gloves, gowns and masks to protect the skin from exposure.

Of the three health-care workers who were infected, only one was wearing gloves — and she was apparently infected when blood splashed into her open mouth. All three of the workers had skin conditions that would have allowed the virus to enter their bloodstreams.

Health officials point out not only that precautions were not followed in these cases, but also that health workers are exposed to far greater quantities of blood than are other persons.

The latter reminder should help to allay fears about the likelihood of being infected by the virus through much more casual contact — say, shaking hands with an infected person who has a cut on his hand. Medical officials have yet to report a single case of transmission of the virus through casual contact.

Even the sort of incident described last week is an extremely rare occurrence. According to the National Institutes of Health, 103 workers have accidentally stuck themselves with needles infected with the AIDS virus, and 229 others have splashed blood on mucous membranes, usually in their mouths. No one in either group tested positive for the virus.

There is a great deal to worry about in connection with the spread of AIDS. Especially vital is education about the way the disease is transmitted in the vast majority of cases — through sexual contact. Yet, even after last week's announcement, there are no grounds for taking a leper-colony attitude toward those infected with the AIDS virus. Sensible precautions in special situations are another matter.

The Union Leader

Manchester, NH, June 8, 1987

Of all the statistics presented in Washington last week at the Third International Conference on AIDS we regard as the most chilling the report that 69% of hospital doctors believe they can get AIDS from their patients and **one in four** would refuse to treat AIDS patients if given a choice.

In our view, those statistics challenge the argument that, absent a cure, education is the only answer to controlling the spread of the acquired immune deficiency syndrome and that all other responses are a waste of money and are violative of the right to privacy of such people as prisoners, prostitutes, about-to-be-married couples, intravenous drug users and persons being treated for venereal disease.

Surely the reasonable assumption is that doctors working in hospitals are educated on the subject of AIDS contamination!

Do these statistics constitute evidence of hysteria on the part of these doctors, or are they simply reasonably cautious when confronted with the unknown? After all, at this stage of the AIDS controversy at least, it would appear that there might be a vast category of "facts" we "know" that are not so.

Even with basic precautions, there are still certain risks attendant in taking care of such patients, and the statistics cited above may reflect doctors' understanding of those risks. A prominent New Hampshire doctor reminds us there are some important public health issues involved in the question of AIDS testing of prisoners or high risk people such as homosexuals or drug users. He cites the case of a male subject who committed suicide by cutting his wrists and bleeding to death in his cell.

"The list of people who were directly exposed to his blood," he points out, **"included the nurse from the county home, the guards and investigating officers at the jail, the inmates or janitors who had to clean up the cell, the EMTs who transport-**ed the subject to the hospital, the hospital personnel who attended him on admission, the medical examiner and pathologist who had to examine the body, other investigators who were present at the autopsy and the undertakers who had to embalm the body afterwards."

The tests on this man proved negative, but the doctor's point is that any of these people could have had a significant exposure to either hepatitis or AIDS. He questions whether these cases should be brought into hospitals for autopsies. "Hospitals," he says, "are obligated to care of the living but they are not obligated to provide facilities for the state or counties to perform autopsies, especially on potentially contaminated cases or bodies that are decomposed. In some cases the contamination is limited to the autopsy room, but many bodies also have to have x ray studies, which adds to contamination outside the autopsy room. This is one of the major reasons the state needs a separate facility for the chief medical examiner."

The doctor favors, as do we, routine testing of prisoners for hepatitis and AIDS. It would, he reminds us, "provide at least some forewarning of a serious hazard so that the medical personnel and others could take precautions to minimize the risk of attending these people when they are injured."

Indeed, it's a question of balancing risks. People who take care of members of high risk groups at considerable risk to their own personal health and well-being vs. what the doctor candidly calls "a new category of social lepers among the positives."

"In questions of public health the rights of society have always taken precedent over the rights of the individual," he points out.

But must we wait for public hysteria, increasing in direct proportion to the growth of an AIDS epidemic, to cause that principle to come back into vogue?

CHARLESTON EVENING POST

Charleston, SC, July 16, 1987

A small but growing number of physicians around the country are refusing to treat patients who are carriers of the AIDS virus. (A study released in May by the Centers for Disease Control reported that three health care workers had been infected with the virus through brief exposure to contaminated blood, apparently through breaks in their skin.)

Dr. C. Everett Koop, the surgeon general of the United States, has stated his belief that even if all reasonable precautions are taken, it is likely that other casual or accidental infections will occur. This, however, he sees as a necessary risk of the physician's job. Others do not agree.

As reported in The New York Times, two well-known heart surgeons in Milwaukee are but the latest to refuse to operate on carriers of the virus. Said one: "Today, I had to clean specks of blood off my glasses twice. Nobody can tell me how many specks of blood it takes to transmit the disease. There are simply too many unknowns, too many questions."

"His words carry a great deal of weight," said Jeffrey S. Akman, the director of the National Institutes for Mental Health's AIDS Education Program for Health Professionals. "He scared the hell out of most of the country."

Meanwhile, in Massachusetts, Gov. Michael S. Dukakis, a presidential candidate, has had to reverse an earlier policy forbidding insurance companies from testing prospective policyholders for AIDS. The governor's insurance commissioner resigned in protest, saying that "testing is not needed at this time and it may not be in the future," a position widely disputed by many insurance companies.

There surely must be some middle ground between those who see testing as a form of discrimination against homosexuals and intravenous drug users, and health care professionals who see AIDS as an infectious, fatal disease about which everything is *not* known.

Part II: AIDS and the Reagan Administration's Response

Since the AIDS virus was diagnosed, distrust has heightened between the gay community and the Reagan administration. Critics have accused the federal government of delaying its response to AIDS because those primarily affected by the disease have been homosexuals, saying that efforts began in earnest only when officials became afraid that AIDS might spread to the general community. With every budget cycle, Congress has prodded the Reagan administration to increase funding to combat a disease the administration itself has labeled the nation's "Number One health priority." In presenting the President's fiscal 1987 budget proposals, for instance, the administration claimed it was asking for $20 million more in AIDS spending than in 1986. But critics said this was a deception because the administration had proposed $51 million in budget cuts for fiscal 1986. From 1981 until 1986 Congress had not only to overcome the unwillingness of the administration to increase the level of funds the Public Health Service (PHS) required but also to actually battle proposed cutbacks.

The House Intergovernmental Relations and Human Resources Subcommittee, which has been investigating the federal response to the AIDS epidemic, released a report in 1987 that found a continued reluctance of the current administration to deal adequately with this crisis on a number of levels. The result, said the report, is that the agencies and programs that must lead the fight against AIDS have been continuously underfunded, making budgetary constraints the major problem at the federal level.

Traditionally, public health officials have exerted leadership in the fight for action and funds. Critics of the administration have suggested that this has not been the case with AIDS. The Department of Health and Human Services (HHS), for example, did not request additional AIDS funds until two years into the epidemic. Instead, it opted to transfer funds from other health programs. In addition, the Reagan administration was until recently criticized by members of Congress and gay rights groups for spending too little on public education and risk reeducation, leaving these efforts exclusively to local organizations.

Despite the controversial federal response to AIDS, funding for combating the epidemic has increased from $5.5 million in 1982 to President Reagan's hailed $1.3 billion budget request for fiscal 1989, up from $951 million appropriated for fiscal 1988. Of those funds requested for 1989, the largest portion, about $900 million, would go for research activities, including the search for vaccines. The remaining $400 million would be spent on public information and education efforts, including $15 million for a congressionally ordered informational mailing to all 108 million U.S. households. The new budget request seems to reflect the growing awareness among federal officials of the urgent need for a well-coordinated, efficient, and sufficiently funded program to fight this deadly disease.

Responding to an inquiry from the HHS concerning the application of federal antidiscrimination laws to persons with AIDS, the Justice Department issued an opinion holding that such people would not have the discrimination protections afforded other disabled persons. The opinion distinguished between "the disabling effects of the disease on its victims" and "the ability of the victims to spread the disease to others." Though the opinion acknowledged the medical consensus that AIDS was in all probability not spread by the sort of casual contact found in the workplace, it questioned the finality of that consensus, asserting that the "risk of medical uncertainty must be borne" by those who allege discrimination. Critics, including members of the House Intergovernmental Relations and Human Resources Subcommittee, argue that the decision, in effect, downplayed the medical opinion repeatedly endorsed by the PHS that AIDS is not transmitted by casual contact, thus allowing the fear of getting AIDS in the workplace to be used as the basis for discriminating against persons suffering from AIDS or AIDS-Related Complex.

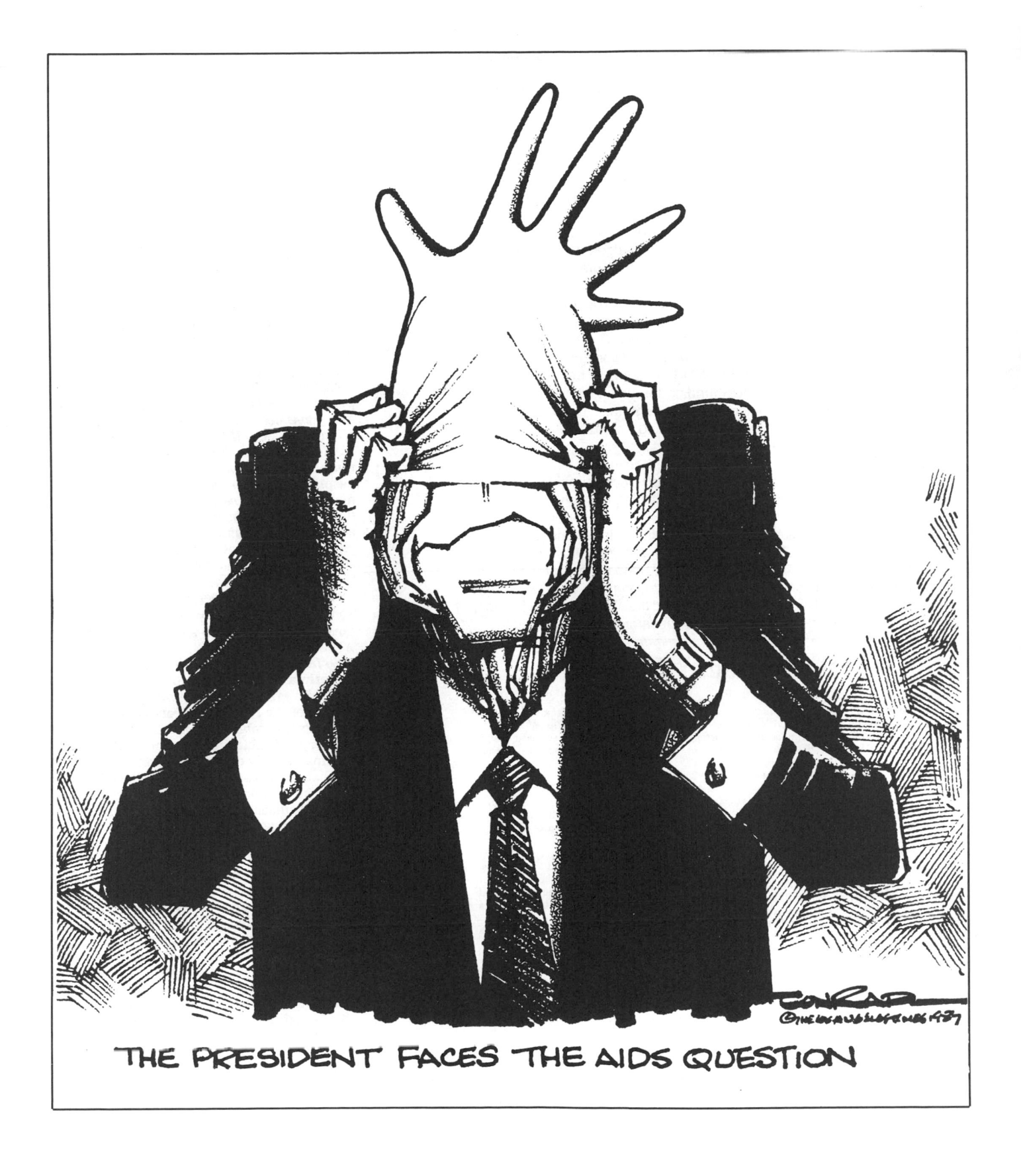

THE PRESIDENT FACES THE AIDS QUESTION

45

AIDS Called No. 1 Priority; Heckler Defends Admin. Effort

The investigation of AIDS was labeled the "No. 1 priority" of the U.S. Public Health Service by one of the government's top health officials May 24, 1983. Edward N. Brandt Jr., an assistant secretary of health and human services, told reporters that the government was engaged in a "nonstop pursuit to identify the cause of AIDS so that effective treatment and prevention measures can be developed and put in place." He announced a number of new research grants connected with his effort, and said that approval had been given for a new heat treatment for blood products, seen by some as a means of transmission of the disease.

Margaret Heckler, the secretary of health & human services, told a meeting of the U.S. Conference of Mayors June 14, 1983 that she intended to increase her department's spending on AIDS research to $26.5 million for 1983. This total included the $14.5 million already budgeted for the research and $12 million to be drawn from other departmental programs. Heckler also said that she had ordered a national toll-free "AIDS Information Hotline" to be set up to help promote public understanding. The measures were intended to demonstrate that the administration was sincere in stating that it viewed AIDS as the leading health priority in the U.S. The U.S. Mayor's Conference, however, took issue with the administration June 15 by calling for new money to be budgeted for AIDS research. The mayors were concerned that an increase in AIDS funding through shifting money from other areas would damage other needed programs. The mayors also unanimously passed a resolution June 15 backing increased efforts by state and local officials to promote AIDS research.

In her comments June 14, Heckler also reiterated the administration view that "for the overwhelming majority of Americans, there appears to be little or no risk of falling victim to the disease, in particular, through normal, daily social contacts."

The Reagan administration had been too tightfisted in funding research to combat AIDS, according to a report issued February 21, 1985 by the Office of Technology Assessment. The report by the nonpartisan congressional agency claimed that "except when prodded by Congress, the Department [of Health and Human Services] has maintained that [Public Health Service] agencies should be able to conduct AIDS research without extra funds."

St. Petersburg Times

St. Petersburg, FL, May 23, 1983

The magnitude of the threat of acquired immune deficiency syndrome (AIDS) continues to take on frightening new dimensions.

The number of AIDS victims doubles every six months, an exponential growth rate that baffles and disturbs researchers. There is increasing evidence that the disease, once thought limited to male homosexuals, hemophiliacs, heroin addicts and Haitians, is spreading to members of the general population. Medical researchers have not isolated AIDS' cause, and they have discovered no cure.

AND AIDS is a killer. About 40 percent of the more than 1,400 confirmed AIDS victims have died, and the remainder face the continued threat of recurring infections or cancer as a result of the breakdown of the body's natural defenses.

All of those factors have caused medical researchers to acknowledge the very real possibility that AIDS could become the sort of mysterious, widespread killer seldom seen since the plagues of the Dark Ages. Without wanting to be pictured as alarmists, researchers at the Centers for Disease Control in Atlanta are now stressing the need for a coordinated, national program to find a cause, treatment and cure for AIDS before the disease grows further out of control.

AIDS is so new — the first cases diagnosed in this country were reported in 1980 — and its potential effects are so huge that researchers have been caught off-guard. When the disease seemed limited to relatively small subgroups, it was treated as a relatively non-threatening curiosity. But findings from several recent independent research projects have ominous implications for the entire population:

✔ A study published in the *New England Journal of Medicine* found that six of seven women whose sexual partners were AIDS vic-

tims had also developed symptoms of the disease. Previous studies had concluded that only promiscuous homosexual men suffered a high risk of contracting AIDS through sexual contact.

✔ A report in the *Journal* of the American Medical Association, finding AIDS symptoms in children of men who had contracted the disease, suggests that members of the same household could transmit AIDS without sexual contact.

✔ Other victims have reportedly contracted the disease through blood transfusions. A New York City sanitation worker is thought to have contracted AIDS when he was pricked by a used syringe in a garbage bin outside a South Bronx hospital.

✔ There have been eight reported AIDS deaths in Hillsborough County since 1980. Researchers at USF Medical School are studying the potential threat to the general population.

But there is little official coordination or organization of these various research projects. Scientists in Boston, Atlanta, Houston and other research centers are attempting to isolate the virus that is the suspected AIDS culprit, but they do so without the sort of concerted federal backing that the task appears to warrant.

THE SOCIAL Security system this month instructed its offices to speed up the process through which AIDS victims are awarded disability benefits. That recognition of AIDS' effects is surely welcome, but it comes from an agency concerned with the symptoms — not the cause or the cure — of an increasingly frightening disease.

Given the startling medical breakthroughs of this century, a federal war on AIDS has excellent prospects for victory, but the scale of the battle should escalate before the enemy gains more ground.

The Kansas City Times

Kansas City, MO, May 27, 1983

By the time 558 people die from a disease the point for a preventive initiative has passed. Then it's reaction to crisis. The U.S. Public Health Service is doing so, setting acquired immune deficiency syndrome as its top priority.

The appearance of AIDS the past few years has caused alarm among groups apparently most at risk, as well as among health professionals. Although some researchers suspect a virus, the agent is still unknown. Apparently no available therapy has been able to restore immunity once a patient is afflicted.

Although 1,450 cases of AIDS have been reported in the U.S. since June 1981 (106 cases also have been found in 17 other countries), officials haven't officially labeled it an epidemic. Not yet. So the Public Health Service commitment to identify the cause and find a cure is auspicious. What such a priority designation means is that six research grants for study of the disease have been established at a cost of nearly $2.5 million, and approval has been given for a new heat treatment for blood products. The service's attention to the disease has been building over the past year, reflected in spending, number of personnel assigned to the problem and investigations. Altogether the government expects to spend $14.5 million on AIDS this year.

So far, AIDS, fatal in 38.5 percent of the cases, primarily has struck male homosexuals, drug abusers and Haitian immigrants. The diversity of the risk groups confounds pinpointing links that might help identify a cause. The mystery is frightening enough; scattered new victims recently diagnosed among the general population indicate either that selected groups may not be uniquely susceptible to AIDS as originally thought or that it is evolving.

In either case, the country's health leaders have every reason to mount an immediate attack. AIDS leads to a breakdown of the body's immune system, destroying the natural ability to fight off even the most common infectious agents. The personal army that prevents illness and is responsible for as much, if not more, healing than sophisticated drugs is put out of commission. An epidemic potentially could decimate the human race.

Consequently this country has much at stake in the success of the Public Health Service's efforts and those by other private and public scientists. The battle is not one the country can afford to wage half-heartedly with dollars or talent.

Portland Press Herald

Portland, ME, May 28, 1983

The head of the U.S. Public Health Service has finally conceded a new epidemic-disease is sweeping the country. Dr. Edward N. Brandt Jr. has christened AIDS the agency's "No. 1 priority."

That's good as far as it goes. But the public health service, which should be expected to lead the charge against any national disease, has come up late with relatively little in the battle against AIDS.

Why? Rep. Henry A. Waxman, D-Calif., says it's because AIDS primarily strikes homosexual males. Brandt denies it, pledging, "These people are victims of an illness, and we're going to do everything we can to stop" it. What they've done so far, however, is next to nothing.

New cases of the mysterious immune deficiency syndrome are reported at the rate of two a day. Of more than 1,450 reported victims, at least 558 have died. One of them was a Californian under treatment at the Veterans Administration Hospital in Togus. A second Maine case involves a New Yorker visiting here. James R. Novotny, who tracks sexually transmitted diseases for the state's Division of Disease Control, expects Maine to have its first indigenous AIDS case "before the end of the calendar year."

Private research is underway into the prospect AIDS is spread by a virus. While seven out of 10 victims are homosexual males with multiple contacts, the disease also occurs among Haitian immigrants. Concern that AIDS may be transmitted in human blood has led the Red Cross to request members of these high-risk groups not to donate blood until more information about AIDS is uncovered.

Now the National Institute of Health is awarding research grants worth $2 million, and a 100-member public health task force has been detailed to major cities. That's something, but it's still peanuts.

What it isn't is a commitment to deal with the nation's top public health priority.

Detroit Free Press

Detroit, MI, May 23, 1983

AIDS, or Acquired Immune Deficiency Syndrome, is a mysterious disorder that destroys the victim's normal defenses against disease. Of 1,410 persons known to have developed AIDS since 1981, nearly 550 have died, most from rare strains of cancer and pneumonia. No cure is known. Fewer than 14 percent of its victims have survived more than three years after contracting AIDS. Researchers say that the number of cases is doubling every six months and that as many as 20,000 persons could acquire AIDS within the next two years.

So far AIDS and its victims have received more publicity than help. About three-quarters of the victims have been male homosexuals. Seventeen percent are intravenous drug users, usually of heroin. AIDS has also occurred among Haitian immigrants who are neither homosexuals nor drug addicts. These are not groups with which the general public identifies, or with which many politicians wish to be identified The relative indifference that has until recently surrounded AIDS, compared with the public concern over a potential swine flu epidemic seven years ago, or Legion-naire's disease, toxic shock syndrome or even genital herpes, is resounding.

But AIDS is spilling over into the mainstream of American life. Hemophiliacs receiving blood transfusions have come down with AIDS. So have women and children sharing households with AIDS victims. A New York City sanitation worker who fits none of the above classifications, but who may have handled a contaminated syringe while picking up garbage, has been diagnosed as having AIDS. Although most AIDS victims live in New York and California, nearly every state has some cases, including Michigan.

Some research is under way. And the Social Security system has begun instructing its offices to grant nearly automatic disability benefits to qualified persons suffering from AIDS-related diseases because of the high mortality rate. But a national campaign to unravel the cause of AIDS and to discover preventive and curative measures has yet to get under way. A year ago, simple humanity should have dicated some response. Now, as the incidence of AIDS spreads, self-interest demands it.

San Francisco Chronicle

San Francisco, CA, May 31, 1983

THE BAFFLING acquired immune deficiency syndrome is finally, after considerable foot-dragging, receiving appropriate attention at the federal level. The House of Representatives just voted $12 million for AIDS research for the remaining four months of this fiscal year. That quadruples the amount of federal funds for research into this mysterious malady. Mayor Dianne Feinstein and the San Francisco Board of Supervisors have indicated their support for an additional $2 million in city funds.

So the money is on hand to press the much-needed scientific effort to unlock the cause of the most alarming epidemic in America since the days when polio was such a menace.

With that step achieved, it is now important to take a calm, realistic look at just what is happening. A level-headed approach is needed to reduce some of the hysteria that has cropped up among those who are basically ignorant of what is now known about this cruel sickness.

SINCE JUNE, 1981, 1450 cases of AIDS have been reported, more than 70 percent of them in male homosexuals or in bisexuals with multiple sex partners. Others at high risk include intravenous drug abusers, recent arrivals from Haiti and hemophiliacs. Of these cases, 558 people have died, in the main from Kaposi's sarcoma, an unusual skin cancer, or from infections like pneumonia that the victims' immune systems cannot defeat. Four to five new cases are reported every day in the United States — San Francisco and New York are being hardest hit — and 106 cases have been found in 17 other countries.

With this in mind, it should be emphasized that casual contact will not spread the syndrome. That was reaffirmed just the other day by Edward Brandt, assistant health and human services secretary, as he announced that the malady is "our No. 1 priority. . . I feel a great sense of urgency about AIDS."

There appear to be only three ways the syndrome may be passed from one person to another: sexual contact, sharing needles among drug abusers or use of contaminated blood or blood products.

"What I'm trying to suggest to them (the public)," said Brandt, "is they shouldn't be panicked about this. We have no evidence that it is breaking out into the general population in any way. I'm sure enough that I'm not concerned about the risk of AIDS to me or my family."

THIS KIND of reasonable, dispassionate approach contrasts with the unfortunate bulletin issued by the Police Officers Association that public health officials derided because it implied the syndrome might be transmitted casually. And those police officers who wrote Democrats warning them not to come here for their convention were acting childishly.

The more solid information that can be promulgated on this syndrome the better. In this regard, it seems to us that it is time for the San Francisco Department of Public Health to intensify its educational campaign about AIDS. There are certain precautions that are advisable. And the more one knows about a threat of this sort, the less do unfounded fears abound.

The kind of hysteria we have so far seen manifested about AIDS springs probably less from malice — although there is a nasty, anti-gay element to some of it — than from lack of real knowledge. It is this ignorance that feeds panic and prejudice. What is needed now is to confront this terrifying problem with thoughtful candor — and work to put an end to the AIDS threat.

The Dispatch

Columbus, OH, October 7, 1985

U.S. Sen. Alfonse D'Amato, R-N.Y., has proposed that Congress spend $1 million to establish a 24-hour telephone hotline to answer questions and combat "growing public hysteria" over the spread of acquired immune deficiency syndrome.

The idea of a hotline is a good one. Many people have many questions about AIDS, and there are many misconceptions contributing to the fear that some feel about the disease.

However, the argument is not compelling that it is a federal responsibility to fund the hotline. New York, for instance, has 34 percent of all the reported AIDS cases in the nation. California also has a high percentage. If these and other states want to have hotlines, they are certainly free to find their own way to set them up. They don't need the federal government coming in to tell them how to do it. Each state's health director could simply issue a phone number where questions could be answered.

What the federal government may wish to do is to provide information to the state hotlines that can be used so that everyone gets the same information. There are federal agencies that know as much about the disease as anyone, and their resources could certainly be used to fight fear.

But the hotlines themselves would operate better under state, local or private control.

The Atlanta Journal AND THE ATLANTA CONSTITUTION

Atlanta, GA
September 28, 1985

In the grisly matter of AIDS, the government is finally beginning to sound like it means business. The nation's chief health official has told a Senate subcommittee that he's asked the White House to approve a $70 million increase in 1986 spending for AIDS, a 55-percent increase over the $129 million being spent this year — and was promptly assured of strong Senate support.

"Whatever you ask for, you got," subcommittee chair Lowell Weicker (R-Conn.), informed James O. Mason, assistant secretary for health in the Department of Health and Human Services Thursday.

It may not be so simple to determine how the money ought to be spent: For a public education campaign? A national research headquarters? Better coordination and dissemination of the constantly updated research data? All are urgently needed. But the importance of the government making those funds available can't be overstated.

Though Health and Human Services Secretary Margaret Heckler has in the past called AIDS her No. 1 public-health priority, the president has yet to discuss it publicly or assume a leadership role, a sore point with many researchers.

The administration is only now talking and acting as if it's committed to stopping the spread of AIDS — spurred, Mason admits, by reassessment of the threat. A new study, for example, shows the disease being spread to U.S. servicemen in West Germany by prostitutes, a circumstance that virtually guarantees an eventual, increased incidence of it among stateside heterosexuals.

AIDS, which kills its victims by destroying the immune system, leaving the body fatally vulnerable to diseases that could ordinarily be overcome easily, has already afflicted 13,228 Americans and killed 6,758. No one has been cured, and eight out of 10 Americans now consider it as great a threat as cancer, according to a *Washington Post*-ABC News Poll.

Money in itself is no solution, but an all-out commitment from the top levels of government contributes mightily to the sense of urgency, to its importance. A substantial allocation is, at this point, a timely and appropriate expression of that commitment.

Now they're talking.

Los Angeles Times

Los Angeles, CA, July 29, 1985

Rock Hudson's illness has focused renewed public attention on acquired immune-deficiency syndrome, the epidemic that has struck 12,000 people in the United States in the last four years— half of whom have died. President Reagan, recovering from cancer surgery, telephoned his good wishes to Hudson in Paris. Perhaps the President's personal involvement will lead to a greater federal commitment to wiping out AIDS. For although the government has declared AIDS the nation's No. 1 health problem, its efforts to combat it so far have not been adequate.

Washington is the primary source of money for research on AIDS, which destroys the body's ability to fight infections. This year about $95 million will be spent on AIDS research, and the Administration has asked for an additional $45 million for next year. Almost all that money is being spent on efforts to find a vaccine that would prevent the disease, which is certainly important and should be pressed. But hardly any money is being spent on finding a cure for those who already have AIDS.

At the outset, researchers thought that AIDS would be like legionnaire's disease, which was squelched in short order. But AIDS has proved much more difficult. In congressional testimony last week the Department of Health and Human Services said that no effective vaccine or treatment is expected until 1990 at the earliest. The prospect is frightening. Nationwide, the number of new cases is doubling every nine months; in Los Angeles the number of new cases is doubling every six months. At that rate hundreds of thousands of people will be struck by AIDS before medical science figures out what to do for them. The financial cost of caring for patients with AIDS could run into the billions of dollars. The human cost would be even more staggering.

In addition to preventing AIDS, this country needs to aggressively pursue every potential cure, as the French are doing. Rock Hudson went to Paris, as many other AIDS patients have done, because a promising drug, HPA-23, is being tested there. It doesn't cure the disease, but it appears to slow it down. In several weeks, the government says, HPA-23 will be available experimentally in this country. Based on promising work overseas, it should have been here before now.

The federal health agency's relaxed regulations for new drugs will make it easier for experimental drugs to be used. The government should make funds available for researchers to test any anti-viral drug that they think might work. There would be many blind alleys, but one successful drug would justify the effort.

In the meantime the best way to slow down the AIDS epidemic is to educate the public about the sexually transmitted disease and about ways to minimize the chance of contracting it. Gov. George Deukmejian foolishly vetoed more than $10 million that the Legislature appropriated for that purpose. The Los Angeles City / County AIDS Task Force last week recommended that the county begin a $500,000 program for AIDS education. The supervisors should adopt that proposal forthwith.

Though the vast majority of AIDS patients so far have been homosexual men, the disease has begun to spread through society at large. Everyone is at risk. But there remains a lack of urgency in both the government and the public mind. Perhaps Rock Hudson will wake people up. Much needs to be done, and it needs to be done fast.

THE RICHMOND NEWS LEADER
Richmond, VA, October 8, 1985

There appears to be growing support for increased federal funding for the research of the causes and cures of AIDS, the acquired immune deficiency syndrome that is causing concern — and in some cases panic — across the country. The research is an appropriate federal response to a public health problem and increased funding is needed.

The U.S. House of Representatives last week approved spending $190 million for AIDS related research, education, drug development and other programs for the present fiscal year. AIDS-related funding during the 1985 fiscal year was $100 million. The Reagan administration had asked for $120 million in spending.

While it's difficult to say at this point how much spending is enough, it is obvious that AIDS presents a clear threat to the nation's well-being. Leaders of the House and the Senate should work closely with the White House to reach a compromise on the AIDS funding package. There must be a quick and substantive response to the AIDS threat.

The Boston Globe
Boston, MA, March 5, 1985

What is it going to take to wake up the federal government to the absolute health menace now posed by AIDS? While movie stars plan benefits to combat AIDS, and much is made of a blood test that may prevent 2 percent of future cases, the numbers climb all over the world, and the AIDS virus spreads like a deadly spider's web everywhere.

Rock Hudson now joins the sorrowful roster of AIDS victims. It should be borne in mind that he is one of 12,000 persons in the United States stricken with acute AIDS since mid-1981. Half of them are already dead. The list of new cases grows by nearly 200 patients a week.

Lester Maddox is waiting to see if he will develop AIDS. Yet he is but one of the one million Americans apparently exposed to the AIDS virus, but as yet symptom-free. Maddox fears he received injections of an AIDS-contaminated blood product at a cancer clinic in the Bahamas.

Caught between the fatal form of AIDS and the symptom-free carriers are 100,000 Americans with chronic AIDS. Though their symptoms wax and wane, they are in a no-man's land. One in five will advance to full-fledged AIDS.

Atop all of this is the new medical awareness that anyone who has been infected by the AIDS virus – with or without symptoms – is at risk for a wide range of nervous-system disorders. The virus infects the brain and other nerve tissue.

"We are in the midst of a major AIDS epidemic that has already resulted in the deaths of thousands of individuals. Before it is finished, thousands, perhaps hundreds of thousands, more will become victims," Dr. Martin Hirsch of Massachusetts General Hospital told a congressional health committee.

Hirsch and other physicians who testified at Waxman's hearing are not ivory-tower scientists. They are on the front lines – not only searching desperately for a way to cure or prevent AIDS, but also confronting new patients daily with the devastating nature of their illness and trying to do their best by them, despite the absence of any effective treatment No one with acute AIDS ultimately survives.

Rep. Henry Waxman, (D-Calif.), who called the committee hearing, has been sounding a national alarm on AIDS for two years. Largely through his efforts, Congress has consistently authorized more funds for AIDS research than the Reagan administration has sought – although the amount is not nearly enough. Waxman and AIDS scientists know that the lack of sufficient funds for research has slowed the pace of progress against AIDS.

The upshot of his hearing was a request by Margaret Heckler, the secretary of Health and Human Services, for an increase of 50 percent, or $40 million, in funds for AIDS research. The increase would bring the amount to $126 million for 1986.

There's a catch, though. The Reagan administration wants to take the $40 million from other programs – the Indian Health Service, for example, and new laboratories for cancer and heart research.

Last year, part of the AIDS research money was taken out of programs to combat sexually transmitted diseases – a remarkable irony, considering that AIDS is primarily a sexually transmitted disease. It has been a sorry record, overall.

In 1984, the president requested $40 million, the public health agencies requested $60 million, and Congress appropriated $61.5 million. In 1985, the president requested $60 million and the agencies $91 million; Congress appropriated $103 million.

Waxman is right when he calls such funding " a drop in the bucket" and the approach to funding "robbing Peter to pay Paul." Money should be the last thing to worry about in any consideration of AIDS.

Hirsch, in asking for a coordinated research attack to test anti-viral drugs against AIDS, said: "A crash program enlisting the nation's best clinicians, virologists and immunologists is necessary to limit the deadly progression of this disease, and the sooner this is begun, the better. The problem is real. The need for action is urgent."

William Haseltine, a virologist at the Dana-Farber Cancer Institute in Boston, predicted "a conservative half-million cases in the next five to six years." He said that "we lack leadership from the White House and funds from Congress," and that it will take an all-out commitment from both to make any headway in the "man versus microbe" AIDS war.

Dr. James Oleske of New Jersey, who primarily treats children with AIDS, pleaded for new sources of funding to pay for the enormously expensive care of AIDS patients. There are so many fronts on which the AIDS menace must be fought that a commitment on the scale of the Manhattan Project, which produced the atomic bomb during World War II, may be needed.

One thing is certain. Delay and niggardly funding will cost an incalculable price. Unless some way is found to thwart the spread of AIDS, there is no scientific doubt that the number of cases here – and worldwide – will double in a year's time and keep doubling thereafter. AIDS scientists agree with Hirsch that "there isn't a moment to be lost."

ST. LOUIS POST-DISPATCH
St. Louis, MO
August 15, 1985

The U.S. Conference of Mayors has awarded $145,000 to eight cities to help pay for several anti-AIDS projects designed to cut the incidence of the deadly disease. The money is to be used to fund a public education and awareness drive against acquired immune deficiency syndrome, a devastating viral disease that destroys the body's immune system and usually kills its victim.

The grants were awarded at the same time a new Gallup poll showed that 50 percent of the American people believe the government is not spending enough money on AIDS research. More than 12,000 cases of the disease have been diagnosed, and health researchers anticipate 250,000 cases — in the United States alone — by 1990.

AIDS, which initially was perceived to be solely a homosexual disease, has now spread into the heterosexual community. Because of the homosexual stigma that has surrounded AIDS, public officials have been wary of addressing the disease. But that is changing. Although $145,000 is a drop in the bucket when it comes to the amount of money needed to educate the public about the disease, it is symbolic that the issue now is being addressed by the top officials of the nation's cities. Locally, a bill in the Board of Aldermen is aimed at minimizing the risk that the disease will be spread. It would regulate commercial blood banks and mandate blood tests among donors for exposure to AIDS.

Wisely, officials are beginning to address this deadly disease. Increased public awareness of AIDS and intensified research for a cure are the best hope for a decrease in the number of cases or — perhaps more optimistically — elimination of the disease.

Surgeon General Wants AIDS Classes

U.S. Surgeon General C. Everett Koop issued a report October 22, 1986 calling for education of school children "at the lowest grade possible" about sex and the fatal disease AIDS. The unusually explicit 36-page report, available to the public in booklet form, was the federal government's first major statement on how to contain the spread of AIDS. The White House had requested the paper, and Koop himself was the author. He discussed the report at a Washington, D.C. news conference.

Koop said sex education, including material on AIDS, should begin in elementary school. He added that the AIDS epidemic could foster agreement among "diverse groups of parents and educators with opposing views on inclusion of sex education in the curricula." Programs targeting blacks, Hispanics and other groups that showed high rates of infection would be useful, he said. The Reagan administration had been criticized for not providing enough AIDS education funds, but Koop said there was now enough money.

Parents and teachers would have to deal frankly with the subject of AIDS, the Koop report said. "Many people, especially our youth, are not receiving information that is vital to their future health and well-being because of our resistance in dealing with the subjects of sex, sexual practices and homosexuality," the surgeon general wrote. "This silence must end. We can no longer sidestep frank, open discussions about sexual practices—homosexual and heterosexual." Homosexual contact accounted for most AIDS cases, but transmission by heterosexual contact was expected to grow, Koop told reporters. His report emphasized that the disease was "not spread by common everyday contact," such as shaking hands, social kissing or sneezing. Sexual relations and the sharing of intravenous drug needles and syringes accounted for most AIDS cases, Koop said. Koop said "protective behavior" was called for so long as there was any question at all as to the health of the sex partner. "The best protection against infection right now—barring abstinence—is use of a condom," he said. "A condom should be used during sexual relations, from start to finish, with anyone whom you know or suspect is infected." The Koop report urged individuals with high-risk sexual pasts to check for infection by taking blood tests.

But the surgeon general dismissed calls for compulsory testing and said quarantine of AIDS victims would be medically pointless. "It's time to...recognize that we are fighting a disease—not people," he said at his news conference.

A White House advisory commission on AIDS held its first full-scale meeting September 9-10, 1987 in Washington, D.C. Perhaps the most impassioned testimony by a federal official came from Surgeon General Koop. Citing reports that more doctors and other health workers were refusing to treat AIDS patients, Koop Sept. 10 warned that "the ethical foundations of health care itself" were threatened by a "fearful and irrational minority." He suggested that health workers would have little to worry about if they carefully followed "the sensible and rather elementary guidelines" issued by the federal Centers for Disease Control, which prescribed the use of gloves and other protective measures to avoid contamination.

The Augusta Chronicle
Augusta, GA
October 29, 1986

Surgeon General C. Everett Koop, in his long-awaited report on AIDS, has drawn both praise and criticism for calling for sex education in the schools to combat the spread of the fatal disease.

We understand where the critics are coming from. In the past the nation has had some unhappy experiences with sex education — which was used in many cases as a radical forum to promote a "value free" society based on "situation ethics." Under the aegis of being taught about sex, kids were encouraged to engage in it.

Koop makes it clear this is not the kind of sex education he has in mind. He thinks kids should be taught, beginning at an early age, that sex can be fatal to your health. He recommends total abstinence for teenagers.

The surgeon general's report also says the only safe sex is "mutually faithful monogamous relationships" and urges the use of condoms if there is any doubt. That's certainly good advice for adults, particularly since statistics indicate AIDS is beginning to break out of the homosexual and drug communities into the heterosexual community.

Our only quarrel with the report is that it would start sex education in elementary school, which is a little too young. Few 8-year-olds are prepared intellectually or psychologically to deal with the subtle human complexities involved in sex and AIDS.

But the thrust of Koop's report — that leaving our children ignorant about sex will endanger their lives — is right on target. Parents have been terribly remiss in educating their children about sex. The job often falls to schools by default.

What is needed now is for concerned citizens across the nation to work with their local school districts in helping to establish *responsible* sex education courses that will both teach our kids what they need to know and reflect contemporary local standards.

The curricula shouldn't become radicalized again if Koop's advice is taken — and local School Boards keep a sharp eye on how the courses are taught.

The Washington Post
Washington, DC, October 24, 1986

IT ISN'T OFTEN that Planned Parenthood and the Reagan administration see eye to eye, but a national crisis has brought them together on at least one subject: AIDS. A report issued earlier this week by Surgeon General C. Everett Koop drew praise from the family-planning group specifically because it urges sex education in schools at the earliest possible grade. But that recommendation is not the only noteworthy item in Dr. Koop's frank and sensible report.

Wednesday's statement was prepared at the request of President Reagan and is styled "a report to the American people on AIDS." No reader could come away complacent about the statistics presented on the spread and deadliness of the disease, but the report contains more than facts. It exhorts Americans to put aside prejudices they may have against homosexuals and intravenous drug users, to help the victims of this epidemic and to stop talking nonsense about quarantines, universal blood tests and tattoos for those who test positive. Perhaps most gratifying to those who view the surgeon general as a conservative, he approaches this sensitive subject without making value judgments, only medical ones. "It is time," he says, "to put self-defeating attitudes aside and recognize that we are fighting a disease—not people."

On the issue of sex education, Dr. Koop is forthright. "There is now no doubt that we need sex education in schools and that it include information on sexual practices that may put our children at risk for AIDS." This risk applies primarily to homosexuals and intravenous drug users, and the report contains specific instructions on how people in these categories can reduce their exposure. But, as the most recent data on the spread of AIDS confirm, it is not limited to these groups, and the disease is spreading, through sexual contact, to the general population. Abstinence and the maintenance of mutually faithful monogamous relationships, whether homosexual or heterosexual, are the only sure means of avoiding sexually transmitted AIDS. But the report acknowledges that not everyone will accept such restrictions. It goes on to describe the steps that can be taken to reduce the risk.

Dr. Koop's statement sets a standard for other government officials—federal, state and local—in dealing with AIDS and its victims. Without a hint of mean-spiritedness or hesitation, he says three things. We must help and not condemn those who suffer. We must take precautions against the spread of AIDS. We must educate our children about the dangers of this disease. That's good advice, and it should be heeded.

Buffalo Evening News
Buffalo, NY, October 23, 1986

SURGEON GENERAL C. Everett Koop, in his long-awaited report on AIDS, lays great stress on education, which is, indeed, one of the few means so far at our disposal in fighting the dread disease.

The disease, formally known as acquired immunity deficiency syndrome, was discovered only a few years ago, and it has been spreading at a rapid rate. So far, 26,566 Americans have been diagnosed as having AIDS, and 14,977 of them have died. There is no cure and no known survivor.

Koop's reasoned report should put the disease in proper perspective as a serious national health problem but one that is no cause for panic. He dispels some of the mystery about the disease, stressing that it "is not spread by casual, non-sexual contact" and that new infections can be prevented through precautionary measures.

Since AIDS is spread mostly by intimate sexual contact, especially homosexual contact, it is vital that information about the disease be disseminated so that proper precautions can be taken. While heterosexual transmission of the disease is still low in this country, it is rising rapidly in other countries, and Koop warned that "freewheeling, casual sex" is "a dangerous game."

Unfortunately, this much-needed information is not getting through to those who need it, particularly many young people. Koop said there was a reticence about dealing with subjects like sex, sexual practices and homosexuality.

"This silence must end," he said. "We can no longer afford to sidestep frank, open discussions about sexual practices — homosexual and heterosexual." Education regarding AIDS, Koop said, should start at an early age, with both parents and schools taking a role.

Sex education in the schools has always been a controversial subject, and the forthright stand taken by Koop is especially noteworthy because of his conservative background. Koop once described the gay rights movement as "anti-family."

Now, however, in the effort to control AIDS, he said that "there is now no doubt that we need sex education in schools and that it include information on heterosexual and homosexual relationships."

Koop noted that when AIDS was first discovered among homosexuals, some people felt that people from certain groups "deserved" their illness. "Let us put those feelings behind us," Koop said in the report. "We are fighting a disease, not people." He opposed compulsory testing, quarantines or the tattooing of infected persons — all ideas that have been proposed as a means of controlling AIDS.

While the number of people known to be infected is at present comparatively small, they may be just the tip of the iceberg. Hundreds of thousands of people could be carriers of AIDS without knowing it.

With the outlook for a preventive vaccine fairly remote at present, the fight against this insidious disease must be carried on with the weapons we have — education concerning the spread of the disease and how to prevent infection.

The Miami Herald
Miami, FL, November 7, 1986

FIRST THE Reagan Administration's conservative and often-moralistic Surgeon General fired a blast at hysterical and punitive treatment of AIDS victims. Now a special committee from the National Academy of Sciences and the Institute of Medicine has followed with a chilling report that warns of potential "catastrophe" as AIDS seeps into the general population. The academic committee suggests a $2-billion-a-year national campaign of research, education, and treatment to curb the burgeoning epidemic.

Surgeon General Everett Koop issued a report urging education at an early age and dismissing quarantines as useless as well as cruel. He suggests teaching children about anal intercourse and other homosexual and heterosexual practices so they can "grow up knowing the behavior to avoid to protect themselves."

The science groups' report projects that AIDS cases among heterosexuals will increase by 1991 to about 7,000 from the current 1,100. Pediatric cases from *in utero* infection will increase to more than 3,000.

Its rapid spread makes clear that AIDS can strike any sexually active person, even a monogamous person whose sex partner has had even *one* other, infected partner. Clearly, AIDS has the potential to become a modern-day Black Plague.

The Surgeon General and the nation's most respected biomedical experts properly are seeking a balanced approach to AIDS and its victims, an approach grounded in knowledge, compassion, and realism. They deserve the careful attention of every governmental and private agency that is grappling with the ever-increasing threat.

★ ★ ★

South Florida not only is a focal point of AIDS cases, it's also a leading center of AIDS research. Yet such is the fear of AIDS that those trying to help its victims — and potential victims — find theirs at best a frustrating endeavor.

Consider the American Society of Interior Designers' South Florida chapter. The group has enlisted Diahann Carroll and Peter Allen to appear at a Nov. 16 black-tie dinner capping "A Designers Weekend" Nov. 14-16. Profits, if any, will go to the University of Miami's AIDS Research Fund, the Health Crisis Network, and Center One.

Ticket sales are going slowly, says co-chairman Judi Male. She attributes the poor response to people's reluctance to recognize that AIDS — like heart disease, cancer, or other afflictions — can affect *them* too. The evidence cited above attests to that.

South Floridians who wish to support AIDS research couldn't find a better avenue than "A Designers Weekend." For ticket and other information, please call 576-2739.

The Chattanooga Times
Chattanooga, TN, October 29, 1986

With the number of confirmed cases spiraling upward, the dread disease AIDS, or acquired immune deficiency syndrome, is considered an epidemic in this country; the disease is spreading in other countries as well. That makes Surgeon General C. Everett Koop's report on AIDS last week valuable. At a time when so many treat AIDS as a taboo subject, Dr. Koop has addressed the matter with remarkable candor.

So far as is known, AIDS is inevitably fatal, so the only way to combat it now, Dr. Koop said, is by prevention. Despite some slight hints of a breakthrough, scientists have been unable to come up with a cure or a long-term treatment that arrests the fatal deterioration of the body's immune system.

Although the principal victims of AIDS are homosexuals, the disease is now occurring increasingly among heterosexuals as well. Dr. Koop said the AIDS epidemic had already killed nearly 15,000 Americans and that 12 times that number could die by 1991 unless preventive measures are taken. Simple precautions taken by partners during sexual intercourse would drastically reduce, if not eliminate, the incidence of the disease's transmission from one person to another. Granted, that would help neither the relatively small number of hemophiliacs stricken by AIDS through the transfusions of contaminated blood nor users of illegal drugs who contract the disease with unsterile needles. But the number of AIDS cases would drop dramatically if precautions reduced the sexual transmission of the disease.

Dr. Koop's candid recommendations are a breath of fresh air in the public discussion of this matter. He is putting the health of our people, particularly young men and women, above the fears of those who think that instruction in sexual hygiene will encourage sexual activity. He wrote in his report: "Many people, especially our youth, are not receiving information that is vital to their future health and well-being because of our reticence in dealing with the subjects of sex, sexual practices and homosexuality. We can no longer afford to sidestep frank, open discussions about sexual practices — homosexual and heterosexual. Education about AIDS should start at an early age so that children can grow up knowing the behaviors to avoid to protect themselves from exposure to the AIDS virus." (Dr. Koop's report is available from the U.S. Public Health Service by writing to AIDS, P.O. Box 1452, Washington, D.C. 20044.)

Sexual promiscuity, the hopes of some to the contrary notwithstanding, will not disappear if we simply refuse to provide adequate sex education. And the evidence is clear that AIDS no longer infects only those who some say "deserve" it — the homosexuals. The subject is too important in terms of public health to ignore the dangers. Dr. Koop's report is an outstanding public service. The question now is whether its recommendations will be followed.

The Record

Hackensack, NJ,
October 30, 1986

Surgeon General C. Everett Koop is no advocate of alternative life styles. He once called single parents, childless couples, and homosexuals "anti-family." This makes his recent compassionate and wise remarks about AIDS all the more welcome, and it should make them persuasive to even the most traditional-minded citizens.

It's a relief to hear someone in high government office talk sense about AIDS. Dr. Koop, who built a national reputation as surgeon-in-chief at Philadelphia's Children's Hospital, said last week that there's no need to fear the spread of AIDS through casual social contact, and no reason to react to AIDS victims with anything but caring and sensitivity. Nor is there any need, he said, for mandatory testing, quarantines, or tattooing — some of the misguided notions put forth by frightened Americans as the epidemic has spread. The real danger of AIDS, said Dr. Koop, comes from sexual contact — heterosexual as well as homosexual — and from needle sharing in drug use. This is why schools need sex-education courses even in the early grades, with a special emphasis on AIDS and other sexually transmitted diseases.

Dr. Koop is right on all counts. One of his most important messages is that there is no reason, medical or moral, to try to isolate AIDS victims. "We are fighting a disease, not people," his report says. "Those who are already afflicted are sick people and need our care, as do all sick patients." Shaking hands, eating in restaurants, using public toilets, or swimming in public pools will not spread AIDS. That can't be said often enough in a society where fear has led people to treat even young children with AIDS as untouchables. Ostracizing the victims isn't merely inhumane. It makes the disease harder to track, to treat, and, one day, to cure.

Equally important is Dr. Koop's insistence on education. Americans need to know that casual sexual relations and intravenous drug use can put them at risk of a fatal disease for which there's no known cure. They need to know about such basic precautions as the use of condoms. There's a special need to warn teen-agers, who tend to act as if they were immortal. Dr. Koop's report should encourage school boards, teachers, and parents to overcome any squeamishness about talking sex with youngsters. In 1986, it's a matter of life and death.

ST. LOUIS POST-DISPATCH

St. Louis, MO, October 24, 1986

Surgeon General C. Everett Koop is not a man known for his daring. Yet his report on AIDS, the sexually transmitted immune deficiency disease, is remarkable for its candor and forthrightness in addressing a subject that many hold taboo.

Prevention, the surgeon says, is the best way we know so far to avoid AIDS, or acquired immune deficiency syndrome. Scientists are frustrated in their search for a cure or long-term treatment, but simple precautions taken during sexual intercourse can effectively eliminate the possibility of the disease being transmitted from one sexual partner to another. Though this is no comfort to the small numbers of hemophiliacs who may acquire AIDS through transfusions of contaminated blood or to intravenous users of illicit drugs, who contract AIDS when they use unsterile needles, reducing the sexual transmission of AIDS would result in a drastic decline in the numbers of future victims.

Dr. Koop is to be commended for putting the health of the nation's youth above the concerns of those who fear instruction in sexual hygiene will only encourage sexual experimentation. He wrote: "We can no longer afford to sidestep frank, open discussions about sexual practices. . . . Education about AIDS should start at an early age so that children can grow up knowing the behaviors to avoid to protect themselves from exposure to the AIDS virus."

What a refreshing statement is Dr. Koop's, putting in their place those who would stick their heads in the sand, hoping that sexual promiscuity will vanish in the absence of sex education or that the AIDS virus will infect only the deserving. Those who want to read the surgeon general's full report may request copies from the U.S. Public Health Service by writing AIDS, Box 1452, Washington, D.C. 20044.

The Washington Times

Washington, DC, October 27, 1986

U.S. Surgeon General C. Everett Koop, who got his present job at the urging of pro-life forces in and around the fledgling Reagan administration and who has scarcely been heard from on that issue since, had one doozy of a bomb for his old supporters last week. Taking aim at AIDS, he recommended sex education starting in third grade, with detailed information about homosexuality starting in junior high school. A more complete case of mental takeover by the Washington establishment is probably not on record.

By way of introducing his new study on the subject, Dr. Koop observed that many people, especially young people, "are not receiving information that is vital to their future health and well-being because of our reticence in dealing with the subjects of sex, sexual practices, and homosexuality." Hmm. From what we have heard about what goes on in those sex-ed seminars in the public schools, "reticence" is not exactly the word that first comes to mind.

To be sure, Dr. Koop's course would not be the usual "value-free" how-to. "Couples who engage in freewheeling casual sex these days are playing a dangerous game," he warns. Perhaps he expects parents to rally behind a sex-ed program designed to frighten kids into chastity. If so, he misses the point.

Chastity prevents AIDS — agreed. But fear does not produce chastity. Even as Dr. Koop was speaking, a conference sponsored by the Department of Health and Human Services was taking stock of "what works" in preventing teen-age pregnancy (not the same issue as AIDS, obviously, but relevant). There was general agreement that what works is teaching kids self-esteem and resistance to peer pressure — not merely providing information.

A compelling case can be made, on the other hand, that some children are harmed psychologically when given sexual information at too tender an age. As a result of its transfer of parental roles to institutions — which would be a dubious project even if it attained its advertised objectives — the present generation may be raising its children as emotionally handicapped misfits.

Physician, heal thyself.

THE ATLANTA CONSTITUTION

Atlanta, GA, October 27, 1986

Surgeon General Everett Koop is turning out, at least at moments, to be one of the more pleasant surprises of the Reagan administration. His report on AIDS could turn the nation to a thoughtful and reasoned yet compassionate policy toward the disease and its victims.

Certain to be controversial, the report recommends that sex education aimed at preventing the spread of AIDS start as early as elementary school. The report also specifically condemns some of the extreme recommendations that have been bandied in the anti-AIDS hysteria, and it even turns thumbs down on a recommendation that has been favored by some Reaganites: compulsory AIDS testing. Koop says the procedure could be "unmanageable and cost-prohibitive."

In the early years of his tenure, Koop was known mostly for his adherence to right-wing orthodoxy. Since then, however, he has shown himself capable of letting his insights as a man of medicine override his ideology. He urges the nation to show compassion toward AIDS sufferers. "Those who are already afflicted are sick people and need our care, as do all sick patients."

There is a danger that opponents of real sex education will use Koop's report as an excuse to browbeat teens about early sexual activity rather than to teach them about contraception and "safe sex." (By the way, studies show that sex education does not encourage youth to become sexually active. In fact, students given sex education are more likely to delay their first sexual encounters.)

The general outline of Koop's recommendations, though, seems worthy. And beyond its common sense, the report has an added edge: It represents the conclusions of a conservative who is at home with many of the values espoused by the far right. Koop may be able to make some headway with those who don't yet understand the dangers of our national reluctance to teach our children about sex.

The San Diego Union

San Diego, CA, October 24, 1986

To date, U.S. deaths from Acquired Immune Deficiency Syndrome (AIDS) number nearly 15,000. And that mortality rate is expected to increase 12-fold by 1991 because there is no cure for this killer disease. Given these grim statistics, the American people would do well to heed the U.S. Surgeon General's report on AIDS that was released last Wednesday.

Dr. C. Everett Koop's comprehensive report, which was nine months in preparation, is commendable for its unusual candor. It correctly emphasizes the need for education so that individuals are better able to protect themselves against AIDS. Although Dr. Koop concedes that parents are primarily responsible for informing their children about such matters, he urges schools to fill in the blank spaces.

Specifically, he calls for a program in the elementary grades that stresses the prevention of AIDS and other sexually transmitted diseases. Such a program, which could begin as early as the third grade, would certainly be controversial. But the surgeon general's case is especially compelling, considering the estimated 12,000 to 14,000 lives that could be saved during the next five years if everyone at risk from exposure to the AIDS virus took precautions.

Dr. Koop is on target when he warns that this society's free-wheeling attitude toward casual sex has placed the entire nation at risk. Thus youngsters ought to be told the plain truth about the dangers of promiscuity, particularly among homosexual and bisexual men. Students should also be warned that intravenous drug users are another high-risk group for AIDS. Such straight talk beginning in the early grades might dissuade many youngsters from literally jeopardizing their lives by fooling around with sex and drugs.

The surgeon general's report also clears the air by underscoring that casual social contact between children and persons afflicted with the AIDS virus is not dangerous. "We are fighting a disease, not people," Dr. Koop concludes. Consequently, neither quarantine nor mandatory testing for the AIDS virus is called for. To the contrary, such discrimination would only drive the very persons who need help into the shadows.

According to the federal Centers for Disease Control in Atlanta, 26,566 cases of AIDS have been reported in the United States since 1981. Until a vaccine is discovered for this deadly disease, Americans must take every reasonable precaution to protect themselves against being infected. The surgeon general's report spells out some of those precautions that will be ignored at America's peril.

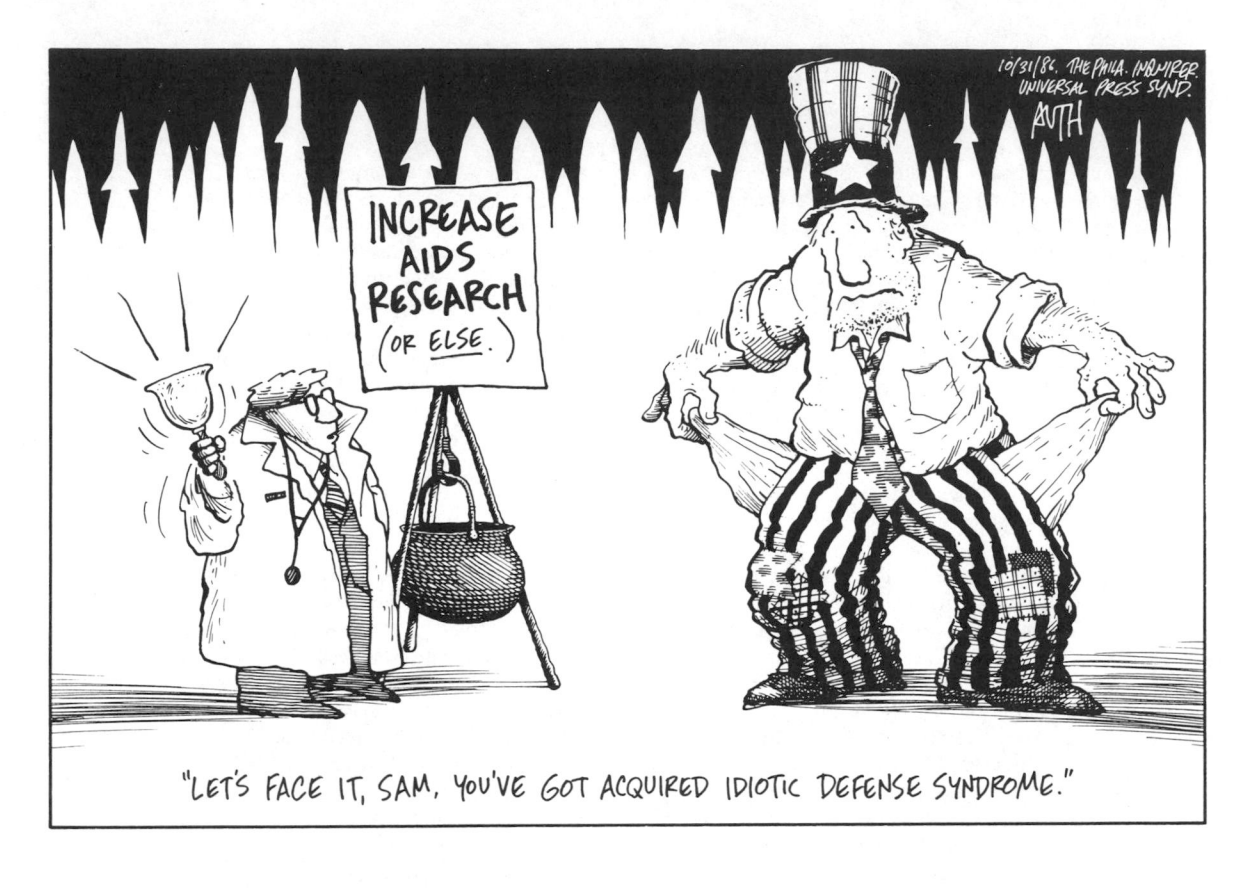

10/31/86. THE PHILA. INQUIRER
UNIVERSAL PRESS SYND.
AUTH

INCREASE AIDS RESEARCH (OR ELSE.)

"LET'S FACE IT, SAM, YOU'VE GOT ACQUIRED IDIOTIC DEFENSE SYNDROME."

The Seattle Times

Seattle, WA, October 24, 1986

IN THE government's first official major policy statement on what Americans can do to curb the spread of AIDS, Surgeon General C. Everett Koop has struck exactly the right tone.

"We are fighting," Koop declared, "a disease — not people. Those who are already afflicted are sick people and need our care, as do all sick patients."

As to preventive measures against the deadly disease, Koop placed top priority on AIDS sex education both at home and in schools "at the lowest grade possible . . . on both heterosexual and homosexual relationships."

Koop's admonition that "we can no longer afford to sidestep open, frank discussion about sexual practices" calls to mind the ill-considered refusal by some Puget Sound-region TV stations to air a Northwest Aids Foundation public-service message designed to discourage sexual behavior that transmits AIDS.

Dr. C. Everett Koop

Coming from a Reagan-administration official long identified with right-wing views (against legal abortions, for example, and the gay-rights movement), Koop's report occasioned surprise — even anger — in conservative circles. The surgeon general also spoke out against such extreme measures as quarantining or tattooing AIDS patients, and stressed that the often fatal virus is not transmitted through casual, nonsexual social contact.

"At the beginning of the AIDS epidemic," Koop says, "many Americans had little sympathy for people with AIDS. The feeling was that somehow people from certain groups (homosexual and bisexual men and intravenous drug users) 'deserved' their illness. Let us put those feelings behind us."

A White House statement said it's hoped the surgeon general's report will inspire more enlightened public thinking about AIDS, just as Koop's statements on the dangers of tobacco have defined the smoking issue. It's an objective well worth seeking.

THE INDIANAPOLIS STAR

Indianapolis, IN, October 25, 1986

The handwriting was on the wall, but the surgeon general has made it official.

Because of the AIDS epidemic, Surgeon General C. Everett Koop said, "Couples who engage in free-wheeling casual sex these days are playing a dangerous game."

Koop said his office is taking the initiative to assure that America's teen-agers get enough information to stay out of harm's way.

At the same time, the Indiana University School of Medicine and the Indiana State Board of Health are undertaking a joint effort to analyze data and coordinate AIDS-prevention programs throughout the state.

These efforts are significant.

Much government response to AIDS has been influenced by groups which downplay the role of promiscuity in spreading the disease. The plain truth, as voiced by one New York public health expert, is: "There is no 'safe sex' with a person who has AIDS."

Heterosexuals are increasingly at risk and the risk escalates with the number of different sex partners.

Koop said education emphasizing sexually transmitted diseases should take place in schools and homes. He has prepared a booklet about AIDS that can be obtained by writing to AIDS, Box 14252, Washington, D.C., 20044.

Reticence and silence must end, Koop declared. "Education about AIDS should start at an early age so that children can grow up knowing the behaviors to avoid to protect themselves from exposure to the AIDS virus."

Because teen-agers tend to act as if they were immortal, young people can put themselves at great risk as they begin to explore their sexuality and perhaps experiment with drugs, he added.

Realizing those same pitfalls, parents should find Koop's booklet both informative and helpful.

Minneapolis Star and Tribune

Minneapolis, MN, November 5, 1986

With a 100 percent fatality rate, acquired immune deficiency syndrome is among the most virulent diseases in medical history. Americans can no longer afford to view AIDS as a disease that afflicts a few unlucky strangers. A new report by scientists from the National Academy of Sciences and the Institute of Medicine warns that the disease now poses some threat to anyone who engages in the activity known to spread it. Echoing the recent plea of Surgeon General C. Everett Koop, the panel's report wisely urges a concerted federal effort to slow its spread and find a cure.

In the five years since the disease was first recognized, AIDS has claimed more than 26,000 victims — more than half of whom have already died. Another 1.5 million people are infected with the virus that causes the illness. Any one of those carriers may transmit the virus through sexual contact or needle-sharing; a third or more of them may eventually fall prey to it. According to estimates from the Centers for Disease Control, the number of AIDS cases may top 270,000 by 1991. In that year alone, caring for AIDS victims could cost up to $16 billion.

Gay men, hemophiliacs and drug abusers will be hardest hit. But sexually active heterosexuals are vulnerable to AIDS as well. Bisexual men and heterosexual drug-abusers who unknowingly carry the virus have introduced it into the general heterosexual population, where it now may spread like other sexually transmitted diseases.

The panel recommends an increase in federal spending on AIDS research and prevention to $2 billion a year — five times the 1986 amount — by the end of the decade. It favors establishment of a national commission to direct the fight against AIDS, as well as a program to train health-care workers to handle AIDS victims.

And the scientists propose several extraordinary tactics to stop the further spread of AIDS. Their report backs Koop's call for a full-fledged sex-education program beginning in the elementary grades. It calls for an explicit, public, poster-and-pamphlet campaign urging people to use condoms to guard against sexual transmission of the virus. And it recommends widespread distribution of sterile needles to drug addicts in an effort to stem the spread of the virus from shared syringes.

Those frank suggestions, along with the recommendations for dramatic spending increases, are bound to raise eyebrows in Washington and elsewhere. But the price of neglecting the proposals is more astonishing still. The country must now prepare for a long war against AIDS. While the disease rages, greatly expanded research and education are the best weapons immediately at hand. Congress and the president should seize them.

St. Petersburg Times

St. Petersburg, FL, November 3, 1986

The nation's most prestigious scientists are alarmed and frightened by the increasing spread of the AIDS epidemic and the federal government's feeble efforts to curb it.

Last week, the National Academy of Sciences criticized the government's dangerously inadequate response to the epidemic and called for a $2-billion-a-year emergency program to educate the public about how to avoid the deadly virus and for intensified research to avert a national catastrophe.

The AIDS threat is so urgent, said the academy's report, that it requires "perhaps the most wide-ranging and intensive efforts ever made

AIDS' terrifying potential and the warnings by the nation's top scientists ought to prompt the federal government's commitment to intensify research to stop this plague.

against an infectious disease."

"This is a national health crisis," said Nobel laureate Dr. David Baltimore of the Massachusetts Institute of Technology. Its magnitude, he said, "requires presidential leadership to bring together all elements of society to deal with the problem."

In only five years, AIDS has gone from an unknown disease to an epidemic. Although it was first discovered among homosexuals and intravenous drug users, the deadly virus that cripples the body's immune system and leaves victims unable to fight infections and cancers is now found in heterosexuals and people who do not use drugs. It is found in women and children. It has become everybody's problem.

As of September, AIDS had been diagnosed in more than 24,500 Americans, 15,000 of whom have died. The U.S. Public Health Service estimates that more than 1-million people are infected with the AIDS virus and projects that by 1991 AIDS will have killed more than 179,000. Other experts predict that, beginning in 1990, more than 58,000 Americans will be killed each year by AIDS. That exceeds the American death toll in the entire Vietnam War.

With no cure or vaccine in sight, scientists say the best hope of controlling the epidemic is a massive, continuing campaign to increase awareness of how persons can protect themselves against infection and intensified research to develop a vaccine and therapeutic drugs.

AIDS is not spread by social contact — such as shaking hands, hugging, social kissing, crying, coughing, sneezing, using swimming pools or hot tubs or eating in restaurants. The AIDs virus is transmitted during sexual contact with an infected person or by sharing drug equipment.

Clear, frank sex education in the schools ought to begin now. "To be effective, educators must use whatever language is required," said the academy report. "We cannot let people die because society finds some words embarrassing."

U.S. Surgeon General C. Everett Koop's recent report to the nation offered similar advice — including frank sex education in the schools, starting as early as the third grade, the use of condoms, avoidance of "freewheeling casual sex," avoiding and certainly not sharing drug injection equipment.

AIDS' terrifying potential and the warnings by the nation's top scientists ought to prompt the federal government's commitment to intensify research to stop this plague.

THE LOUISVILLE TIMES

Louisville, KY
November 3, 1986

FOR most Americans, the terrible disease known as AIDS seems a shadowy and distant threat. The prevailing assumption has been that homosexuals and intravenous drug users are at risk while others, if not totally safe, are unlikely to become infected by the mysterious virus that destroys the body's ability to resist illness.

Such notions should be rapidly dispelled by the growing body of knowledge about AIDS and especially by the findings of a committee that studied the disease and its impact under the auspices of the National Academy of Sciences.

The researchers confirmed that we are indeed dealing with a dangerous epidemic that will claim thousands of lives unless individuals and government agencies begin doing what is necessary to control its spread. About 25,000 Americans are known to be victims. This number could explode to 270,000 cases and 179,000 deaths by 1991.

Heterosexuality is no refuge. Cases among heterosexuals are rare in the United States, but common in Haiti and Africa and expected to increase dramatically here. The disease is also expected to spread geographically. The 60 per cent of cases outside New York and San Francisco is likely to rise to 80 per cent by 1990.

While arguing something must be done, and soon, the scientists properly reject mandatory blood tests, quarantines and other oppressive measures that California voters will consider tomorrow.

But with effective vaccines still years away, the committee called for spending $2 billion annually on AIDS research and the creation of national commission to monitor efforts to combat the diseases.

What's equally important, the report echoed Surgeon Gen. C. Everett Koop's recommendation for a public health education program. Dr. Koop urged that children be educated from an early age about the transmission of AIDS and ways they can avoid it. An effective effort would not only safeguard the health of many people, but also check the immense cost of caring for AIDS victims.

Such ideas do not sit well with Americans who think government has no role in sex education and who blanch at the explicit language experts say must be used to convey a vital message. But preparing young citizens to make wise decisions for themselves and others is far preferable to the alternatives, which are made painfully clear in the academy's report and the California referendum.

San Francisco Chronicle

San Francisco, CA, October 24, 1986

THE SURGEON GENERAL'S report on AIDS is a necessary and welcome contribution to public discussion of the disease which has already killed more than 15,000 Americans.

In his long-awaited report, Dr. C. Everett Koop showed frankness, compassion and a proper perspective of the dread disease. Americans, he said, must set aside any prejudices when dealing with the disease that has hit hardest so far among homosexual and bisexual men and intravenous drug users.

"We are fighting a disease, not people," he said. "Those who are already afflicted are sick people and need our care, as do all sick patients."

DR. KOOP CALLED for sex education as early as elementary school, so that children grow up knowing how to protect themselves from the sexually-transmitted disease. As the first federal health official to recommend AIDS-oriented sex education in the schools, he conceded that the idea is likely to draw opposition. But he said, quite correctly, that the danger is so great that such a program is a public health necessity.

The surgeon general also set the record straight on several issues raised by Proposition 64, the California ballot measure sponsored by followers of political cultist Lyndon LaRouche.

Dr. Koop said programs to quarantine anyone carrying the AIDS virus would be useless "because AIDS is not spread by casual contact" and that requiring blood tests of all gays is "unnecessary, unfeasible and cost prohibitive." He urged defeat of Proposition 64, as we have recommended.

HIS REPORT, along with a new military training film that deals with AIDS in a straightforward, non-political way, are important in the fight against a disease whose death toll may reach 180,000 by 1991.

The Des Moines Register

Des Moines, IA, November 7, 1986

The surgeon general's report on AIDS — acquired immune deficiency syndrome — is one of the most reasoned and compassionate statements to emerge amid a growing hysteria. Coming from the Reagan administration's chief health officer, it might have as much impact as an earlier surgeon general's report on smoking.

It should. Surgeon General C. Everett Koop took a decidedly humanitarian approach in recommending a national policy on AIDS. The report says the nation should begin to treat AIDS victims as people who need help and compassion rather than label them "diseased" and segregate them as modern-day lepers.

It is a refreshing approach toward a disease that has the potential for resurrecting medieval attitudes toward its victims.

Koop wrote: "At the beginning of the AIDS epidemic, many Americans had little sympathy for people with AIDS. The feeling was that somehow people from certain groups 'deserved' their illness. Let us put those feelings behind us. We are fighting a disease, not people. Those who are already afflicted are sick people and need our care, as do all sick patients."

Koop counsels against compulsory testing for exposure to the AIDS virus because of the fear and discrimination that would engender. He instead recommends that AIDS be attacked with education, beginning in the elementary schools so that "children can grow up knowing the behavior to avoid to protect themselves."

Starting AIDS education at the elementary level has sparked predictable controversy. There is some question of how to present facts about sex and homosexuality to such young children. But efforts must be directed at cooling the hysteria about children with AIDS spreading the disease through casual contact.

Despite efforts of some parents who would ban AIDS sufferers from attending school, the surgeon general's report stresses that casual contact with persons infected with the virus poses no danger.

Koop criticized a proposed California law — soundly beaten at the polls Nov. 4 — that would have labeled AIDS victims as suffering from a "communicable disease" and barred them from schools and certain jobs.

The AIDS epidemic is a tragic problem for its thousands of victims. The surgeon general's report should go a long way toward easing their misery by discouraging hysterical efforts to treat them as untouchables.

LEXINGTON HERALD-LEADER

Lexington, KY, November 5, 1986

Expected to kill more than 50,000 Americans a year by 1991, AIDS is as savage and persistent a killer as there is. No cure exists. Without a massive injection of federal aid — at least the $2 billion education and research package now being proposed by the National Academy of Sciences — there is also little hope of finding a cure in the immediate future.

So spending $1 billion on establishing a public awareness of and caution about the AIDS infection is perfectly justified. So is the suggested $1 billion on research. Should the AIDS prevention education begin with 8-year-olds, as U.S. Surgeon General Everett Koop has suggested? Probably not. But it should begin at the onset of puberty.

And it should not be schoolchildren alone who are subjected to a barrage of cautionary tales about AIDS.

All adults should be made aware of how to avoid the AIDS virus: limiting sexual contact, using condoms and avoiding the transfer of body fluids. This is not simply advice that applies to the high-risk groups for AIDS, such as homosexuals and intravenous drug users. It applies to almost all Americans who are sexually active.

For many of them, just saying "no" is not a realistic option. But being careful is.

Warning about AIDS, the plague of the 80s, is not pleasant. Having a government agency dispensing explicit information about tidying up bedroom activities is a proposition not for the faint of heart. And many people will be alarmed unnecessarily, reading every ache for signs that it's more than the flu.

But AIDS is not like a venereal disease, and fighting it calls for more dramatic weapons. There's no need for hysteria, but there is every need for caution.

The $2 billion in research and education suggested by the sciences academy is not overblown. Nor is the $1 billion included for public education simply a trumped-up excuse for a glossy media blitz. AIDS is a problem that shows no signs of disappearing on its own. Fighting such a persistent killer is deserving of all the money that the United States can muster for such an effort.

For the American public, contributing to AIDS research and prevention is self-defense. When the number of AIDS deaths in the United States reaches 50,000 a year, there will be few who will be so isolated as not to feel the impact of the killer virus. That's why the NAS request is more than just reasonable. It's downright modest.

The Honolulu Advertiser
Honolulu, HI, November 2, 1986

U.S. Surgeon General C. Everett Koop has done the nation a real service in issuing a forthright and compassionate report on AIDS, acquired immune deficiency syndrome.

As the disease begins to spread through sexual contact from its original victims — chiefly male homosexuals and intravenous drug users — to the general community, including women and children, the need for blunt but humane talk could not be greater.

AND COMING from the conservative Koop, the non-judgmental, non-condemning attitude is welcome, setting a tone all should emulate. "We are fighting a disease, not people," says Koop. "Those who are already afflicted are sick people and need our care."

Koop's urgent advice is for sex education in schools from the earliest possible grade to alert youngsters to the dangers of AIDS and the means of avoiding it.

He clearly instructs those in highest risk how to protect themselves — including instructions for those who will not abstain from homosexual activity and intravenous drug abuse. And he lays firmly to rest some of the greater panics and wilder responses that have developed around AIDS.

Among the causes for unfounded panic have been rumors that AIDS can be transmitted: by donating blood (it cannot); through casual, non-sexual contact (not even coughing or sneezing will do it); or from one child to another in school or day-care (not a single such case has been identified).

Among the wilder suggested responses for which there are no grounds whatsoever are compulsory AIDS blood testing and quarantining or tattooing those tested positive for the AIDS virus.

SO FAR 26,500 people in this country have been diagnosed with AIDS, and the epidemic is growing by geometric proportions. The present death toll of 15,000 could reach 180,000 in five years unless dramatic steps are taken — and that means a lot of money is spent — to educate the public and research an effective treatment and vaccine, something most everyone agrees is a long way off.

A group of scientists under the auspices of the National Academy of Sciences and Institute of Medicine has called for spending $1 billion each for education and research in the next few years. An effort of that scope appears to be what it will take.

DESERET NEWS
Salt Lake City, MO, October 24, 1986

So far, at least 26,500 Americans are known to have contracted AIDS, and 15,000 of them have died from it. The others will die, too. If present trends continue, the number of Americans killed by AIDS can be expected to amount to a cumulative total of 179,000 by the end of 1991.

So U.S. Surgeon General C. Everett Koop did the responsible thing this week in calling for a massive public information campaign against AIDS. Indeed, at this point, there's not much else that can be done about AIDS. Currently, there is no known cure for the disease. The only treatment developed so far merely delays the ravages of the illness but doesn't conquer the AIDS virus. Researchers don't expect to be able to find an AIDS vaccine until the turn of the century, if then. That leaves knowledge and prevention as the only remedies.

In essence, here's what is known about AIDS: Though it is most prevalent among homosexuals and drug users, AIDS isn't confined to those groups. Heterosexuals can get it, too. For instance, Dr. Koop reports, someone having sex with a drug user is at "signifi-cant risk." The immune-crippling disease is transmitted only by intimate sexual contact and the sharing of contaminated hypodermic needles. But there's a danger the virus could spread widely among the general population.

The new report from Koop also contains this vital piece of information: The risk of infection increases as the number of sexual partners — man or woman — increases. As the surgeon general put it, "Couples who engage in free-wheeling casual sex these days are playing a dangerous game."

The message should be unmistakably clear: There's still no substitute for traditional morality. It's a message, however, that should be accompanied by a large measure of compassion for the victims of AIDS.

Meanwhile, until the U.S. can get underway with the information program being urged by Dr. Koop, Americans wanting to know more about AIDS and how to deal with it can find out from the new report he issued this week. It can be obtained from the U.S. Public Health Service by writing to: AIDS, Box 14252, Washington, D.C. 20044.

The Kansas City Times
Kansas City, MO, October 25, 1986

Acquired Immunodeficiency Syndrome is long past the stage where anyone looks at it lightly. Now Surgeon General C. Everett Koop has outlined recommended attitudes toward AIDS. He urges compassion for victims, restraint from a rush to compulsory testing and public school education.

The first two are honorable. The latter sounds better than it is.

In the first place, far too much of a load with every social, personal and moral problem human beings must deal with already has been dumped in teachers' laps. Resources are stretched too thin to cover any of them. It's little wonder such basics as reading and writing also get squeezed. Responsibility for AIDS is one more job the schools don't need.

This is augmented by what's happened to sex education courses. Watered down and targets of animosity, classes have had larger ambitions than most have accomplished. Funding for added programs, including new classwork, usually is not forthcoming from those who demand them. There's little likelihood AIDS education, by the time all the layers of review, criticism and sanitizing were finished, would be very effective.

Good arguments exist for integrating sex information and lessons on AIDS and other venereal diseases in health courses, biology and other appropriate disciplines. A new project with great expectations is another matter.

Moreover, to focus on educating youth, particularly children in elementary grades, as an effective answer to the problem is misguided. To date, the government has not been an outstanding leader in adult education about AIDS.

A recent edition of *The Journal of the American Medical Association,* has a long discussion of ways to avoid infection or reduce its likelihood. It contains the kind of frank information people need to know and believe such as the fact that gay men with AIDS and heterosexual victims reported larger numbers of sexual partners than control groups. Hence, the more sexual contacts, the higher the risk.

And there are ways to prevent transmission. Avoid sexual intercourse. Or use condoms.

If you think it's too frank for a family newspaper, would you promote it in grade school? Yet less than that is of little value to anyone.

DAYTON DAILY NEWS

Dayton, OH, April 17, 1987

When Dr. C. Everett Koop was appointed surgeon general of the United States, the main public fact about him was that he was an active opponent of abortion. This caused some to wonder whether his office might be used for the furtherance of some political or ideological agenda, which would have been a shame. The position must be a non-partisan, non-ideological one if the public is to have any confidence in its pronouncements. And making authoritative pronouncements is perhaps the main thing the surgeon general does.

Dr. Koop's performance has put those concerns to rest. He has gone wherever the medical evidence — not political ideology — has taken him. He has been more actively and staunchly anti-smoking than a member of a conservative administration would normally be expected to be. He has not simply gone through the motions of saying smoking is bad for you, and kids shouldn't do it. He has pushed the anti-smoking cause farther than it has ever gone before, making clear that smoking is a threat to the health not only of smokers, but of people near them. He cannot be one of North Carolina Senator Jesse Helms' favorite Reagan administration people.

More importantly, Dr. Koop has handled the extraordinarily sensitive AIDS (acquired immune deficiency syndrome) problem in a thoroughly professional and responsible manner, keeping in mind always that he is the nation's public health officer, not its moral leader. He has emphasized the need for education about AIDS and sex generally and the need for the use of protective measures in sexual activity. Some members of the Reagan administration — including Secretary of Education William Bennett — would like to see Dr. Koop taking a more moralistic, less pragmatic approach to the problem, but Dr. Koop has remained focused on the goal of saving lives, his job.

Dr. Koop has pushed for the availability of tests for AIDS that could be accomplished not only with confidentiality for the patient, but with anonymity. His idea is that some people have viewed the taking of an AIDS test as an admission of certain kinds of sexual behavior. If an anonymous test proves negative, he points out, then nobody has to know a person was even tested. Of course, as time passes it becomes clear that an AIDS test is a good idea for an enormous number of people, not just homosexuals and the very active sexually. Nevertheless, if anonymity encourages more people to be tested, then it should be used widely.

Dr. Koop has performed his job correctly. He is the kind of person the next presidential administration should consider keeping on, whatever its party.

The Washington Post

Washington, DC, May 20, 1987

WE AMERICANS have a lot to give thanks for. Among the many things are an abundance of moral guidance and the steadfastness of our politicians. Consider, for example, the testimonial dinner scheduled to be held last night by the National Alliance of Senior Citizens for Surgeon General C. Everett Koop.

Dr. Koop has been much in the news of late on the subject of AIDS. Last October he wrote a frank report on that dread and controversial disease not from the perspective of a moralist, but from that of the nation's chief public health officer. He was careful to say that the best defense against AIDS is abstinence, the second best a "mutually faithful monogamous" relationship. But mere admonition was not his goal; he called as well for sex education "at the lowest grade possible" and said "the best protection against infection right now—barring abstinence—is use of a condom." He later urged that condoms be advertised on TV.

The doctor has taken a fair amount of heat for the report from those, including some in the administration, who feel it was not reproving enough, that in advocating sex education and the use of condoms it acquiesced in behavior that the government should only condemn. There is now a further dispute on whether testing for AIDS should be mandatory at certain points—application for a marriage license, for example—or remain voluntary, as Dr. Koop believes, and whether results should be disclosed.

The testimonial was organized by friends as a show of support in this difficult moment, not for the doctor's views on AIDS but for the doctor himself. There were 57 cosponsors, a pretty fair who's-who of conservatives. That's when the moral guidance began. Two well-known figures from the political right, Paul Weyrich and Phyllis Schlafly, sent a letter to the cosponsors, asking them to withdraw because "This dinner will clearly play right into the hands of those promoting the gay rights agenda, which is to teach children to use condoms for premarital promiscuity with either sex while opposing the measures that are desperately needed to protect the uninfected from the infected."

Then came the steadfastness. Eleven of the sponsors withdrew. Among them were presidential candidates Jack Kemp—aides say he withdrew before he received the letter—and Bob Dole. Others stood their ground—Sen. Orrin Hatch, for example. Secretary of Health and Human Services Otis Bowen has also spoken out for Dr. Koop, and a good thing too. AIDS is epidemic enough, without demagoguery as a side effect.

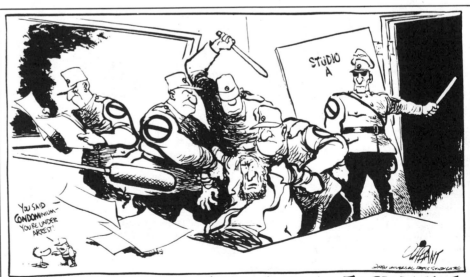

FCC RADIO POLICE TODAY ARRESTED SURGEON-GENERAL KOOP FOR BROADCASTING AIDS WARNINGS WHICH CONTAINED SEXUAL INNUENDO.

THE DAILY OKLAHOMAN
Oklahoma City, OK, May 25, 1987

ADVISERS to the state education department obviously have a tough assignment developing an AIDS instructional program that will satisfy all sides of this highly emotional issue.

In walking a narrow line, the council has properly chosen to stress the practice of abstinence — avoidance of sexual intercourse — as the most effective way not to contract or spread the acquired immune deficiency syndrome virus. That may be all right as far as it goes, but it still falls short, in the view of many, of the message that should be presented to schoolchildren.

Work on the new curriculum results from a legislative mandate that information about the threat to public health posed by AIDS be made available this fall to Oklahoma students between grades five and 12.

Judging by a rough draft of the curriculum, the instructors, while emphasizing to the pupils that they should "learn to say 'No,' " will still avoid any attempt at moral teaching. Presumably, the curriculum planners fear, as do public schoolteachers generally, that any moral content in their instruction will leave them open to charges of violating the Constitution by bringing religion into the classroom.

This reflects the controversy raging at the national level. Dr. C. Everett Koop, U.S. surgeon general, has been in the eye of the dispute because of his insistence on treating AIDS as a public health rather than a moral problem. His fellow conservatives accuse him of playing into the hands of those promoting "homosexual rights" by stressing the use of condoms.

Oddly, Koop in a recent speech spoke approvingly of guidelines laid down by Dr. Otis R. Bowen, secretary of health and human services: Any federally developed health information to be used for education should encourage responsible sexual behavior - based on fidelity, commitment and maturity and placing sexuality within the context of marriage.

Yet Koop's own standard doesn't go quite that far. He believes children should be taught to be abstinent until they grow up, assume the role of a responsible adult and find a "mutually monogamous relationship." That may mean marriage but it could apply to other arrangements.

Some say Koop speaks as a doctor concerned about a public health problem and that morality has no part to play in this context. But what is bad about teaching moral values in school? Even those who may rationalize their own unorthodox lifestyle cannot argue that it is morally wrong to confine sex to marriage.

The Orlando Sentinel
Orlando, FL, May 26, 1987

Five chickens flew the Koop in Washington, D.C., last week.

The Koop was U.S. Surgeon General Everett Koop, whose courageous candor about the AIDS menace has alienated some right-wingers. The chickens were the five presidential candidates who lent their names to a Tuesday night dinner honoring Dr. Koop, then pulled out to avoid the wrath of Koop-bashers.

It was quite a spectacle by five Republicans: Rep. Jack Kemp, Sen. Bob Dole, ex-Sen. Paul Laxalt, ex-Gov. Pete du Pont and the Rev. Pat Robertson. A quintet of people supposedly ready to stand up to Mikhail Gorbachev, who wouldn't face down right-wing rabble-rouser Phyllis Schlafly. Pitiful.

What the episode says about these gentlemen is bad enough. What it says about the AIDS issue is equally odious: The way Washington is responding to this crisis is being shaped as much by politicos as by health professionals.

As surgeon general, Dr. Koop is the government's No. 1 doctor. Yet his crusade to give the public sound medical facts about AIDS has run afoul of simplistic moralizing by such non-experts in the administration as Education Secretary William Bennett, whose doctorate is in philosophy, and White House policy adviser Gary Bauer, a doctor of laws.

Some conservative activists really have hit the low road. Dr. Koop has insisted that schools must teach about the deadly risk of AIDS, which can be spread through sexual contact. Dr. Koop wants young people to know that condoms can reduce the risk. In response to that levelheadedness, critics recklessly have slandered him as a Pied Piper of Prophylactics for third-graders.

Dr. Koop has been turned into too hot a political commodity for respectable GOP candidates to be associated with. Or at least that was the collective wisdom of the Fearsome Fivesome. Considering that such stalwart conservatives as Sen. Orrin Hatch not only lent their names to the dinner but showed up as well, the five's skittishness looked ridiculous.

If Dr. Koop runs into any of these egg-layers again, he might examine them for a missing part. Sure, it's clear they have wings, but what about a backbone?

The Wichita Eagle-Beacon
Wichita, KS, April 13, 1987

THE epidemic spread of AIDS and the policies needed to combat the lethal disease have forced themselves into the arena of public debate. The man entrusted with the collective health of 280 million Americans, Surgeon General C. Everett Koop, has taken strong criticism from many conservatives who once praised him. Dr. Koop suggests that the same conservatives who now oppose him are being intellectually dishonest.

He's right.

Phyllis Schlafly and William F. Buckley, among others, have criticized Dr. Koop for his advocacy of sex education as a realistic method of curbing the AIDS epidemic, and for his recognition that abortion is one way that AIDS-infected mothers may decide to handle pregnancy. Although both are controversial positions, both are in the best interest of public health.

Dr. Koop's sex education plan calls for frank discussion about anatomy, sexual relationships (including homosexuality) and the transmission of sexual diseases, and his plan outlines what schoolchildren should learn at what ages. While agreeing that parents must be involved in teaching children about AIDS and sexuality, the surgeon general suggests that conservatives who advocate limiting the teaching of sex education to the home often fail to follow through with their own plan.

The lack of a cure for AIDS puts infected mothers in a terrible situation. A pregnant woman who tests positive for the disease has a one-in-three chance of transmitting the disease to her child, and about half of these women opt for abortion. Not an advocate of abortion under most circumstances, Dr. Koop believes that women in this situation should be able to terminate their pregnancy.

Dr. Koop came into office with strong backing from right-to-life and other social conservative groups. He may have ruffled the feathers of the political right-wing, but he's taking responsible positions in fighting the AIDS epidemic. His honesty and pragmatism have forced the Reagan administration to confront, rather than to avoid, the problems surrounding this dread disease.

The News and Observer
Raleigh, NC,
September 16, 1987

U.S. Surgeon General C. Everett Koop has displayed repeated courage in speaking out about the deadly AIDS virus. Koop publicly has opposed some Reagan administration testing proposals, and has advocated more education instead. He has visited an AIDS hospice. Now he has taken on another issue guaranteed to win him no friends among his professional colleagues.

During a meeting with the president's commission on AIDS, Koop blasted doctors and others health care professionals who have refused to treat AIDS victims. He reported hearing about increasing instances of care denied, though such incidents are not believed to be widespread. Koop rightly believes that if more doctors and nurses were to follow that pattern, it "threatens the very fabric of health care in this country."

With AIDS already causing widespread fear and even hysteria — much of it based on a lack of knowledge about the disease — the last thing the country needs is for professionals who are supposed to be well-informed to fall victim to unwarranted prejudice. That will only compound the problem of misinformation and lend a misplaced credibility to the hysteria.

Doctors who would turn away AIDS patients don't just hinder the battle against prejudice. They walk all over their Hippocratic oath. Certainly no one expects them to risk their lives. But as Koop noted, precautions have been well-established — the use of gloves, for example — and following those precautions minimizes risk.

A responsible doctor would not walk away from a heart attack victim. Nor would informed physicians or nurses shun AIDS sufferers — victims of a disease that needs all the enlightenment the medical community can provide.

The Seattle Times
Seattle, WA, June 25, 1987

THOSE "newsletters" that most senators and congressmen send home to their constituents — for which taxpayers foot the mailing cost — are often self-serving pieces of political puffery.

Because it's so different from that custom, the latest mailing by Rep. Mike Lowry, D-Seattle, deserves note. It's a worthwhile newsletter filled with valuable information about AIDS.

Sample sentence: "Couples who maintain mutually faithful monogamous relationships (only one continuing sexual partner) are protected from AIDS through sexual transmission . . ."

That and an array of other facts in the Lowry newsletter were extracted from the report of U.S. Surgeon General C. Everett Koop on the Acquired Immune Deficiency Syndrome. In a preface to residents of the 7th District, Lowry notes that "Dr. Koop's report is the most credible and comprehensive information on AIDS the federal government has produced."

Not enough copies of the Koop report were printed to send to everyone, says Lowry, so he used his newsletter to relay the highlights. Medical authorities agree that the best weapon available to fight the spread of the disease is education. Yet the federal education effort has been weak and controversial.

If every member of Congress followed the Lowry lead, information about AIDS would reach every postal patron in the nation. *That* would be a true education campaign.

The Hartford Courant
Hartford, CT, September 16, 1987

Superior Court Judge John P. Maloney only served to intensify the fear generated by AIDS when he ruled last week in Hartford that evidence stained with the blood of a victim of the disease could not be handled by the jury in a sexual assault case.

The evidence — a gun, handcuffs and some clothing — was stained with dried blood more than a year old and it would have been encased in plastic — a safeguard that would bring the risk to the jury "as close to zero as possible," Dr. Edward L. Pesanti, a specialist in infectious diseases, told the court.

Even so, Judge Maloney, noting a "high degree of fear of infection" among the public, ruled that worry about the disease might distract jurors from "coolly and rationally" coming to a decision in the case. He ordered that the jurors be shown photographs of the evidence instead.

Judge Maloney's banning of the blood-tainted evidence points up one of the greatest dangers posed by the AIDS epidemic: giving a greater value to fear than other factors in making important decisions, rather than basing the decisions on the best available information. Fear does exist, and it can't be ignored, but it shouldn't be the dominant factor in making policy.

Dr. Pesanti, who treats AIDS patients every day and claims he safely uses plastic bags to dispose of possibly infected material, says he can't figure out why the year-old dried blood, sealed in plastic, "is such a big deal." There is "rather extensive, well-written source material" on AIDS available to inform the judge, he said. Hartford State's Attorney John M. Bailey said, "If this decision by Judge Maloney is based on fear, I'm worried."

The state Judicial Department is developing a policy on AIDS. We hope that those who formulate the policy take into account the best scientific knowledge about the transmission of the AIDS virus and write guidelines that won't needlessly cater to the fears of jurors, witnesses and court employees.

Decisions like the one made by Judge Maloney are being made every day in courts, schools, government agencies, hospitals and businesses throughout the country. More of them will have to be faced as the number of AIDS cases grows. It will be difficult for people to react rationally to victims of the disease and to those infected with the virus if those who should be the best-informed and most judicious are calculating their decisions on a scale of fear.

U.S. Surgeon General C. Everett Koop tells parents who worry about children attending school with youngsters infected with the AIDS virus that he would hold a child with a full-blown case of AIDS on his lap. He has said that he would feel confident being treated by a physician who had AIDS. Dr. Koop has tried to allay public fears about the disease, but he meets resistance.

Last week, he brought up the issue of the "fearful and irrational minority" of doctors who refuse to treat AIDS patients, calling their conduct "extremely serious" because it "threatens the very fabric of health care in this country."

"In some ways," Dr. Koop said, "the purely scientific issues [of AIDS] pale in comparison to the highly sensitive issues of law, ethics, economics, morality and social cohesion that are beginning to surface."

In seeking guidance on AIDS issues, the public should look to professionals like Dr. Koop, who give caution its proper weight but also base their advice and decisions on science, reason and compassion.

THE KANSAS CITY STAR

Kansas City, MO, September 11, 1987

It's not so much what people don't know about AIDS but what they won't believe that's the shameful part of this epidemic.

First and foremost, you have to look at the cruel—and criminal—behavior involved with children who have AIDS.

The three boys harrassed out of a Florida school come first to mind. Bomb threats and name calling and parental boycotting pretty well cover the continuum from illegal to inhumane. A court order got the children back in school. But an immense amount of damage has already been done to innocent children because they were sick. It'll be a wonder if they learn about much beyond meanness and what a miserable master fear is.

Dr. C. Everett Koop was right to fume and lash out at the public. He's renewed the issue of discrimination in appearing before the presidential AIDS commission. It's one result of ignorance, the surgeon general notes, hammering away at the need for accurate information. He has from the beginning put the weight of his profession and his position into promoting education about the disease as the best public health course.

This endless chatting about what the nation's policy should be is delaying prevention efforts. So is egotistical disagreements among disciplines, and experts within them, about funding and management.

Such nonsense as keeping children out of school is one example. Unlike other dread contagious diseases, AIDS doesn't go through the air or sit on the hands, ready to leap to the first person who passes by. Adults who remember polio or even longer ago, tuberculosis, are wrong to assume similarity in disease processes. With those, there was reason to avoid the physical presence of victims.

With AIDS, every major health source, from the surgeon general to private organizations, emphasizes that transmission is through body fluids, primarily blood and semen; the channels are overwhelmingly sexual activities and using dirty needles to inject illegal drugs. Surely we can assume that these things aren't going on in the classrooms. What is going on, however, is the cruel and ignorant wounding of innocent children who already have been dealt a mortal blow through no fault of their own.

THE BLADE

Toledo, OH, June 30, 1987

WARNING: the surgeon general may be hazardous to complacency. And also to conventional wisdom and labels.

C. Everett Koop, a distinguished surgeon from Philadelphia became a public figure as an outspoken critic of abortion. He went on to become something of a darling to the right wing. This in turn, jeopardized his confirmation by the U.S. Senate when President Reagan nominated him to be surgeon general.

Would Dr. Koop use this position, asked the legislators to foist his views on others? The doctor answered that he would do his duty and hold to his convictions; he saw no conflict. As surgeon general he would attempt to protect public health.

It was not to be abortion that kept Dr. Koop in the spotlight as a government servant, but smoking. To him the evidence is plain and so is his duty. Tobacco kills, and it can harm the non-smoker. So Dr. Koop has labored tirelessly to do all he can to restrict smoking and to slow its spread.

That has not made him greatly popular with the tobacco institute or the Marborough men of the nation, but it did, for a time, make him fashionable in Washington. He was the liberals favorite right winger and the conservatives' own man of compassion.

Then Dr. Koop got a little too much compassion. He begin to speak about the subject of AIDS. Now, political bigwigs stay away from dinners in his honor, William Bennett questions his judgment and dues-paying Reaganites avoid mentioning his name.

The surgeon general will not say what his personal feelings about AIDS victims are. But he is not afraid to do what he sees as his duty. There he was a couple weeks ago in news magazine photos holding the hand of a hospitalized AIDS patient. It must have driven Jesse Helms to his bourbon bottle.

Dr. Koop has lobbied hard for AIDS research money and opposed punitive forms of testing. Here is a Reagan appointee both competent and courageous, one who offends almost everyone on the political spectrum and who seems to have no firm place on the spectrum to call his own. He is something of a mystery man, unless it is actually possible that he takes the Hippocratic oath seriously.

THE ATLANTA CONSTITUTION

Atlanta, GA, September 24, 1987

It is a peculiar brand of "federalism," if that's what it is, that pits the Reagan administration against the American Medical Association, the American Nurses Association, the American Hospital Association, the American Psychological Association and the Health Association of America in its consideration of AIDS sufferers.

With its opposition to a bill protecting the confidentiality and basic rights of people who test positive for the AIDS virus, the administration stands practically alone.

There are compelling reasons, of course, for testing federal prisoners and people convicted of sex crimes, and for making the results available to surgeons and other health professionals on a need-to-know basis.

But there are equally compelling reasons for insuring that no "otherwise qualified individual" is denied employment, housing, public accommodations or governmental services solely because of infection with the virus, as Rep. Henry Waxman (D-Calif.) proposes, with the backing of almost every major health organization. His bill would set penalties of up to $2,000 for each instance of bias, and for each unauthorized disclosure of names and other information about those tested or counseled for AIDS.

Only a fraction of the people whose tests show they have been exposed to the virus exhibit symptoms, and experts are still unsure what proportion will develop AIDS, which is not transmitted through casual contact. But fear and ignorance have led some employers, school principals, landlords and even doctors to shun AIDS carriers — and a no-nonsense federal law is needed to keep others from closing ranks against them.

In deciding that the states "should be free" to make their own rules, Health and Human Services Secretary Otis Bowen argues in effect for their right to discriminate. The stand also could have the ominous consequence of undermining voluntary testing, which the administration ought to be doing everything in its power to encourage.

Widespread voluntary testing remains the best hope we have of curbing the spread of AIDS, by reaching those who need to make lifestyle changes — but it has fallen off in states, such as Colorado, that have made AIDS reportable, along with information identifying the patient. There have been declines even in states where such changes are only being considered.

For all these reasons, the Waxman bill deserves to pass over the administration's objections. The pity is, it may have to.

Justice Dept. Says AIDS Victims Can Be Fired

The U.S. Justice Department June 23, 1986 said federal civil rights laws did not forbid the firing of employees afflicted with AIDS. The department's 49-page opinion addressed whether AIDS victims were protected by Section 504 of the 1973 Rehabilitation Act. The section barred discrimination against the handicapped in any program or activity that received federal funds. (See pp. 164-167.)

The opinion distinguished between "the disabling effects of the disease on its victims" and "the ability of the victims to spread the disease to others." According to the opinion, an employer could not fire an AIDS victim because of an erroneous assumption that the employee's illness would keep him from doing his job. But an employer could fire an AIDS victim if he acted solely out of fear that the employee might spread the disease. The opinion acknowledged the medical consensus that AIDS was in all probability not spread by the sort of casual contact found in the workplace. But it maintained that federal laws to fight discrimination against the handicapped did not constitute "a general prohibition against irrational decision-making by employers..." The opinion also questioned whether the medical consensus was indeed final and asserted that the "risk of medical uncertainty must be borne" by those who alleged discrimination. Finally, the opinion challenged an appeal by the U.S. Court of Appeals for the 11th Circuit in September 1985, ruling that contagious diseases should be considered handicaps in themselves under the 1973 act. The Justice Department opinion conceded fear of contagious disease could cause carriers "adverse social and professional consequences," but insisted that "a person cannot be said to be handicapped simply because others shun his company."

The department opinion also argued that in enacting the measure, Congress had given no indication that it meant to "disturb the venerable body of federal and state laws giving public health officials broad powers to prevent the spread of communicable diseases."

The opinion had been requested by the Department of Health and Human Services and drawn up by Assistant Attorney General Charles J. Cooper, head of the Justice Department's Office of Legal Counsel. It was publicly released the day after the *New York Times* reported on its contents.

The Washington Post

Washington, DC, June 25, 1986

IN RESPONSE to a request from the Department of Health and Human Services, the Justice Department has issued a thoughtful memorandum on the question of disability rights and AIDS. HHS had received complaints from workers employed in hospitals and clinics alleging discrimination because they have AIDS or AIDS-related complex or because they test positive for AIDS antibodies. The question posed to the Justice Department was this: how does Section 504 of the Rehabilitation Act of 1973, which prohibits, in federally funded programs, discrimination based solely on handicap, relate to AIDS?

This question requires that two deeply held values be balanced against each other. AIDS patients deserve compassionate care and protection against discrimination based solely on their affliction. At the same time, the public justifiably relies on the government, as in the case of all contagious diseases, to take steps to contain its spread. The Justice Department memorandum reconciles this apparent conflict by advising that while an AIDS victim cannot be discriminated against *solely* because of his handicap, the law does not prohibit discrimination on grounds that his disease might be transmitted to others.

Is it reasonable for an employer or coworker to be afraid of an AIDS victim when it is so difficult to contract the disease? There are no certainties with AIDS, only probabilities. As recently as last November, for example, the Centers for Disease Control reported evidence of transmission only by blood or semen. Now scientists speculate that breast milk, saliva and other body fluids may be implicated. Estimates of the time the virus remains active outside the body have been revised upward. And researchers are still not certain how the disease is transmitted in such places as Africa and Haiti, where it is far more widespread than here.

The probabilities of contracting AIDS through casual contact remain minuscule but, as the Justice Department memorandum notes, "the extent of the harm that would be caused by a contagious disease bears an inverse relationship to the degree of risk of transmission that a normal person . . . can be required, to assume." A cold is easily transmitted, but its symptoms are temporary and relatively mild, so most people would not go to extraordinary lengths to avoid getting one. AIDS, though, is incurable, painful and invariably fatal. Medical knowledge about the disease and its transmission is incomplete. In this situation most people will go to extraordinary lengths to avoid risk of infection.

The Justice Department's interpretation of the law will surely be tested in court. But the memorandum is a good faith analysis of an extremely difficult legal and human problem. Now efforts must be accelerated to find other ways to help those who may not be able to rely on the 1973 law for protection.

The Miami Herald

Miami, FL, June 30, 1986

THE JUSTICE Department's Alice-in-Wonderland new ruling about AIDS and discrimination may play well in some mythical Peoria, but it does little to further public understanding of AIDS. And it does less to guide employers in their treatment of afflicted employees. Its major impact may be the muddying of public discussion and the cluttering of the courts.

Justice has said that AIDS victims — and carriers of AIDS antibodies — cannot be fired from Federal jobs or excluded from Federal programs because they have the disease. But they *can* be excluded because of fears of contagion unless those fears are a "pretext" for discrimination. The Justice opinion further declared that Federal law does not prohibit "irrational decision-making," that an employer lawfully can decide that "persons with curly hair make better employees than persons with straight hair." Say what?

Justice Department career staff had recommended that AIDS (acquired immune-deficiency syndrome) be treated as a handicap. This recommendation was similar to an April ruling by the Florida Commission on Human Relations in a Broward case. Broward's county government had fired a junior budget analyst after being tipped by his dentist that he suffered from AIDS.

The Supreme Court may decide the issue of disease as a handicap. It is reviewing a case involving a Florida school teacher fired in Nassau County because of a chronic susceptibility to tuberculosis. The Eleventh Circuit Court of Appeal ruled that her disease is a handicap and that, while it might disqualify her from teaching, the school system ought to try to place her in another job. Tuberculosis, however, is airborne and somewhat easier to contract than AIDS.

Now the Justice Department has given credence to irrational employment decisions and substituted its judgment about AIDS contagion for that of the U.S. Public Health Service and the Federal Centers for Disease Control. Its ruling affects all Federal agencies and programs and other entities such as hospitals and schools that receive Federal funding. This ruling should be tested in the courts, and promptly, before it further complicates an already difficult public concern.

The Hartford Courant

Hartford, CT, June 28, 1986

A U.S. Justice Department ruling that limits civil rights protection for AIDS victims could help spread, rather than contain, the deadly disease.

That unwanted result, in addition to the prospect of unjustified job discrimination against possibly scores of thousands of people infected with the AIDS virus, makes an early court test of the department's ruling a must.

The Justice Department's opinion, written at the request of the Department of Health and Human Services, said that carriers of antibodies to the AIDS virus are not necessarily protected by the Rehabilitation Act of 1973. The act prohibits discrimination solely on the basis of handicap in any program conducted by the federal government or receiving federal money.

According to the Justice Department, an AIDS victim is entitled to protection if he can show he was discriminated against "solely by reason of his handicap." But, under the opinion, a healthy person carrying antibodies to the virus does not necessarily have a handicap and could be fired legally if an employer believed he could transmit the disease.

The ruling is at odds with the recommendation of career civil rights attorneys in the Justice Department, who wanted greater protection from discrimination for those carrying the AIDS virus. It is also at odds with the weight of medical opinion, which agrees that AIDS is not spread through casual contact.

The Justice Department said it is impossible to rule out the possibility that AIDS is spread by means other than those identified to date. Those alleging discrimination must prove that the risk of their transmitting the virus is acceptably low, according to the department. That places an impossible burden on people who lose their jobs because of an employer's stated concern for public health. All they can do is cite the opinion of most researchers and public health officials that AIDS is not transmitted through the kind of activity that occurs in most work places.

A case can be made for imposing extraordinary measures in certain circumstances to protect public health. Transferring an AIDS victim from a job in a hospital lab would be prudent, for example.

But giving employers and administrators wide latitude to fire those carrying the AIDS virus irrespective of their work situation and without regard to accepted medical opinion about the transmission of the virus is wrong. Many people who represent no threat to their colleagues in the work place stand to lose their jobs. Because up to 1.5 million people have been infected by the virus, the ruling, if unchallenged, could have devastating economic and social consequences.

The department's ruling could actually harm public health. It's a safe guess that even more people in the high-risk groups will now refuse to be tested for the AIDS virus out of fear that they will lose their jobs. Some of them who otherwise might have been tested may transmit the virus, not knowing that they carry it.

The opinion nourishes a climate of prejudice and will probably hinder the fight against AIDS.

The Oregonian

Portland, OR, June 25, 1986

Acquired immune deficiency syndrome — AIDS — is bad enough on medical grounds. There is no known cure, and its victims invariably die.

But now the Justice Department, on shaky legal grounds, wants to make it even worse.

Current law says that private employers cannot discriminate against handicapped persons just because they are handicapped, and the Justice Department agrees that AIDS qualifies as a handicap. Nonetheless, the department now holds that employers can discriminate against AIDS victims if they believe that doing so will prevent the spread of the fatal disease.

Sounds reasonable. No one wants to see the spread of AIDS, and every employer has a responsibility to protect its unaffected workers.

But there's a Catch-22, and it's some catch.

The department would shift unfairly the burden for proving that AIDS is not contagious onto the victims themselves. Scientists agree that there is no evidence to suggest that the disease is spread through casual contact in the workplace. But proving this once and for all, and convincing employers of it, would be like proving that there is no Bigfoot. When we actually see Sasquatch, we'll know he exists; but if we never see him, we can't be absolutely sure that he's not out there hiding someplace.

So the victims of AIDS have a lovely choice. Either they can prove that they are contagious, in which case they rightly are discriminated against. Or, they can show at best that there is as yet no clear evidence of contagion, in which case — according to the Justice Department — they can still be discriminated against.

Injustice, like AIDS, is a disease. Unlike AIDS, it can be cured. Until AIDS is shown to be communicable through casual contact, its victims should have the same rights as other handicapped persons.

The Justice Department's ruling should be purged from the body politic, like any other virus.

THE ARIZONA REPUBLIC

Phoenix, AZ, June 30, 1986

THERE is much hysteria abroad these days on all sides of the AIDS epidemic.

Take, for example, the ruling of Charles J. Cooper, head of the Justice Department's Office of Legal Counsel, that employers can fire AIDS victims if there is *legitimate* reason to believe they pose a public health risk.

Hysteria flowed freely in the wake of the decision. *The New York Times* editorialized that the opinion "invites employers to dismiss people who have (AIDS)." The *Times* said the decision would allow firings if employers rightly, wrongly or irrationally believe a worker might spread AIDS.

The decision does no such thing. It specifically prohibits an employer from using a false fear of AIDS contagion as a pretext to dismiss a worker. The decision argues with a good deal of common sense — something in short supply in the public debate about the syndrome — that AIDS is not a handicap, but is a disease capable of being spread.

Present evidence seems to indicate the disease is spread only by the exchange of bodily fluids, such as semen or blood, and not through casual contact. But the scientific jury is still out. There is some conflicting evidence, so the Justice Department ruled that generally AIDS is not a handicap, but is a communicable disease. It makes sense to exclude AIDS victims from some jobs — such as food preparation — until the disease is better understood.

If the Justice Department had ruled AIDS victims are handicapped and protected from discrimination by the 1973 Rehabilitation Act, inevitably an AIDS sufferer would have brought suit under current affirmative action guidelines against an employer to force him to hire a worker with the syndrome or the virus.

Critics argue the decision will foster the spread of the disease by discouraging people in the high-risk groups — homosexuals, bisexuals and intravenous drug abusers — from taking the AIDS antibody test. This is a tired argument used against nearly every public health effort to isolate the disease and stop its spread, which in the absence of a vaccination or cure is the only way to control the deadly syndrome.

The Cooper decision is cautious and prudent, but has been subject to deliberate misinterpretation by gay-rights activists who want to transform AIDS from a public health into a civil rights issue.

AKRON BEACON JOURNAL
Akron, OH, June 24, 1986

A JUSTICE Department ruling on the legal rights of AIDS victims will open up a Pandora's box of problems in the workplace. The department says that those afflicted with the fatal disease are not fully protected by the nation's civil-rights laws. By saying that, the Reagan administration is almost sanctioning widespread discrimination against people suffering from AIDS.

The Justice Department is not taking away all rights. It would be illegal to fire a qualified employee simply because that person has AIDS. But the Reagan administration is also saying that employers can discriminate against AIDS victims if their motive is strictly to prevent the spread of disease.

In doing so, the Justice Department is really demanding that fired AIDS victims prove that they pose no health danger in the workplace, instead of making employers prove that they do. There are still many unknowns about AIDS, but medical scientists — including the government's own experts — repeatedly have said the illness is not spread through casual contact.

Apparently Justice Department administrators don't buy prevailing medical opinion. Nor do they give much weight to the legal opinions of their own lawyers, who had recommended that people with AIDS be broadly protected by civil-rights laws that prohibit discrimination against the handicapped.

The danger, of course, is that the Justice Department's ruling will further fuel fears and prejudice toward AIDS victims. It will become much easier for employers to fire employees with AIDS. They will merely say that they got rid of a worker in the interest of public health. It will be up to the fired worker to prove he was wrongly dismissed.

There is another potential problem that the government has overlooked. Limiting the civil rights of AIDS victims may in fact work against the public that is being protected. If people with AIDS are denied broad legal rights, they will understandably be reluctant to admit to their disease. Homosexual-rights groups predict that many people in high-risk groups will refuse to take the blood test to detect AIDS for fear they will lose their jobs. They may be walking time bombs, but public health officials will never know.

One thing is almost certain; the Justice Department ruling will be challenged. Even before the department's action, a federal appeals court ruled that contagious diseases such as AIDS constitute a handicap, and its victims are fully protected by law. The Reagan administration chose to ignore the law and to play with the facts. It has labeled a group of Americans who deserve help and sympathy as little more than second-class citizens.

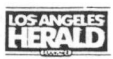

Los Angeles, CA, June 30, 1986

The facts about AIDS and how it is spread are well-documented by medical authorities. The disease cannot be transmitted through casual contact, such as sharing an office with a fellow worker. Neither does an AIDS patient or carrier of the virus permanently contaminate housing; disinfectants easily kill the disease on contact. Still, AIDS patients and carriers face losing their jobs or housing simply for having the disease or having come in contact with it.

Los Angeles and West Hollywood, along with a handful of other California cities, have adopted ordinances to fight such discrimination. With AB3667, introduced by Assemblyman Art Agnos, D-San Francisco, the Legislature could send a signal that the state will not tolerate unfair treatment of AIDS patients.

The bill would add little to state law, which already prohibits discrimination based on physical handicaps, including AIDS. But such symbols seem more necessary than ever, with the federal Justice Department's recent ruling that employers may legally discriminate against AIDS patients.

That decision, which disregards the fact that AIDS is not easily transmitted, shows that AIDS *hysteria* is highly contagious.

Discriminating against AIDS patients won't provide employers or landlords any more protection from the disease. But it may increase its spread, since those at high risk might avoid being tested for fear of losing their jobs or housing.

Education remains the best defense against the epidemic. To that end, AB3667 also would provide easier access to AIDS patients' records, given the consent of the patient, for doctors studying the disease. But without protections against discrimination, the educational effort is doomed.

Discrimination may add not only to the number of California's AIDS cases, which will soon top 5,000, but also to the state's Medi-Cal expenses. After all, when a worker is fired, and subsequently denied employer-paid medical benefits, Medi-Cal is often the only resource available.

The response to AIDS proves once again that discrimination is an expensive form of fear. AB3667 could be a useful weapon against that fear. The Senate this week should follow the Assembly's lead and approve it.

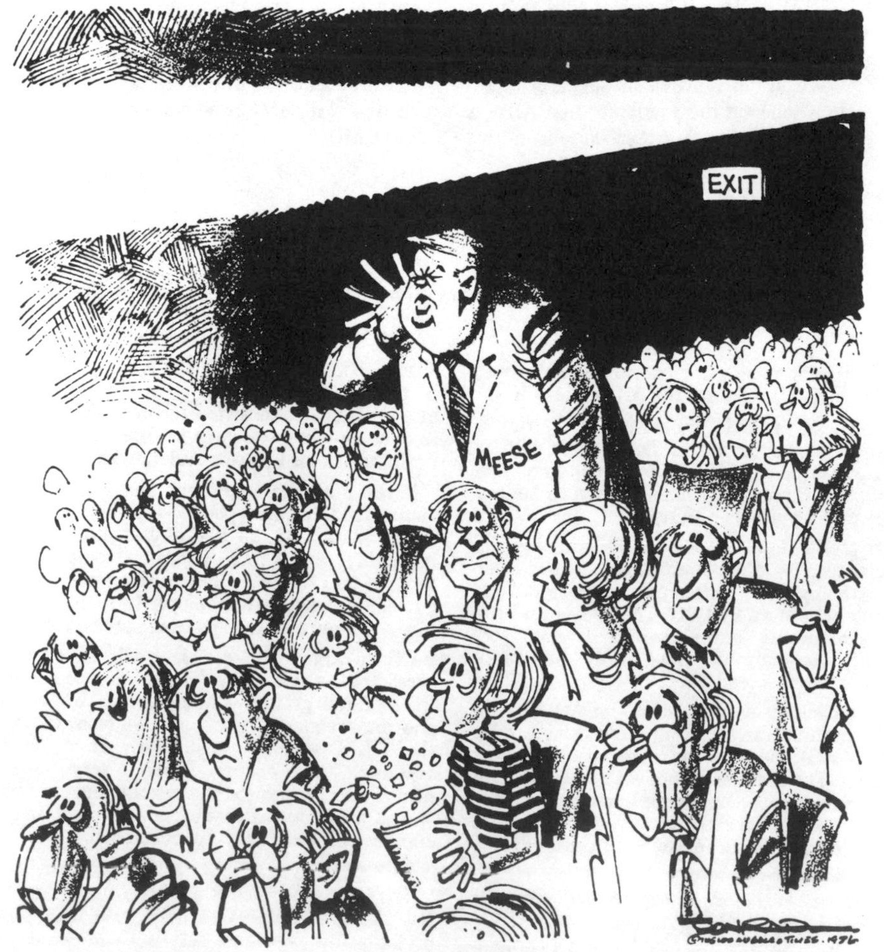

From the Los Angeles Times

'AIDS!'

The Providence Journal

Providence, RI, June 17, 1986

The acronym AIDS, familiar in general parlance for only the last five years, conveys little of the national calamity that this disease may cause in the next five years even if a major campaign is undertaken to combat it.

That does not mean that public hysteria is an appropriate response although there are indications that many Americans have been unable to view acquired immune deficiency syndrome dispassionately. The nature of the disease and its transmittal (neither through the air nor by casual contact) ought to reassure most people not in the high-risk groups that they are not susceptible.

Still, irrational fear persists in many quarters. Because it does, lawyers in the U.S. Department of Justice have tentatively concluded that people who have AIDS are "handicapped individuals" entitled to federal protection against discrimination under the Rehabilitation Act of 1973.

With about 21,000 cases of AIDS diagnosed since 1981, more than half of which have already been fatal, officials are using the term epidemic. In a report last week, the U.S. Public Health Service (PHS) said that in the next five years the figures would grow rapidly. By the end of 1991, the agency says, some 270,000 will have been diagnosed leading to a cumulative 179,000 deaths.

The full extent of the disease, which actually takes a variety of forms, lies beneath the surface of epidemiological statistics. Because it takes an average of four years for those with the virus to develop the disease, health officials believe that between a million and 1.5 million have already been infected by the virus and are potential carriers. In 20 to 30 percent of those cases, AIDS will manifest itself.

Further complicating the epidemic, clinicians across the country have concluded that AIDS is not a single syndrome as was thought originally. It is a complex of virus-caused infections and cancers that now come under the heading ARC (AIDS related complex). These include tuberculosis, pneumonia, hemophilus influenzae, Hodgkin's disease, squamous cell carcinoma of the mouth, psychosis, seizures, paralysis, and severe pain in the legs.

While research is continuing in an effort to develop a vaccine, and PHS is spending $234 million on the disease this year, officials say a vaccine for general use may not be available until 1993. Meanwhile, the cost of treating an AIDS patient is expected to reach an average $46,000 a year in the next five years or a total of between $8 billion and $16 billion.

"The numbers . . . are staggering," said Donald Ian Macdonald, acting assistant secretary for health in the Department of Health and Human Services. "This a major problem, probably bigger than the Public Health Service . . . These numbers make it very clear that our work must be intensified."

With the first hospital devoted exclusively to AIDS treatment and research tentatively planned for Houston, Tex. and federal concern escalating, it's incumbent upon state and local health agencies to place greater emphasis on public education aimed at preventing the spread of this devastating virus. Panic is not the answer, knowledge is.

Detroit Free Press

Detroit, MI, June 28, 1986

THE JUSTICE Department's recent ruling on acquired immune deficiency syndrome elevates fear above scientific knowledge. The evidence is increasing, researchers meeting this week in Paris said, that AIDS is not transmitted by casual contact. Not one such case has been recorded. Yet the Justice Department says that an employer may discriminate against AIDS victims if an employer believes they might somehow spread the disease to co-workers.

The government's ruling means that workers who are dismissed or otherwise discriminated against because they have AIDS must prove they don't pose a health threat. "The risk of medical uncertainty," the opinion said, "must be borne by the person alleging discrimination."

A judge can overrule that interpretation — the final version of which was contrary to recommendations from the department's civil rights lawyers. But meanwhile, it may be used by employers, especially those that receive federal funds, as a license to harass AIDS victims.

In addition, the opinion may actually discourage efforts to get people in high risk groups to take the AIDS antibody test, by increasing their concern that test results could be used against them. Anything that interferes with the public health goal of gaining the co-operation of people who test positive in order to help limit the spread of the disease is bad policy and ought to be reversed.

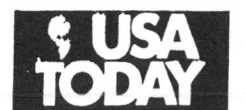

Washington, DC, June 26, 1986

The news is in from the scientists meeting at the international AIDS conference in Paris, and it is scary:

■ Around the world, there are an estimated 5 million to 10 million people carrying the virus; they can infect others.

■ By 1991, if current trends continue, 179,000 people in the USA will have died from this dread disease. By then, AIDS will be one of nation's top 10 killers; it will have killed three times as many people as the Vietnam War. So far, no one who has developed the disease has been cured, although three patients show signs of recovering.

■ Originally thought to be limited to homosexuals, it is now clear that AIDS can be transmitted by heterosexual sex — from man to woman, and from woman to man. In many countries, prostitutes are spreading AIDS; sexually active heterosexuals are at high risk.

■ Although research shows promise, no sure cure or effective treatment is likely in the near future.

In the USA, the epidemic has hit many cities hard. In San Francisco, more than half the gay men and 10 percent of heterosexual drug users are infected. In New York, 53 percent of gay men are infected; in Omaha, 14 percent.

So far, 22,000 people here have come down with AIDS; nearly 12,000 have died. This fearsome malady is a modern-day plague.

Society is struggling with difficult issues: Can people be fired if they contract AIDS? Can insurance companies deny high-risk groups medical coverage? Who will pay the enormous costs for care, which run $147,000 per patient?

While we struggle to find the answers, a second plague threatens to rear its ugly head — AIDS panic.

Last week, the Justice Department said it could be legal for employers to fire AIDS victims if they fear the victims will spread the disease. And Justice added that assurances from the U.S. Public Health Service that AIDS cannot be spread by casual contact are "too sweeping."

That's an ill-advised opinion that opens the door to abuse, discrimination, and panic. Instead of fomenting fear, the Justice Department, and government in general, must work harder to give the public the facts:

AIDS is a hard disease to catch. It is spread by sexual contact, homosexual or heterosexual.

It is also spread by blood-to-blood contact. Drug users have gotten it from needles used by infected people; hemophiliacs have gotten it from blood transfusions. No medical worker has caught AIDS through casual contact.

Some fear is understandable. But under proper medical supervision, some victims of AIDS can continue to work, attend school, and lead reasonably normal lives as long as they are well enough.

Instead of labeling victims as lepers, we must treat them with compassion.

Instead of fanning hysteria, we must face the facts.

Instead of promoting panic, we must push for a cure.

Instead of surrendering to fear, we must attack this vicious disease — and vanquish it from the face of the Earth.

Rockford Register Star

Rockford, IL, July 2, 1986

In the wake of 22,000 registered cases of AIDS and 12,000 deaths, the U.S. Department of Justice might have addressed the disease — and its impact on workers paid from federal funds — with clarity and concern. Instead, moralistic bias seems to have prevailed and botched the job.

Do federal civil rights laws protect those infected by the disease?

The Justice Department says, in effect, yes and no.

Yes, says the department, these civil rights laws protect the AIDS-infected worker if the worker is able and qualified and AIDS is simply an excuse for an employer to get rid of that person.

No, says the department, these laws do no protect that same worker if the employer sees AIDS as a potentially contagious disease that threatens others in the same work place.

So it's yes and no, until somebody blows the whistle and hauls this kind of thinking into court where a less murky reading of the laws must be sought.

Said Marvin Goldstein, an attorney who advises corporate clients, "To say it's not illegal to terminate an individual because of fear of contagion, but it's illegal to terminate because a person has the disease is a distinction without meaning." He added, "What this has done is to confuse ... everybody."

Amen to that.

ST. LOUIS POST-DISPATCH

St. Louis, MO, July 5, 1986

The Department of Justice's Office of Legal Counsel has ignored both government and court precedents in ruling that employers may fire some victims of AIDS. The ruling has created much confusion among employers and may well touch off unreasonable demands by co-workers that victims of AIDS be dismissed.

The problem of AIDS raises any number of legitimate health concerns in and out of the work place. But the Justice Department has given a reactionary response, not a rational approach to these concerns. The ruling says a company can't dismiss or refuse to hire a person solely on the ground that the person has AIDS. But it says the fear that the disease may spread — no matter how irrational that fear — gives a company a legitimate reason to discriminate against the victims.

That ruling by Charles J. Cooper, head of the agency's Office of Legal Counsel, is bound to create problems. It is unfortunate that Mr. Cooper apparently paid little or no attention to government and court precedents in putting together the agency's position. The Department of Health and Human Services, for instance, has issued regulations that specifically protect AIDS victims who are discriminated against in response to the attitudes of others. And a ruling last year by the 11th U.S. Circuit Court of Appeals said, in effect, that a contagious disease qualifies as a handicap under federal law. The ruling prohibited school officials from firing a Florida teacher who was diagnosed as having tuberculosis.

Mr. Cooper has sounded an irresponsible alarm in the absence of proof that victims of AIDS pose a health threat simply by working alongside others. His ruling focuses on emotions, not reason; it protects nobody's interest, least of all the public's.

The Record

Hackensack, NJ, July 21, 1986

Edwin Meese's Justice Department can be called many things, but dumb is not one of them. Consider its recent ruling denying AIDS victims protection against job discrimination.

It is an ingenious opinion — cruel, but ingenious. The Rehabilitation Act of 1973, which forbids job discrimination against the deaf, the blind, and others, defines a handicap as "a physical or mental impairment which substantially limits one or more ... major life activities." You might think that AIDS constitutes just such a handicap, and therefore ought to fall under the act. The Justice Department says no.

Why? Because, the department ruled, of the fear of *catching* AIDS. This affects not the victim but those around him. It is not, properly speaking, an impairment as defined by law. Therefore, it is still *within* the law to discriminate against AIDS victims on this basis. Even though the federal government's own Centers for Disease Control in Atlanta say there is no evidence that AIDS can be spread through workplace contact, the Justice Department has decided that it is not illegal to fire a victim because of the unjustified fears of his coworkers.

But if scientific evidence is irrelevant, then what about the even more baseless prejudices that some people may harbor about other disabilities? Take blindness. An employer who refuses to hire a blind person because, as he tells her in front of a dozen witnesses, "I just don't like your type," risks prosecution, denial of federal contracts, and a hefty civil suit. But if he tells the blind person that her job application was rejected because someone once sidled up to him in a bar and whispered that blindness is contagious, then he is apparently home free.

This is the absurd logic that the Justice Department is now pushing. No matter what the department seems to think, the irrationality of such prejudices is far from irrelevant. Allowing employers to penalize AIDS victims on the ground that the contagion issue is somehow outside the law's purview means permitting them to dodge the law on the basis of a silly and irrational side issue.

Mr. Meese should take a hint from the Centers for Disease Control and act accordingly. The federal government's job is not to spread panic and prejudice, but to discourage them.

The Washington Post

Washington, DC, July 13, 1986

SUPPOSE THAT YOU are an employer, and you learn that one of your employees is carrying the AIDS virus. Should you fire him to protect other employees' health? The answer to that one is no. No one has ever caught the disease through normal contact in the office, shop or school. But suppose that his presence bothers you and, medical risk or not, you want to get rid of him. There's a federal law prohibiting discrimination against handicapped people. Does it prevent you from firing him? In a memorandum last month the Justice Department argued that it does not.

That memorandum has been met with a great deal of sharp rebuttal, including a column by Charles Krauthammer in this newspaper. On the op-ed page today we publish the department's response to Mr. Krauthammer. Earlier, when the memorandum appeared, we commented on the law and the balance it needs to strike. But the Justice Department is asserting a policy that has deeply troubling implications, especially the status that it would provide for irrational fears of the disease and of the people who are infected. That is the point made by Mr. Krauthammer and, on Friday, by the American Medical Association in a suit now before the Supreme Court.

The Justice Department holds that, when Congress enacted protection for handicapped people, it did not intend to include those who carry communicable diseases. The law forbids discrimination on a long list of grounds—race, gender, age, handicap and so forth—but, Justice says, infection with AIDS or any other disease is not on the list. Since carriers aren't protected, Justice argues, it doesn't make any difference whether people's fears of contracting the disease by casual contact are rational or irrational. And if it's not illegal to discriminate against genuine carriers, then it's not illegal to discriminate against people only suspected of being carriers.

The courts will be asked sooner or later whether the department's reading of the law is correct. Sooner would be better.

In effect, the memorandum provides a rather explicit set of directions for discriminating against not only AIDS victims but anyone who might be suspected of carrying the disease—homosexuals in general. And perhaps, in addition, people afflicted by diseases other than AIDS. The case now before the Supreme Court involves tuberculosis. How about cancer? Until now, the discrimination statute has protected people suffering from it. The Justice Department thinks that it can distinguish between AIDS and cancer, but its logic is not compelling. An employer could claim that he feared catching an employee's cancer. Remember, Justice says that fear of the disease need not be rational.

The memorandum makes the further mistake of suggesting heavily that the danger of infection through casual contact is an open question. The same administration's Department of Health and Human Services quickly pointed out, uneasily, that Justice was not making a medical judgment and was offering no new medical findings. There are only three known ways to get the disease: sexual intercourse, direct introduction of infected blood into a person's bloodstream, and birth from an infected mother. More than 22,000 cases have been diagnosed so far, and not one of them has been shown to have been contracted any other way.

The Chattanooga Times

Chattanooga, TN, July 9, 1986

In a ruling that ignored legal and government precedents, Charles Cooper, head of the Justice Department's Office of Legal Counsel has now said that employers may fire some AIDS victims. One result of the ruling is that it has created confusion among employers; another, more pernicious possibility is that we may now see demands by some workers that colleagues with AIDS be dismissed.

The growth in the number of AIDS cases and the nature of the disease itself raise legitimate concerns, in the work place and elsewhere. But Justice's response in this instance was at best irrational and at worst hysterical. The department conceded that employers cannot fire, or refuse to hire, a person simply because he has AIDS. But it nevertheless said a fear that the disease could spread — and never mind if the fear is baseless — gives the company the right, in effect, to discriminate against those afflicted.

Mr. Cooper's ruling virtually invites problems, in part because he apparently ignored other precedents in forming Justice's position. The administration's Department of Health and Human Services, for instance, has published regulations specifically protecting AIDS sufferers who are discriminated against solely because of others' attitudes. And last year, the 11th Circuit Court of Appeals held essentially that a contagious disease can be treated as a handicap under federal law.

AIDS is, no doubt about it, a controversial matter, the more so because the principal victims are homosexuals. There is no proof, however, that AIDS victims constitute a health threat merely because they work with those who don't have the disease. Hospital workers who tend to AIDS victims and family members who visit them do so without contracting the disease themselves.

That makes Mr. Cooper's alarm all the more irresponsible. It rests on the premise of emotion, not reason, and works against the public interest.

The Seattle Times

Seattle, WA, June 25, 1986

AFTER an intense internal debate among its staff, the Justice Department has handed down a legal opinion that in effect wrongly invites employers and public-program administrators to violate the civil rights of AIDS victims.

The ruling grew out of department studies of whether a patient suffering from AIDS (Acquired Immune Deficiency Syndrome) can be classified as handicapped under federal statutes prohibiting discrimination on account of an-otherwise-qualified person's disabilities.

Acknowledging that AIDS patients have "some" protection under civil-rights laws, the opinion said those rights are not absolute — that there's "a distinction between the disabling effects of AIDS on its victims, and the ability to spread the condition to others."

Translation: An AIDS sufferer could be fired or denied benefits under a federally supported program if there was a "concern" the disease might be spread. Unless contradicted by a future court ruling, the department's statement potentially will affect countless employers and institutions operating in all or in part with federal funds.

The department's position was taken despite repeated assurances from government scientists and the medical community that AIDS cannot be transmitted through casual contact. The kinds of situations where the disorder can be spread — through sexual intimacies or blood transfusions, for example — are not likely to occur in a workplace or classroom.

Clearly, public fears over the dramatic nature of the fatal disorder and its links to homosexuality have led the department to a conclusion based more on political motives than on scientific fact. Too bad the department's top brass overruled staff civil-rights attorneys, who had advocated a much broader interpretation.

What the nation needed from the Justice Department was an enlightened statement on a public-health issue of enormous dimensions. What it got instead was a document reflective not of reason, but of emotion — hardly a basis for sound public policy.

Reagan Speaks Out on AIDS

Making his first extensive public comments on AIDS, President Ronald Reagan April 1, 1987 endorsed AIDS education in the schools but insisted that such programs should remain under local control and teach sexual abstinence and fidelity. Speaking before the College of Physicians in Philadelphia, at the college's celebration of its 200th birthday, the President pledged an all-out war on AIDS, which he labled as "public health enemy Number one." He said the federal government would spend $766 million to fight the disease in fiscal year 1987 and $1 billion in fiscal 1988.

The AIDS education approach advanced by the President was in contrast to recommendations of some advisers, such as Surgeon General C. Everett Koop, who had called for explicit instruction in the schools on how to use condoms to reduce the risk of transmitting the AIDS virus. Other advisers such as Education Secretary William J. Bennett, had argued for the need to emphasize sexual restraint.

The President said, in response to questions from reporters, that Bennett's views were similar to his. But, at the same time, he said that he was not opposed to Dr. Koop's position. "I don't quarrel with that, but I think that abstinence has been lacking in much of education," he said. "One of the things that's been wrong with too much of our education is that no kind of values of right and wrong are being taught in the education process.

"And I think that young people expect to hear from adults of what is right or wrong," he said.

Newsday

Long Island, NY, April 2, 1987

Whether at international medical conferences or intimate family dinners, the menace of AIDS has been on people's minds and in their conversations. Yet President Ronald Reagan — the person who, more than any other, should be speaking out about this epidemic — had remained noticeably silent.

Finally yesterday the president made his first formal statement on AIDS. But the long-awaited speech was a disappointment.

While the president branded the disease as "public health enemy number one" and promised $1 billion of next year's budget for AIDS research and education, he failed to demonstrate strong and decisive leadership. Instead he chose to sidestep some of the controversial questions raised by the spreading AIDS virus: He said nothing about encouraging the use of condoms or other "safe-sex" techniques or about AIDS testing priorities.

Nor will the speech satisfy those who worry that White House conservatives are trying to muzzle U.S. Surgeon General C. Everett Koop, one of the most thoughtful and forthright spokesmen on AIDS. Koop has relentlessly campaigned for frank sex education as a key to preventing the virus' further spread.

Reagan's silence on AIDS had fueled speculation that he wanted to distance himself from the nation's top public health official. The speech did not go far enough in quelling that speculation. Certainly no one disputes the idea that abstinence should be part of any school sex-education curriculum. But a prevention program that focuses only on abstinence and monogamy is, as Koop has said, unrealistic. Reagan's insistence on moralism as well as his emphasis on the limited federal role in sex education throws his proclaimed support of Koop into doubt.

If Reagan indeed believes that AIDS is the nation's number-one public-health problem, then he should act like it. That requires getting behind his own surgeon general and staying out front on this critical issue.

Post-Tribune

Gary, IN, April 17, 1987

The federal government must fight AIDS by spending big money on research and a great effort on education, not by presidential emphasis on sexual abstinence. The administration cannot create a national policy on morality. Neither can the states.

President Reagan is not wrong about abstinence and the need for moral instruction, but he is wrong in not taking a strong leadership role in trying to conquer the disease. He did, finally, call AIDS "Public Health Enemy No. 1." His reluctance to discuss the controversial issue in depth is linked to the failure of his administration to agree on how to handle it.

Our opinions

Surgeon General C. Everett Koop is outspoken — he wants to emphasize medical advice. Others in the Reagan administration, notably Education Secretary William Bennett, call it a problem of national morality. The president keeps saying that Koop is his man, but he has not met with the surgeon general to talk about AIDS.

Ending his silence last week, the president did elevate the issue's priority, but he did not offer strong hope that he would get vigorously involved. Caution is politically wise, but it is not good leadership. Several social issues are linked to AIDS, including testing as a condition of employment and insurance eligibility and the presence of infected children in the public schools. Those issues demand top-level attention and guidance.

There is some ambivalence in Indiana, too, although progress is being made. The State Board of Health is distributing an AIDS prevention booklet to schools. State Sen. William Costas of Valparaiso has proposed a law that would prevent the board of health from educating children about AIDS if a local school board disapproves of the material. He wants more focus on morality.

The senator is right about a need to emphasize morality. But that is not a health board's function. Doctors and health officials must deal with the urgency of reality.

A state health board spokesman said employees already work informally with teachers and principals to tailor materials to specific districts. That is the fair way to do it.

Federal and state public policies should pound out the message on health dangers and the risks of sexual encounters and they should provide guidance on all kinds of prevention methods. The threat of AIDS transcends ideology. It is larger than moral issues. It is first a major health issue and that is where the emphasis must be put. The national morality demands it.

The Hartford Courant

Hartford, CT, April 17, 1987

President Reagan's endorsing AIDS education in schools and his declaring that AIDS is "public health enemy No. 1" signal welcome and needed White House leadership in the fight against the fatal disease.

Nothing matches the power of the presidency in its ability to focus public attention and to direct resources to solve a problem.

Although the administration has requested more money for AIDS research each year since 1981, Mr. Reagan has refrained from exerting leadership in the AIDS education effort. Factions within his administration argued about whether the disease should be considered a moral issue or a health issue.

Surgeon General C. Everett Koop has been the point man in advocating early, and specific, education in the schools about how AIDS is transmitted. Dr. Koop has done a splendid job, but Mr. Reagan's voice was also needed.

The president now says he wants an "all-out campaign" against AIDS, and he should be commended for it. It's hoped that the speech in Philadelphia Wednesday was only the beginning of his leadership on the issue.

Mr. Reagan's caveat on AIDS education in the schools — that it include advising sexual abstinence — should offend no one. That's good advice.

The administration is asking for more than $600 million for research and other programs to fight AIDS for the 1988 fiscal year. Congress, however, has appropriated more money each year than the president has requested. That likely will be the case when the 1988 budget is approved, given the activism of Sen. Lowell P. Weicker of Connecticut and other lawmakers.

Now that Mr. Reagan has taken a more active leadership role, he should ascertain whether the federal agencies involved in AIDS work are cooperating sufficiently, and whether his administration is asking for enough money to fight the disease.

The doleful statistics — more than 50,000 deaths predicted in 1991, for example — undoubtedly have raised the president's consciousness about the seriousness of the epidemic.

St. Petersburg Times

St. Petersburg, FL, April 4, 1987

The battle against AIDS finally has the commander in chief aboard. President Reagan's belated pronouncements this week do give renewed urgency to the need for an adequate national effort in AIDS education and medical research.

The President called AIDS "Public Health Enemy No. 1," but didn't call for an adequate array of forces to cope with it. He told the College of Physicians of Philadelphia that AIDS deserves "an all-out campaign," but he didn't adjust his own meager budget requests to finance a forced march to attack the disease.

At least, the President did recognize the need for education in public schools on the epidemic. When asked whether children should be taught about AIDS, he said, "Yes, I think so — as long as they teach one of the answers to it is abstinence." He emphasized the need for values education along with medical information. That is reasonable.

How much less hollow his words would have been had he committed the nation to providing the resources for the battle in education and medical research. The AIDS epidemic as of March 23 had killed 19,021 persons in the United States. Another 33,158 have been identified as stricken, while public health officials estimate the number of persons who have contracted the fatal disease at anywhere from 400,000 to 4-million Americans.

The President also has a responsibility to lead the world's campaign against the disease, which is history's first global epidemic. The World Health Organization estimates 100,000 persons are dying worldwide and 5-million to 10-million afflicted.

Within four years, the cost of treating and caring for U.S. AIDS victims alone could be $70-billion, according to the Palo Alto Medical Research Foundation. The U.S. Public Health Service says that need may be only $16-billion. In any case, it will be a whale of a lot more than the Reagan administration seems prepared to spend.

So far, the administration has proposed only $534-million in its fiscal 1988 budget. A national task force on the disease urged that a reasonable annual expenditure would be about $2-billion, including a minimum of $1-billion of new money not a mere reallocation of current public health service funds.

Yet the Reagan budget adds only $117-million in new funds, while shuffling others from the National Institute of Health budget, which it proposes to cut by $649-million. This is shortsighted.

The fundamental lack of prudent investment in research and prevention begs criticism. How much wiser to spend more up front to educate and to research medical solutions than merely to make a token response now and be faced with staggering care costs later. The problem won't go away; pursuit of its solution can either be financed or delayed.

Reagan has been criticized for months now for not making a major statement on the subject. He has left the difficult task of leadership on the AIDS issue to the surgeon general, Dr. Everett Koop, who to his credit has attempted to educate the nation and the world about the pandemic proportions of the problem. Koop's candor has been greeted by catcalls from the far right. Perhaps the President's belated recognition of the gravity of the issue will help redirect public energies.

Still, the President would have been more credible if his call for an "all-out campaign" had been backed by a more realistic appropriations request. The Congress, which has had to increase Reagan's AIDS requests every year, will have to act responsibly again.

BUFFALO EVENING NEWS
Buffalo, NY, April 3, 1987

PRESIDENT REAGAN has placed needed stress on the seriousness of the current AIDS epidemic, calling the disease "public health enemy No. 1."

In his first major speech on AIDS — or acquired immune deficiency syndrome — the president called for determined research efforts to find a cure or vaccine for the dread disease, which is always fatal and has so far killed nearly 20,000 Americans. The Reagan administration is seeking a 28 percent increase in spending for AIDS research and education in the coming fiscal year.

In educating children and the public in general concerning the danger of AIDS, Reagan said that both medical and moral considerations should be emphasized. He said the schools should discourage sexual promiscuity, which could help to spread the disease. So far, the disease has been largely limited to homosexuals and intravenous drug users, but it is now spreading into the heterosexual population.

Reagan said the government should give educators accurate information concerning AIDS but that the dissemination of the information should be up to the schools and parents. He stressed that "AIDS information cannot be what some call 'value neutral.'"

He differed in emphasis but not in substance with his surgeon general, Dr. C. Everett Koop, who, while warning about "freewheeling, casual sex," also realistically stressed the need for condoms if abstinence or monogamy were not practiced. He urged "frank, open discussions about sexual practices" and education concerning AIDS at an early age.

Some persons on the political right were troubled by the stress being placed on "safe sex," preferring that more emphasis be put on abstinence. But a realistic program should emphasize both, and the surgeon general has correctly presented such a program. The president said he had no quarrel with Koop's position, but he felt that the importance of abstinence and morality had been lacking in the educational process.

AIDS was unheard of until a few years ago, but it has already become a major health threat. Because of the long incubation period of the disease, no one knows how many people are in danger of contracting it, possibly years from now. Medical authorities are estimating deaths in the hundreds of thousands.

Beyond the human tragedy, there is likely to be a staggering financial burden in health care. Thus the president's address, pinpointing AIDS as the nation's No. 1 health problem, should help to intensify action against AIDS in many ways — through prudent changes in sexual habits, education and redoubled efforts in medical research.

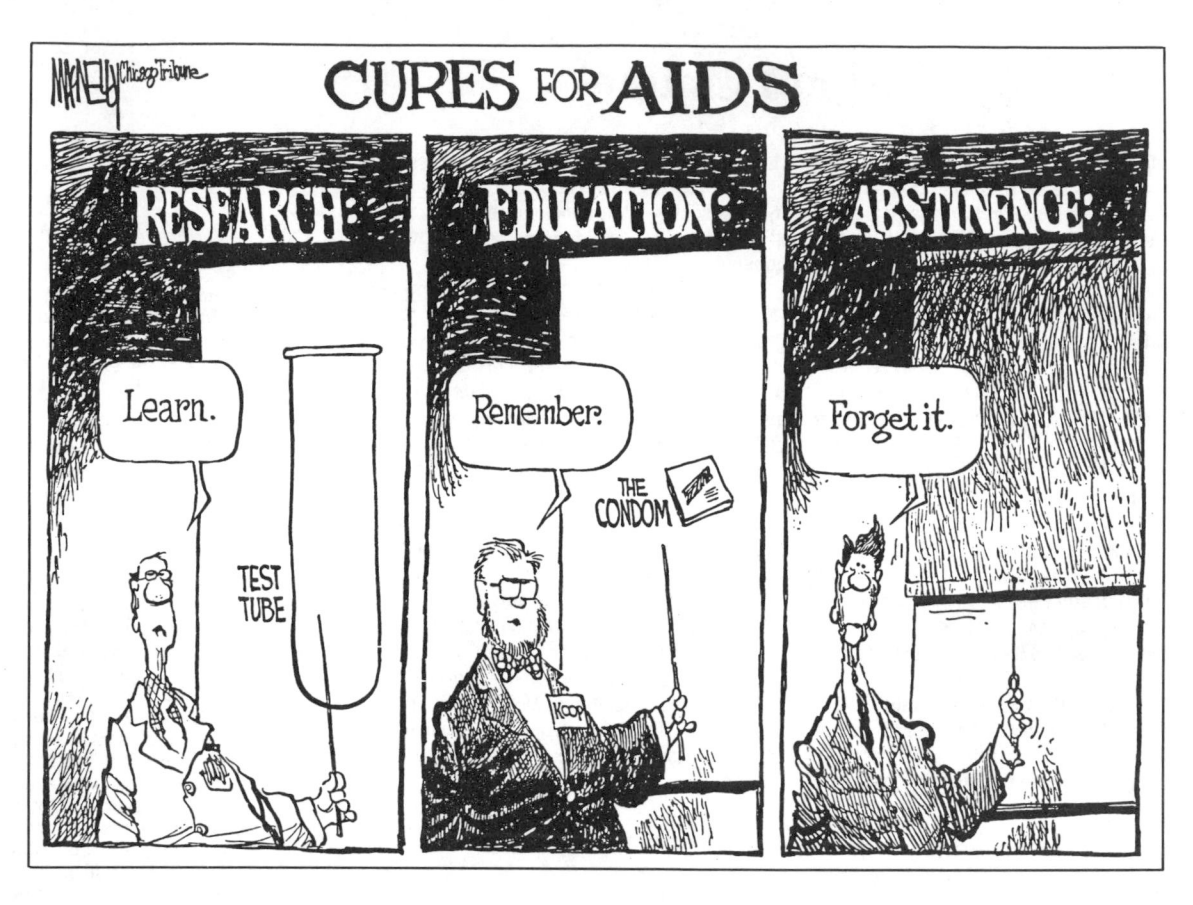

The Boston Globe
Boston, MA, April 10, 1987

In his first extensive commentary on AIDS a week ago, President Reagan asserted that "we've thrown everything we have into it." But the president's fight against AIDS has been more like a schoolboy skirmish, with a lot of dust kicked up and little else.

The president pointed to the $416 million for AIDS research and education in this year's federal budget, but certainly did not mention that he had requested only half that amount. Nor did he note how much of the federal money that is being spent on AIDS is being extracted from other medical and research programs in a rob-Peter-to-pay-Paul fashion.

Perhaps the most ironic diversion of funds is seen in programs to control the spread of sexually transmitted diseases. Since AIDS is spread sexually, diminished efforts to fight other venereal diseases also dilute AIDS control.

Moreover, venereal diseases themselves constitute a serious health problem. The incidence of drug-resistant gonorrhea has increased 30-fold since 1980, cases of congenital syphyllis increase every year, and the caseload of genital herpes is still rising dramatically.

Sen. Lowell Weicker (R-Conn.) called the president's AIDS speech a "damaging piece of deception." The president's claim that he is asking for $100 million more for AIDS research, Weicker said, sounds good only until it is also known that Reagan is asking for a $600-million cut in funds for basic medical research through the National Institutes of Health.

Because of the complexity of the AIDS virus, it is widely felt that the best hope for conquering the disease lies in the kind of advances in knowledge that can only be found in basic research. "The net of all this," Weicker said, "is that he [Reagan] has cut $500 million for AIDS."

What is needed to fight AIDS in any meaningful sense was spelled out months ago by the National Academy of Sciences: one billion dollars a year for research, plus a billion more per year for public education. A hollow speech by the president, coupled with budgetary sleight of hand by his administration, does not measure up to the task.

BUFFALO EVENING NEWS
Buffalo, NY, March 26, 1987

WITH NO CURE in sight, the only way to fight AIDS now is with prevention. The spread of the disease in the population has to be tracked, as well it can be, so people most at risk can be warned. And since prevention is primarily a battle individuals have to fight, the public needs the widest possible knowledge of what it is dealing with.

The Reagan administration has come out with a belated plan for a public information campaign. It calls for a national media blitz and coordination of educational efforts by a coalition of public and private organizations.

The program would be aimed at all Americans and would deliver practical and accurate information. Congress may want to make some changes, but there must not be major delays in getting the effort funded and under way.

Some officials within the administration want to stress monogamy and abstinence as preventives — sound advice but not prescriptions everyone is likely to follow. Since those who don't follow it are at greater risk, information must also be widely distributed on using condoms to prevent the spread of AIDS. The government recommends providing this information and also stressing the danger of drug abusers' sharing of needles.

Surgeon General C. Everett Koop wants the campaign designed to target groups most at risk, as determined by the pattern of the disease's spread. This makes eminently good sense. While everyone needs accurate AIDS information, education should be delivered in extra large doses where AIDS is spreading fastest.

The report recommended extra help in geographical areas where there are the most cases. Special programs are also suggested to target black and Hispanic young people, many of whom live in poor areas where there is a relatively high incidence of drug abuse.

A question health officials soon will have to confront is that of wider voluntary testing for the AIDS virus, another important prevention step.

The federal Public Health Service is expected to recommend soon that testing be made available to people who received blood transfusions between 1977 and 1985, the years before procedures were in use to protect the blood supply. While no one should be made to take the tests, those who received blood in that period should be contacted. Those who had transfusions in areas with the most cases, especially toward the latter part of those years, should be high on the list.

Any carriers who are found must be given counseling on the danger to themselves and the necessity of protecting others.

Some states are also considering requiring AIDS testing as part of the application process for marriage licenses. Since many AIDS victims now are babies born to infected parents, this step is also worth serious consideration. So is the advice of Surgeon General C. Everett Koop, who says anyone planning a pregnancy should have an AIDS test.

The Atlanta Journal
THE ATLANTA CONSTITUTION
Atlanta, GA, April 15, 1987

Ronald Reagan has marshaled the moral authority of the presidency to deliver a strong message: AIDS instruction to young children cannot be "value-neutral." One way of avoiding the fatal disease — indeed, the best way for youths — is abstinence.

Some may be tempted to tell Mr. Reagan to crawl back into the Neanderthal hole dug by his generation. That would be a mistake. The president has a right, indeed, an obligation, to set moral tones on issues of our time, and he has done so with courage and wisdom on AIDS.

Moreover, the federal government has more than a moral interest in preventing the spread of the disease. Hundreds of millions were spent this year for research on AIDS cures. More than $1 billion will be allocated next year. Medicaid costs associated with AIDS have skyrocketed, as more and more AIDS patients have turned to the health program for the poor to seek treatment. Too, the government is spending millions to treat some AIDS patients with Retrovir (formerly AZT). Those costs are expected to skyrocket next year.

Should the president keep his old-fashioned view to himself? Hardly. It is a message students need to hear. And it is a message teachers must heed as they go about the sensitive task of teaching young children about AIDS.

AIDS has put consequences back into sexual promiscuity, consequences that for a time appeared to have been rendered largely avoidable. AIDS means that a possible consequence of sexual activity is a slow, painful death.

Failure to impart that message is a failure to teach. We applaud the president's courageous stand.

THE SPOKESMAN-REVIEW
Spokane, WA, April 4, 1987

When President Reagan spoke out this week in favor of monogamy and sexual abstinence prior to marriage, the critical response from some quarters offered discouraging evidence of the nation's moral confusion.

On the other hand, the fact the president commented on sexual habits offers encouraging evidence that the sexual self-indulgence and promiscuity of the last two decades is falling out of favor.

But the change has relatively little to do with traditional values of self-control, responsibility and respect for the well-being of others.

Rather, the change has to do with self-preservation — specifically, the fear of AIDS.

In his first extended public comments on the disease, Reagan recommended sexual abstinence and monogamy and declared, to an audience of several thousand health professionals, that "When it comes to preventing AIDS, don't medicine and morality teach the same lessons?"

Fortunately, Reagan did not stop there. Sexual promiscuity does place people at risk of AIDS and so does needle-sharing by intravenous drug abusers. But morality lectures, even by the president, will not in all cases deter either promiscuity or drug abuse.

There lies the value of another Reagan remark. He said this week that "I don't quarrel with" the advice of Surgeon General C. Everett Koop, who advocates telling those who may not abstain from high-risk sex — particularly young people — how to protect themselves by using condoms and otherwise following Koop's explicit "safe sex" guidelines.

Koop has had to endure virulent criticism from his fellow conservatives for taking this stand, which he rightly believes to be in the best interest of public health. Although Reagan's endorsement was less than ringing, it was welcome and necessary nonetheless.

The nation needs an approach to AIDS prevention that strikes a balance between two extremes. On one side are the gay rights activists who lambasted the president for advocating traditional morality. On the other are the moral guardians of the religious right who have attacked Koop for his unflinching realism.

Reagan came close to the proper balance with his remark that "AIDS information cannot be what some call 'value-neutral.' "

In clinical settings, moral neutrality should be expected; not so in sex education programs. Although educators must begin to tell young people precisely how to protect themselves from sexually transmitted disease, they should, as Reagan argues, convey responsible moral values as well.

Young people cannot easily distinguish moral neutrality from moral apathy. To advocate condom use without discouraging promiscuity sends a message that promiscuity is expected and condoned.

AIDS is not the only national problem that sometimes can be attributed to irresponsible, indiscriminate sex. Teen pregnancy is another. So is abortion. So are unwanted children who often end up as victims of abuse and poverty.

Thoughtful educators will challenge young people to consider these consequences and the values that can prevent them.

Chicago Tribune
Chicago, IL, April 4, 1987

Like abortion, AIDS is turning into a political albatross. There is nothing a politician can say that won't make him the target of an angry attack by one group or another. It's not even politically safe to ignore the growing epidemic, as President Reagan has tried to do, despite charges that he doesn't know enough, care enough, spend enough, do enough or lead enough when it comes to AIDS.

Demands from the political right run toward mandatory testing for a growing list of groups, including prisoners, marriage license applicants, immigrants, prostitutes, drug users, patients admitted to hospitals and health care workers. Most of all, they don't want children taught in public schools how to practice what Phyllis Schlafly calls "safe sodomy" or any kind of education implying that premarital sex is all right and probably the norm. They also fear AIDS is getting more than a fair share of research appropriations and attention.

Other groups, including those most at risk of AIDS, want more money for AIDS research, money for patient care, money for new drugs (the only medication to get federal approval so far costs $7,000 to $10,000 a year), faster approval for new AIDS drugs, more legislation to protect the civil rights and privacy of AIDS victims and more obvious evidence of caring by the federal government.

The President's aides have been sharply divided on what the administration's stand should be beyond keeping the federal money flowing in AIDS research pipelines. His education secretary, William J. Bennett, opposes explicit sex education in the schools. His surgeon general, Dr. C. Everett Koop, has moved to a more pragmatic approach, recommending that children, from the early grades on, get straight talk about using condoms to reduce AIDS risks.

When the President was finally prodded into speaking out, he took a buck-passing, have-it-both-ways straddle that did him—and the battle against AIDS—little good. The federal role, he said, must be to give educators accurate information about the disease. "How that information is used must be up to schools and parents, not government."

Then he deferred to the political right and urged that elementary school children be taught to abstain from sexual relations as the best way to protect themselves from AIDS. He added, "When it comes to preventing AIDS, don't medicine and morality teach the same lessons?"

Sure. Abstinence—from intravenous drug abuse as well as sex outside of a long-term, monogamous relationship—would be an effective weapon against most further spread of the AIDS virus. But the President's version of his wife's just-say-no campaign against drug abuse isn't enough—not now, not in the real world, not against this new killer disease. President Reagan is not off the hook on this problem. Neither are all the other candidates for his job who are still trying to dodge the issue.

Reagan Seeks Wider AIDS Testing; Third Annual AIDS Parley Held

President Ronald Reagan May 31, 1987 in Washington, D.C. called for a range of AIDS testing at the federal and state levels, saying that AIDS was "spreading surreptitiously through our population" and that we have a moral obligation not to endanger others." The President's call for wider testing came in prepared remarks at a benefit dinner sponsored by the American Foundation for AIDS Research (AmFAR), a two-year-old organization whose national chairperson is actress Elizabeth Taylor. The President's speech, his first devoted exclusively to AIDS, called for mandatory testing of all federal prisoners and said he would ask the states to require testing in state and local prisons. The President said he would ask for a review of other federal programs, such as veterans' hospitals, to see if testing might be appropriate there too. The President also called for mandatory testing of new immigrants and announced that he had approved adding AIDS to the list of contagious diseases for which immigrants and aliens could be denied entry. The President called for "urgency, not panic" in battling the epidemic, and "compassion, not blame" for its victims. However, Reagan issued no call for legislation or state action to protect AIDS victims against discrimination. Nor did he discuss the widely perceived need for counseling in conjunction with AIDS testing.

Although guests at the AmFAR banquet frequently applauded Reagan during his speech on AIDS, the President also drew scattered boos and hisses, particularly while outlining his testing proposals. AmFAR advocated voluntary, confidential testing procedures accompanied by counseling. Furthermore, the group favored an increase of federal funding for research, treatment and education, rather than an emphasis on testing. After Reagan concluded his speech, Taylor said that "while there are differences of opinion" about AIDS testing, the President's remarks were "basically in concurrence with what we hope and pray for: a cure to AIDS." Taylor's statement met with thunderous applause.

The Third International Conference on AIDS met June 1-5, 1987 in Washington, D.C. More than 6,000 scientists and health professionals from 50 countries attended, making it the largest scientific meeting yet devoted exclusively to the disease. In the nearly 250 formal presentations, no major breakthroughs were reported—only significant steps. However, in contrast to earlier such gatherings where highly technical discussions dominated the agenda, the Washington conference reflected the growing politicization of the AIDS epidemic.

Vice President George Bush was booed June 1 during his keynote address to the conference when he pushed for broader testing at both state and federal levels to detect individuals who were infected with the AIDS virus. Bush, however, was applauded when he went on to stress the need for strict confidentiality of testing results, in the strongest statement yet made by any top Reagan administration official on protecting the civil rights of AIDS victims. After the speech, Bush, obviously angered by the booing, said, "Who was that? Some gay group out there?" The comment was picked up by some microphones and recording devices on the podium and was later widely reported.

Before the vice president's speech, an estimated 350 protesters, some of them suffering from AIDS, had staged a noisy demonstration in front of the White House to protest the Reagan administration's AIDS policies. Local police, wearing yellow gloves to protect against possible AIDS-virus infection, arrested 64 of the protesters. Among those arrested was Leonard Matlovich, who had become a public figure in the 1970s by proclaiming his homosexuality while serving as an Air Force sergeant. Matlovich had recently been diagnosed as having AIDS. "If I can spend three years fighting for democracy in Vietnam, I can spend an hour in jail fighting for our lives," he said.

The conference ended June 5 the way it began, with boos and jeers for the Reagan administration, as closing remarks were being delivered by Dr. Otis Bowen, secretary of health and human services. Bowen was booed when he invoked the President's stands on mandatory testing and AIDS education, which stressed abstinence rather than "safe sex" techniques. But he drew applause when he said AIDS wasn't "a them-versus-us thing; this thing is truly just an us thing."

Rockford Register Star

Rockford, IL, June 8, 1987

President Reagan's first major address on the topic of AIDS revealed true compassion for those who suffer from the disease, but it also is cause for concern on some fronts.

Speaking to the American Foundation for AIDS Research gathered in Washington, D.C., he said about the epidemic: "This calls for urgency, not panic. It calls for compassion, not blame. And it calls for understanding, not ignorance."

Yet, some of his actions and those of other officials contradict those words.

We have seen panic — President Reagan proposing widespread mandatory testing of various groups, high-risk as well as low-risk, against the advice of leading health professionals. Health officials say such testing would be tremendously expensive while yielding a very low rate of identification of carriers. Meanwhile, the needs for education and prevention and research into treatment would suffer.

We have seen blame - Vice President Bush remarking when he was booed at the convention that the dissenters "must be a group of gays." Recent reports show transmission rates among heterosexuals to be higher than that among homosexuals.

We have seen ignorance — police wearing rubber gloves to arrest demonstrators who may or may not be homosexuals, may or may not have AIDS, even though research has shown that the disease cannot be transmitted by casual contact.

However, some of the testing proposed by the president is logical and has merit. President Reagan has asked that AIDS be added to the list of diseases for which immigrants can be denied entry or permanent resident status. He also has asked the Justice Department to plan for requiring testing of all federal prisoners.

Testing immigrants only makes sense as an effort to curb the influx of persons with dangerous, contagious diseases. Prison testing is only fair so that prison officials can better protect a captive population from becoming infected.

The other categories the president advocates for testing are patients visiting public health clinics and persons seeking marriage licenses. Mandatory testing in some of these areas would be a violation of individual rights. It also would be expensive and health professionals believe the money could be much better spent on research.

In addition, there are serious questions about how the testing information would be used. What guarantees would there be of confidentiality? Could the information be used to discriminate against individuals in jobs, housing or education? People who advocate widespread, mandatory testing wave those questions aside with vague assurances that confidentiality would be guaranteed and discrimination would be prevented, but they don't give details.

In spite of concerns about some elements of President Reagan's AIDS proposals, we are pleased to see him at last acknowledging this threat to the health of our nation. Federal attention is required if AIDS is ever to be brought under control.

SYRACUSE
HERALD·JOURNAL
Syracuse, NY, June 7, 1987

What do we do about AIDS? They are calling it one of the most perplexing social policy dilemmas ever faced by a president.

That's simply not accurate. It's not that AIDS is not a problem, because it is every bit as gigantic a health problem as we have faced. But that's what it is ... a *health* problem. AIDS is not a socio/health problem, if indeed it ever should have been limited to that status. It is not a problem facing only a clearly defined segment of our population.

AIDS is a matter of life and death for *all* of us. It is readily transferrable from gay to gay, from gay to heterosexual, from heterosexual to heterosexual. Whenever two people have sex together, there is a chance one of them is passing the AIDS virus to the other, particularly if one or both has sex with one or more partners. This is no longer a disease associated exclusively with aberrant behavior. It is no longer, as some like to think, "punishment for those who disobey the rules of God."

No, we *all* are susceptible to AIDS. And, as we all know by now, once the virus has established itself in our system, an early, probably painful death is inevitable.

In other words, we are looking down the road at a possible health crisis unmatched in our time.

In a very few short years, for instance, AIDS will be the No. 2 cause of premature death of young men, considering the alarming increase already evident in the death rate. And the increase in women contracting the disease and dying from it is increasing alarmingly as well.

At this point, with a presidential election year just over the horizon and the well-known fact this disease is best known as a disease of the gay — passed from man to man — AIDS also is being called a "political nightmare." Many politicians feel that to voice concern for the victims of this horrible disease is to offend a huge portion of the populace that would consider it the same as endorsing the gay lifestyle.

We're at the stage now, however — regardless of the political repurcussions — where brave men must step forward and recognize this scourge for what it is. Politicians must accept the premise there is no way they can *not* commit whatever national resources are necessary to defeat this plague.

The president said the other day in outlining the administration's "policy" on AIDS that we should not panic. If by panic he means the kind of reaction exhibited by New York City Mayor Ed Koch in suggesting everybody who comes into the country should be tested, the president is right. However, if he is seeking to downplay the urgency of the situation, he is making a mistake.

Testing, of course, of certain high-risk groups is part of the answer. Education will be helpful, as well, as long as we don't oversell the idea of "safe sex." (There is no such thing, in this case.)

The real answer to the problem will not come, however, until we find a cure. To that end, we should be making a 100 percent national commitment, regardless of the cost, to research until the cure is found. In the meantime, the same commitment should be made to the care and treatment of those now afflicted.

Houston Chronicle
Houston, TX, June 5, 1987

President Reagan's proposals for AIDS testing are minimal and deserve wide support. The negative reaction to his program shows how far the country has yet to go to get the battle against AIDS out of politics and into the field of communicable diseases where it belongs.

One part of the president's program is traditional. He added AIDS to the list of contagious diseases for which immigrants and aliens can be denied permanent U.S. residence. Denying entrance on health grounds has long been the practice.

Testing federal prisoners for AIDS certainly fits into the "routine" category the president mentioned. He called for a review of whether it might be appropriate to make testing for AIDS routine at Veterans Administration hospitals.

President Reagan urged states to "offer" routine tests for couples seeking marriage licenses. The Texas Legislature Monday passed a bill requiring such tests if the incidence reaches a certain point. The bill also would allow the Texas Department of Corrections to test new prisoners for the AIDS virus.

All of these steps comprise a moderate approach to what is now recognized as a world health threat. Voluntary AIDS testing should be encouraged. The benefits of mandatory testing for a greater segment of the population were questioned by experts at the recent Washington conference. At least there is unanimity on increasing funding for research.

Locally, Dr. James Haughton, city of Houston Health and Human Services Department director, makes an important point. Testing is useless, he said, unless there is an effort to counsel and educate. People must learn to modify their behavior to prevent the spread of the disease.

President Reagan and Vice President George Bush were booed during their speeches at the Washington meeting. Politicians are wary about statements on an issue that combines health, civil rights, sexual practices and social standards. One of the major problems in the fight against AIDS is to reach the point where it is dealt with strictly as a public health issue.

The News and Courier
Charleston, SC, June 5, 1987

The boos and hisses that greeted Vice President Bush when he announced the administration's plans to make AIDS testing more widely available were indicative of deep-seated resistence to not only mandatory testing, which is understandably controversial, but to any testing at all.

It is questionable, however, whether, merely because the boos and hisses emanated from an international conference on AIDS, they deserve more consideration than they would at a sporting event.

Medical opinion is divided on whether tests should be mandatory. The administration appears to have responded to this concern by recommending mandatory testing in prisons and for would-be immigrants and proposing that tests be routinely available in other instances — for example, when people apply for marriage licenses. The intent behind wider testing is to protect people from catching or passing on AIDS.

Expressions of repugnance, similar to the boos and hisses that Mr. Bush received in Washington — compensated, later, by applause for his pledge that the results of the AIDS tests must be treated with confidentiality and fairness — tend to follow efforts to provide more information about AIDS. The column by George F. Will that is printed elsewhere on this page is a case in point. It contains descriptive passages that might, in another context, be considered offensive. The intent, however, is to provide information that will help people avoid contracting AIDS.

Mr. Will is not — as a reader (whose letter is printed below Mr. Will's column) charges another columnist — "homophobic." Certain homosexual practices are known to cause AIDS. These practices, if they were widespread among heterosexuals, would be equally risky. As Mr. Will points out, "not all homosexuals are promiscuous or given to high-risk behavior. However, even some who are not are dismayed by dissemination of information about those who are." As he says "insufficient information about homosexual practices has impeded understanding of the epidemic."

It is healthy that homsexuals can now come out of the closet, as Rep. Barney Frank did the other day. But it is not healthy if certain behavior remains closeted. Avoidance of practices that Mr. Will is necessarily explicit about will save lives.

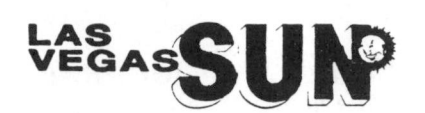

Las Vegas, NV, June 12, 1987

The Charlotte Observer

Charlotte, NC, June 10, 1987

There are two critical tasks in controlling the spread of AIDS, says Dr. Donald Hopkins of the Centers for Disease Control. The first is to find and counsel the carriers, which is difficult and often controversial. Not everything that is politically attractive makes medical sense. There is danger that energy and resources will be absorbed by sideshows.

That is one reason health professionals refuse to board the bandwagon for routine testing of everything that moves. They fear clogging an already jammed system, while driving away the people who most need to be reached. Testing is important, but needs to be used intelligently.

The second task is to persuade the uninfected to avoid putting themselves at risk, which is also difficult and controversial. The groups most at risk are male homosexuals and intravenous drug users, and their sex partners. The very behavior that places them at risk is the behavior that had already placed them outside mainstream society's historic norms. Persuading them to abandon the behavior is difficult. Advising them how to carry it on with greater safety seems, to many, like condoning it.

Still, society has the duty to spread the message of safety as forcefully and honestly as possible. If condoms, clean needles and blunt talk in public places can slow the spread of AIDS, then squeamishness is both bad policy and immoral.

But campaigns for "safer" sex and drug abuse are only half the truth. Drug abuse is inherently unhealthy and unsafe, as is promiscuous sex — homosexual and heterosexual. Any partner willing to engage in such high-risk behavior is, by definition, a risky partner.

Educational efforts, particularly among young people, should stress those things. AIDS is largely an avoidable disease. Real safety does not lie in using condoms or sterilizing needles, but in avoiding risky behavior altogether. In this case, as Surgeon General Everett Koop says, "Science and morality are walking the very same path."

Society can protect itself by stressing healthful behavior and re-instituting it as the cultural norm. Safe sex is what Dr. Koop calls "faithful, monogamous" sex. He puts it that way instead of just saying "marriage," we suppose, because marriage is not *medically* necessary. But continuing epidemics of unwanted pregnancy, sexually transmitted diseases and, now, AIDS all suggest that marriage and the ethic of faithfulness are *socially* necessary.

The frightening fact about the AIDS virus stands out sharply in the heartbreaking picture of California anti-tax crusader Paul Gann, tears welling in his eyes and voice breaking, saying "I'm going to die. I don't want to."

Acquired Immune Deficiency Syndrome doesn't discriminate. Once in the bloodstream, it overpowers any body and eventually leads to death.

In his last campaign, Gann will wage a frustrating battle against a deadly disease that crippled his immune system after the virus attacked him following open heart surgery five years ago.

That was the critical time before health officials tested blood supplies. How many more like Gann will be stricken with AIDS? There have been children who need blood transfusions to control their hemophilia and a case of a Roman Catholic nun in San Francisco who contracted the disease — all through blood transfusions.

Routine screening of blood from donors for the AIDS virus began in 1985. Nationally, about 2 percent of the 36,000 known AIDS cases have been scientifically traced to blood transfusions. So far, none of Nevada's 90 confirmed AIDS cases resulted from a blood transfusion.

By 1991, Nevada health officials predict that there could be 1,000 cases of AIDS statewide and several thousand cases at the turn of the century in this state.

The Reagan Administration has taken a first step in a long, agonizing process that this country will endure to survive this 20th century epidemic, calling for routine testing of federal prisoners and immigrants.

Gann already has vowed to campaign for more openness about the disease and endorsed legislation proposed in California to require wider testing for the virus, including those requesting a marriage license.

There are very serious questions facing policy makers as the AIDS virus spreads. Some scientists have called for voluntary testing only, since mandatory exams could drive high-risk groups away from screening clinics. Others, like Gann, can't understand why the AIDS carriers are not known to the medical community. That's an ethical question of privacy still facing not only the medical community, but society.

Since AIDS cannot spread like a cold — through sneezing, coughing, handshakes — not many have an appetite for quarantine or any kind of restriction on afflicted patients.

And because AIDS is not easily transmitted, more testing to define the distribution of this ever-increasing disease is the best possible measure at the moment.

Certainly, cases like Paul Gann will raise the fears of many people who do not have the virus. Such public attention demands more education and information, a facet of the war on AIDS that the United States, and each of its state and local governments, cannot ignore.

If we are serious about declaring war on AIDS, then the first volley of shots have been fired at this unseen enemy through President Reagan's call for testing. The next fusillade needs to be accurate information provided to everyone, not only homosexuals, bisexuals and intravenous drug users.

And Nell Gann, Paul's wife, set the example for compassion when confronted by the victims of this deadly virus. She hugged and kissed her husband after his hour before the television cameras.

Minneapolis Star and Tribune

Minneapolis, MN, June 3, 1987

After years of silence on AIDS, President Reagan last weekend finally acknowledged the modern-day plague, expressed concern for its victims and promised to help stem its spread. Unfortunately, his proposals for controlling the disease would aim expensive arrows at some unlikely targets.

The president favors mandatory AIDS-antibody testing for all prison inmates and immigrants. He recommends that states enact "routine" but voluntary testing for marriage-license applicants and patients at Veterans Administration hospitals and drug-abuse and venereal-disease clinics. His reasoning is straightforward: Hundreds of thousands of Americans are carriers of the AIDS virus and don't know it. Why not test the masses to find and warn that dangerous minority?

Sound reasons do exist for some of the president's screening plans. Testing prisoners makes sense because of their proclivity for drug abuse and their vulnerability to rape. Testing aspiring immigrants for AIDS is in keeping with the longtime practice of checking them for communicable diseases. Offering tests to individuals seeking treatment for drug addiction and sexual diseases also is sensible — so long as the offer doesn't drive people from the clinics.

But Reagan's call for testing VA hospital patients and marriage-license applicants deserves no support. Even if voluntary, the plan may not grant credible promises of confidentiality and protection from discrimination. And even with such guarantees, mass screening would be pointless. As the Centers for Disease Control has emphasized, such tests would identify only a handful of virus carriers at tremendous expense. Testing Minnesota's annual crop of 72,000 brides and grooms, for instance, would uncover just one or two carriers. Screening VA hospitals' disproportionately elderly patients would yield even fewer positive tests. The few carriers identified would almost certainly belong to groups especially susceptible to AIDS.

If AIDS reaches further into the general population, well-focused screening may be necessary. But for now, mass testing is as promising as searching for a needle in a row of haystacks. It would consume resources better spent on efforts Reagan's premiere speech on AIDS neglected to mention: encouraging voluntary AIDS tests for those at high risk and discouraging all Americans from engaging in behavior known to spread the virus. Before those tactics are tried, widespread testing would be wasteful and fruitless.

The Register-Guard

Eugene, OR, June 3, 1987

President Reagan's first speech devoted entirely to the subject of AIDS offered a variety of proposals for testing people for exposure to the disease. Most of the discussion of the speech has centered on whether those proposals go too far or not far enough toward identifying AIDS victims and carriers. But the most important words the President spoke Sunday had little to do with testing:

"America faces a disease that is fatal and spreading," Reagan said. "This calls for urgency, not panic. It calls for compassion, not blame. And it calls for understanding, not ignorance. It is also important that Americans not reject those who have the disease but care for them with dignity and kindness . . . . Final judgment is up to God; our part is to ease the suffering and to find a cure. This is a battle against disease, not against our fellow Americans."

If those words could find a place in people's hearts, much of the concern about the details of testing programs would cease to exist. A primary aim of efforts to stop the spread of AIDS must be to reach people who have the disease but do not know it, so that they can be educated to change or refrain from the practices that transmit the disease. Effective programs to reach such people — whether they involve education, testing or both — demand the humane understanding Reagan urged in his speech.

The fact that AIDS usually spreads through sexual contact or the shared use of intravenous needles has raised formidable barriers to such understanding. Many who are in the greatest danger of contracting the disease are fearful of the discrimination that could result from being identified with the at-risk groups. Such fears are well founded, given some people's tendency to blame homosexuals and drug abusers for the disease.

Against that background of fear and distrust, Reagan's testing proposals are moderate. He did not call for universal, mandatory AIDS testing for any group. He proposed that AIDS tests be routinely administered to immigrants and federal prison inmates. He asked that states adopt routine testing for people who visit drug and venereal disease clinics and for inmates in state prisons and local jails.

These steps are defensible, either in terms of the opportunity a testing program offers for educating members of at-risk groups or in terms of the nation's long-standing interest in denying entry to immigrants who suffer contagious diseases. Surgeon General Everett Koop, the administration's voice of reason on the subject of AIDS and an opponent of mandatory testing, endorsed Reagan's proposals.

Some of Reagan's proposals may be ineffectual. He urged states, for instance, to require AIDS tests of people applying for marriage licenses — a step that promises to do little to stop the spread of AIDS. The President also ordered a study of whether to test patients treated in federal Veterans Administration hospitals. The study is likely to show that there would be little public health benefit to such testing.

Reagan's approach has been criticized by public health officials who feel that AIDS education should be the nation's top priority. But testing and education can be complementary. It is essential that people learn how to stop the transmission of the disease. At the same time, testing can yield valuable information about the spread of AIDS and can bring that information to those found likely to need it most.

Neither education nor testing will succeed without the compassion and understanding that Reagan stressed in his speech. Slowing the spread of AIDS is an unprecedented challenge for the nation, and fear will compound the difficulty of the task. The most important part of the President's message — that Americans must fight the disease, not each other — was highly encouraging.

The Des Moines Register

Des Moines, IA
June 12, 1987

AIDS is a deadly, incurable disease. But it is not yet clear that it is another Black Death, as some public-health officials and writers would have you believe. It is spread primarily through homosexual acts and sharing of drug needles — not by casual contact — and the overwhelming majority of its victims are those who engage in one or the other high-risk activity.

That means that testing to identify those who have the disease or are carrying the virus that causes it should be limited.

The top public-health priorities should be finding a cure, warning people about the disease's dangers and how to avoid it or limit their exposure to it, and getting a solid fix on the disease's spread.

Today's available evidence clearly does not call for the mandatory testing of the population at large. Some testing is in order now. The Reagan administration order for mandatory testing of all immigrants and federal prison inmates is an appropriate step. The United States should not admit AIDs-carrying immigrants, nor allow the spread of the disease within prisons, where homosexual acts are common.

Also appropriate is the government's plan to get a statistical projection of the disease's spread beyond the high-risk groups — homosexuals, bisexuals and drug-users — by spot-testing some 45,000 persons on a voluntary and anonymous basis.

These steps do not downgrade the severity of the disease or the need for educational programs and voluntary testing. They are aimed at getting some perspective, finding out what we're dealing with.

As part of the public-education and prevention effort, the states should offer free AIDS tests to people applying for marriage licenses. Iowa and other states should urge all couples contemplating marriage to take the test, and should make the tests widely available at no cost.

These tests should not be mandatory. But they should be offered to every couple applying for a license, and the couple would have to consciously reject the offer of a test. The test results should be provided only to the two persons planning to marry.

Most prudent people, if offered a free, confidential test and if told of the dangers of AIDS, probably would accept the test. The program would save some people from the horror of finding out — too late — that their mate carried the AIDS virus, perhaps unknowingly.

News-Tribune & Herald

Duluth, MN, June 6, 1987

Every day, the medical, social and political importance of AIDS becomes more obvious.

Columnist Sandy Grady writes elsewhere on this page of the rising political profile of AIDS. The medical significance of a disease that kills most or all of its victims is obvious.

And the social significance of AIDS is shown by the news items of just one day on one wire service. Friday offerings of the Associated Press included word that:

● Insurance firms are cutting the amount of insurance they'll write without a medical exam because they believe victims are applying for insurance after becoming infected.

● Because of the high costs of AIDS treatment, some insurance companies are trying to weed out homosexual applicants.

● The number of AIDS-related lawsuits is likely to rise from a few hundred to 4,000 in the next few years.

● The number of AIDS-related discrimination cases have increased yearly, and most involve minority group members who already suffer from other social problems.

● AIDS infections are twice as likely among Navy and Marine Corps personnel as those in the Army and Air Force.

These and other stories arriving Friday show the need for a broad, compassionate, generous (in money and spirit) AIDS policy.

As we've said in this space before, it's not enough to endorse sexual fidelity or urge mandatory testing of certain people. The federal government *must* get involved.

In dealing with AIDS, American society needs to provide compassion for its victims, research on a cure, education as a preventive measure and a wide range of programs — some of which are not even obvious now.

To accomplish this, we need an active federal government. And we need it soon.

Omaha World-Herald
Omaha, NE, June 3, 1987

THE ATLANTA CONSTITUTION
Atlanta, GA, June 5, 1987

President Reagan announced two sensible responses recently to AIDS: The mandatory testing of federal prisoners (the same should be done in state and local lockups, too, so the infected population could be segregated and the others protected) and the addition of AIDS to the list of contagious diseases for which immigrants and aliens can be denied entry to this country.

But in his zeal to step up testing of other groups, Reagan continues to confuses morality — and a dubious, homophobic morality, at that — with medical practice.

The president now proposes to "routinely offer" the costly test to marriage license applicants and Veterans Administration hospital patients. That is a welcome and substantial softening of his earlier call for widespread mandatory testing, but it would be a questionable use of funds even so.

The payoff is likely to be slight, given the low incidence of homosexuals and intravenous drug users applying for marriage licenses or checking into veterans' hospitals. (These are still the most vulnerable groups, though AIDS is now spreading more rapidly among heterosexuals than among homosexuals.) And testing could be counterproductive if it becomes standard — without absolute guarantees of confidentiality and protection from discrimination.

In fact, the prospect of testing has already emboldened homophobes, like Conservative Caucus Chairman Howard Phillips, to speak openly of quarantines — the surest possible means of dissuading those at risk from any action, such as voluntarily taking the test, that might identify them.

"I say there should be a stigma attached to homosexual behavior, it's an abomination," thunders Phillips, seemingly unconcerned about the loss of gay lives — or the potential for saving them through counseling, voluntary testing, strict confidentiality and the teaching of safe sex.

These must be the centerpieces of any serious strategy for combating AIDS, as Surgeon General C. Everett Koop maintains and as Vice President George Bush seemed to recognize Monday in a speech calling for "an all-out war against the disease ... not the victims." Yet they are things to which the Reagan administration gives short shrift.

Perhaps it was inevitable that AIDS would take its place along with Central America and nuclear power as an issue that generates shrill rhetoric and street demonstrations. Almost since the day the disease was identified and given a name, some of the spokesmen for victims and homosexual rights groups have cast the matter as a confrontation between their organizations and the U.S. government, or American society in general.

At times, the rhetoric has descended to the level of nonsense. At a fund-raising walk for AIDS research in Massachusetts Sunday, Gerry Studds, a homosexual and member of Congress from Massachusetts, praised the participants, saying that they were doing a job that the government should be doing. Perhaps no one told him that President Reagan was speaking the same day at a fund-raising dinner for the American Foundation for AIDS Research in Washington. The event in Massachusetts raised $500,000. The dinner at which Reagan spoke raised $1.5 million.

Too seldom is it mentioned, moreover, that the government is spending $400 million this year in search of a cure for AIDS and that federal spending may reach $900 million next year. Reasonable people might disagree over a few million dollars one way or the other, but this year's expenditures and next year's projected expenditures aren't exactly piddling amounts, considering that the government is under a mandate to reduce deficit spending.

Reasonable people might also disagree about what conditions would be appropriate for mandatory testing. But federal immigration law bars the admission of "aliens afflicted with a dangerous, contagious disease." It would be patently illogical to turn away prospective immigrants with tuberculosis, which can be treated, while failing to test for AIDS, for which no known cure exists.

Likewise, it would be illogical for federal prison officials to screen inmates for other things that can be transmitted from prisoner to prisoner, from head lice to ringworm, while failing to screen for AIDS.

Yet Reagan was booed at the fund-raising dinner Sunday when he proposed testing immigrants and federal prisoners for the virus. Surgeon General C. Everett Koop, who opposes mandatory testing, said he had no objection to the Reagan proposals.

The government's role in the battle against AIDS is the public's business. The use of testing deserves debate, as do the appropriate level of spending and the role of education. It would be too bad if a civilized debate were drowned out by the boos and catcalls of a group that, for reasons of its own, demands to have this dangerous, communicable disease treated differently from other dangerous, communicable diseases.

The Salt Lake Tribune
Salt Lake City, UT, June 10, 1987

President Reagan, one day, called for "urgency, not panic . . . compassion, not blame" in the fight against acquired immune deficiency syndrome. A day later, Washington police officers donned plastic gloves before breaking up a demonstration of gay activists in Lafayette Park across the street from the White House.

Sadly, the president's message didn't even get through to constituents in the capital of the country he leads. The situation only confirms the need to intensify AIDS education efforts.

Scientists are quite satisfied that the AIDS virus is not spread through casual contact. Transmission, they agree, is conducted primarily by sexual intercourse, the sharing of dirty needles and blood transfusions. Even hospital workers exposed to the blood of AIDS patients have only a remote risk of infection.

Lending credence to the misconception that AIDS can be acquired through touch, as Washington police did, does not convey the compassion President Reagan encouraged. Rather, it further stigmatizes and shows contempt for the victims and high-risk groups.

Instead of calming the public, as was their responsibility, those law enforcement officers contributed to the kind of irrational alarm that will prevent, instead of foster, solutions to the AIDS problem.

Panic-driven public policies undoubtedly would be enacted at the expense of the facts and personal rights. If some AIDS victims are treated irresponsibly — unnecessarily fired from jobs, quarantined or otherwise discriminated against — others with a high risk of infection will refuse to cooperate with public health officials in testing for the disease. And it will be that much more difficult to control its spread.

With the Washington Police Department flaunting its ignorance of the facts only hours after President Reagan tried to put the AIDS crisis into perspective, there's obviously a critical need for the nation to learn more about the threat and how best to cope with it. If scrupulously and immediately supported with money and action, the administration's promise to "wage an all-out war against the disease, not against people" will help.

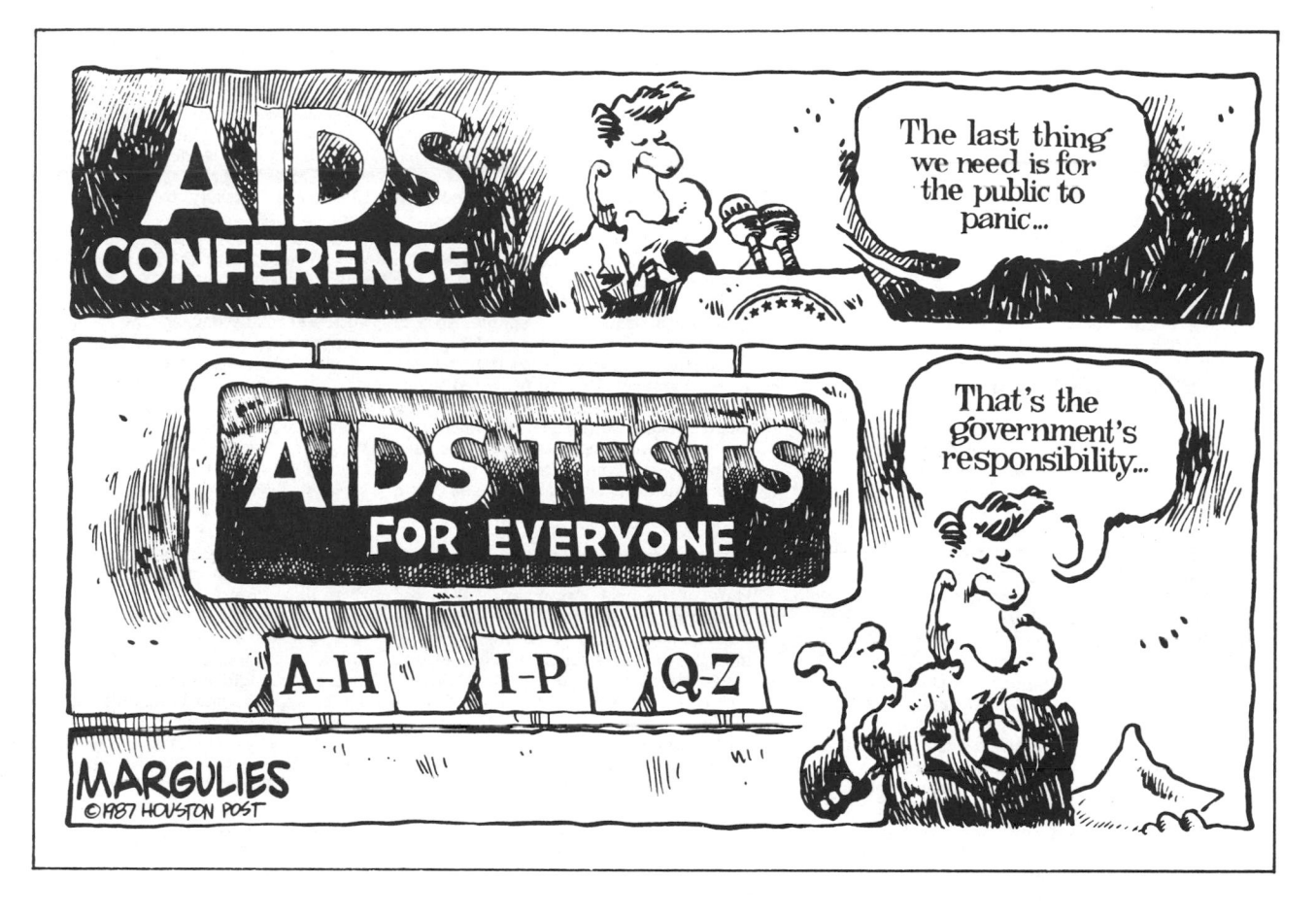

TULSA WORLD

Tulsa, OK, June 6, 1987

ON one hand, homosexuals want to portray the AIDS epidemic as having "crossed over" into the heterosexual population; thus, the dread disease is the business of everyone; no longer can "straights" smugly refuse to worry about gays and their problems.

On the other hand, however, homosexuals fight every effort to identify those carrying the AIDS virus. Such identification through testing, they contend, would be ineffectual. Testing, they fear would discriminate against gays and lead to further stigma for homosexuals.

Now, AIDS is either a disease affecting the general heterosexual community or it isn't. It is, of course, although most publicity as to the extent of the "crossover" appears to be highly exaggerated.

While gay leaders were complimenting Gov. Henry Bellmon on vetoing a bill that would have required testing of some high-risk citizens for AIDS, at least two articles appeared in the same edition of the Tulsa World with impressive arguments to the effect that AIDS still is primarily a disease of the homosexual world and drug users.

This is not to suggest that AIDS is not one of the most horrifying health problems of the 20th century.

But homosexuals cannot have it both ways on this issue. If AIDS had remained a disease peculiar to gays, cries of discrimination and unfair treatment should have been taken seriously.

But now that it is clear that AIDS threatens heterosexuals and conceivably is a danger and economic burden to everyone, then society has the right to treat it like it has treated dread, communicable diseases of the past.

That might mean mandatory testing and steps to protect the uninfected from the infected. Unfortunately, there is a stigma that will accompany those infected — be they homosexual or heterosexual. But there was a time when that was true of citizens with typhoid, diphtheria, even cancer.

Attitudes change and they are changing about AIDS. But the immediate question that should remain before the public — regardless of attitudes — is whether society can do what is medically feasible to protect itself from a dread disease.

In every other instance of the past, the answer has been yes.

The Seattle Times

Seattle, WA, June 2, 1987

MANDATORY testing of the general population for the AIDS antibody is a bad idea whose time, one hopes, will never come. Yet there is merit in the expansion of compulsory testing to select groups under federal jurisdiction, as urged by President Reagan the other day.

Universal AIDS screening should be dropped from consideration for a number of reasons, including the fact that facilities for such mass testing do not exist. To put such a program in place would amount to pouring a vast amount of resources into an unworkable program.

Many of the high-risk invididuals who are of prime concern would not only find means of avoiding testing, but would be driven away from the counseling and treatment of which they stand in greatest need.

In addition, of course, any attempt to apply compulsory measures to the general public would involve complex and agonizing civil-rights issues.

Yet Reagan's request that AIDS be added to the list of diseases for which immigrants can be denied permanent-resident status in the United States, and his call upon the Justice Department to plan for the "routine testing" of all federal prisoners, are, as Surgeon General C. Everett Koop put it, "eminently reasonable." Koop is opposed to any push toward universal testing.

Immigration law has long listed the presence of "a dangerous contagious disease" in an applicant as grounds for denying permanent-resident status. AIDS obviously is such a disease.

As for the prisoners, their status automatically consigns them to categories both of limited rights and of higher-than-normal risk of AIDS.

Wider screening is needed to learn more about the deadly disease. AIDS-virus testing of applicants for military service already has yielded valuable information. Testing of immigrants and prisoners would add to that knowledge.

For the nation as a whole, a three-sided response to the AIDS menace is in order: expanded research in seeking a cure, highly amplified public education as to safe sex practices, and voluntary confidential testing, accompanied by sympathetic professional counseling.

Newsday

Long Island, NY, June 2, 1987

It was in 1981 that the Centers for Disease Control first diagnosed AIDS as a major threat. Since then, 35,518 people in the United States, including 3,307 in San Francisco and 10,332 in New York City, are reported to have come down with AIDS. By 1991, it is predicted, 1 million people in New York City alone will harbor the virus. Last fall the surgeon general issued an AIDS report unprecedented in urgency and detail. Yesterday in Washington the World Health Organization's Third International Conference on AIDS opened — the most heavily attended AIDS parley to date. Next week, at the western economic summit in Italy, AIDS will be at the top of the agenda.

Against this backdrop, President Ronald Reagan on Sunday made his first public statement devoted wholly to the AIDS issue. His speech was as short on inspiration as it was long in coming. Perhaps the president was simply out of his depth, but the complexities of the epidemic were just not addressed. Reagan was vague or uninformative in areas where presidential leadership could prove extremely helpful (such as a big federal push on AIDS education). And when he did get down to cases (on the now-politicized issue of AIDS testing, for instance), one somehow wished that he hadn't strayed from generalities.

Testing is no end in itself but a means to an end: epidemic control. Regrettably, the president offered no hint as to where testing might lead. Nevertheless he proposed testing all Americans planning to get married, all foreigners applying for permanent residency and all prisoners — a curious list. Perhaps his pitch was meant to sate the appetite of conservatives (who seem to want to test everybody) while not seriously offending health professionals. They argue that testing is best targeted at the at-risk population (e.g., intravenous drug users and homosexuals, who must be helped to cope with the reality of their medical problem — and to avoid spreading the disease to others).

If an AIDS test could pave the way toward a cure-all — if there were some medicine to prevent those who test positive from infecting others — then widespread mandatory testing would be defensible. But until a genius comes along with a Salk-like vaccine for AIDS, the only hope against this epidemic is preventive medicine. A dual and nuanced approach — to educate the general population and to test and counsel, with guarantees of total confidentiality, the at-risk population — is at the moment the only honest prescription.

THE CHRISTIAN SCIENCE MONITOR

Boston, MA, June 2, 1987

AIDS has become a public policy issue of wide currency. But care should be taken that the official response not overwhelm the rights of individuals to privacy in health, occupational, and other matters.

Without doubt, the burden in personal suffering and in economic and health service demands has contributed to the political saliency of the issue, requiring government leaders to respond. AIDS is the subject of a five-day conference in Washington this week, at a fundraiser for which President Reagan proposed wider testing for the disease among immigrants, aliens seeking permanent residence, federal prison inmates, patients in veterans' hospitals, and couples seeking marriage. AIDS policies will be on the agenda of the seven-nation Western economic summit in Venice next week.

At the more extreme end of political response, the conservative West German state of Bavaria last month called for regular quarterly testing for AIDS among male homosexuals, prostitutes, intravenous drug abusers, and foreigners seeking visas. Elsewhere as in the United States, "education" programs are proposed, with mailings of information about the disease, its transmission and prevention.

The Reagan administration as a whole has been rather slow to react, whether in terms of funding for research or in formulating a comprehensive response. It has hesitated to follow the more vigorous lead of its own surgeon general, C. Everett Koop, out of fear of appearing to condone nonmarital sexual relations by advocating prophylactic measures. The administration's tendency to treat AIDS sufferers as culprits rather than as victims led it initially to consider vastly wider testing.

Because testing is not foolproof, widespread mandatory testing could lead to false "positive" results for as many as one-fourth of those tested, critics say, with potentially devastating employment or personal consequences. To the health issue of AIDS would be added the intrusive and oppressive posture of government, which could lead many citizens to avoid public health officials entirely. Voluntary testing programs – which are favored by many health officials – would be less effective if citizens feared their privacy would be violated.

Room should be maintained for individual response. For some citizens, abstinence from sexual relations outside marriage, or a voluntary test before marriage, seems the obvious recourse for protection. For some who believe an intense public focus on disease is itself unhealthy, information and educational campaigns can be kept to what is required to assure an informed citizenry. For some who believe that the individual is not helpless even before a generalized health threat, the public clamor over AIDS should underscore the need to keep thought, practices, and conduct in line with their conviction, so as to support the general resistance to the challenge as well as their own exemption.

THE TENNESSEAN

Nashville, TN, June 3, 1987

IN his first major speech on the acquired immune deficiency syndrome, President Ronald Reagan said the AIDS epidemic "calls for urgency, not panic" but his answer was expanded testing and little else.

Some boos were heard in the audience of the American Foundation for AIDS Research, when he said he was asking that AIDS be added to the list of diseases for which immigrants can be denied permanent residence status.

Mr. Reagan also encouraged states to offer routine testing for those who seek marriage licenses and for those who visit sexually transmitted disease or drug abuse clinics, as well as local prison populations. He said he had asked the Justice Department to plan for required testing in the federal prisons.

Although Mr. Reagan didn't call for mandatory testing, he did call for increased testing. That should be done with great care. Testing itself is not a guaranteed procedure. Between the time of exposure and time when the virus is present in blood levels is uncertain. One might test negative at the time and then after a few weeks or months become positive. Yet that person would assume that everything was just dandy and continue on with past sexual practices.

Although Mr. Reagan mentioned Surgeon General Everett Koop, he avoiding getting into some of the surgeon general's recommendations, such as education of the general public and the use of condoms.

It would have been better had the President publicly embraced a measure introduced by Sen. Edward Kennedy, which calls for spending some $900 million on AIDs. It would increase education on the disease, recruit and train more medical personnel and let AIDS victims be treated at home.

Mr. Reagan is right in saying the epidemic "calls for urgency." Testing may be necessary in some specific cases, but it should be used in conjunction with education, particularly education on ways to avoid sexual transmission. There should also be a greater and immediate expenditure of funds by the government, as well as from private sources. It is an urgent problem and it requires a broad range of ways to deal with it. ■

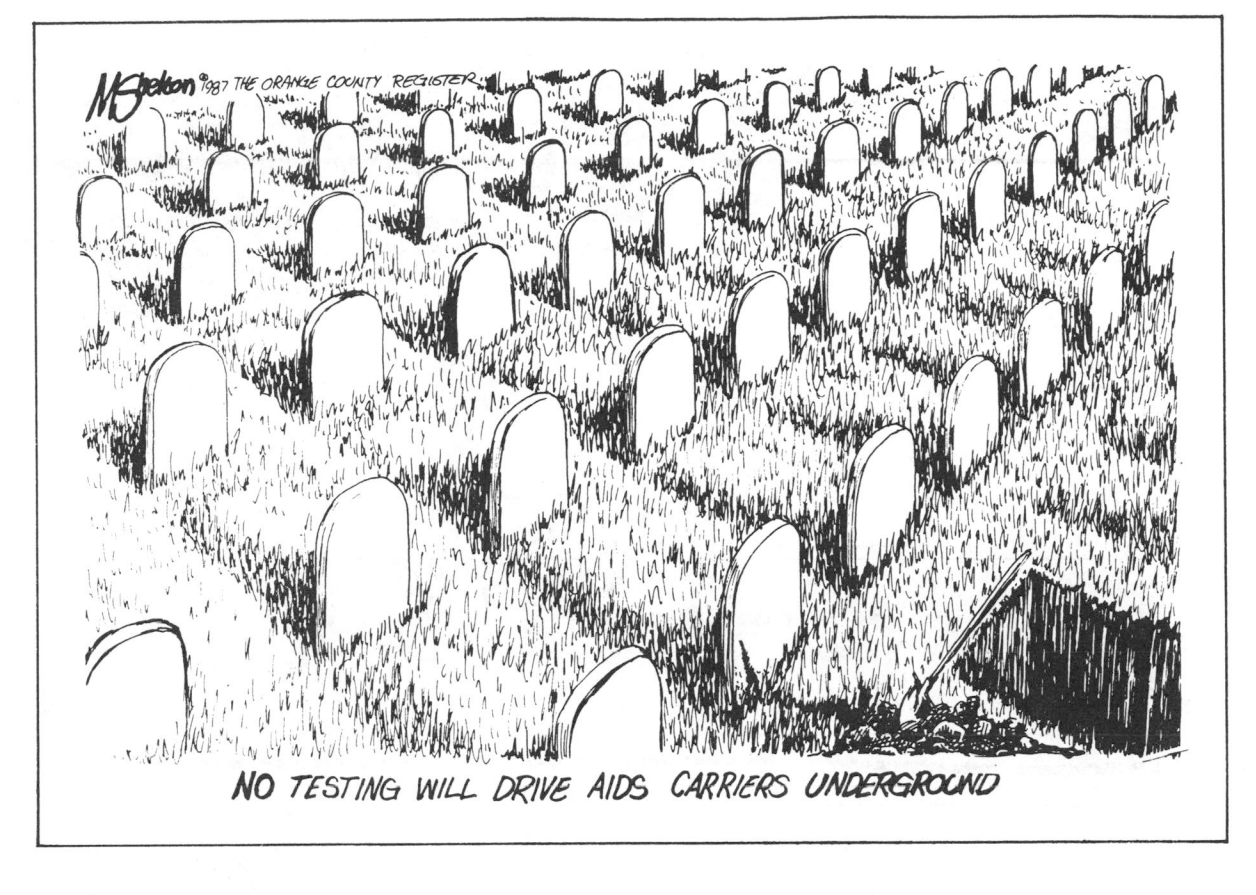

NO TESTING WILL DRIVE AIDS CARRIERS UNDERGROUND

The Evening Gazette

Worcester, MA, June 12, 1987

The storm of protest that has met the Reagan administration's new policy on testing for acquired immune deficiency syndrome illustrates the difficulty of separating the science of AIDS from the politics of AIDS.

The administration endorsed a limited program of testing for certain groups, including immigrants and federal prisoners, and recommended that states include AIDS screening in pre-marital blood tests. The policy on immigrants and prisoners was spelled out this week by Attorney General Edwin Meese.

Although some have dismissed the recommendations as a political ploy, the scientific value of testing is beyond dispute. If nothing else, it would provide a valuable epidemiological data base for understanding and tracking AIDS, even if no cure is yet available.

Yet, it was the political aspects of AIDS, not the thousands of scientific papers on virology, epidemiology, drug treatments and vaccine development, that took center stage at the Third International Conference on AIDS in Washington, D.C. last week. Even some public health professionals who generally favor broad testing criticized the mandatory testing urged in the administration policy.

Fears have been raised that testing might lead to infringements on the civil rights of infected people, including the registering of victims, restrictions on travel rights and even quarantining.

But testing itself could actually benefit victims of the disease. Most people infected with AIDS are not aware they have the disease, since the slow-working virus may take seven years or more to produce symptoms. At the very least, testing would enable AIDS victims to seek early treatment and to avoid spreading the virus.

Clearly, guarding the civil rights of AIDS victims must be an integral part of any national policy. But no one is served by attempts to downplay uncomfortable truths about AIDS — including the fact that its spread in the United States has been associated primarily with a promiscuous homosexual lifestyle — that run counter to the social agendas of some advocacy groups.

Denial of the facts about AIDS, from whatever motivation, poses an obstacle to devising a fair, workable national policy to combat the disease. The administration's limited-testing policy falls far short of being a comprehensive solution, but it is a responsible step in the right direction.

The News and Courier
CHARLESTON EVENING POST
Charleston, SC, June 6, 1987

Participants in the Third International Conference on AIDS, which was held recently in Washington, have called on world leaders at next week's seven-nation economic summit in Venice to endorse a coordinated global campaign against AIDS. They noted that the AIDS virus already has killed 51,535 people worldwide and has infected as many as 10 million more.

A spokesman for the World Health Organization urged the government leaders to establish an AIDS trust fund that would help economically strapped countries, particularly those in Africa. Such a fund makes sense. There is no question that the fight against AIDS will be expensive, and a well-managed trust fund that targets the African continent would be in everyone's best interest.

However, the United States should not be expected to carry the lion's share of the expense as it has in so many other international humanitarian endeavors. As many as 400,000 people in the United States will contract AIDS by 1991, according to a study commissioned by the U.S. Health Care Financing Administration. Costs of treating those patients could well exceed $37 billion for the five-year period from mid-1986 to mid-1991, according to the study. About a third of the AIDS-related medical costs are expected to be borne by Medicaid, with private insurance companies and state and local governments covering the remainder.

AIDS will consume about 1 percent of the total national health spending by 1991 and about 3 percent of Medicaid costs, researchers say. The question that must soon be answered in this country is how the burden will be distributed among taxpayers, employers, employees (through health insurance premiums) and AIDS patients. While it may be prudent for the United States to assist in establishing a world trust fund to help fight AIDS in Africa and elsewhere, it would be foolish to do so at the expense of the national effort that is sure to come.

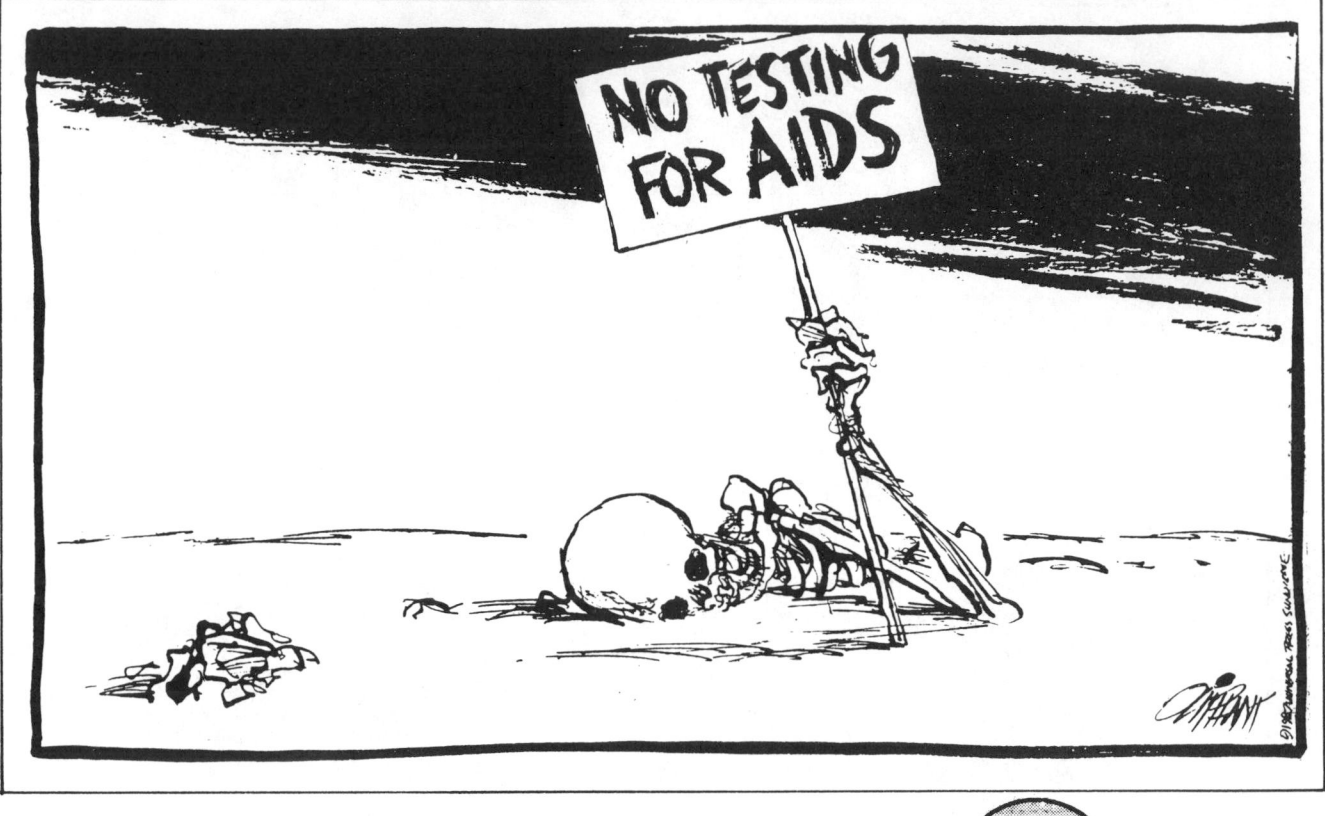

The Birmingham News

Birmingham, AL, June 4, 1987

President Reagan drew mixed reviews earlier this week when he called for mandatory AIDS testing of all federal prisoners and those seeking to immigrate to the U.S. We thought his plan a good one, and Tuesday the U.S. Senate concurred.

As part of a supplemental appropriation bill, the senators voted 96-0 to have the president add AIDS to the government's list of dangerous contagious diseases and to require that immigrants be tested for it before being allowed to come to the U.S.

The Senate and the president are wise to be cautious about the deadly AIDS virus. At present, AIDS is 100 percent fatal and it is spreading beyond those groups which first seemed most vulnerable to it. AIDS is no longer a disease of only homosexuals or those who inject drugs.

Testing will not "cure" the disease. It is no substitute for scientific research or for counseling and care. But it may help slow the spread of AIDS. The AIDS virus requires a very long incubation period. It may be years before the disease begins to take it toll. In the meantime, a person may be infected and not know it and may be spreading AIDS to others.

Calling for testing of federal prisoners and immigrants is hardly unreasonable. Those prisoners are in the custody and care of the federal government. The federal government is responsible for their health. When a person seeks to take up residence in this country, we ought to know if he will bring with him a dangerous disease — whether it's AIDS or others the government has long tested for, such as tuberculosis.

The president also recommended that AIDS tests be given by state governments to those who apply for a marriage license. There is ample precedent for that. Many states, such as Alabama, have long tested for venereal diseases as part of the license granting process.

The Alabama Legislature should consider requiring such tests, but it should also consider how to follow up on the testing. Will those who test positive be advised of the incidence of "false positive" tests and be given additional tests? Will those who truly have the AIDS virus be directed to appropriate health care and counseling? How will the confidentiality of the tests be protected? The testing must be handled responsibly.

We hope the continuing, intensive AIDS research program will someday point to a way of curing or controlling the killer disease. In the meantime, all we can do is show compassion for its unfortunate victims and take reasonable, precautionary steps like those directed by the president and the Senate.

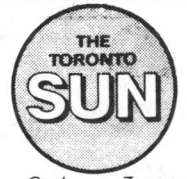

THE TORONTO SUN

Toronto, Ont., June 2, 1987

Let's state it clearly: Testing for AIDS, especially among high-risk groups, isn't an infringement of anyone's civil or human rights.

It's a basic step toward guaranteeing that the rights of *all* citizens are protected. Just as when tests for TB or VD are carried out, as they have been for decades.

Society has rights too!

The fundamental idea is to prevent the spread of devastating diseases — which AIDS certainly is.

A "star-studded" audience booed Ronald Reagan on Sunday when he announced a plan to test millions.

Clearly they equate AIDS bashing to gay bashing. Wrong! This "liberal" attitude risks lives.

The president might have expected more understanding from an audience donating funds for AIDS research. They know that AIDS is contagious, incurable and always fatal.

Reagan's plan calls for testing immigrants, prisoners and applicants for marriage licences. Sound ideas.

Canadian authorities should follow the U.S. lead.

True, the spread of the disease here is less dramatic than in the U.S. where 20,000 people have died.

Only 500 have died here. But we'd be fools to wait till it's as bad here as south of the border before launching an all-out drive to find a cure.

We test would-be immigrants for tuberculosis, a disease that's far less threatening now than AIDS.

Many states wisely test persons wishing to marry for VD as a condition for receiving a licence. Yet most potentially fatal forms of VD are curable.

Until there's a cure for AIDS, governments must spare no expense backing the necessary research.

We just can't bury our heads in a trendy dune.

Right on Reagan's front door, the largest-ever conference on AIDS began yesterday.

The best promise that's emerged so far is a vaccine to prevent acquired immune deficiency syndrome by the mid-1990s.

Meanwhile, countless millions of lives are in danger.

The AIDS virus plays no favorites. Once it's in the bloodstream, the lethal work begins — regardless of race, creed, sex or sexual preference.

The Honolulu Advertiser
Honolulu, HI, June 2, 1987

The AIDS testing question is going to severely challenge our ability to balance public health and civil liberties with compassion and common sense.

It's no surprise President Reagan is for routine, mandatory testing. His administration's response to the drug crisis is testing and to security leaks it's lie detectors and loyalty oaths.

But a key question about mandatory AIDS testing is: What will be done with the results? Vice President Bush yesterday said testing must be accompanied by confidentiality and non-discrimination, stipulations Reagan notably omitted from his speech plugging mandatory testing at an AIDS fundraiser Sunday.

But realistically, what's the point of required testing if no action is taken on results?

For example, if all marriage license applicants are tested, will those found positive be denied the right to wed? Can they be prevented from having sex without a license?

It's important to realize the limited usefulness of mandatory testing, even without questions about the tests' reliability. If testing is mandatory, some with reason to fear a positive result will avoid testing situations rather than face the repercussions.

Mandatory testing has its place for those in prison, the military, the foreign service and would-be immigrants, especially those who might be in highly vulnerable groups. In such cases, in so far as possible, AIDS should be treated like other communicable diseases, with clearly defined responses to positive results designed to help the victim and protect others.

Also, voluntary testing with stringent privacy protection should be widely available. People who take a test voluntarily are more likely to be responsible about safe sex if found positive than those caught in ever-wider mandatory testing programs.

Over-broad testing has another danger. AIDS resources are always limited and putting the priority on expensive testing will inevitably drain funds better used for research and education.

A cure is the ultimate solution to the AIDS dilemma. Teaching people to protect themselves and avoid passing the virus is next best, and in the absence of a foreseeable cure, the most important right now. Trying to find out who has AIDS, with the inevitable dangers of discrimination and stigmatization this entails, is a poor third.

Detroit Free Press
Detroit, MI, June 9, 1987

DR. OTIS BOWEN, secretary of Health and Human Services, heard booing and hissing and saw many people turn their backs on him as he addressed an international conference on AIDS last week. The federal AIDS testing plan that the secretary announced from the speaker's platform deserved a warmer reception.

The government's plan to test 45,000 randomly selected Americans is as good as testing plans come. It would be absolutely voluntary and strictly confidential. Statistical analysis of the tests' results could produce some of the critical information that epidemiologists, striving to curb the spread of the disease, now lack.

As outlined by Dr. Bowen, the program does not appear to violate our liberties; it certainly doesn't offend our sense of fairness and civic decency. The only question is whether the government can develop guidelines and procedures for the actual testing that would make the program as foolproof as originally presented.

The protesters, who included defenders of homosexual rights and critics of the Reagan administration's policies in general, insisted that the government should focus on finding a cure for the disease instead of trying to monitor its victims. The critics have a point when they warn against fanning homophobia, already disturbingly evident in places when AIDS has become a major public health problem. Those who oppose random testing, however, fail to realize that it is uncertainty stemming from the lack of reliable statistics on AIDS that makes the public nervous in the first place.

Publicly funded research to find a cure for the disease must be accompanied by vigorous public efforts to protect as many people as possible from contracting it. Studying the spreading pattern of AIDS is one of the most urgent tasks that our health officials face today.

THE ANN ARBOR NEWS
Ann Arbor, MI, June 11, 1987

As with any war, the objective is to know the nature of the enemy and then wipe him out. Knowledge, or in the case of war, intelligence-gathering, will do that.

With AIDS, ignorance only feeds an incipient public panic. The perception of AIDS as a disease of homosexuals, drug users and prostitutes tends to show how far perception is removed from reality, as news reports chronicle the slow march of AIDS into the ranks of heterosexuals.

Knowledge about AIDS begins with the certainty that this is not some 20th century equivalent of the Black Death. The Black Death in Europe so many centuries ago killed indiscriminately; AIDS is largely controllable because behavior — sexual behavior — is controllable.

No battle plan against AIDS is complete without behavior counseling programs. And let's face it, the temptation to moralize about AIDS while administering behavior counseling is going to be strong. But moralizing about AIDS will be just so much after-the-fact scolding unless it is accompanied by care and compassion toward AIDS victims.

"We must not," said President Reagan, "allow those with the AIDS virus to suffer discrimination." It follows that doctors who take the Hippocratic Oath seriously will not refuse to treat AIDS victims.

President Reagan used his recent speech on AIDS to call for "routine testing" of immigrants, federal prisoners, patients being treated for drug abuse and sexually transmitted diseases and applicants for marriage licenses. The controversy is over what Reagan meant by "routine." In this case, it appears he means "mandatory."

The president's administration is badly divided on the issue. Education Secretary William J. Bennett and presidential policy adviser Gary L. Bauer have called repeatedly for mandatory testing.

They argue that the interests of those not currently infected with the AIDS virus outweigh anyone's right to privacy, and that the nation urgently needs to know exactly how many people are carrying the virus.

The other position is taken by Health and Human Services Secretary Otis R. Bowen and Surgeon General C. Everett Koop. They argue that mandatory testing would drive underground those who are most likely to be carrying the disease and that testing low-risk groups would waste precious resources.

The privacy aspect is pivotal. Does anyone, asks columnist William Safire, have the right to refuse to find out whether he or she has AIDS? Does anybody have the right to have this disease without telling anybody else about it?

It sounds like something for the American Civil Liberties Union to take up in earnest, except that we're talking epidemic here and lengthy, inconclusive debates over mandatory versus voluntary testing do not serve a rising public health emergency.

Testing alone won't defeat AIDS. It can, of course, help to identify people who register positive that they may be carriers of the virus. Testing also adds to the epidemiologists' store of knowledge in tracking the spreading pattern of AIDS.

As always, education is the key. We have to get word to children and young people who are sexually active that promiscuous sex can be deadly and that AIDS may lurk in any sleeping partner whose sexual history is unshared information.

High-risk groups need behavior counseling. Accurate, forthright AIDS information needs wide circulation among junior high and high school students. Medical science needs to do research. The government and the drug companies need to feel the urgency of developing a vaccine. The public needs to keep its cool.

Testing has its benefits, but it puts the cart before the horse in that it only determines where the damage has been done instead of focusing on education in the beginning and a cure at the end. Testing is a one-front war when the situation clearly calls for a multi-front campaign.

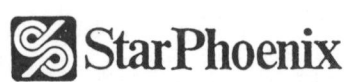

Saskatoon, Sask., June 6, 1987

With each day, more evidence mounts on the growing threat of acquired immune deficiency syndrome (AIDS) and the drastic impact the deadly disease is having on people all over the world.

Like all major issues, the debate over AIDS and how to slow its spread is often marked by extremes. In Calgary, two entrepreneurs who advertised plans to open an "AIDS-free" private club were swamped with more than 300 applications in just three days. Each applicant appeared willing to pay about $300 for a membership and submit to regular AIDS tests in return for the opportunity to meet others free of the disease.

In reality, the promoters and the potential club members are fooling themselves by pretending they can avoid the disease and shut out the rest of the world. As various AIDS support groups point out, the test for the AIDS virus is only good on the day it is conducted. Unless daily tests are required, it can never be guaranteed that no club members will have the disease. Indeed, liberal sexual conduct which might result from the presumption that all members are AIDS-free could actually mean the disease will infect and spread among members more rapidly than among the general population.

But while the Calgary proposal illustrates a desperate fear of AIDS, others almost casually disregard the risks and court illness and death by exposing themselves to known carriers. For example, thousands of Quebec business executives and office workers annually flock to the French-speaking Caribbean island of Haiti for a vacation filled with sun and sex. The island has legal prostitution and visitors intent on living out sexual fantasies can have their choice of partners from huge red light districts. Although it is well known that at least half, and perhaps as many as two-thirds, of Haiti's prostitutes carry the AIDS virus, business continues to boom. As a result, the killer disease comes to Canada in even greater numbers each year.

Somewhere between such extremes is where the proper approach to dealing with AIDS lies. Sticking our heads in the sand and pretending the disease can be avoided does as little to help check its spread as does liberal carousing with little thought of the attendant risks.

World Health Organization officials estimate as many as 10 million people may be infected with AIDS and they say the epidemic has just begun. Panic won't serve any useful purpose, but it's clear public education and abundant precautions are in order, together with ongoing support of research into ways to combat this killer disease.

The Oregonian

Portland, OR, June 7, 1987

President Reagan should resist temptation and listen to his White House adviser Gary Bauer and not his old Hollywood friend Elizabeth Taylor.

Taylor, actress and national chairman of the American Foundation for AIDS Research, has joined gay rights advocates in demanding that Reagan specifically appoint a homosexual to his national commission on AIDS. Bauer, in putting together the commission for the president, has resisted calls for the creation of a special gay seat — or special seats for anti-gay or other groups that might want representation.

Instead of a commission that includes every possible group interested in the AIDS problem, Bauer is working to assemble a group of 10 to 12 thoughtful citizens who can periodically advise the president on AIDS public policy questions. The commission will make no policy and will present the president with recommendations or a mix of competing recommendations, depending on the level of consensus in the group.

Bauer envisions a commission made up of, among others, medical experts who have worked directly with AIDS, child development specialists with experience in teen-age sexuality, and even ethicists who can sort out the ethical implications of various AIDS matters.

Proponents of specially designated gay representation on the presidential commission correctly argue that AIDS is a predominantly homosexual affliction and that the homosexual perspective is necessary. They incorrectly conclude that only a designated homosexual commission member can assure the kind of understanding necessary.

Would a special seat therefore be needed for other affected groups — intravenous drug users, for instance? Of course not. There is no lack of available information on the particular dynamics of such worlds or experts for the commission to draw on.

But neither should a homosexual be explicitly excluded from the commission, and the White House maintains that it has never inquired into the sexual preferences of possible appointees. That's as it should be.

A disinterested weighing of public policy options is needed in the face of this scourge. A commission of individuals committed to exploring AIDS issues with depth and sensitivity can provide this. A commission of special representatives from gay groups or anti-gay groups is likely to degenerate into a politicized and quarrelsome debating society that at best becomes irrelevant.

DAYTON DAILY NEWS
Dayton, OH, June 10, 1987

The other groups that some have said should be subject to mandatory tests are those who visit drug treatment centers and clinics for sexually transmitted diseases.

Testing for these people should be voluntary.

Although these are precisely the persons who are most likely to have AIDS, if an AIDS test were required as a condition for treatment, a lot of addicts and prostitutes wouldn't seek help for their health problems.

It's generally recognized that people with substance-abuse and behavioral problems have to want help before it can be given effectively. They probably need to want help and counseling about AIDS, too, if it's to matter much. Moreover, some studies show that some addicts were more reckless after they were told that they had AIDS than before. Without counseling that gets through to people, testing won't stop the AIDS epidemic.

Education about AIDS and tests for it need to be easy to get at these centers, but society has to understand that not everyone responds to offers of help in the same way. Strategies to fight AIDS have to be crafted according to whom the professionals are trying to reach.

THE DAILY OKLAHOMAN
Oklahoma City, OK, June 2, 1987

TO test or not to test has developed into one of the major controversies in the whole business of dealing with the AIDS epidemic.

President Reagan drew scattered boos from the audience when he told a fundraising dinner of the American Foundation for AIDS Research he will seek expanded testing for the disease. He did receive frequent applause, but some listeners took exception to his idea of adding AIDS to the list of diseases for which immigrants can be denied entry or permanent resident status.

He was booed, too, when he said he had asked the Justice Department to plan for requiring testing of all federal prisoners. And he encouraged states to offer routine testing for marriage license applicants and in state and local prisons.

The fact Vice President George Bush also was booed when he spoke later and supported Reagan's plans suggests the hostile reaction was political. It would be unfair to tar all researchers with a single brush but undoubtedly many in the audience were Reagan haters and would oppose almost anything he said.

Another explanation, even less complimentary, would be that the researchers have a selfish pecuniary interest in the government spending its money on their pet projects rather than on a practical testing program to identify and isolate AIDS victims and carriers.

Why all the stir over screening immigrants for AIDS when they are already tested for other diseases that pose considerably less public health danger?

LOS ANGELES HERALD
Los Angeles, CA, June 2, 1987

AIDS finally has the attention of the president. That was obvious from his speech last weekend, in which he called for expanded testing for the infection. What also became clear is that the White House has no plan for confronting this crisis.

Instead of a comprehensive approach to AIDS, the president simply suggested that states offer testing for those wanting to marry and for people seeking treatment in drug abuse and sexually transmitted disease clinics. He also proposed mandatory testing of federal prisoners, patients in veteran hospitals and immigrants.

He's right that prospective spouses, sexually active people and intravenous drug users should have the opportunity to find out if they've been infected with AIDS. It's also not unreasonable to *require* tests for criminals in prison. Whether immigrants should be tested poses far more difficult problems, and the president went off the track in targeting patients in veteran hospitals.

Most troublesome, however, is what the president left out of his speech: If testing is going to be more widespread, those undergoing the exam must be offered counseling and some greater guarantees that the confidentiality of their test results will be protected. If the White House wants to encourage those in high-risk groups and others to come forward to be tested, there must be better protections against AIDS discrimination. If the federal government is committed to staunching the epidemic, the president should boost the current $250 million appropriation to $2 billion.

The president undoubtedly has heard all of these recommendations from public health officials, including his own surgeon general, Everett Koop. In fact, it was probably Koop's influence that toned down what probably would have been a reactionary response engineered by Reagan's health policy adviser, Gary Bauer.

In developing a desperately needed national AIDS strategy, the president would do well to listen more to Koop and other professionals working on the front lines of this epidemic and less to administration operatives like Bauer whose first concern is some ill-advised political agenda.

The Kansas City Times
Kansas City, MO, June 4, 1987

The Senate, led in a sinister way by Jesse Helms, has charged right into an AIDS minefield. When the explosions cease, one may find that very little has been done to curb the spread of Acquired Immune Deficiency Syndrome beyond legislators' "Amens" to presidential sermons. Senators who unanimously approved AIDS testing for immigrants, without forethought of what to do with those who test positive, demonstrated remarkable short-sightedness and an inability to maturely confront a serious global health problem. Rather than approach the AIDS problem sensibly and scientifically, 96 senators merely circled the wagons.

Only now are they asking what, beyond the paperwork involved in restricting legalization, will become of immigrants who test positive for AIDS? What of those who otherwise would qualify for legalization under Simpson-Rodino? Should nations of origin be notified and in detail? Suppose their countries refuse to accept them? Given the Senate's dangerous attitude about such humane concerns, immigrants may as well be put on a barge like the Islip garbage waiting for some nation to accept them.

Sen. Alan K. Simpson has proposed that Congress immediately create a committee to determine what is to be done with AIDS-positive aliens. This laudable plan suffers for its tardiness. Senators should have looked at this idea before they leaped. The House must not mimic the Senate but look beyond its vote. In the meantime, aliens seeking legalization and federal agencies established to work with them are in limbo.

Many of the senators probably approved the proposal with the intent of protecting U.S. citizens from becoming any more susceptible than necessary to the dangerous contagion. But one biased, brazen assumption stands out. The Senate assumes that Americans who travel abroad are less likely to spread AIDS than people who travel here, and that the U.S. citizen who returns does not have it. While it is likely that foreigners have contracted the AIDS virus at home, certainly, given the statistics, some immigrants living in the U.S. have come in contact with Americans with AIDS. Dr. Jonathan Mann, director of the World Health Organization, has warned that realistic approaches to AIDS are being hampered by prejudice about race, religion, social class and nationality. The Senate may verify. The federal government does have a statutory right to protect citizens from dangerous and contagious diseases. But AIDS cannot be cured by politics based on prejudicial hysteria.

Reagan Names AIDS Adviser Panel

President Reagan July 23, 1987 appointed a 13-member commission to advise him on combating AIDS. The panel included Roman Catholic Cardinal John J. O'Connor of New York, an outspoken opponent of explicit AIDS education campaigns and of promotion of the use of condoms, as well as prominent political conservatives and medical professionals who were not generally associated with AIDS treatment research. It included one avowed homosexual.

The medical members included the panel's chairman, Dr. W. Eugene Mayberry, chief executive of the Mayo Clinic. Others were Dr. William Walsh, cofounder of Project Hope, a hospital ship; Dr. Woodrow Myers Jr., the Indiana state health commissioner; Colleen Conway-Welch, dean of nursing at Vanderbilt University; and Dr. Burton Lee III, a New York City cancer specialist. The panel included several outspoken political conservatives: *Saturday Evening Post* publisher Dr. Cory SerVass; Amway Corp. founder Richard De Vos, a prominent Republican fund-raiser; and Rep. Penny Pullen (R, Ill.), an associate of antifeminist activist Phylis Schlafley.

Against the urging of conservatives inside and outside the White House, the panel included one avowed homosexual. He was Dr. Frank Lilly, a geneticist at the Albert Einstein Medical Center in New York City and a chairman of Gay Men's Health Crisis. Lilly said he would endeavor to "forcefully represent the gay community as well as the biomedical community as a member of the commission." Reports in late May that the panel would not include any homosexuals had brought protests from AIDS researchers and gay activists since the disease had first been identified among homosexual men, who remained a primary risk group.

Prominent AIDS researchers expressed puzzlement at the qualifications of some panelists and suggested that the panel had been selected to achieve a political consensus, not to find scientific or medical answers. San Francisco public health official George Rutherford noted that the original pool of candidates had included several people with a track record in AIDS research. The fact that none of them was chosen, he said, seemed "peculiar, and very purposeful." News accounts said the panel was chosen by White House officials with little consultation with the federal AIDS experts. President Reagan said he had relied heavily on the advice of Dr. Richard Davis of Philadelphia, the brother of First Lady Nancy Reagan.

The Record
Hackensack, NJ, July 31, 1987

Here are a few tips on how not to appoint a blue-ribbon panel:

1. Instead of qualified professionals, seek out citizens from widely differing backgrounds with no particular expertise in the area under review.

2. Make sure the panelists adhere to a wide range of philosophies, so that achieving a common point of view is all but impossible.

3. Although the subject may be complex, give panel members only 90 days to come up with a preliminary report.

If you follow these steps one by one and avoid cutting corners, you will come up with something very much like President Reagan's new Advisory Commission on AIDS. Relying heavily on advice from his wife's stepbrother, a Philadelphia physician, Mr. Reagan has assembled a rather motley crew heavily weighted with conservatives. Few of them are qualified to render advice on the most pressing medical emergency of our age.

To ensure ideological incompatability, for instance, the president has enlisted Dr. Frank Lilly, chairman of the genetics department at Albert Einstein Medical College and an acknowledged homosexual, and Cardinal John J. O'Connor, a leading opponent of gay rights. He has also appointed:

● Richard M. De Vos, co-chairman of the Republican Leadership Council, former finance chairman of the Republican National Committee, and co-founder of the Amway Corporation, a sales concern that has been widely criticized for the cultlike loyalty it demands of its employees.

● Cory Servaas, editor and publisher of the Saturday Evening Post, a magazine now devoted to preventive medicine. Last year, Ms. Servaas announced the development of a cure for AIDS using an amino acid called lysine; the anti-viral drug acyclovir, which is used to treat herpes; and various vitamins. No recognized AIDS experts have stepped forward to substantiate Ms. Servaas's report.

● Woodrow A. Myers Jr., Indiana commissioner of health, who is in favor of isolating AIDS carriers who engage in prostitution or drug abuse.

A panel like this can be called many things, but an effective, productive commission is not one of them. Any AIDS panel that includes Cardinal O'Connor can hardly be expected to be sympathetic to gays, the chief victims of the disease. One that includes both the cardinal and Dr. Lilly, a former member of the board of the Gay Men's Health Crisis, is likely to be at loggerheads. Actually, the commission is a reflection of the Reagan administration's confusion over how to handle the AIDS problem. It seems torn between relatively enlightened voices such as Surgeon-General C. Everett Koop and hard-line rightists for whom any suggestion of safe sex for homosexuals is anathema.

Unfortunately, while the Reagan administration dithers, thousands of AIDS victims, most of them gay men, die. The president's new AIDS commission may well be part of the problem, not part of the solution.

The Burlington Free Press
Burlington, VT, July 30, 1987

Eyebrows went up when President Reagan announced two of his appointees to the new AIDS commission.

Wisely, we think, Reagan rejected the hysterical opposition from the political right by choosing Dr. Frank Lilly, an acknowledged homosexual, as one of the panel's 13 members.

Also named to the committee — the proper name is the Commission on the Human Immunodeficiency Virus Epidemic —was New York's Cardinal John O'Connor, an outspoken opponent of homosexuality.

There are those who say Reagan bowed to political pressure from the left by selecting Lilly. Let's understand two things: 1) Lilly as head of the Department of Genetics at the Albert Einstein College of Medicine in New York is supremely qualified; his appointment should not be regarded as a token gesture to the gay community although representation by at least one homosexual on the panel was certainly appropriate; and 2) the panel's purpose is to study the status of research on AIDS rather than to make judgments about the lifestyles of homosexuals.

So why was O'Connor named to the group? Like many Catholics, O'Connor objects to homosexuality on religious grounds. Still, O'Connor's diocese has provided medical care to many homosexuals who suffer from AIDS. He brings another informed view to the panel.

Reagan also deserves praise for something else he did last week: He held an AIDS baby in his arms. By doing so, Reagan sent the clear message that the rumors concerning the spread of AIDS are false. It was a gesture of compassion, and perhaps more than any speech or report can help ease the hysteria about AIDS.

Late though Reagan may have been in recognizing AIDS as a national problem, it is appropriate to applaud his interest and welcome his leadership.

The Washington Post

Washington, DC, July 25, 1987

DR. FRANK LILLY, head of the Department of Genetics at the Albert Einstein College of Medicine in New York, is an expert on biomedical research. He is also an acknowledged homosexual and a founding member of the Gay Men's Health Crisis Center. On Thursday, President Reagan appointed him to the newly constituted Commission on the Human Immunodeficiency Virus Epidemic. The panel was created by executive order last month and will report in 90 days on the status of research on AIDS and the plans for addressing the epidemic in the future.

More than 40,000 Americans have already been diagnosed as having the disease, and more than half of these have already died. About three-fourths of those afflicted have been homosexual or bisexual men, and the gay community has been particularly supportive of AIDS victims, very successful in promoting education on the disease and admirably effective in prompting the government to mobilize resources in the effort. Because homosexuals have been both active and successful in the campaign against AIDS, it is wise to include at least one person from this group on the panel. This is not an entitlement or a quota that must be met; it is simply good sense. The White House has done well to name a man who is doubly qualified to serve—not only because he is gay and can reflect the experience and concerns of that group but because he is a medical expert as well.

The panel is broadly representative and also includes New York's Cardinal John O'Connor. He is opposed on religious grounds to the practice of homosexuality, but he also leads a diocese in which the church has provided important services—from hospital and hospice care to foster-care facilities for children—to those, including homosexuals, who have AIDS. Retired Adm. James Watkins, who participated in the Defense Department's decision to test armed forces recruits for AIDS, brings another perspective. So does John Creeden, president of the Metropolitan Life Insurance Company, who has special knowledge of the economic costs and civil liberties problems connected with the disease.

The commission is not charged with studying homosexuality or making a judgment about it. Its task is to make recommendations about a deadly disease, and each of the 13 members will bring a special perspective and expertise to the study. The choice of Dr. Lilly makes clear the administration's decision to be inclusive in seeking advice and developing plans for the future. The commission would have been flawed from the start if the important homosexual group had been ignored.

The Wichita Eagle-Beacon

Wichita, KS, July 27, 1987

PRESIDENT Reagan didn't seek the advice of the federal public health hierarchy in impaneling a 12-member national commission on AIDS Thursday. That raised questions about the commission's potential usefulness. But Mr. Reagan has left no question that AIDS, at last, will get major-league attention.

Some conservatives charge the presence of a homosexual medical researcher among the commission members could send young people the wrong message about homosexuality. Some, including homosexual activists, argue that the panel's general lack of AIDS expertise will render whatever findings it may reach of dubious value. Neither strain of thought is appropriate.

The commission's mission is to recommend measures that federal, state and local officials can use to stop AIDS' spread, and to assess current AIDS research and to seek better ways to care for those who've contracted the disease. Commission members will have sufficient resources to command whatever expertise they need. Considering that, Mr. Reagan's decision to put together a panel of levelheaded citizens of diverse political, religious and professional backgrounds makes sense: Whatever recommendations the commission ultimately makes must be capable of attracting broad support.

The commission members, who will have 90 days to complete their initial report and a year to complete their final report, would do well to study the comprehensive AIDS program proposed recently by Sen. Edward M. Kennedy, D-Mass. The measure would establish a national AIDS prevention program focusing on the risks of drug abusers using dirty needles and making better use of advertising and the press. It would step up the search for a cure. It would encourage research into ways to give AIDS victims better care without overtaxing hospital capacity.

As for AIDS testing, perhaps the most controversial AIDS-related subject, Mr. Kennedy separately has proposed outlawing AIDS-based discrimination and a national voluntary testing program. Mandatory testing, in his view, is the surest way to drive AIDS carriers underground.

The nation needs a program along those lines, and the commission could prove invaluable in building public support for one. Considering that as of last week 37,807 AIDS cases had been reported, with 22,328 deaths, and that those numbers are expected to grow in coming years, the nation needs to unite quickly behind a workable AIDS plan.

EVENING EXPRESS

Portland, ME, July 27, 1987

When President Reagan last week named Frank Lilly, a prominent geneticist, to a national commission to study AIDS, the choice came in for some criticism. Lilly is an avowed homosexual.

Republican Sen. Gordon J. Humphrey of New Hampshire, for example, complained that inclusion of Lilly on the 13-member panel puts the government in the position of condoning homosexual behavior.

That's the sort of knee-jerk polemic nonsense which only serves to detract from the important — and positive — role which government must play in the fight against AIDS.

Reagan's move in forming a commission to develop a "full-fledged strategy" for coping with the AIDS menace deserves support and encouragement, not pointless kibitzing from the moralistic right.

Government is in a position to move against the spread of AIDS in any number of legitimate ways.

Setting the machinery in motion for the formulation of a national policy is just one step taken by the administration last week.

The Labor Department announced it would begin enforcing what had been voluntary guidelines for the protection of the nation's health care workers against contagious blood diseases. Under the new policy, hospitals and other health care facilities can be fined for violations.

Coordination and enforcement of sensible health policies — along with public education — is exactly the sort of positive approach the government should be taking in the struggle against AIDS.

Debating moral irrelevancies is not in the least bit helpful at this point.

LAS VEGAS REVIEW-JOURNAL

Las Vegas, NV, July 30, 1987

Some homosexual activists are objecting to President Reagan's naming of only one gay to the newly constituted Commission on the Human Immunodeficiency Virus Epidemic.

The presidential panel was established to assess the status of research on AIDS and to suggest methods of dealing with the deadly disease. It is to report to the president within 90 days.

The panel includes a retired admiral who participated in the Defense Department's AIDS testing program for armed services recruits; a Catholic cardinal from New York; a businessman, civil libertarians, and others.

The panel also includes Dr. Frank Lilly, who heads the Department of Genetics at the Albert Einstein College of Medicine in New York. Lilly is also a gay rights activist.

But for some homosexual pressure groups, the naming to the panel of a single gay-rights activist was not enough.

It must be stated that the panel was commissioned — not to study gay rights issues or make some kind of judgment about homosexual lifestyles — but to study the issue of the AIDS epidemic and suggest national policies designed to deal in a rational manner with this murderous disease that has already touched 40,000 victims, killing half of them.

It is tragic, though probably it was inevitable, that the AIDS issue has become so intertwined with the homosexual-rights issue that governmental bodies seem paralyzed, unable to address the epidemic as an epidemic for fear of offending well-organized gay pressure groups.

It seems that gay rights groups have managed to set the limits of public discussion, managed to dictate to the scientific community, to the political community, what it is permissible to talk about and what it is not permissible to talk about. Witness the way President Reagan was shouted down, hissed and booed by gays when he dared suggest widespread blood tests for AIDS.

Witness the outrage demonstrated by gay groups when a Los Angeles man was arrested after he repeatedly attempted to donate his AIDS-infected blood to a plasma center. Gay activists seem to have determined that it is permissible for society to discuss AIDS education and "safe-sex," but it is not permissible to suggest that a promiscuous homosexual lifestyle is in itself dangerous in the present context of the AIDS epidemic. Nor is it acceptable to even mention the word "quarantine."

So AIDS rages on. Society has done nothing worth mentioning to stop it, and it will do nothing until it decides that the matter is too serious to allow rational discussion to be stymied by those who think AIDS and homosexual rights are one in the same issue.

The Morning News

Wilmington, DE, July 29, 1987

THE CENTERS for Disease Control began keeping count of AIDS cases in July 1981. By now the total of confirmed AIDS sufferers in the United States exceeds 38,000, of whom more than 22,000 have died.

AIDS clearly is a national health problem. But that's not all. AIDS also has significant societal impact.

There is fear of contagion, though scientific data so far show that AIDS is not transmitted through casual contact such as being in the same office or classroom.

Then there is the cost factor — AIDS patients require extensive medical care to control their infections. Health insurance underwriters find they face high claims. Many AIDS victims have neither insurance nor financial resources; government programs such as Medicaid come to their rescue. That in turn strains federal and state budgets.

Life insurance underwriters, too, are faced with more claims than had been actuarially predicted.

When one takes these factors into account, the 13-member AIDS panel named by President Reagan last week is appropriately representative. The chairman, Dr. W. Eugene Mayberry is head of the distinguished Mayo Clinic. The expertise brought by other panel members includes nursing, medicine, insurance, spiritual matters, knowledge of developing countries, sexual counseling and marketing.

Some were quick to find flaws in the panel's composition. One of the panelists, a respected scientist, is a homosexual. Some find that offensive. Others object that a Catholic cardinal is on the panel because he views homosexuality as a sin. Then there are those who deplore the absence of leading AIDS researchers on the panel.

These critics obviously don't understand the panel's function, which is to study the extent of the AIDS problem, recommend measures to stop the spread of AIDS and suggest ways of improving AIDS research and care of AIDS patients. The panel will have access to experts within and outside of government; its role will be to weigh conflicting and overlapping factors and come in with its recommendations.

The panel will make an initial report in three months and a full report in a year. It is hoped those reports will form the basis for a unified national approach to AIDS and end the present confusion, with the education secretary putting the emphasis on morals education and the surgeon general stressing the need for sex education. Then there are some state legislatures voting to ban discrimination against those with the AIDS virus while others concentrate on mandatory premarital testing.

How we deal with AIDS affects the entire country. A carefully developed, unified policy is overdue.

The Courier-Journal & TIMES

Louisville, KY, July 27, 1987

PRESIDENT Reagan was timely and sincere when he called last week for a "national strategy" to make AIDS as rare as "smallpox and polio." A visit to a hospital ward where children suffering with the disease are treated convinced him, he said, of the need for a breakthrough.

What's less certain is whether the national commission he appointed to find answers will help him realize those goals. Members were chosen from a number of fields, which is characteristic of national commissions. And a homosexual seems to have been named to the group as an afterthought, and only after the size was expanded from 11 to 13. Critics also complain that the group does not include experts on the disease, and that most members do not have a background for such a study.

That's unfortunate, because a strong commission could have been an important asset in shaping policies to combat the disease and help its victims. But then it's somewhat consoling to recall that while presidential commissions sometimes produce constructive ideas, those that don't are generally harmless.

DAILY NEWS

New York, NY, July 22, 1987

The word from Washington is that President Reagan will be appointing Dr. Frank Lilly to his new AIDS panel tomorrow. A first-rate choice. Dr. Lilly is chairman of the Genetics Department at New York's Albert Einstein College of Medicine. He has *two* doctoral degrees—one in organic chemistry and one in biology. He's a member of the National Academy of Sciences. And he's a former board member of Gay Men's Health Crisis, the well-known New York AIDS support group.

Publicly, the White House has been saying all along that it would ignore demands from gay rights groups that a homosexual be named to the AIDS panel. Privately, the message is different. Dr. Lilly's sexual preferences, it seems, *were* taken into account—but he was nominated strictly on the basis of his academic credentials.

Word play? Maybe. But there can be no doubt that Frank Lilly's resumé qualifies him for membership on the AIDS panel. Nor can there be any doubt that a gay belongs on the presidential panel dealing with a disease that is ravaging the homosexual community, among others. If the White House wants to mince words on the subject of Dr. Lilly's sexual orientation, that's President Reagan's business. Either way, the outcome is satisfactory.

AKRON BEACON JOURNAL
Akron, OH, July 27, 1987

PRESIDENT REAGAN has named a 12-member national commission on AIDS that is significant for a couple of reasons. For one thing, an appointee — Dr. Frank Lilly, a medical researcher who is a homosexual — is, as he points out, "among the first openly gay persons to have been appointed to a significant position in any U.S. administration."

For another thing, it appears to be a commission that is short on medical expertise but long on political diversity. So if the members can come up with a coherent, unified policy on AIDS, there may be hope for cooperation within the rest of the nation.

The first reactions to the panel were critical. Conservatives objected to the appointment of a homosexual; gay-rights groups objected to the heavy weighting of conservative social activists; health organizations objected to the absence of any real AIDS expertise on the panel.

A homosexual member is certainly warranted; that group has the most at stake in the AIDS threat. The White House defends the professional makeup of the panel by saying all are "thoughtful people" who know where to go to find AIDS experts.

As for politics, perhaps there is some value in exposing conservative activists to the real dilemma of AIDS and AIDS victims, and in letting the other side hear the social concerns of conservatives. It might turn out that ideology won't stand up to reality. In any case, all should understand that developing a sound AIDS strategy is important enough so that ideology should be checked at the meeting-room door. Perhaps then, the nation can get an AIDS policy that will help fight this deadly threat.

ST. LOUIS POST-DISPATCH
St. Louis, MO, July 27, 1987

President Reagan has appointed 13 people to a commission he has charged with the task of sending AIDS "the way of smallpox and polio." But had those maladies been addressed in the same way — had such unlikely committees as this one been set up to fight them — the human race just might be extinct by now.

The commission includes no one who possesses expert knowledge of the way the AIDS virus wreaks its havoc on the human body. It has just one acknowledged homosexual, although homosexuals are the group most affected by AIDS. Of those with preconceived ideas against the victims, however, there is no want: Penny Pullen, an Illinois state representative who believes that requiring engaged couples to be tested before marriage might help control AIDS; Cardinal John O'Connor of New York, who thinks AIDS is primarily a problem of sinful living; and Richard M. De Vos, co-founder and president of Amway, whose views on AIDS aren't a matter of public record but who can be presumed, the White House says, to inject the opinion of "the average American" because of his expertise in door-to-door sales.

Possibly the panel will produce some positive results. Maybe discussions and debates among its members can serve a cathartic purpose for the nation as a whole, performing as a stage on which widespread fears, suspicions and ignorance can be confronted and exposed for what they are.

But we are less than hopeful that this assortment of people will send AIDS packing. For that, dispassionate, dedicated researchers alone can light the way — and a representative of that group hasn't found a place on Mr. Reagan's panel.

The Orlando Sentinel
Orlando, FL, July 24, 1987

With the appointment of Frank Lilly to the presidential advisory board on the AIDS epidemic Thursday, the Reagan administration backs away from a very wrong policy.

Dr. Lilly's scientific credentials are up to the task: He's chairman of the genetics department at New York's Albert Einstein College of Medicine. But his sexual orientation — Dr. Lilly is a homosexual — would have kept him off the panel as it originally was designed.

That is both absurd and wrong. The Reagan people tried to cloak their resistance to a gay man on the advisory board in the usual palaver about no quotas, etc. That reasoning was transparent from the beginning. Even Ronald Reagan wouldn't think of forming a panel on, say, poverty among blacks without including black members, or a panel on women in the workplace without including women.

Stripped of its shaky ideological justifications, the no-gays policy was little more than open homophobia. Dr. Lilly's appointment corrects that, and it helps to assure — as must be the case — that gays, who have suffered the brunt of the awful epidemic, will be heard. That should have been a goal from Day One.

Newsday
Long Island, NY, July 23, 1987

The White House's initial refusal to put a homosexual on its national AIDS commission shows what can happen when politicians put ideology before public health — and symbolizes its overall ineptitude on AIDS policy.

Imagine ignoring the group that has not only been hardest hit by the deadly virus but is most experienced in providing education, outreach, home care and counseling. Well, the outcry from the medical community has finally reached some ears inside the White House: It looks as if a respected New York geneticist and gay-rights activist, Dr. Frank Lilly, is being asked to join the panel.

Unfortunately, the White House bungling on AIDS policy hasn't ended. Some time ago, to the astonishment of the federal health community, Reagan called for an AIDS survey, to be completed in six months, to show how prevalent the virus is in the U.S.

Maybe such a request sounds reasonable. But a survey of this magnitude and complexity is anything but. Although the federal Centers for Disease Control says it hasn't figured out the tab yet, insiders believe the project could cost as much as $30 million and take as long as two years (way over the president's six-month deadline). And what would we get from this expenditure of resources? At best, mildly interesting but at bottom useless data.

The CDC already has a good fix on the prevalence of the AIDS virus among high-risk groups (especially homosexuals and intravenous drug abusers). It also has a good working estimate that 1.5 million Americans are infected with the AIDS virus.

Sure, more exact information would be nice — but not at this cost. A $30-million bill isn't exactly petty cash, even for the federal government. The total CDC budget for surveys this year is $8 million; its entire AIDS program gets only $19 million. Where is the money going to come from?

Moreover, it's hard enough getting this administration to act quickly and responsibly without giving it a possible excuse for delay. And an AIDS survey of this sort would be a technical nightmare. It's doubtful that the president or any White House officials realize what is involved in this type of endeavor; researchers would have to take blood tests from perhaps 45,000 people — anonymously.

Embarking on an AIDS survey might prove helpful to politicians eager to look as if they're doing something meaningful about AIDS. But it's less useful to the scientific community, which has more pressing tasks on its AIDS agenda. If the White House wants to do something significant to combat AIDS, it could fund education initiatives or drug treatment programs. It could also listen to the advice of those with the most to offer in the fight against AIDS, such as the medical profession and the homosexual community.

Leaders Quit Reagan AIDS Panel

Dr. W. Eugene Mayberry, chairman of the presidential advisory commission on AIDS, October 7, 1987 resigned as chairman of President Reagan's 13-member AIDS advisory commission. Several hours later the panel's vice chairman, Dr. Woodrow A. Myers Jr., announced his resignation as well. Mayberry, chief executive officer of the Mayo Clinic in Rochester, Minnesota, declined to say why he left. Myers, health commissioner of the state of Indiana, said that he quit the panel partly because of his close association with Mayberry but also because of a "lack of support" from the Reagan administration and "significant" clashes of personality and ideology within the commission that rendered it unable "to move the agenda forward." Myers had been the panel's only public health expert and only black member. He had been appointed vice chairman by Mayberry without consultation with the other commissioners. The commission was scheduled to make its first report in December 1987.

Previously, Linda Sheaffer, the executive director of the presidential advisory commission on AIDS, was ousted September 11, 1987 by Dr. Mayberry. Sheaffer Sept. 14 issued a brief statement saying that Mayberry asked her to resign "because of internal disagreements within the commission that had nothing to do with my overall performance as the executive director." Asked to elaborate on those disagreements, she replied: "To discuss it further will only do further damage to the commission. It proves to me how frightened everyone is that they won't be able to complete the job assigned to them."

Only three of the 15 permanent staff members had been hired as of Mayberry's resignation. One of those, Dr. Franklin Cockrill 3rd, a Mayo Clinic AIDS specialist who had been serving as senior staff adviser for medical and research affairs, resigned Oct. 7 along with Mayberry and Myers.

The White House Oct. 7 announced that Mayberry would be replaced as chairman by Adm. James D. Watkins (retired), a panel member.

Los Angeles Times

Los Angeles, CA, October 12, 1987

Resignation of the leadership of President Reagan's national AIDS commission measures the disarray of both the commission and his Administration's own policy. The President, like so many other public officials, has not engaged the problem with the commitment and determination that it urgently requires.

As constituted by the White House, the national commission was long on concessions to political forces that do not grasp the public health implications of the pandemic and short on the professionals that already understand the problem and are enlisted in finding solutions. It is far from clear that a couple of substitutes for the resigned members can resolve that.

More important than repairing the commission, however, is providing vigorous leadership. The President's reluctance to be involved at all was a setback that cannot readily be overcome. What matters now is that no more time be lost. Reagan needs to pick up where he belatedly began on April 1 in Philadelphia, when he spoke authoritatively on the problem for the first time. He needs above all to take a central role in the education of the nation and in committing the federal government to providing adequate resources for research and for public health programs.

In education alone, the President could play a significant role. Education is the only defense against the deadly disease, with no vaccine or cure in sight. The President has every right to moralize, if he so chooses. But moralizing must be matched with the facts so that all Americans understand the risks of their sexual behavior, understand ways to reduce the risks and share that information with all potentially at risk.

Surgeon General C. Everett Koop has been the most effective spokesman in the Administration. He was the first to speak out, and he has consistently been the most candid. He has made clear that abstinence from high-risk sex is the only safe course. He has, however, felt free to advocate the use of condoms to reduce the risks. And, as research has shown the unreliability of condoms, particularly in the practice of anal intercourse, he has been willing to revise his counsel.

But none in the Administration has been candid enough about the inadequacy of funding. More is needed for research, including the search for a vaccine. More also is needed to serve existing institutions that are unable to expand services because of budget squeezes. One of these is the national drug-treatment program, the essential contact point for reaching the intravenous drug users who are second only to homosexuals as the population most impacted in the United States. In many areas, AIDS is having its most rapid spread among drug abusers, and from drug abusers into the heterosexual community. Yet in city after city there are no funds to expand drug-abuse services or even to offer adequate voluntary AIDS testing programs to trace the disease and help plan its containment.

Reagan is not the only leader who has failed to deal vigorously with AIDS. Gov. George Deukmejian has also failed to provide leadership and has allowed efforts to create a state commission to be sabotaged by a partisan political wrangle. In Los Angeles County, however, there are encouraging developments. The Los Angeles County Medical Assn., has launched a forthright billboard campaign, in both Spanish and English, to encourage the use of condoms by those at risk. An AIDS commission is now in place. The Board of Supervisors already has referred some critical issues to it for recommendation, with the likelihood that the commission can play an important role, the kind of role the federal commission could have played had the President been more respectful of balance and professional ability.

The Philadelphia Inquirer

*Philadelphia, PA
October 12, 1987*

With the presidential commission on AIDS in full self-destruct mode last week, the question arises: Can this venture be saved? And *should* it? Nothing is really wrong with its agenda, of course — to advise the White House on the "medical, legal, ethical, social and economic" impact of the deadly virus. But its conception has been, if not doomed, at least suspect from the start.

The resignation of its chairman, Dr. W. Eugene Mayberry of the Mayo Clinic, and vice chairman, Dr. Woodrow A. Myers Jr., the commission's only public-health expert, have only further eroded confidence in the commission's ability to get past its internal bickering and to shape an effective national policy on AIDS.

The necessity for a policy isn't in question. In fact, as members of the National Gay and Lesbian Task Force descended on Washington for a week of lobbying and protest, their leader, Jeffrey Levi, spotlighted the disparities in the quality of care for AIDS victims when state and local governments are left to operate without strong federal committment. "If you are a gay white man in San Francisco," he observed, "you are going to receive better care than a black IV drug user in Harlem."

Fairness, to be sure, is not the only issue in the fight against AIDS — public education, drug research, care compensation are among the many others. These are issues that can benefit from being coordinated on a national level. And while the surgeon general urges the nation's physicians to take a more active role in warning their patients about safe sexual practices and while the infection of another laboratory worker underlines the insidiousness of the disease, the coordination of a national response languishes.

The fault-finding is in high gear. Dr. Meyers was quoted as saying that "strong ideological perspectives, strong personalities and differences in leadership style" have set the AIDS commission at war with itself. And without a full degree of support from the administration, he said, the problems have only grown. More resignations are rumored to be imminent.

There is abundant evidence that the White House, in trying to have various political views represented on the commission — including some highly inflammatory ones — failed to consider whether the members could work together productively. In trying to achieve diversity, there is a good case to be made that the President instead has achieved ineffectiveness.

The commission's credibility, at this point, appears beyond redemption. Perhaps looking to the National Academy of Sciences, or another existing group with a track record on the public health implications of AIDS, would be more worthwhile than trying to salvage this fractured and factioned commission.

THE KANSAS CITY STAR

Kansas City, MO, October 9, 1987

The President's AIDS Commission is still getting attention for what it isn't. Appointments were far behind the disease's advances. AIDS expertise was thin. Dr. W. Eugene Mayberry wasn't a popular choice for leader.

Now he's quit. Mayberry, chief executive office of the Mayo Clinic, resigned abruptly. Dr. Woodrow A. Myers, the vice chairman, followed him. Then Dr. Franklin Cockerill 3rd, a Mayo Clinic physician specializing in AIDS who was serving as senior staff adviser for medical and research affairs, left the commission.

The men couldn't hide past incidents and turmoil that seemed to have been daily routine. These included ignorance and bickering over turf, personality clashes, tattletaling to the White House and conflicting ideologies

The commission was to make recommendations about public protection from AIDS, fighting the disease and treating victims.

From the commission's inception, few were convinced the fight had leadership. These mighty battles being fought now before the commission does anything illustrate the reason there's a credibility problem which simply gets bigger.

Worse, what medical expertise the commission had is now gone. Efforts to deal with AIDS have been hampered by a lack of national leadership and a lack of focus as well as uncertain policy and research funding. What faint hope was held that the special panel might eventually help fill those gaps now is gone.

THE INDIANAPOLIS NEWS

Indianapolis, IN, October 14, 1987

If a problem causes too many meetings, the meetings eventually become more important than the problem.

— Murphy's Laws On Justice

Infighting on the presidential AIDS commission recently prompted a walkout by commission Chairman Dr. Eugene Mayberry and Vice Chairman Dr. Woodrow Myers Jr.

While the tiff made for some good headlines the makeup of the AIDS commission is of little import as long as the commission has no defined purpose. Indeed, one wonders if the commission does have any legitimate role other than to satisfy some political demand for the government to do SOMETHING about the spread of AIDS.

AIDS is a serious problem. According to the most recent figures from the Federal Centers for Disease Control, 41,770 AIDS cases have been reported in the United States. The Public Health Service estimates that an additional 1.5 million Americans have been infected with the HIV virus but have not yet shown symptoms.

There are limited areas where federal involvement is warranted.

Federal funds must be — and are being — provided in the search for a cure of this dread disease or for medicines to prolong lives and ease suffering. There also needs to be more research into the means by which AIDS is spread and accurate data on the extent to which it is spreading.

There are already federal agencies — the Centers for Disease Control, the Department of Health and Human Services and the Surgeon General's office — in place to deal with these matters.

Congress is going to have to deal with some AIDS issues that are international in scope. It has already determined that all immigrants, refugees and individuals seeking residency in the United States must be tested for AIDS. But what about tourists or foreigners here on business for more than a few months? What about military personnel stationed abroad?

There are some vexing international issues involving AIDS that are clearly federal in scope.

They don't, however, need a commission to be sorted out.

It is appropriate for top federal officials — President Reagan, Surgeon General C. Everett Koop, Education Secretary William Bennett or Health and Human Services Secretary Otis R. Bowen — to use their bully pulpits to quell hysteria, impart information about AIDS and the conduct that spreads it.

But in most respects, AIDS is an issue that is best dealt with at the state and local level.

To begin with, what clearly borders on an epidemic in some urban areas, such as New York or San Francisco, is much more of an abstract concern in Butte, Mont., or Anderson, Ind. The possible need for mandatory testing, for special insurance regulations, for quarantines or for a host of other laws, regulations or policies varies throughout the nation.

Outside of some major urban areas and certain groups of individuals — intravenous drug users, prostitutes, homosexuals or hemophiliacs — AIDS does not appear to be the galloping plague it is often portrayed to be. On the other hand, it may prove to be a very intractable disease that defies a magic cure.

The battles on the AIDS commission may be but a diversion from the real attention that needs to be focused on this disease and all of its ramifications. But in the end, these internal disputes may be much to do about nothing.

Arkansas Gazette

Little Rock, AR, October 9, 1987

The administration's campaign against AIDS is in still more disarray, but it probably matters little. The thing has seemed mostly smoke from the beginning, as far from reality as Reaganomics.

The commission appointed by President Reagan to recommend how the government should cope with the AIDS epidemic has been in continual turmoil, beset by internal bickering and external criticism for its lack of medical specialists in AIDS. Wednesday, the commission's chairman and vice chairman resigned, with the commission's first report due in two months. The chairman, Dr. W. Eugene Mayberry, chief executive officer of the Mayo Clinic, gave no reason for his resignation. The vice chairman, Dr. Woodrow A. Myers Jr., the Indiana state health commissioner, said he resigned because of the internal squabbling and inadequate White House support for Dr. Mayberry in particular and the commission in general.

Mr. Reagan accepted Dr. Mayberry's resignation "with regret," didn't acknowledge Dr. Myers' (hearing the truth always makes the president cranky), and elevated retired Admiral James D. Watkins to the chairmanship of the commission. Admiral Watkins is a former chief of naval operations; Mr. Reagan evidently thinks sea power is the key to defeating AIDS.

Who needs medical expertise anyway? Not Education Secretary William J. Bennett. On Tuesday, Mr. Bennett again challenged the nation's top health officer by issuing a guide to AIDS education that frowns on the use of condoms and emphasizes the teaching and practice of sexual restraint as the proper safeguard against the disease. Dr. C. Everett Koop, the surgeon general, is something of a right-wing ideologue himself, but as a physician he's been compelled to acknowledge that AIDS can't be whipped by preaching alone. He has advised the use of condoms. Dr. Koop is a realist. Mr. Bennett is not.

★ ★ ★

Mr. Bennett and Mr. Reagan are optimists. Where others see in AIDS a horrible plague, Mr. Bennett and Mr. Reagan see opportunity to make political hay and to promote the ideology they share. Mr. Bennett even panders to the hysterics who run AIDS-infected children out of school and out of town, despite physicians' assurances that AIDS is not spread by casual classroom contact. Mr. Bennett's booklet admits that school districts must educate children with AIDS. But, it says, the schools should "take into consideration bona fide medical considerations about the likelihood of the risk of infection to other children" in deciding whether to keep an AIDS-infected child in regular classes. This is as unnecessary as advising people in a burning theater that they should consider moving toward the exit.

It appears the president and the secretary of education will be of little assistance in the fight against AIDS and the panic that accompanies it. Another chance for leadership lost, and tragically so.

The Ann Arbor News
Ann Arbor, MI, October 13, 1987

AIDS is a disease that is relatively difficult to contract, but once acquired almost certainly means a slow, painful death.

The numbers of reported cases in Washtenaw County have not been large so far (18 cases of AIDS have been reported, seven this year), according to Washtenaw County Health Director Dr. John Atwater. Still, the county is threatened, not only because reported cases will grow into the hundreds in the next few years, but also because of the growing AIDS hysteria.

Atwater has been among the leaders in the area attempting to deal with AIDS now, through public education sessions and programs such as the county's free AIDS testing clinic. What he and others are doing here, however, seem in sharp contrast to what's going on at the national level.

It appears as though the Reagan administration is not persuaded AIDS constitutes a public health menace of growing proportions, judging from the inaction of the commission Reagan appointed last July to draft policies for protecting Americans from AIDS.

After three months, the commission is a shambles. It is has not even begun to deliberate its goals of setting policies to keep AIDS from spreading, to care for victims with "love and respect" and to set priorities for spending limited money on research and other programs.

The commission's staff director has been fired, and last week the panel's chairman and vice chairman quit abruptly amid allegations of infighting and deep ideological differences. Another panel member, Amway Corp. President Richard DeVos, said Reagan should avoid placing AIDS-involved people on the commission, instead choosing members who can apply "common sense intelligence (to) look at the problems and solve them without being so emotionally involved."

DeVos also criticized homosexuals and AIDS victims for wanting to control the commission and "capture the agenda." He was critical of a homosexual rights rally in Washington, D.C., over the weekend, in which appeals were made for more funds for AIDS research and treatment. "When they march in the streets and all that garbage, the whole thing stops," he said.

His narrow views contrasted sharply with new commission chairman James D. Watkins, who responded to the weekend gay/lesbian rights demonstration by saying that his group intends to deal with the "concerns and apprehensions" of homosexuals and other affected groups. Still, Watkins is a retired Navy admiral who, The New York Times said, "knows even less about AIDS than his fellow commissioners."

The near self-destruction of President Reagan's AIDS commission dramatizes the need to reconstitute this body with public health professionals, researchers and people with AIDS expertise, and to support this group with a strong staff.

The commission is supposed to be developing a "national AIDS policy." But while they're bickering, the number of AIDS cases keeps growing. In September, the Centers for Disease Control in Atlanta said it has received reports of 42,354 cases, an increase of 4,000 since July. (The center also reported that by September, 24,412 victims had died.)

Also, other problems related to the AIDS issue are developing. Homosexual rights activists say the AIDS crisis has spurred an increase in violence and discrimination against the nation's male and female homosexual communities. Statistically, this may be hard to prove but certainly the perception is that of frustration and anger with homosexuals over the AIDS phenomenon.

Call it scapegoating or whatever, but homosexuals are feeling the sting of the haters and the moralists.

Clearly, education and new knowledge gained from research are powerful weapons against ignorance and AIDS-fueled hysteria. A White House AIDS commission with a stronger mandate and a clearer sense of what it hopes to accomplish needs to put ideological bickering behind it and get on with the real business of preparing the country to control the spread of AIDS.

With, we might add, more medicine, education and less preaching.

Buffalo Evening News
Buffalo, NY, October 14, 1987

THE 13-MEMBER presidential AIDS commission named last July was supposed to provide strong leadership in fighting this dread disease, to assess the nation's AIDS programs and to coordinate action by federal, state and local health agencies.

Now just as the panel was scheduled to give its initial report, its top leadership has resigned and the panel is in disarray.

In fact, the commission by all indications has accomplished hardly anything in the past three months, and we are back to Square One. Meanwhile another thousand or more Americans have died of AIDS.

President Reagan was slow to provide national leadership in the AIDS crisis, taking a year to appoint the presidential commission after it was recommended by the U.S. Public Health Service.

The commission, once named, got off to a slow start, with the first executive director forced out after a power struggle. Now three key people have thrown up their hands and left, including an AIDS specialist who was serving as the senior medical adviser.

The chairman, Dr. W. Eugene Mayberry, head of the Mayo Clinic, did not comment on the reason for his abrupt resignation, but the vice chairman, Dr. Woodrow A. Myers, said: "I don't feel the commission, as currently constituted, would be effective." Myers, who is the Indiana health commissioner, cited clashes of personalities and ideologies, lack of support by the Reagan administration and the lack of doctors and health officials on the commission.

The new chairman, retired Adm. James D. Watkins, is a former chief of naval operations and has obvious leadership qualities. But in view of the reports of bitter factional disputes within the commission, he appears to face a formidable challenge in getting things moving. It will take time for the panel to establish credible leadership in the national fight against AIDS.

No commission or research group can find any easy answers to the problem of AIDS, a fatal disease for which no cure or vaccine has yet been found. But there are so many aspects to the AIDS problem that the presidential commission could perform a valuable service by recommending action in various areas.

Education to curb the spread of AIDS, research to cure or curb the disease, the proper care of AIDs victims, the advisability of testing programs, the control of intravenous drug use (a major means of spreading the disease) — all these should be reviewed by the commission to provide guidance for health agencies as the disease continues to spread inexorably across the nation.

Los Angeles Herald
Los Angeles, CA, October 14, 1987

In January 1981, while Ronald Reagan was taking his first oath of office as president, doctors around the country were just discovering the pattern of symptoms and infections in patients that comprise what is now recognized as AIDS. From that first isolated cluster of cases, according to the latest figures from the federal Centers for Disease Control, the epidemic has grown to more than 42,000 cases nationwide, more than half of whom have already died. Applying the CDC's recently broadened definition of the disease will raise those depressing statistics even higher.

The health-care and social-service communities have learned a great deal about AIDS since then, from the virus that causes it to the high-risk behavior that spreads it. The president, meanwhile, seems to have learned almost nothing. So it can be no surprise that seven years into the epidemic, the hollow public-relations gesture of appointing a presidential panel to recommend a national AIDS policy is collapsing in disgrace.

Last month, the panel's executive director, on loan from the Department of Health and Human Services, was forced to resign. Last week, the chairman, vice chairman and the senior staff adviser for medical affairs followed her out. After three months of false starts, the new acting chairman, Adm. James Watkins (ret.), former Chief of Naval Operations, now inherits the unenviable task of producing an initial report by early December, and the final version by next July. Putting it mildly, expectations are modest.

As former Secretary of State William Rogers demonstrated in heading up the commission investigating the Challenger space shuttle disaster, proven administrative ability may be more important in a chairman than technical expertise. But Rogers at least had a qualified panel. The Reagan AIDS commission appointees are not only lacking in stature, many are lacking any direct experience in dealing with AIDS at all.

What's needed is not another AIDS panel, but a major commitment of federal funding for education and research. In the near term, the administration could best demonstrate its concern by supporting the efforts of Surgeon General C. Everett Koop. But as one of the most credible national figures speaking out on the problem, Koop has been drowned out by more strident administration voices. Attorney General Edwin Meese says it's all right to discriminate against AIDS victims in the workplace, while Secretary of Education William Bennett recommends in a new pamphlet to just say no.

It's past time for the amateurs to quiet down and let the public hear what a federal expert says about stopping the spread of AIDS.

The Miami Herald

Miami, FL, October 12, 1987

PRESIDENTIAL commissions can inspire wise policy that shapes response to an issue via legislative action and public reaction. They can also be a poor excuse for doing nothing. The commission appointed to guide President Reagan on the medical, legal, ethical, social, and economic impact of the deadly disease AIDS must inspire. The country can afford no less in dealing with the epidemic of acquired immune-deficiency syndrome.

Since the commission was appointed three months ago, AIDS has claimed at least another 1,000 victims. Meanwhile, the commission has mired itself in unproductive squabbling that this week culminated in the resignations of three physicians with expertise in AIDS treatment and public health. W. Eugene Mayberry resigned as chairman. This triggered the resignation of vice chairman Woodrow A. Myers, Jr., whom Dr. Mayberry had appointed without consulting other commissioners. Franklin Cockerill, a Mayberry associate at the Mayo Clinic, resigned as staff consultant to the commission.

President Reagan showed awareness of the importance of keeping the group from foundering by quickly appointing retired Adm. James Watkins chairman. A commission member, Mr. Watkins is a former chief of naval operations who helped formulate the military AIDS-testing policy. His appointment is acceptable to the commission majority, which is important if real work is to get done.

The commission is supposed to report its findings to the President in June 1988. In order to make them credible, physicians with experience in treating AIDS patients and with an understanding of public-health policies must be part of the team. AIDS is a vicious, frightening disease. Fear and ignorance have hindered progress in disseminating reliable information to the public, in formulating fair testing policies, and in ensuring humane and adequate medical treatment for victims.

An antidote to fear and ignorance is wise counsel. The commission must meet the task assigned without delay. There must be no poor excuses about why the nation hasn't reacted responsibly to the AIDS threat.

St. Petersburg Times

St. Petersburg, FL, October 9, 1987

When scholars write the history of America in the 1980s, they are likely to conclude that the greatest leadership failure of our times was in not recognizing and combating the AIDS epidemic.

Almost seven years after the first AIDS cases appeared in 1981, the late-starting presidential commission in the fight against AIDS is in chaos.

In human terms, the dimensions of this national failure are staggering. AIDS is a behavioral disease. If people know how to avoid the behavior that transmits the virus, they can protect themselves against it. If a vigorous national educational campaign had been organized early in the epidemic, the size of the epidemic could have been reduced, perhaps contained. In six years of doing almost nothing to educate the public, the wild fire has spread rapidly. More than 24,000 persons already have died in this country. Experts now believe that between 1-million and 2-million Americans already are infected by the disease. Most of those people will die. Many of those Americans would have lived if the federal government had launched the right kind of campaign against AIDS years ago.

Dr. Paul Volberding, who diagnosed some of the very early cases of AIDS and who helped devise San Francisco General Hospital's model treatment program, described the tragedy in these words: "If there is one thing we can really be ashamed of it is that we did not develop a national response that educated the general population about the disease. We did not see the leadership at the federal level that allowed the creation of an educational program. Now we have to follow the lead of other countries, such as Great Britain, which have clearly overtaken us."

The epidemic never has been mentioned in any State of the Union Address. President Reagan made his first detailed policy statement on AIDS in April of this year. In that statement to a group of physicians in Philadelphia, he said that abstaining from sexual relations was the best way to prevent the spread of the disease. He did not appoint a presidential commission to guide federal policy until August, and when he did he stacked it heavily with ideologues.

The commission began to disintegrate on Sept. 11 when Linda D. Sheaffer, its executive director, was forced to resign. On Wednesday it lost its leadership and medical expertise. Three top members resigned: Chairman W. Eugene Mayberry, chief executive officer of the Mayo Clinic; Vice Chairman Woodrow A. Myers, Indiana health commissioner; and Dr. Franklin Cockerill III, the commission's only physician specializing in AIDS.

The House of Representatives declared its lack of confidence in the presidential commission shortly after it was appointed by voting 355 to 68 to create a congressional commission. That commission offers the best hope that the late-starting effort will be carried forth as a medical and scientific project in conjunction with the efforts of Surgeon General C. Everett Koop, the most effective leader so far.

Senate Majority Leader Robert Byrd should act immediately to bring the bill creating the congressional commission to a vote on the floor. The tragic delay in this nation's fight against AIDS already has cost far, far too many lives, and the dying has just begun.

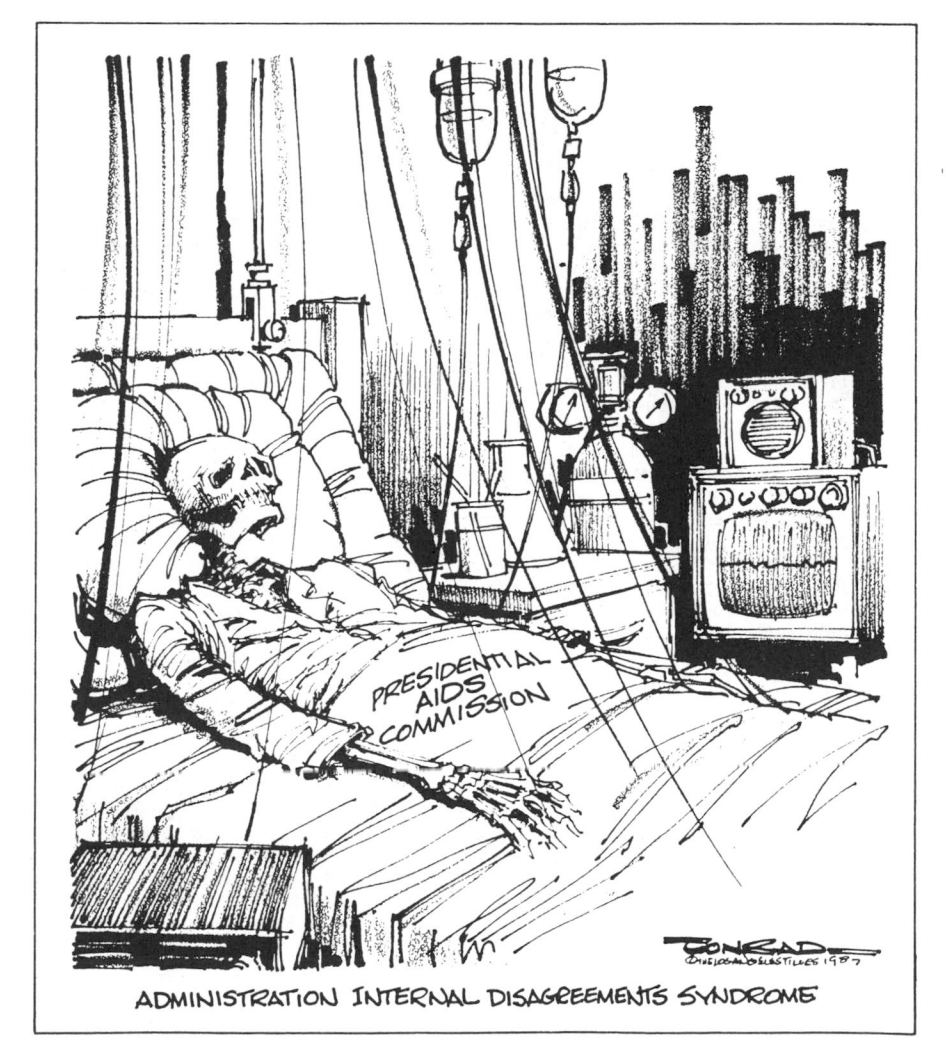

ADMINISTRATION INTERNAL DISAGREEMENTS SYNDROME

Chicago Tribune

Chicago, IL, October 11, 1987

With the resignation of its two top leaders, the Presidential Advisory Commission on AIDS is in disarray, its already murky future further clouded by the defections.

Probably a bad idea from the start, the commission by all accounts has limped through three unproductive months marked by bitter internal wrangling only to be faced with virtually starting over.

If its goals to produce comprehensive findings and recommendations on all aspects of the AIDS epidemic by next June were unrealistic before, as many believed, they are all but impossible now.

In resigning, Dr. W. Eugene Mayberry, chief executive officer of the Mayo Clinic, said he had not realized the job would be so time-consuming. Others said he was just papering over the differences that had torn the commission apart. His appointed deputy, Dr. Woodrow A. Myers Jr., the health commissioner of Indiana, said he resigned as vice chairman because he did not "feel the commission as currently constituted would be effective."

Weeks ago, opponents on the commission forced the resignation of the executive director appointed by Dr. Mayberry. She has yet to be replaced. Another senior staff adviser, a physician from the Mayo Clinic, left with Dr. Mayberry and Dr. Myers.

The commission, officially named the Presidential Commission on the Human Immuno-deficiency Virus Epidemic, was controversial from the start. After years of struggling to find a politically acceptable public stance on a spreading fatal disease that primarily infected homosexuals and intravenous drug users but was increasingly frightening the wits out of unaddicted, heterosexual America, the White House finally settled on the all-purpose solution—a commission.

So far so good, although some critics thought it was a little late to be getting around to studying the problem to see if a national policy could be set forth. Then the members were named, and the controversy began in earnest. There was one acknowledged homosexual in the group, but no known AIDS victims and not many persons—even among the doctors appointed—who had much, if any, experience with the disease. Moreover, there were protests that several members were ideologues who might, at best, consider the epidemic a plague sent forth to punish society's aberrants. For those, the argument went, the commission might well be little more than a platform from which to preach salvation through their own view of morality.

The split, when it came, appeared to be along some subterranean ideological fault line that remained obscured to the casual outside observer. And perhaps it is a temblor in a teacup.

Surely, the superstitious among us will ascribe the panel's troubles to President Reagan's mischievousness in naming a 13-member commission on the 13th day of the month of July.

But the rest of us, realists all, know that no matter how inconclusive your polls are, you can't always deal with every sticky political problem by sending a commission to postpone a President's tough decisions.

Commissions usually buy time, not wisdom.

Detroit Free Press

Detroit, MI, October 12, 1987

PRESIDENT REAGAN'S most visible response to the growing AIDS epidemic was the creation earlier this year of a commission to advise him what to do about it. That long-awaited action by the White House seemed very limited and, from the start, there was criticism that the commission, as a whole, lacked the objectivity and expertise to make a major contribution to public policy.

The critics have reason for increased pessimism with the resignation last week of the panel's two top members — the chairman, Dr. W. Eugene Mayberry, chief executive of the Mayo Clinic, and the vice-chairman, Dr. Woodrow A. Myers, Indiana's health commissioner. In addition, a Mayo Clinic physician who specializes in AIDS quit as an adviser. Another highly qualified panel member, Dr. Frank Lilly, chairman of the genetics department at Albert Einstein College of Medicine, has indicated that he is considering resigning.

In stepping down, Dr. Myers specifically cited his belief that the commission "as currently constituted" can't be effective and said "lack of support" from the administration and "significant" conflicts of ideology have gotten "in the way of getting the work done." Personality clashes are said to have contributed to the commission's turmoil, which also was marked by the firing three weeks ago of its executive director.

If we had greater faith that the president really considered the AIDS commission's work a high priority, we would urge him to thank the remaining members and say goodby, then seek new and better appointees with greater emphasis this time around on public health professionals, physicians and researchers. But this is the president who only last spring broke his long silence on AIDS. That unconscionable delay and the disagreements within the administration that caused it give us little reason to think this White House is willing — or able — to put together a stronger panel.

The new chairman, James D. Watkins, a retired admiral, likely will find the skills he developed during his naval career put to an even tougher test. His priorities must be attracting a top-notch staff, restoring some sense of purpose to the commission and doing much needed public relations work on behalf of a panel whose credibility — limited from the start — is now at about zero.

We wish him well. One thousand or more people have died while AIDS commission members have been bickering.

ST. LOUIS POST-DISPATCH

St. Louis, MO, October 10, 1987

Despite massive publicity over the last few years, fear of AIDS remains largely a fear of the unknown. People often try to calm such fears with a test, something that can anchor a free-floating anxiety with a yes-or-no answer. Many government officials have put their faith and their resources into AIDS testing instead of mounting educational efforts to keep the disease from spreading. Results of newly released studies on AIDS should shake that faith.

First came a study last week in the *Journal of the American Medical Association* on the use of AIDS tests for couples seeking marriage licenses — tests already approved in Illinois and two other states. Researchers at the Harvard School of Public Health said such tests not only are ineffective, inefficient and costly — they will do little to retard the spread of the disease.

The researchers estimated that the potential cost for screening, testing and counseling the 3.8 million people nationwide who plan to marry each year would exceed $100 million. That money would be spent on a population at a very low risk of getting AIDS in the first place. Of the 3.8 million people tested, researchers said, 9,000 would test positive on an initial screening test, and only 1,200 of those would show up positive on a second test.

Their conclusion: "The more resources we devote to such marginally effective ventures, the fewer we will have to develop truly effective public health programs."

Some people may feel such money — $83,000 just to identify one AIDS case, with no treatment involved — would be well spent. But a second report, from Finland, shows that people infected with the virus may go for a year or more without developing the antibodies the tests detect. Previous estimates had been that the antibodies show up no later than six months after someone is infected with the virus.

In other words, not only will tests show false positives, disrupting many lives needlessly; they will miss many real positives, because people who take the test and come up negative could actually be infected with the virus but not have developed antibodies yet.

If governments had unlimited funds to fight AIDS, these studies may not make much difference. But such money is not unlimited. A recent report in *The New York Times* said AIDS was spreading quickly in poor neighborhoods among drug addicts who share infected needles. Counseling and treatment in drug programs could help check the spread, experts said, but hard-pressed treatment centers cannot accommodate all those who need help.

With no cure in sight and tests that are unreliable at best, responsible government officials should admit that testing is not the answer to combatting AIDS. Education is. Both the Public Health Service and the Department of Education have released booklets about AIDS, and organizations such as the National Education Association are doing the same. These efforts — not tests that invade privacy and give no definitive conclusions — are the best way to help stop both the spread of AIDS and the fear that surrounds it.

The Hartford Courant

Hartford, CT, October 12, 1987

Resignations last week by the top leaders of the presidential commission on AIDS probably ensure that the panel will be irrelevant in the government's response to the epidemic.

The commission is to recommend a federal strategy on how to protect the public from the disease, find a cure and treat victims. A final report is scheduled for next July. But the panel has been divided by ideological differences and personality clashes, has accomplished next to nothing in its three months of existence, and is unlikely to meet its first deadline, Dec. 7, with a report of any substance.

Turmoil on the commission, moreover, aptly reflects the disjointed and generally ineffective approach to the epidemic thus far taken by the Reagan administration.

Dr. W. Eugene Mayberry, chief executive officer of the Mayo Clinic, quit as chairman without offering a formal explanation, but was said to have called the White House often to complain that other members were undercutting his authority. The resigned vice chairman, Dr. Woodrow A. Meyers, was one of only two members who have actually treated AIDS patients and was the commission's only public-health expert. Dr. Franklin Cockerill, a physician specializing in AIDS who also resigned, was the commission's only medical staff member.

Dr. Mayberry will be replaced as chairman by retired Adm. James D. Watkins, a panel member. He's said to be an effective administrator, but he has his work cut out for him. The commission has been without an executive director since last month, when Dr. Mayberry's choice for the job was forced out. Only three of 15 permanent staff members have been hired, and one of them, Dr. Cockerill, has resigned.

The commission is divided between members who see AIDS as a public-health issue — which it is — and those who treat the disease also as a moral and political issue. Unless the bickering stops and a consensus is formed, the commission can't gain credibility.

Hopes for an effective response to the AIDS crisis by the presidential commission had not been high at any rate. The president had not devoted a public speech to the epidemic until April — even though more than 20,000 people had already died from AIDS and an estimated 1 million had been infected by the virus. Mr. Reagan's annual requests for funds for AIDS-related programs have increased each year. Congress has voted additional money but even with that, some experts claim that not enough has been devoted to AIDS education and research.

In addition, Mr. Reagan has distanced himself from one of the few officials in his administration who has responded to AIDS with the urgency it requires: U.S. Surgeon General C. Everett Koop. Dr. Koop's apolitical attitude and his call for candid sex education, even for schoolchildren, as a means to stop the spread of the disease has put off the president and many of his conservative supporters. With that background, having an AIDS commission absorbed with ideological infighting is not surprising.

Congress should go ahead and create an AIDS commission to take up the work that should have been done by the disintegrating presidential panel. Legislation is pending to do that.

And if the president patches up his commission with new members, let them try to listen to public-health professionals rather than following their political compasses.

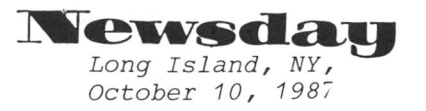

Long Island, NY, October 10, 1987

The AIDS debate in Washington is degenerating into a morality play scripted for a conservative audience. This could prove a serious menace to public health.

In the world according to the White House, those on the side of the angels preach sexual abstinence as the perfect prophylactic AIDS program. The bad guys advocate measures like condom use to reduce AIDS transmission; they're denounced as promotors of sexual promiscuity.

At least this seems to be the way administration ideologues, especially Education Secretary William Bennett and domestic policy adviser Gary Bauer, are framing the issue. By so doing they undermine responsible medical authorities like Surgeon General Everett Koop, who have outspokenly supported frank AIDS education.

More than personalities are clashing here. The overall direction of the federal AIDS educational effort may be at issue. Though the Health and Human Services Department was specifically directed by Congress to send AIDS information to every household, so far there have only been selected mailings of a moderately informative pamphlet rather than Koop's definitive report on AIDS.

Now Bennett has decided to issue his own AIDS education booklet. It completely ignores Koop's advocacy of sexual education for grade-school children and recommendation of condoms as appropriate AIDS-prevention measures.

This week the two top officials on the president's AIDS panel resigned. Not surprisingly, they cited lack of White House support as one of their reasons. The public may rightly wonder whether the Reagan administration is going to play any role in the struggle against AIDS that isn't either ideological or nonsensical.

The Washington Times

Washington, DC, October 9, 1987

LAST JULY when the White House announced the names of those chosen to serve on the Commission on the Human Immunodeficiency Virus Epidemic, we expressed high hopes for a commission so "broadly representative." Perhaps we spoke too soon, for it is now apparent that the diversity of the AIDS panel members is producing more conflict than cooperation. Two commissioners have already resigned, the executive director has been forced out, and the only physician with AIDS experience on the staff has quit.

The panel received a broad mandate from the White House. It was to study the "medical, legal, ethical, social and economic impact" of AIDS and make an initial report to the president by Dec. 7. While a variety of reasons have been given for the resignation of the chairman, Dr. W. Eugene Mayberry, the head of the Mayo Clinic, he has not explained his decision. The vice-chairman, Dr. Woodrow Meyers, who also resigned, was more candid: "I felt that there was no way that anybody else [except Dr. Mayberry] could coalesce this group and make it work efficiently. There are strong ideological perspectives, strong personalities and differences in leadership style" on the commission.

Adm. James Watkins now takes over as chairman of the commission, and if he is to prevent a total fiasco he must act quickly. The open slots on the commission need to be filled immediately, and there should be less emphasis on political agendas and more on AIDS expertise. Panel members who can't subordinate egos and personal causes to a larger public-service interest should resign. It would be better to extend the life of the commission if the work has to begin again with new members than to continue the squabbling and the stalemate. A first-rate staff is urgently needed too. There are now only two people working for the commission, though 15 slots have been authorized. Can't staff be borrowed temporarily from one of the many federal agencies that know something about this epidemic?

This weekend, many thousands of gay and lesbian activists are expected to come to this city in a March on Washington. Millions of other Americans share their concern about AIDS and the government's plans to meet the crisis. This is the time for a strong statement from the White House on the commission's future and a hard-headed reassessment of its membership and its task.

Part III: AIDS, Education and Schools

The September 1985 announcement that a single child with AIDS would enroll in a New York City public school sparked an angry boycott in two city school districts. After parents vowed to "stand in the schoolhouse door" to keep children with AIDS out of school, between 9,000 and 11,000 children stayed home in protest on the first day of classes. Parents posted a sign saying "Enter at Your Own Risk" at the entrance to one school. Against this backdrop, boards of education and departments of health have struggled to formulate policies that will protect the rights of the few children who are ill as well as the vast majority who are healthy. The issue has raised formidable questions: Do children with AIDS have a right to attend school? Who should decide which children cannot enroll? What precautions should the schools take?

Many of the infected children have since gained admission to classes on the strength of data showing the risk of casual transmission of the disease to be apparently nonexistent. Their presence in school has, however, provoked a new set of considerations: By what means should these children be protected from harassment and ostracism? To what extent do these children have a right to privacy? Who has a right to know their identities? The policy makers grappling with these issues are finding the legal and ethical dimensions of the disease in children sometimes as difficult as the medical questions.

Education has been one of the most effective ways of combating AIDS-related discrimination. According to Peggy Clark, a public health educator of the New York City Department of Health, "education is the key tool used to allay fears about AIDS by providing accurate information and clarifying misconceptions." The Health and Public Policy Committee of the American College of Physicians has published a report encouraging education for the general public. The committee views education as an appropriate way to stem the fear of AIDS and control the epidemic spread of the disease. Researchers who conducted an attitude study in San Francisco, New York City and London found that the less informed people are about AIDS, the more likely they are to harbor unreasonable fears about the disease.

Despite the efficacy of educational programs, very little funding has been allocated them. The National Academy of Sciences says that "AIDS education should be pursued with a sense of urgency and a level of funding that is appropriate for a life-or-death situation." It recommends that the total budget for AIDS education from public and private sources should approximate $1 billion annually by 1990. In 1986 Surgeon General C. Everett Koop estimated that a comprehensive educational program could prevent as many as 12,000 to 14,000 deaths by 1991.

State and local health departments must comply with numerous conditions established by the federal government in order to qualify for federal funds. This has been a point of contention between AIDS education proponents and its critics. Perhaps the most disputed of these is the establishment of local review panels to consider the "bounds of explicitness" of risk-education materials. Although these review boards are to be made up of no less than five persons representing a reasonable cross section of the community, they are not to be drawn predominately from the target groups. The guidelines for a review panel require that any written materials be understood by a broad cross section of educated adults, but be judged by a reasonable person not to be offensive. The federal government requires that audio-visual materials be put to even greater scrutiny, demanding that they communicate by "inference rather than by display of the anogenital area of the body or overt depiction of performance of 'safer sex' or 'unsafe sex' practices." Critics of such requirements argue that they are self-defeating and create a bureaucratic obstacle to the swift production of effective materials. In addition, proponents of AIDS education suggest that one of the reasons why public dollars have been hard to come by for AIDS education is that the federal government would be forced to directly fund educational programs that don't make homosexuality taboo. Supporters of the requirements argue that educating people about safe sex and safe needles use may increase or insufficiently discourage sexual activity, particularly homosexual activity, and drug use.

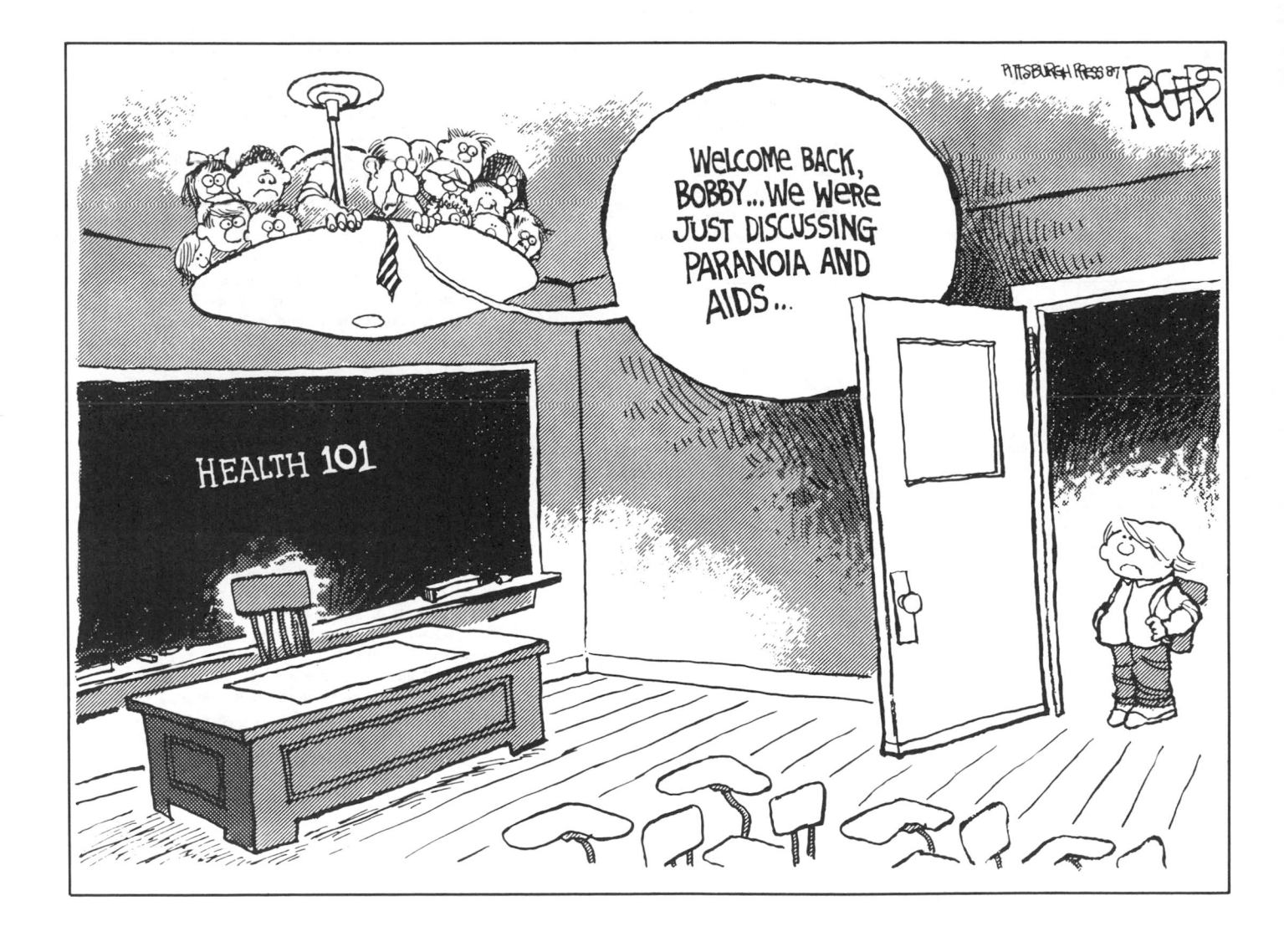

Public's Fear of AIDS Clouds School Attendance Issues

About 12,000 New York City children were kept out of school by their parents September 9, 1985 because an unidentified seven-year-old girl thought to be afflicted with AIDS had been given permission by the city to attend classes. The boycott, launched on the first day of the school year, kept home 25% of two city school districts' students. The fatal virus has touched schools in other states as well. Ryan White of Kokomo, Indiana Aug. 26 began the 1985 school year by learning his lessons over the telephone; local authorities had barred the 13-year-old AIDS victim from attending classes. By contrast, an unidentified boy suffering from AIDS was in attendance at a junior high school in Swansea, Massachusetts., with the support of the school board.

The National Centers for Disease Control August 29, 1985 issued nonbinding guidelines recommending that young AIDS victims be allowed to attend school. Most of these children—about 50 in number—had been born to mothers with AIDS, or had contracted it through transfusions of contaminated blood. Unlikely as it is that children in a schoolroom could thus pass the disease back and forth, the public's fear of AIDS is so strong that many parents feel that children who are victims of the disease should not be allowed back in school. According to the health agency, "Casual person-to-person contact, as among schoolchildren, appears to pose no risk" of contagion. Because of the nature of AIDS, however, it has been suggested that it is actually safer for the infected child not to be exposed to minor illnesses and childhood diseases of his or her classmates, and that AIDS children should therefore not attend school for their own protection. The question of how to protect the rights of both the "AIDS kids" and their classmates had blossomed into an highly emotional issue in 1985, as reports of the near epidemic status of AIDS had fueled parents' fears about the safety of their children.

The Record
Hackensack, NJ, September 1, 1985

It's time to stand up to the AIDS panic and let children with the disease go to public school. There's no medical reason why they shouldn't be there, and strong humanitarian reasons why they should. Careful controls and a case-by-case scrutiny are needed. But 5-year-olds should not be victims of fear.

There are only 17 AIDS children in all of New Jersey. This means that most districts will never encounter these tragic children, who get the disease either from blood transfusions or from their mother in the womb. But the number is likely to grow, and the state Departments of Health and Education have now issued school-admission guidelines — which, as they should, call for allowing children with AIDS to attend New Jersey schools.

There is no absolute guarantee that a healthy child can't catch AIDS from a school-mate. As Dr. Martha Rogers of the U.S. government's Centers for Disease Control puts it, "I can't guarantee that the sun will rise tomorrow." But the risk seems infinitesimal. Of 12,000 cases over the last four years, not a single one stemmed from casual contact. All were traced to sexual acts, transfusions, or contaminated drug needles. It is conceivable that, say, blood from an AIDS child could get into a wound on a healthy child's arm during a fight; but, says the CDC, blood would have to enter a wound in very large quantities to cause a problem. Other scenarios are equally far-fetched.

Indeed, the greatest hazard is to the AIDS sufferers themselves. Without an adequate immune system, they risk fatal infections from flu, colds, or earaches. And, because strict confidentiality is impossible, they risk being harassed or ostracized. But these are chances many parents of AIDS victims may choose to take — as do many parents of hemophiliac children, who attend school even though a bad fall or bloody nose could be lethal.

Children need to see a world outside their home. They need to be with other children, to feel their minds stretched in a classrooms, to laugh and talk and have the broad range of stimulation that children find in school.

Fear should not cheat AIDS children out of such experiences. And society must not give in to unreasoning terror toward those with AIDS. Unless we stand firm against panic, we may turn AIDS sufferers into the lepers of the 1980's. That would be tragic; especially if the victim of our panic is a 5-year-old.

The Miami Herald
Miami, FL, September 20, 1985

THE KNOTTY issue of whether to permit children — and teachers — known to have acquired immune-deficiency syndrome (AIDS) to attend school will not go away. The Centers for Disease Control have urged school boards to review individual cases and to admit some afflicted children to class. Most boards, however, are balking or, as in New York City, facing protests. While there is no evidence that AIDS would be spread by classroom contact, accepting the fears of parents does a community no service.

AIDS is a recent phenomenon — the first cases were reported in 1981 — and a frightening one because at least half of its victims have died and there is no known cure. So the public's fear of contact with AIDS victims is hardly surprising. If there is great concern about accepting adult AIDS victims as co-workers, there is bound to be even greater concern about accepting young victims, especially toddlers, as classmates for one's children. But the issue will not remain as isolated cases. New York City has 300 children afflicted with AIDS and expects that 700 more will be born this year.

These children are infected either at birth or through blood transfusions. The risk of transfusions has been all but eliminated by the development of a screening test for donated blood. Far more common is infection through the exchange of body fluids such as in sexual contact or sharing of contaminated needles by drug addicts.

That is not reassuring to parents who argue that young children share food, cut themselves, vomit, and cry. While no household members or health-care professionals have contracted AIDS from these body secretions, there are not the guarantees that parents demand.

Those fears must be addressed. In Florida, Dade and Lee counties have skirted the issue by opting for separate instruction of afflicted children. Contrast that with the Swansea, Mass., reaction. There, both the faculty and the parents of children at a junior-high school were invited to discuss the admission to classes of a 13-year-old suffering from hemophilia and AIDS and to question his doctor. While officials believe that some parents are keeping their children home, most are not.

The age of the child no doubt was a factor in the acceptance by the Swansea community. The point, however, is that Swansea's care in providing a forum should be a model for the nation. Parents have the right to be informed not of the young AIDS victim's identity but of the extent of the disease and of the precautions that school authorities will exercise. The disease is frightening, and the only way to displace that fear is with that most powerful weapon: accurate information.

Pittsburgh Post-Gazette

Pittsburgh, PA, September 18, 1985

The toll of Acquired Immune Deficiency Syndrome goes beyond the more than 6,700 people who have died so far in the United States. Across the country, healthy people have been infected by a virus of fear and irrationality.

In one of the saddest examples of this mental contagion, parents in Queens, New York, have protested vehemently a decision to allow a child with AIDS to attend public school. By their own testimony, these people sincerely believe they are acting responsibly.

That is part of the sadness. Parental protectiveness is one of the noblest virtues of humanity; propelled by a good impulse, the actions of the New York parents are understandable and forgivable — but forgivable precisely because they are wrong.

If the mob has its way, any child facing eventual death with AIDS will be banished from the companionship of young friends just at a time when he most needs emotional support. As if dying young were not tragedy enough, such a child must hear from society, gathering its sterile skirts protectively about it, that he is a 20th-century leper, too unclean even to sit for a while in a schoolhouse.

Yet isn't paternal prudence justified? Isn't it a fact that we don't know enough about this thing?

In fact, quite a lot is known about AIDS. The virus has been identified, and there have been enough cases — 13,228 since 1979, a figure that includes those who have died — to identify the people who are most at risk. And they are not schoolchildren sitting in the classroom.

Enough about AIDS is known to say that it is not spread by casual contact. In fact, even people living in the same house with AIDS sufferers have *never* contracted the disease through casual contact. Hospital workers, police officers and ambulance personnel regularly manage to handle AIDS patients without becoming sick themselves.

Science may not know all the answers, but this much it knows: Overwhelmingly, AIDS is spread by sexual contact, needle sharing, or less commonly, through blood or its components. While the AIDS virus has been found in saliva and tears, there have been no documented cases resulting from exposure to those liquids.

According to the Centers for Disease Control in Atlanta, Ga., 94 percent of AIDS cases occur in specific groups: Sexually active homosexual and bisexual men (73 percent), present or past abusers of intravenous drugs (17 percent), persons with hemophilia or other coagulation disorders (1 percent), heterosexual contacts of someone with AIDS or at risk of AIDS (1 percent), persons who have had transfusions with blood or blood products (2 percent).

That leaves just 6 percent of patients who do not fall into any category, but even here researchers believe that the disease was contracted in similar ways. Typically, children or infants who get AIDS — 167 cases under the age of 13 have been reported nationwide — do so by being exposed to the virus before or during birth or shortly thereafter, or else they have a history of transfusions.

But all this evidence is beside the point if anxiety blinds you to it. There is no reasoning with the angry and aroused parents of Queens who have set a burden of proof that is impossible to meet — at least in the short term. They want their children indemnified from harm, absolutely and beyond a shadow of a doubt. Back in the real world, of course, these same children face greater threats every day — from drunken drivers, from child molesters, from a fall off the swing. Yet it is the theoretical danger of AIDS that gets the pickets out.

Nobody in authority is saying that prudence is not called for; on the contrary. Indeed, an insistence that every child with AIDS — no matter what his condition — has a right to go to school is just as inflexible and foolish as calls for a complete ban on AIDS children in schools.

The Centers for Disease Control has 11 sound recommendations. Basically, the CDC suggests that each case be looked at individually, weighing the infected child's welfare against that of others in the classroom. In most cases, the CDC says there will be no reason to keep a child out of school.

In special cases, those of children who are very young and may bite, or who are neurologically handicapped and cannot control their bodily functions, or who have uncoverable lesions, the CDC recommends a more restricted setting, at least for the time being.

In Pittsburgh, the Board of Public Education wisely has set up a task force to consider the question and recommend guidelines. It comes not a moment too soon. Although there are no known cases of AIDS among schoolchildren in this area currently — or, indeed, in the state — the mathematics of the situation now seems to make such a development inevitable.

The CDC expects the number of cases nationwide to double in about 12 months. The trend can be seen locally: In Allegheny County, there were two cases in 1982, nine in both 1983 and 1984, and 16 so far this year.

This increase also makes more hysteria inevitable. Yet before the first AIDS child arrives in the schools here, local communities must reach a consensus about what to do — one that balances decent parental feelings with the need to treat a doomed child in a compassionate manner. We know enough about AIDS to do that much.

THE LINCOLN STAR

Lincoln, NE, September 26, 1985

U.S. Surgeon General C. Everett Koop owes the American people a statement on AIDS.

Several years of study have confirmed the ways in which it is spread, as well as identifying the people at high risk of catching the deadly illness. It is an infectious disease, but it isn't highly contagious. People not in high-risk groups have a one in a million chance of getting AIDS.

And this is what Koop ought to say before panic paralyzes some and stampedes others into ill-thought laws and actions.

Education is our best defense. A vaccine and cure are desperately needed, but elusive. Meanwhile it is knowledge vs. ignorance.

IGNORANCE IS winning out in much of the nation. In the New York City borough of Queens, 12,000 grade-school students are kept home because one girl with AIDS is sent to school. In Dade County, food service workers will have to be certified free of communicable disease if a proposed ordinance becomes law.

In the Washington Post, a doctor advocated quarantine as a tool to fight the disease. His lengthy opinion did not mention who should be quarantined nor how.

Even well-intentioned efforts, such as Los Angeles' hasty law prohibiting discrimination against AIDS victims, do not meet our needs. The double victim of AIDS and discrimination may die before getting his case resolved. Meanwhile, discrimination continues because education and reason have failed.

Nebraskans are not insulated. Doctors have diagnosed seven cases of AIDS here since 1983. Researchers at the Centers for Disease Control said the greatest increase in the next several years would come outside of the metropolitan areas where AIDS is now concentrated. Like everywhere else, the incidence of AIDS is likely to increase before it subsides.

We should be concerned.

We should keep it in perspective.

AIDS is not spread by casual contact. Families living with AIDS victims are not getting it, except through sexual contact.

Health care workers treating AIDS victims are not getting it, unless they are members of an identified risk group who contract the disease outside of the medical setting.

IT ISN'T SPREAD by sneezes or handshakes. The virus isn't transmitted through food or on toilet seats. Gay men and drug addicts remain the disease's main targets. The precautions they take should be more drastic. Most of us need excerise only the obvious rules of hygiene, which serve us well against all communicable disease.

AIDS is a horrifying, mysterious disease throttling segments of our population. It came suddenly to our attention and began killing almost before it had a name. Disinformation, some borne by prejudice, spreads faster than illness.

Some of that probably has spread to Nebraska, too.

The federal government was slow to respond to AIDS. Now AIDS research is getting the overdue federal dollars it deserves. But the surgeon general had better read the handwriting in the headlines. People are afraid. People are overreacting. Sick people are suffering needlessly because of it.

Koop's educational effort is past due.

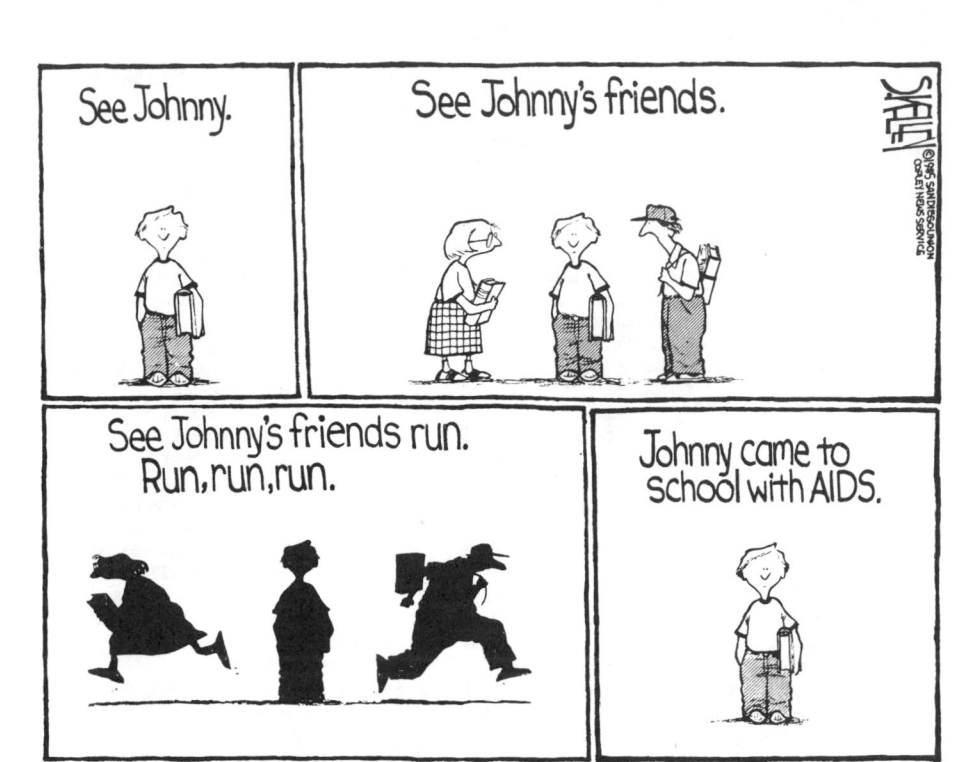

See Johnny.

See Johnny's friends.

See Johnny's friends run. Run, run, run.

Johnny came to school with AIDS.

THE TENNESSEAN

September 4, 1985
Nashville, TN

ALTHOUGH the serious medical threat of the deadly AIDS virus cannot be overstated, the public's reaction to the disease has become, in some instances, a menace in its own right.

The fear of AIDS has already caused tremendous discrimination and threatened the constitutional rights of privacy, not just for AIDS victims but for the groups most likely to contract the virus — homosexuals, intravenous drug users, recipients of blood transfusions, and Haitians. The ripple effect of AIDS has lapped over into some ancillary aspects of health care industry, such as the insurance industry and blood donation centers.

At least 183 juveniles have been diagnosed as having AIDS, and specialists estimate that many hundred more children have been exposed to the virus. Those children with AIDS have raised even more perplexing problems, particularly for public school officials.

Officials at the federal Center for Disease Control said last week that in most cases, children with AIDS should be allowed to attend regular school, and that school officials should attempt to protect those children's confidentiality. So far, the health officials know of no AIDS victim in the nation who has been admitted to a public school.

They suggest that schools admit young AIDS victims on a case-by-case basis, considering factors such as the child's physical and emotional condition. Those specialists emphasized that casual contact will not spread the disease, and in no cases have children acquired AIDS in day care centers, kindergardens, or schools.

Most children with AIDS are children of AIDS victims, or have other medical conditions which require blood transfusions.

AIDS is certainly a mysterious disease that was too long ignored by the government. Now much effort is being put into finding a cure, and in the past few months, the scientific community has had several promising research breakthroughs. Until a cure is found, the public would be best advised to stay calm, stay informed, and treat AIDS victims of all ages with compassion and not scorn.

DESERET NEWS

Salt Lake City, UT, September 21, 1985

As elsewhere in the nation, the numbers of AIDS cases in Utah keep growing — 23 confirmed victims at last count. Of those, 12 have died, including two children, who were added to the list this week.

The spread of AIDS has been described as an epidemic. Certainly, the growth has been rapid, from an unknown malady five years ago to about 12,000 diagnosed cases nationwide. Yet there is no need for public panic.

Statistically, the number of AIDS cases is still small, much research is being done, and a great deal is already understood about AIDS. However, there is no vaccine and no cure yet. The disease is invariably fatal.

AIDS itself does not kill anyone. What it does is break down the body's immune system so that the victim becomes susceptible to a variety of illnesses that the body cannot fight. Cancer is often a result.

But the AIDS virus is not a free-floating virus that can be easily passed along like the flu. As far as scientists can tell, there are only three ways to transmit the disease: (1) by sexual contact, particularly among homosexual men, (2) by use of contaminated needles, a problem among drug abusers, or (3) by receiving infected blood or blood products.

Females may be infected through sexual contact with males who have AIDS virus, but the opposite apparently is far more rare. Those factors ought to help limit the spread of AIDS.

In Utah, as is the case nationally, about 70 percent of AIDS cases are in homosexual or bisexual males, 20 percent in intravenous drug users, and 10 percent from transfusions or blood products.

Unfortunately, there has been almost a panic in some states where children have been diagnosed as AIDS victims, with parents demanding the AIDS child be removed from school. Those reactions are understandable, but they have little to do with reality.

Of the two children who died in Utah, one contracted AIDS from a blood transfusion out of state. The other case is still under investigation.

Utah Department of Health officials are careful to explain that it does not appear AIDS is transmitted by casual kissing, by using the same eating utensils, or touching objects such as doorknobs or toilet seats. Family members of AIDS victims do not come down with the disease by living in close proximity on a daily basis with the victim. Neither have doctors and nurses caught AIDS while treating the sick.

Of course, none of this means that AIDS can be lightly dismissed. An estimated two million people have been exposed to the AIDS virus. Most of those will never come down with the disease, but some may be unwitting carriers.

Because the incubation period for AIDS can be as long as five years, victims may be stricken long after the initial exposure. Such time elements keep the risk level fairly high. And there's always the danger that AIDS may find a way to invade the general population if an answer to the disease is not found soon.

In the meantime, as spokesmen at a Salt Lake City-County Health Department seminar pointed out this week, the safest course for people in high-risk categories is to adopt a more conservative lifestyle.

As for the rest, people should avoid hysteria, rumors, or a plague mentality that treats AIDS victims as some kind of lepers.

The San Diego Union

San Diego, CA, September 18, 1985

Across the country, school districts and administrators are moving to establish policy about school-age children with AIDS. This emotion-laden issue has already reached the classroom doors in California, Connecticut, Florida, Indiana, Massachusetts, New Jersey. New York and the District of Columbia.

Predictably at this early stage, the response by school authorities to the AIDS dilemma varies dramatically.

In Miami, triplet girls who contracted AIDS from their mother, now dead, are being given first-grade instruction by a volunteer teacher in a largely empty old building, removed from the general school population.

In Kokomo, Ind., a 13-year-old boy with hemophilia, who contracted AIDS from contaminated blood, has been barred from school and can only monitor classes by telephone from his home. Several neighbors, upset that he continues his newspaper route, have canceled their subscriptions.

Pre-school children with some form of AIDS have been rejected for schooling in Redondo Beach, Calif., and Plainfield and Washington Borough, N.J.

Only two communities — one tiny, and one enormous — have publicly admitted AIDS victims to the classroom. In Swansea. Mass., a 12-year-old with AIDs contracted from a contaminated blood transfusion has been admitted to class. This after a thorough discussion by school authorities and the boy's physician, who is a professor at the Brown University Medical School. No public protest has followed.

But in New York City, 18,000 students — a quarter of the children in two Queens Districts — stayed home from school last week as parents protested the city's decision to permit a child with AIDS to attend second-grade classes. Even as the protest raged, a state judge rejected a petition to bar the child from school. The boycott is subsiding, although hundreds of protesting parents continue to storm Board of Education meetings.

The New York policy calls for each child with AIDS to be screened by a special panel of health experts, an educator, and a parent to determine whether instruction should be in the classroom or at home. Victims admitted to class will not be identified.

Meanwhile, mixing toughness with tenderness, the New York schools last week ordered five employees, including teachers and a food-service worker found to have AIDS, to depart on permanent medical leave. Additionally, all New York students from kindergarten through high school will get information about AIDS as part of courses on drug abuse, family living, and sex education. And, beginning immediately, there will be workshops on AIDS for parents and employees.

New York's approach bodes to become a model for school authorities around the country, who must grapple in time with the AIDS issue. Time and additional medical knowledge may make decisions easier than they are today. As of now, the Federal Centers for Disease Control, the most knowledgeable authority on AIDS, recommends that most children with AIDS be admitted to public schools. Even so, it urges a significant precaution: That preschoolers who bite or have open lesions be separated from other children who could be exposed. New York's screening of each child with AIDS would provide for this one known exception to the known rule that the virus can be transmitted only by sexual contact, and by contaminated needles and blood transfusions.

Physicians have diagnosed 120 cases of AIDS in San Diego, resulting in 55 deaths to date. The most recent was a 29-year-old prostitute who had been confined at the Las Colinas Detention Facility.

Although there are no known youngsters with AIDS in San Diego, almost certainly there will be. School boards in San Diego County should formulate an AIDS admission policy now and announce it publicly before public panic and protests arrive with the first case. New York City, we repeat, has provided a model policy that is thoughtful, cautious, and humane.

The Seattle Times

Seattle, WA, September 11, 1985

NO MATTER how deep the fear of AIDS (acquired immune deficiency), denying blameless young victims of the mysterious killer the right to attend public schools is cruel and unreasonable.

Just how cruel is evident in New York City where frightened parents are protesting a 7-year-old boy's presence in a Queens classroom. The child, an AIDS sufferer since birth, had attended school for two years, but panicky authorities now want to bar him from classes.

In Indianapolis, a young hemophiliac who contracted AIDS after treatment with contaminated blood, no longer is allowed in school. As similar issues arise elsewhere, school officials need to remember there's no evidence that AIDS is transmitted through casual contact.

St. Paul Pioneer Press & Dispatch

St. Paul. MN, September 26, 1985

Children with AIDS should not be barred from school; neither should they be identified, except to the school nurse and the principal. Furthermore, AIDS guidelines should be uniform throughout the state, to discourage transfers of students motivated by fears not based on fact.

Sensible guidelines were set forth by the Minnesota Department of Health this week. Those guidelines advise against quarantine. They also correctly urge the formation of an advisory committee to help parents, school districts and doctors decide when children with active AIDS need to be at home because of their own risk of catching life-threatening infections from others.

Quarantine of AIDS victims is simply not necessary. Terrifying as the disease may be, no one that researchers know of has ever caught it from casual contact — even contact every day, even when the victims are children whose diapers and scrapes and runny noses are tended by other family members for years and years.

With the tragic exception of babies who get it from their infected mothers, AIDS comes from deliberately chosen, specific behavior. People get it by injecting drugs with contaminated needles; or else they get it by having sex with an infected partner. The latter risk zooms when the sex is with multiple partners, especially with homosexual or bisexual men, especially with anal sex.

AIDS contagion does *not* lurk in sneezes or shared sandwiches or drinking glasses or toilet seats or mosquito bites. Because a reliable test was developed last spring to screen donated blood, people don't get it from transfusions, either. Sadly, most children with AIDS today picked it up from transfusions before that time.

Dr. Frank Rhame, director of infection control at University of Minnesota Hospitals, told us that it is "frustrating as all get out that people are worried about little schoolkids, when the virus is killing us through sexual transmission."

AIDS is starting to show up in prostitutes and in the general population. Sowing facts about AIDS will help stop the spread not only of the virus itself, but also of irrational fears about it. Adults must first educate themselves and, when appropriate, modify their behavior. Then, urgently, they must educate teen-agers about the extreme hazards of promiscuity and of specific sexual practices.

If ever adults needed to face the fact that sexual behavior, including homosexual behavior, begins in high school for many, they need to face it now. If ever sex education was needed in schools, it is needed now. Far more is at stake than an unplanned pregnancy or a curable venereal disease.

It is fortunate that education, not quarantine, is the key to controlling AIDS. How would such a quarantine be possible? The quarantine would be lifelong. Some 13,228 active cases are on record in this country, but people infected with the virus, yet not showing symptoms, can spread it at least as easily as the sick. Estimates of the number of infected people range from 500,000 to 2 million. How does one set up a leper colony for 2 million Americans?

Behavior is to be shunned, not victims.

The Union Leader

Manchester, NH, September 16, 1985

The controversy over AIDS intensifies, especially in New York City, the nation's largest school system. There, it is being fueled by a physician's testimony on behalf of protesting parents that an AIDS-afflicted child in a school does indeed pose a danger to other children, by the disclosure that five school employes are on medical leave because they contracted AIDS, and by the recent report that three others have died from the deadly disease.

Before this backdrop, Brooklyn school board member Walter Johnson angrily called last week for the indictment of Schools Chancellor Nathan Quinones for "endangering the lives" of children by failing to notify parents that Donald Baldwin, the former *food-services supervisor* at a Brooklyn junior high school, had AIDS.

It is becoming more and more apparent that, rather than calming public hysteria, some of those in positions of responsibility are unintentionally inciting it by submerging the rights of the non-afflicted majority to those of the tragically afflicted minority.

As long as authorities, reacting largely to demands from homosexual activists, view AIDS primarily as a political issue, rather than a medical one, and as long as even justified expressions of parental concern are contemptuously dismissed as "hysteria" by officials who seem to lack even a basic understanding of human nature, for just that long will this controversy grow more bitter. ——Jim Finnegan

ST. LOUIS POST-DISPATCH

St. Louis, MO, September 1, 1985

A new hysteria is developing among many Americans today who are frightened about AIDS, acquired immune deficiency syndrome. In one case in Kokomo, Ind., a 13-year-old boy with AIDS has been kept out of school. He is a hemophiliac who contracted AIDS because of contaminated blood in transfusions.

But the federal government now says that children with AIDS should be allowed in the classroom and that school officials should do their best to protect the pupils' privacy. No evidence has shown that the disease can be transmitted through casual contact in the classroom, school showers, day-care centers, gymnasiums or elsewhere.

That should end the hysteria right there. But it probably won't, because the disease remains a mystery. It is reminiscent of years ago, when many parents refused to allow their youngsters to go to school if another child at that school had polio. Children were kept in their homes by parents who wanted to make sure they didn't "catch" the disease. Of course their fears were unwarranted, as are those of school systems that refuse to allow children with AIDS to attend school. In addition to being a violation of the civil rights of youngsters with the disease, refusing to allow such students to attend school is an unreasonable posture. And, says the federal government, it is also an unfounded one.

A vaccine was eventually found to prevent polio, and today the disease is virtually nonexistent in the U.S. Let us hope that something similar will happen with AIDS. Until then, the public must practice tolerance and realize that the rights of the well do not supersede the rights of the ill.

THE ATLANTA CONSTITUTION

Atlanta, GA, September 18, 1985

School officials in Georgia have an opportunity that eluded their counterparts last month in Massachusetts, New York and Washington: to formulate AIDS policies in the absence of a crisis.

Forced by the demands of parents to admit or bar students suffering from AIDS, educators elsewhere took widely divergent approaches to the problem: admitting them in one school district, rejecting them in another. There has been little in their scattershot responses to guide others.

But more is known about the deadly disease with each week that goes by: how it's transmitted, how it's not transmitted, the tremendous odds against its being transmitted through casual (that is to say, non-sexual, external) contact.

Of the more than 13,000 Americans afflicted with AIDS, 216 have been in Georgia. None of the Georgia cases involves a school-age child, but two groups — the Bibb County School Board and a task force of the state Department of Human Resources — are meeting to consider their options.

The Bibb County board plans to vote Thursday on a proposal to ban AIDS sufferers from attending or teaching classes in its schools. It would be wise to await the report of the state DHR task force, but if the Bibb board feels for some reason that it must act now, it at least should take into account the recommendations of the Atlanta-based Centers for Disease Control before it does.

Until the DHR task force issues its recommendations, State School Superintendent Charles McDaniel sensibly has advised local districts to follow the CDC recommendations. The CDC, holding that most children with AIDS should be allowed to attend classes, recommends barring only those who are suffering from skin eruptions or lesions that cannot be covered, are habitually incontinent, tend to bite others or are in advanced stages of the disease.

Meanwhile, proposals to add an AIDS test to the premarital blood test in Georgia, protect the confidentiality of AIDS victims and channel public funds into AIDS treatment programs must also be dealt with on an expeditious, if not yet urgent, basis. The cooler the heads brought to the debate, and the calmer the atmosphere, the better.

The Burlington Free Press

Burlington, VT, September 15, 1985

AIDS (acquired immune deficiency syndrome) is a mysterious ailment which inhibits the body's ability to fight disease with generally fatal consequences.

Doctors and researchers who are familiar with the disease say it can only be transmitted through homosexual contact, intravenous drug use or transfusions of contaminated blood. It cannot be contracted through casual contact with victims, they say.

Editorial

But parents of public school students in New York City are so alarmed by the announcement that a second-grade pupil with the disease will be allowed to attend school that they have organized a boycott of classes. In Queens, more than 11,000 elementary and junior high school students were kept home by concerned parents when city schools reopened Monday. Parents and children picketed the school buildings, demanding that the child not be allowed to mingle with other pupils. While the number of absentees was but a fraction of the 946,000 children in the city's public schools, the parents' action indicated that they have genuine fears about the possibility of the spread of the disease through contact.

A solid case may be made on the basis of available medical evidence for allowing students with AIDS to attend classes. But the qualifying phrase in that sentence is "available medical evidence." Researchers cannot yet have a clear idea about the ways in which the disease spreads. It is, after all, a virus. In the past, misconceptions about the transmission of other viruses have only been corrected by lengthy and thorough research. Even today, some viruses still are inexplicably complex. It is possible, for instance, that AIDS is transmitted by as-yet undiscovered means. In fact, AIDS victims who bite or have open sores will not be allowed to attend classes in New York City with other children. That, in itself, is an indication of some doubt about the possibility of transmitting the disease in other ways.

Children in kindergarten or the first grade have a tendency to disregard some of the basic rules of hygiene, often sharing drinks and food during lunch periods. Body fluids tend to flow freely in younger children.

Thus it is not difficult to understand why parents are so concerned about the health of their children when they learn that a child with AIDS may be in the classroom with them. And parents will not be reassured by statements from school administrators or doctors who claim that children are not in jeopardy under those circumstances.

Certainly children who have AIDS should not be denied the opportunity to attend public schools.

At the same time, however, those in charge must take extraordinary precautions to ensure that healthy students do not contract the disease.

The Providence Journal
Providence, RI, September 11, 1985

Amid the fear and confusion surrounding the disease AIDS, some are able to keep clear heads and reasonable perspective. An outstanding example is Swansea, Mass. school officials and teachers at Case Junior High School there. Case may be the first school in the nation to knowingly enroll an AIDS victim.

When it became known that a teenage boy who suffers from hemophilia had contracted AIDS (acquired immune deficiency syndrome) school officials consulted medical experts.

The Star-Ledger
Newark, NJ, September 11, 1985

One child—a seven-year-old girl with the misfortune of being born with AIDS—was the cause of a boycott that kept thousands of students out of New York City schools because of their parents' concern that she might transmit the dreaded disease to other youngsters. This is the latest and most disturbing public protest, a pattern of escalating hysteria that threatens to become epidemic.

Parental concern is, of course, an understandable protective reaction. But unless all medical knowledge concerning this life-threatening disease is completely misleading, there is little danger of it being transmitted by casual social contact.

Making a single second-grader afflicted with acquired immune deficiency syndrome a pariah can only further intensify this highly emotional controversy. A school boycott deepens and complicates a problem that should be dealt with in a rational manner, based on medical research.

Instead, there are widespread public misperceptions and unfounded rumors about AIDS that have grossly distorted factual information which medical scientists have developed through research.

* * *

The little girl who has become a *cause celebre* in New York has attended school for two years without endangering her classmates. But that has not quelled the fears of the parents who staged the New York boycott. And similar concern is surfacing in New Jersey, where there are several known cases of AIDS among school-age children. A court suit has been filed to admit three students suffering from AIDS back into class.

In this instance, a court challenge may be premature—an action before the fact. New Jersey's top education and health officials have recommended that children with AIDS be permitted to attend school. But the crucial decision about whether they should be admitted has been left to local school boards.

The state has set guidelines drawn from the most recent medical findings on AIDS. Whatever formula that evolves may not allay the fears and concerns of parents, but at the very least it should provide a starting point in dealing with this complex, emotional medical-social problem. It should be evident, at this stage, that there are no easy answers.

Because the boy "has no unusual behavioral problems or uncontrollable lesions," said George F. Grady, Massachusetts state epidemiologist, "there is no reason why he should not attend classes as long as his general health permits."

Mr. Grady noted that the only significant means of AIDS transmission is through blood or blood product injections and sexual contact. It is this point that arouses so much unnecessary concern. Some believe AIDS is contagious — that by merely being in the presence of an AIDS victim one can "catch" the disease. Scientists say this is not so. That information comes from the federal Centers for Disease Control, the Governor's Task Force on AIDS in Massachusetts and numerous other sources.

But uncertainty still exists in many professional and lay quarters. School officials knew that teachers, school personnel and parents would be concerned if the boy were admitted. Wisely they called a meeting earlier this summer attended by the school principal, nurse, teachers who would be instructing the boy, the boy's father and physician, a social worker and a nurse from the Hemophilia Center of Rhode Island. Later a larger meeting was held to allay fears, with more teachers present.

The upshot is that school officials now report a generally supportive attitude toward the boy. Such enlightenment should be an inspiration to others caught in the grip of fear. AIDS is not the black plague. While there is much about it that is not known, efforts are under way to develop a vaccine and only simple precautions need be taken to avoid virtually all danger of developing the disease.

As Dr. Peter Smith, the boy's physician and director of the hemophilia center, told Case Junior High teachers, there is no such thing as 100 percent assurance in the biological sciences. But he added, "You face greater risk getting into an automobile. And I can't promise you that no one is going to plant a bomb in the school or you are not going to fall out a window."

Bravo to Dr. Smith and school officials and teachers at Case Junior High. Fear of AIDS is perfectly understandable. What is not is a tendency, even after danger signals have been responsibly lowered, to treat AIDS victims as untouchables to be ostracized as a societal threat. The travesty of barring a 13-year-old AIDS victim from school in Kokomo, Ind. has been offset and then some by the intelligent approach of Swansea's pioneers.

Birmingham Post-Herald
Birmingham, AL, September 4, 1985

Just the mention of the disease AIDS is enough to arouse fear in a large segment of the public. And that fear is adding unnecessarily to the tragedy faced by victims of Acquired Immune Deficiency Syndrome.

Victims find themselves shunned, treated as lepers. Nor does the ostracism stop with victims. Relatives and friends of those with the disease as well as individuals in high-risk groups face the same stigma.

Perhaps the hardest hit of these new social outcasts are children. At a time when they should be with others of their own age, they are being isolated. School officials across the country are refusing to let children with AIDS into regular classrooms.

Recently, a federal judge in Indiana upheld the decision of Kokomo school officials to bar 13-year-old Ryan White from Western Middle School. Ryan, a hemophiliac who caught AIDS through a blood transfusion, is being taught by telephone. Other children with AIDS face similar isolation.

Now, there is no doubt that AIDS is a horrible disease. Despite identification of the virus that causes a victim's immune system to break down and despite tests that can identify presence of the disease before symptoms appear, AIDS has no cure at this time. Over half of this country's 12,736 identified victims have died since AIDS was first diagnosed in 1981. The prognosis for the others and future victims remains bleak.

But the hysterical attempts to avoid contact with its victims do not make sense. AIDS is not transmitted through casual contact. Sexual intercourse, other intimate contact involving the exchange of body fluids or injections are required to transmit it. These do not normally occur in a school setting.

In light of these facts, the national Centers for Disease Control says that school-age children with AIDS should be allowed to attend school or day-care programs. The centers' guidelines do make exceptions for very young children and some handicapped children. And obviously, a child for whom the ravages of the disease are far advanced will not be physically able to attend classes with other children.

But for many children with AIDS, the words of Dr. Martha Rogers, one of the center's AIDS specialists, apply. "I don't see any need to keep them out. They have enough suffering without it being made more so by the rest of society."

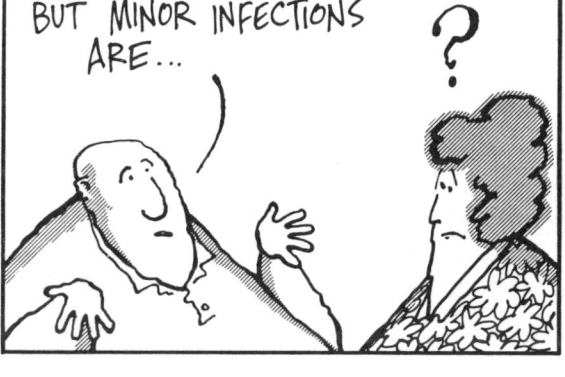

DAILY ● NEWS

New York, NY, September 15, 1985

AIDS IS NOT the Black Death, or smallpox or influenza. Those were plagues that spread rapidly by casual contact and killed millions. Almost all known AIDS cases in the U.S. have been traced to sexual contact, exchanges of blood by intravenous drug users, blood transfusions or inheritance—babies born to infected women.

There have been 13,074 cases of AIDS in the U.S. but no known cases where the disease has spread to their families. AIDS has been known for five years. Incubation can range from two or five years. So if casual contact could transmit AIDS, it would probably have been detected by now.

The danger it can be passed between children is tiny: It has never happened, so far as anyone knows.

But that's the sticking point. If there's a risk, however slight, parents won't let their children run it.

A study in Science magazine said saliva carries the AIDS virus but "is not thought to be an efficient transmitter of the disease." It is reasonable to refuse to submit children to even very inefficient transmitters of AIDS.

The city has placed an unnamed second-grade pupil with AIDS in a New York school. Her condition is in remission, there are no symptoms, and most medical opinion is sure she is no danger to other children.

The reaction of Queens parents who have boycotted local schools was unjustified. But that doesn't mean the city was right to put the child in school. The object of public policy must be to fight the epidemic—and to stop the plague panic before it turns into a witch hunt against homosexuals.

BUT THE CITY MUST PICK the right battles. It will lose its attempt to keep this child in school. And it will lose any attempt to keep school personnel with AIDS. With children, authorities must err on the side of caution.

There are about a dozen children in the city with AIDS. It's manageable—so far, though it will get worse. The problem of adult patients is incomparably more serious.

It's not a "gay disease." It's a horrible, always fatal disease that can be transmitted sexually—and in the U.S. it happened to break out first among the gay population.

Now it's spreading to heterosexuals through prostitutes and casual promiscuity. It could spread very far indeed.

The school boycott was mistaken but understandable. The protest over the proposed AIDS clinic in the Rockaways was unjustified. The city made a serious mistake giving in to it. That was the fight to pick and win, and the failure could come back to haunt the Koch administration.

There may be anything from 100,000 to 250,000 AIDS cases in the U.S. by 1990, a third of them in New York. It's time to get ready—in the right places and in the right ways.

ARGUS-LEADER

Sioux Falls, SD, September 17, 1985

In Indiana, a 13-year-old boy is barred from school. He sits alone in his bedroom, listening to teachers and classmates over the telephone.

The boy became ill when treated for hemophilia. Now, he is among at least 165 children in the United States known to 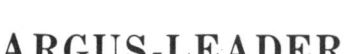 suffer from AIDS — acquired immune deficiency syndrome.

The teen-ager suffers a double misfortune.

AIDS is a mysterious disease that is tearing down his body's immune system and probably will leave him susceptible to deadly infections and cancer. So far, unfortunately, that can't be prevented. There is, as yet, no cure for AIDS.

There is no justification for the boy's second problem: rejection by society.

AIDS is a serious and growing health problem in the United States. But fear of the virus does not justify panic.

There is no reason to make AIDS victims outcasts. There is no reason to ban children with AIDS from school.

Researchers believe that AIDS is transmitted through the exchange of body fluids, mainly blood and semen. Three-fourths of those in the United States known to suffer AIDS happen to be gays and bisexual men, but the disease is not a "gay plague." Victims include drug users who have used contaminated needles, hemophiliacs who have received blood transfusions and children born to infected mothers.

AIDS may spread into other segments of society. But all evidence indicates the virus is not easily spread, that AIDS is not spread through casual contact and touching. So there is no reason to overreact.

We do not label cancer victims outcasts. We do not ban children with venereal diseases from attending school. Why the special vengeance against AIDS victims?

It's especially unfortunate that children have become victims of this shabby treatment. They contract AIDS passively. Most get it from infected parents. The disease apparently can be transmitted during pregnancy.

But even that does not justify the infectious fear that is spreading across the nation. Hysteria is spreading faster than the disease.

Some worry is understandable. But let's not allow fears to get in the way of facts. And let's quit freezing out victims.

Instead, let's freeze out the rabble-rousers who are too ignorant to keep their minds open to the facts about AIDS.

THE SAGINAW NEWS
Saginaw, MI, September 18, 1985

In an emergency, the first rule is: Don't panic.

The spread of AIDS certainly qualifies as an emergency. The disease is deadly, it is infectious and it is not confined only to the high-risk groups of homosexuals, drug addicts and hemophiliacs.

The epidemic raises two points of response. One is finding a cause and cure for acquired immune deficiency syndrome. The other is what to do in the meantime.

On the first point, there can be no argument. AIDS justifies a full-scale research campaign, with accelerated funding. The frightening prospect is that millions of Americans may be at risk.

The fear, however, is verging on panic. It has led to extremes, from different directions, on how society should try to deal with AIDS and, more to the point, its victims and possible carriers.

The Los Angeles City Council did not act in panic when it put AIDS patients under the protection of civil rights laws. But it did go to an extreme. However the disease is transmitted, it is still infectious. "Gay rights" does not mean AIDS rights.

From Kokomo to New York City, however, public feeling is equally high on the opposite issue: Should AIDS victims be, in effect, ostracized from society?

In the small Indiana city, school officials said yes. A hemophiliac child was barred from classrooms. His lessons were sent by telephone.

In New York, Superintendent Nathan Quinones refused to either identify or expel children born with AIDS. Outraged parents kept 10,000 children home in one district. When it was disclosed that a food-service employee had kept working while dying of AIDS, a local board member demanded the indictment of Quinones.

The reactions reflect deep uncertainty about AIDS. They demand, first, public education, and second, a measure of rationality.

A New York Times-CBS poll shows more than half of Americans think AIDS can be transmitted by ordinary contact. Yet doctors say AIDS is spread only by sexual contact, use of contaminated needles, or tainted blood transfusions.

That means you cannot contract AIDS by giving blood. It means school children with AIDS cannot spread the disease. Until the recent disclosures, some of the afflicted New York children had been attending classes for years without incident.

Fear is not justified. Concern, however, is.

Until its precise nature is identified, AIDS victims probably should not work in certain occupations — such as medicine — where blood exchange is possible. The Center for Disease Control urged men who have had homosexual contact within the past eight years to refrain from giving blood. That should be more than a recommendation. The donation of blood that may carry AIDS should be a crime.

Such legal measures cannot eliminate, but may alleviate, a justifiable source of public anxiety. Meanwhile, the health community should stress the total lack of evidence that casual contact spreads AIDS.

Its victims deserve sympathy and scientific assistance. Society deserves reasonable protections. But panic never conquered any disease.

The Boston Globe
Boston, MA, September 9, 1985

The decision to allow an AIDS-stricken Swansea schoolboy to attend class was difficult but right. Great credit is due state Human Services Secretary Philip Johnston and Swansea school superintendent John McCarthy who stood by him — on solid public health ground. They faced down widespread misunderstanding, often bordering on hysteria, about the disease.

Their admirable stance, however, does not diminish the need for an all-out research effort to combat AIDS. If anything, it illustrates the growing threat of AIDS, a threat that has been paid little more than lip service by the Reagan administration.

AIDS, an acronym for Acquired Immune Deficiency Syndrome, is a major and complex disease, caused by an exotic and little understood new virus, that has spread worldwide since it was first recognized in June 1981.

The manifestations of the disease are hard for the public to grasp, but therein lie the best grounds for preventing panic. At the same time, what is already known about AIDS is so worrisome, not a moment should be wasted in marshaling a full-scale attack against it.

In the United States and other countries with high standards of living, the pattern of AIDS is relatively constant. It still is most commonly spread by sexual contact with virus-infected semen, primarily among homosexuals; and by exposure to AIDS-contaminated blood — through blood products needed by hemophiliacs, blood transfusions and the exchange of dirty needles by drug addicts.

Spread into the heterosexual population remains slow, accounting for one percent of the 13,000 cases of acute — and deadly — AIDS confirmed over the past four years in the United States. That statistic is both reassuring and misleading. While the percentage stays the same, the numbers grow. When there were only 6,000 cases of acute AIDS, only 60 heterosexuals had the disease. Now there are 130.

Most important, however, is that there is still no evidence that AIDS can be spread by casual contact — at least, not in First World countries. Even in the Third World, where AIDS occurs equally among men and women, that spread is believed to be largely due to primitive folk-medicine practices.

Massachusetts' new policy allowing school-age children with AIDS to attend class is well founded. It is impossible to simply "catch" AIDS, like measles or a cold. Because the AIDS virus can exist in body excretions, such as tears, saliva, urine and feces, the state's policy, following CDC guidelines, would exclude AIDS-afflicted schoolchildren who have behavior problems such as biting or incontinence. For the same reason, pre-schoolers with AIDS who are not yet toilet-trained may be excluded from nursery school or day-care centers.

"Both the child's right to an education and the importance of recognizing the concern of school officials and parents have been taken into consideration," said Philip Johnston. "Where other children in classroom will not be endangered, a child with AIDS is entitled to receive an education. We will not succumb to unnecessary fears."

The policy tries to protect the rights of all — the stricken schoolchild and his classmates — during a time when there is great anxiety over AIDS. Anxiety, however, does not legitimize irrational discrimination. Officials in New York City and Kokomo, Ind., who recently took the easy way out, barring AIDS-afflicted children from school, should be ashamed.

AUGUSTA HERALD
Augusta, GA, September 25, 1985

Is the most amazing aspect of the current hullabaloo over admission of youthful AIDS victims to public schools being overlooked?

Parents and school administrators ponder in perplexity the possibility of the condition being passed on to other children. Health authorities cannot say with finality that there is no such danger, although apparently they strongly think there isn't.

Meanwhile, however, there is no doubt whatsoever about danger to the AIDS-afflicted children themselves. AIDS is, if we need a reminder, acquired immune deficiency. Its victims have no natural immunity defense against a multitude of infections which could fasten their talons on the luckless patient.

This being so, and infections being as widespread as they are among school-age children who have not yet acquired an adult level of precautions in hazardous contacts, it gives one pause.

It would seem that the chances for an AIDS child to acquire a fatal infection are too great to risk that child's presence in school.

Isn't that a factor which ought to be considered seriously by parents of the few child victims who have been identified?

Public Education Stressed as AIDS Prevention Measure

Public education has come to be recognized as an effective method to stop the spread of AIDS. Critics have argued that the amount of education the public receives is inadequate. In its 1986 report *Confronting AIDS* the National Academy of Sciences (NAS), stated that education is the most persuasive way to reduce the spread of the AIDS virus. The report urged that much stronger efforts be made to educate the public about the effects of the AIDS virus. The NAS suggested that educational efforts be expanded and diversified to reach as many groups as possible: those who are infected or at risk of infection, those in a position of public opinion, and those who interact with AIDS victims. Surgeon General C. Everett Koop has stressed the importance of education as a necessity in stopping the spread of AIDS. His own *Report on AIDS* stresses the responsibility of all adults to educate the young. He points out that "the lives of our young people depend on our fulfilling our responsibility." The report calls for AIDS education to begin "in the lowest grade possible."

Education can work to prevent the spread of AIDS by altering the behavior through which the AIDS virus is transmitted. Because no medical means such as a vaccine has been developed to contain the spread of AIDS, many educators say people must be taught how to isolate the spread of the virus through their own activity. Some existing evidence suggests that educational programs have been successfully undertaken.

Gay rights groups and civil rights attorneys have also argued that education is an effective way to halt AIDS-related discrimination. Unfounded fears about the transmission of AIDS through casual contact have resulted in the controversies over attendance of school children with AIDS, and employment discrimination. A 1985 NBC poll, for instance, revealed that some people believed that they could catch AIDS by being in the same room as a person with AIDS. In addition, polls have shown that as much as one-third of the general population falsely believed that donating blood can infect them with the virus. It is argued that an aggressive educational program aimed at the general public explaining how AIDS is transmitted will diminish both fear and the reasons for discrimination.

The Oregonian
Portland, OR, October 2, 1985

Neither a vaccine nor a drug is on the horizon as a cure for AIDS, the deadly acquired immune deficiency syndrome. This bad news leaves only one current weapon to fight the spread of AIDS: a public educational campaign aimed at countering the spread of AIDS by ensuring the population is aware of the risks and possible precautions.

The discouraging news came from the United States Public Health Service, which on the positive side has set a goal of slowing the increase of AIDS cases by 1987 and a long-range goal of finding a vaccine or drug cure by the year 2000.

The new pessimism on a more immediate cure or vaccine is a rollback from the optimistic predictions made last year by Margaret Heckler, departing secretary of Health and Human Services, that a vaccine might be available in two years.

The difficulty, scientists have learned, is that the AIDS virus changes its outer coating so rapidly that immune systems have trouble recognizing it.

Scientists need to find an unchanging feature with which a vaccine may couple. Since viruses as a group have not responded well to drugs, there is not much optimism that AIDS can be knocked out with a drug treatment.

An educational campaign on AIDS — both to convey up-to-date information on preventive precautions and to fight unwarranted fears — clearly is as much a continuing responsibility of the federal government as is the funding of research to develop a cure or vaccine.

The government should not be stingy on either front.

THE ARIZONA REPUBLIC
Phoenix, AZ, November 20, 1985

IN recommending that schoolchildren afflicted with the deadly AIDS virus be permitted to remain in the classroom, a statewide task force has come to grips rationally with a hysteria-causing subject.

The state Board of Education should adopt the recommendation when it meets on Nov. 25. That is the next critical step in framing a workable public education policy on acquired immune deficiency syndrome, one that is cognizant of local school district prerogatives while sensitive to innocent pupils and their right to receive a public education.

There is nothing mandatory about the task force recommendation. It is strictly a guideline for setting policy in each local district, leaving the specifics up to districts. Local boards, in anticipation of state Board of Education approval, should begin preparations so that a plan is in place before AIDS cases arise.

The guidelines are patterned after those drafted by a similar task force in Connecticut which permit an AIDS-infected youngster to attend regular classes unless a school medical examiner determines there is a risk of disease transmission due to a child's behavior.

"If it's possible to leave them in a regular classroom setting, they should be left there," commented Dennis Van Roekel, a task force member and president of the Arizona Education Association.

It was a view shared by task force chairwoman Karin Kirksey Zander, who stated that the guidelines send a "real important message" to local districts which, properly so, are "in the driver's seat."

About half of the more than 14,000 individuals afflicted with AIDS have died from the disease, for which there is no known cure. There are some 160 children under age 13 with the disease and it is believed child victims contract the killer disease from their mothers during pregnancy or via blood transfusions. In Arizona, only one pupil is known to have AIDS. The individual receives instruction at home based upon a physician's recommendation.

Appointed by the Board of Education to avert the panic evidenced elsewhere in the nation over the admission of AIDS-infected children, the task force is to be commended for showing compassion in structuring guidelines, yet leaving implementation at the local district level.

THE PLAIN DEALER

Cleveland, OH, July 17, 1985

In too many social services and educational specialties, Ohio has been a follower of trends, not a national leader. But in at least one area the state has won praise for progressiveness. Ohio has budgeted funds and hired a homosexual consultant to educate people about Acquired Immune Deficiency Syndrome (AIDS). The action is significant because there is no known cure for AIDS, which is fatal within five years. Prevention is paramount.

Fifty-two Ohioans have died because of AIDS; more than 100 others are afflicted. They are among 11,000 Americans who have a complex virus that attacks a body's nervous system so it cannot fight off other diseases. AIDS itself does not kill, but allows other illnesses, such as pneumonia, cancer, or a combination of disorders, that become fatal.'

Because the majority of victims are homosexual or bisexual males, some other states have done little or nothing out of fear that education about AIDS might be construed as condoning homosexuality. Some conservative religious and political figures are not eager to promote a cure that they say would enable victims to continue their sins safely.

However, faced with an incurable, spreading disorder—like polio once was—Ohio's health department has chosen to deal with it and leave the moralizing to others. The budget of $60,000 is a relative pittance, yet more than many other states spend. Ohio's consultant has pioneered such things as training bartenders in drinking establishments frequented by homosexuals to inform patrons about safeguards against AIDS.

Credit for the educational effort goes to Dr. David Jackson, state health director, who also has fought unneeded hospital expansions, skyrocketing health care costs and drug abuse. Together, the record has made Jackson one of the bright lights of the Celeste administration

THE ATLANTA CONSTITUTION

Atlanta, GA, November 30, 1985

In a move that should help dispel some of the hysteria surrounding AIDS, the Atlanta City Council's Public Safety Committee has allocated $10,000 for a program to educate the city's police, fire and corrections workers about the deadly disease. Several incidents in other cities involving rescue workers and firefighters hesitant to assist AIDS victims, and the recent confusion here over what should be done to cleanse a patrol car after it had been used to transport an AIDS victim, confirm the wisdom of the decision.

The program will include literature as well as seminars, reinforcing the U.S. Centers for Disease Control's findings that AIDS is a blood-borne disease that is not transmitted through casual contact. Using routine precautions that would be recommended when dealing with any infectious disease, city workers should be able to perform their duties without unnecessary fear of risk even when dealing with people who may have the AIDS virus.

The full council is expected to take up the matter Monday. It should approve it without hesitation. The more accurate information disseminated about this puzzling disease, the better.

DAILY NEWS

New York, NY, July 21, 1985

AIDS is a national epidemic. It crosses state lines: New York and California lead, but cases are mounting in Florida, New Jersey and Texas. Lots of money is going into research. There's still no cure. More than half the people ever diagnosed are dead. The others, most likely, are dying.

AIDS stands for Acquired Immunity Deficiency Syndrome. More than 11,000 cases have been identified. That's not all that many. But health officials predict the numbers will double within a year. A fatal disease, with no cure, spreading like wildfire. Why isn't *everyone* petrified?

There's an obvious answer. AIDS has been billed as hitting only "them": male homosexuals mostly, plus intravenous drug users. Other people have come to believe—and with reason up to now—that they're not in danger.

There's another, less obvious reason. A more painful one. A fair number of folks believe gays and junkies *deserve* it. That AIDS is the wrath of God—righteous punishment.

All that flies in the face of a plain fact—new, but still certain. Everyone is in danger, including "normal" people. More than a hundred small children have it. Some were born with it, to a parent who is a drug user or a homosexual or who had sexual contact with a carrier of the virus.

All three members of one Pennsylvania family have AIDS: the father, the mother and their baby. The father received a transfusion of infected blood, probably from someone who didn't know he had been exposed. He passed AIDS to his wife, unknowing. She got pregnant. The whole family's dying.

America can't hide from AIDS. It won't go away. Sen. Daniel Patrick Moynihan is sounding an alarm. He's calling for $35 million in federal funds for public education about AIDS and for early testing to determine exposure. He's right.

AIDS will be conquered. But before it is, it will claim many lives. Fewer will die before science triumphs, as it eventually must, if people force themselves to learn the habits of this killer—and learn that everyone is vulnerable. That *will* take money.

Newsday

Long Island, NY, October 17, 1985

In recent months, communities across the nation have leaped for the panic button when faced with the prospect of an AIDS-stricken child attending school with their sons and daughters.

Angry parents in Queens kept thousands of children home from school for a while when it was learned that a second-grade pupil with AIDS was enrolled somewhere in New York City. In Kokomo, Ind., a judge backed the local school board's decision to bar an afflicted 13-year-old from the classroom.

But when Swansea, Mass., recently had to deal with the problem, it chose a much different course. Insisting that the community's fears were unfounded, officials quickly launched a program to educate the public about AIDS. And apparently it was effective. Parents in Swansea — despite their initial alarm — now support the decision to let a boy with AIDS attend high school.

"We should be an example to the rest of the country," says Swansea resident Jodi Donnelly, and she's right. Acquired immune deficiency syndrome is a deadly, incurable disease. But adults should not be so swept up in a wave of hysteria that they needlessly deny children fundamental rights.

Educating the public could be the answer.

In Swansea, school and health officials held a town meeting that some 700 worried residents attended. The experts told the crowd that the preponderant evidence shows that AIDS can be transmitted only through sexual contact, unsterilized hypodermic needles and blood transfusions. After hearing the facts, the residents loudly applauded a plea to let the victim go to school.

There's a lesson to be drawn from Swansea: When the public is informed about AIDS, fears born of ignorance can disappear. Maybe Queens is learning that lesson too.

The Birmingham News

Birmingham, AL, May 7, 1985

SO FAR, Delaware has been lucky. There are no known cases of AIDS (Acquired Immune Deficiency Syndrome) among Delaware school children or those working in the schools. But some day there may be.

What should school officials do when they learn that a child is suffering from AIDS or perhaps just carries the virus? School people in other states have had to confront that problem on a case-by-case basis and they have not found it easy. Indeed the opposite is the case — they have been caught between their commitment to fairness to the ailing student and understandable fears of parents and teachers who wanted to have nothing to do with any AIDS sufferers.

Delaware educators have tried to look ahead to the day when AIDS appears at the schoolhouse door. They have come up with a policy, adopted by the state Board of Education, that would permit students with AIDS to attend school unless they have open sores, have a history of biting and harming others, or themselves are so weak that by attending school they face the risk of catching a communicable disease.

Based on today's knowledge about the transmission of AIDS that is a sound policy. It is also a policy that can be applied in an even-handed manner.

The policy's test will come, of course, when the first known AIDS victim comes to school. Parents' natural wish to protect their children against any conceivable harm may make the policy difficult to uphold. In New York this school year parents protested the presence of a suspected AIDS pupil in school. In Indiana, a youngster who contracted AIDS from transfused blood was excluded from school as a result of public demand. And, as happened in Maryland, teachers too may object to having an infected child in their class.

Those difficulties do not invalidate the policy adopted by the state board. But they do forebode the troubles that may arise when the policy is put to the test. That's when local advisory panels of physicians and school officials will have to review specific situations and make recommendations.

Even with a state policy in place, these will be tough calls to make. But they would be even harder to make without the guidance that the board has provided.

The Morning News

Wilmington, DE, December 30, 1985

The information contained in a study of acquired immune deficiency syndrome (AIDS) in New York City signals the need to take stronger measures against the disease.

AIDS is now the leading killer of men between ages 30 and 44 and of women 25 to 29 in New York City, says Dr. Alan R. Kristal, who reported on the study in the *Journal of the American Medical Association.*

Kristal said AIDS in 1984 surpassed homicide as the No. 1 cause of death among New York City males between ages 30 through 39. Last year, the disease surpassed heart disease as the chief killer of men between 40 and 44 years old in the city and rose above homicide and cancer as the prime cause of death among women 25 through 29. For the second year, it was the No. 2 killer of women 30 to 34.

If the early deaths were not threat enough, the impact on medical care for the general population may be considerable in a very short time. AIDS does not kill quickly. Victims usually survive from between 18 months to two years. The cost of treatment and care is tremendous, running as much as $150,000 per patient. Sharp increases in the number of victims could very well force re-allocation of financial and hospital resources from treatment and care of curable diseases to AIDS victims.

Kristal reported that nearly 3,800 New York City residents had died of AIDS or AIDS-related diseases since 1980. About 2,000 AIDS victims died in 1985 alone. Those figures indicate the progressive rate of infection. However, the study still indicates that the disease is confined almost exclusively to homosexual men and intravenous drug users.

That conclusion may be reassuring to heterosexuals and those who do not use drugs, but the public is certain to feel the impact eventually. Judging by the costs of care for AIDS victims, those who suffer from other ailments may receive a lower level of care, and the taxpayer is certain eventually to have to pick up the costs for care of AIDS victims.

The lessons implicit in this study are obvious. A more intense education program on the dangers of AIDS is needed. Health departments around the nation also must devise some additional strategy to combat the disease. At the present rate of doubling every year, a million AIDS victims possible in a few years could put big city hospitals under tremendous pressures leading to unpredictable disruption.

The Star-Ledger

Newark, NJ, December 6, 1986

An informed and compassionate light has been thrown on a life-threatening medical prroblem that many Americans would prefer to remain deep in the dark recesses of the national psyche. In a candid assessment, Surgeon General C. Everett Koop has urged schools and parents to shed their widespread inhibitions about AIDS and to begin "frank and open discussions" with children and teenagers about the insidious spread of this terminal disease

Dr. Koop's report, drafted at the request of the Reagan White House, brings a rigorous official element of credibility and medical realism to the controversy that has been precipitated by AIDS. "It is time," the surgeon general counseled, "to put self-defeating attitudes aside and recognize that we are fighting a disease—not people."

And it is time, Dr. Koop cautioned, that Americans become informed about a medical problem that has caused almost 15,000 deaths and most assuredly will have similar grim implications for more than 26,000 Americans who are victims of AIDS. Being fully informed is the only available option, since at this time there isn't any cure for the disease or a vaccine to prevent its spread.

The pervasive public reticence, as Dr. Koop noted in his report, stems from the reluctance to address in an open, forthright manner with "subjects of sex, sexual practices and homosexuality." Homosexuals and drug abusers who use intravenous devices are the principal victims of AIDS.

"AIDS," Dr. Koop properly emphasized, "is not spread by casual, non-sexual contact. It is spread by high-risk sexual and drug-related behaviors—behaviors that we can choose to avoid." This informed medical opinion should help put to rest baseless fears—in some instances, hysteria—among many Americans, particularly parents of school children, about this highly controversial aspect of AIDS.

As an essential preventive safeguard, Dr. Koop's report to the nation on this dread disease provides valuable medical and social guidelines. It puts a sensible, realistic emphasis on the need of strong sex education, both at home and in the schools, as a necessary precautionary step.

And it should set humane, informed standards for official attiudes at all levels of government in dealing with victims of AIDS: Helping, not condemning, the afflicted; taking precautions against the disease's spread, and educating our children about its inherent dangers.

THE ≈ SUN

Baltimore, MD, November 17, 1986

In recent years, the worst consequence of uninformed teen-age sexual activity has been pregnancy. Now Surgeon General C. Everett Koop warns of more dire consequences — AIDS, which almost always results in death. Dr. Koop insists that society no longer can sidestep the issue, that children must have access to sex education that includes open and honest discussions about heterosexual and homosexual sexual practices, and the potential dangers of some sexual encounters.

With the deadly disease spreading throughout the population, he says, the only way to slow its escalation among the young is to teach children about high-risk sexual and drug-related behaviors that spread AIDS — behaviors that can be avoided. Dr. Koop makes an urgent point. If children are to protect themselves from exposure to the virus, AIDS education must begin at a young age — before kids become sexually active.

THE ANN ARBOR NEWS

Ann Arbor, MI, December 29, 1985

With the death from AIDS of U-M Law School professor Jim Martin, the disease has struck home in a real way and awareness of it has been dramatically increased.

Martin was the first Washtenaw County resident to die of AIDS — the Acquired Immune Deficiency Syndrome. Health officials report at least four cases of AIDS among county residents.

AIDS, obviously, is no respecter of persons or class. The idea that it is a disease of "people out of the gutter is absurd," as U-M Public Health School dean Dr. June Osborn recently characterized it. Osborn, a specialist in AIDS-related health factors, said the disease is claiming some of the nation's finest people.

Now we know that for a fact. Jim Martin was one of those people of prominence and distinction.

There are, of course, high-risk groups. Homosexual men and intravenous drug users are especially susceptible. People who don't fall within these groups are extremely unlikely to get AIDS. It's important AIDS be kept in the proper informational perspective.

That's why it's hard to understand the Washtenaw County Health Department's reluctance to date to take a more active role in educating the public about AIDS.

Health department officials understandably don't want to feed hysteria and rumors. But these elements are present, and their circulation in the community argues strongly for the need to dispel them, promptly. Just as the sunlight is the best disinfectant, to quote Justice Brandeis, more of the right kind of information about AIDS will do much to allay fear and dampen prejudice.

And not just more information is needed. Support groups for persons with AIDS play a useful role and their efforts should be encouraged. Money for AIDS research is an obvious need, as are the human traits of understanding and sympathy as applied to AIDS victims.

There are some positive indications of coming to grips with the problem. The Michigan Corrections Commission is in receipt of a preliminary policy for handling AIDS-afflicted inmates in state prisons — a policy that may eliminate differences between prison guards and the department over the segregation of AIDS victims.

Many people are looking to such public agencies as the health department and other sources for both reassurance and the information they need to better assess AIDS. Parents are looking to the schools and the state's education establishment to develop an AIDS policy that protects victim and non-victim alike.

Can information about AIDS in such places as public school health classes and in doctors' offices possibly not be a public service? Clearly, the more we understand and can form intelligent judgments about AIDS, the better off we'll all be. And the sooner the medical community can develop a vaccine, with the necessary public support.

Edmonton Journal

Edmonton, Alta., December 16, 1986

School boards and parents should welcome a provincial plan to teach children about the deadly virus that causes Acquired Immune Deficiency Syndrome (AIDS).

Edmonton Public School Board chairman George Luck is right to support the program, which would be included in a 10-hour curriculum on human sexuality. AIDs can't be ignored. It's not going to go away.

Teaching Grade 9 students about the dangers of sexually transmitted diseases is a moral obligation society has to the future. Only in recent years has human sexuality been formally taught in schools. Education about venereal disease is part of that process.

The Chattanooga Times

Chattanooga, TN, April 10, 1987

There are 130 members of the General Assembly, so how many do you suppose showed up last week in the House chambers for a forum on AIDS? A hundred? Seventy-five? Twenty-five? Nope: five. A three-hour educational presentation might be tough going, but an understanding of this disease is crucial if the Legislature and other state agencies expect to respond to it effectively. The apparent lack of legislators' interest is not encouraging.

Four groups sponsored the forum — the Vanderbilt AIDS Project, Meharry Family Medicine Center, the Nashville chapter of the American Red Cross and Nashville CARES (Council on AIDS Resources, Education and Services) — but theirs was common message: Legislators must push education as the only major weapon against the spread of this deadly disease.

That does not mean, of course, that education must focus only on instructing how to have "safe sex"; instruction must be much broader than that. Dr. William Schaffner, chairman of preventive medicine at Vanderbilt University Medical Center, says that in talking about the transmission of AIDS, "we must talk about human reproduction and sexual intimacy in a direct but delicate, circumspect way."

According to Surgeon General Everett Koop, users of intravenous drugs make up 25 percent of AIDS cases, with the disease chiefly spread through multiple use of the same needle. The majority of AIDS cases, however, occur as a result of sexual contacts, homosexual and heterosexual, especially the former. As you might expect, this part of the AIDS issue has provoked the most controversy.

Most people agree that education is the key to dealing with sexually transmitted AIDS but there are differences over what kind of education. Some argue that the education should focus on the importance of sexual abstinence from homosexual and indiscriminate heterosexual activities, for health as well as moral reasons. Others insist that it is enough to disseminate information about the precautions that should be taken in conjunction with those activities. In fact, both approaches are needed.

President Reagan correctly said the other day that AIDS information cannot be "value neutral," for the simple reason that a change in one's sexual habits is dictated by a concern over the consequences of those habits, whether the concern derives from moral or health considerations.

The fact remains, however, that since many will not change their habits, either out of ignorance or unconcern, education is necessary to ensure against contracting the AIDS disease. That information must be straightforward, not euphemistical, no matter how disconcerting it might be to some. State health officials took precisely the wrong approach the other day in withdrawing six AIDS education brochures, although they denied it was done in response to pressure from some who objected to the brochures' explicitness.

Despite intensive research, AIDS remains incurable; the recently approved experimental drug, AZT, only prolongs a patient's life. That being the case, it is irresponsible in the extreme for any government agency to suppress the dissemination of any information that could inhibit the spread of the disease. Yes, teach teenagers and adults alike the value of abstinence or monogamy as means of avoiding AIDS. But don't shirk the responsibility to educate others in ways to avoid the disease if they are sexually active.

THE KANSAS CITY STAR

Kansas City, MO, May 27, 1987

Teaching teen-agers or other adolescents about health *without* including reproductive information is a sure way to promote what already is widespread ignorance about important aspects of the body. It is a sure way to continue the high rate of births to unwed children who are ignorant about reproduction. In an age of AIDS, it is also dangerous to children not to protect them with information about sexually transmitted diseases.

That is why it is important that a proposed Missouri task force which will undertake review and improvement of existing health education programs for schoolchildren through 12th grade be permitted to consider family planning, reproductive health and sexuality among other health-related topics.

The legislation to create the task force has undergone the scrutiny of the usual frightened groups determined to kill anything that smacks of family planning and sex education. The bill, as it passed the Missouri Senate, excludes the subjects of sexuality and reproduction to fit these groups' wishes. It also would keep the health task force from considering during its deliberations the recommendations of other statewide study groups on topics such as AIDS and teen-age pregnancy.

A House committee has developed a substitute proposal, however, which would include these other studies and subject matter within the task force's mandate. This is the proposal which the General Assembly should adopt.

The task force is charged with developing proposed comprehensive health studies for young people and promoting model programs the schools should adopt. The group should be able to look at anything that is relevant to a child's or teen-ager's health, and reproductive information certainly falls into that category. The report isn't going to be very comprehensive if these big chunks of education are left out.

The Virginian-Pilot

Norfolk, VA, March 22, 1987

The nation's war against an epidemic of acquired immune deficiency syndrome is a fight on two fronts: medical research and public education. On the research front, one anti-AIDS drug is nearing federal approval and others are showing promise in the laboratory. Despite progress, however, the only prospect for AIDS patients today is certain death — no cure, no vaccine. Experts agree that the AIDS crisis is going to get much worse before it gets better. That deadly prediction holds for the nation and for Hampton Roads cities, as well.

That leaves education as the front where the biggest and quickest advances can be made. Last week's inauguration of the federal government's long-awaited AIDS education campaign is welcome.

Debate over the content of the campaign stalled its start. Prior to last week's initiative, the government's only education effort had been a report written by Surgeon General C. Everett Koop and issued in October. "There is now no doubt that we need sex education in schools and that it must include information on heterosexual and homosexual relationships," the report declared.

That caused a stir at the Department of Education, where officials long have argued that sex education is best left to parents and local authorities. One Education Department official complained that the Koop report "de-emphasizes moral considerations."

The interdepartmental debate delayed the plan. But the compromise evident in its contents should not slow its widespread and immediate application.

To meet moralistic concerns, the plan emphasizes sexual abstinence, allows local moral values to determine what information is offered in local school curriculums and advertising campaigns, and recommends "placing sexuality within the context of marriage," a phrase inserted at the insistence of Attorney General Edwin Meese III, who previewed the report.

But, fortunately, that's only part of the plan. Politicians can pontificate all day about the morality of certain sexual practices, but nationwide abstinence is hardly a realistic possibility. Beyond morality, the report is explicit about prevention. "If it is not possible to practice sexual abstinence until infection status can be determined," the report prominently recommends, "always use condoms during sex, because use of condoms can reduce the risk of transmission of the AIDS virus."

The spread of AIDS allows little time for bureaucratic squabbles over morality or squeamishness about frank, even explicit language. The epidemic has grown from virtually no diagnosed cases in 1980 to more than 30,000 today. Projections for 1991 dwarf current figures. Experts predict an exponential spread of the disease over the next several years, with more than a quarter of a million cases expected by 1991. In Southeastern Virginia — where two cases were reported in *all* of 1982 — health experts predict two new diagnosed cases of AIDS *per day* by 1990.

Until a cure or a vaccine is discovered in the laboratory, the federal AIDS-education prescription, combining moral and amoral considerations, forms a practical approach to use in combat against this deadly enemy.

CHARLESTON EVENING POST
Charleston, SC, March 21, 1987

The statistics are grim: AIDS has been diagnosed so far in almost 30,000 Americans, of whom about half have died since 1979. The federal Centers for Disease Control in Atlanta estimates there will be at least 21,000 new cases of AIDS in 1987 and that 13,000 to 15,000 more of the victims will die within a year. That averages out to three deaths every two hours. There is no known cure for AIDS.

Certainly, a vigorous public education program combined with an intense but voluntary testing program to determine who is carrying the AIDS virus is necessary in the fight to hold down the spread of the disease. The public education program, meanwhile, should not be the responsibility of public school teachers, especially those in the elementary grades, as suggested by the U.S. surgeon general.

AIDS is a health problem. The dissemination of information on how the disease in contracted and precautions that young people should take to avoid being infected is a job for parents, with the help of their family doctors, and federal, state and local health authorities. The public schools already are saddled with too many extracurricular responsibilities at the expense of the quality of general education.

That's not to say, however, that schools should be off limits to AIDS education programs. School facilities are ideal locations for presenting the facts, as long as the programs are conducted after school hours and the children who participate do so along with their parents or with parental consent.

Biology courses on anatomy and reproduction belong in school. Reading, writing, arithmetic and all the other standard courses do too. AIDS education does not, especially in the elementary grades.

San Francisco Chronicle
San Francisco, CA, August 31, 1987

THE BEST HOPES for dealing with the AIDS horror, according to the medical authorities, are education and information. Everyone agrees it is of the gravest importance that accurate information on avoiding contact with the AIDS virus be spread as widely and as quickly as possible.

This need to convey information as quickly and as candidly as possible may step on some finicky toes, but the battle against AIDS is no place for the squeamish. It's more than a battle over taste; it's a battle over life and death.

This is why we strongly urge Governor Deukmejian to approve, as soon as it hits his desk, the bill requiring AIDS education for public school children in grades 7 to 12. It will direct state health director Dr. Ken Kizer and state schools superintendent William Honig to select the materials that will go into the schools.

SAFEGUARDS built into the legislation ought to answer critics of the program. The school kids will be taught that abstinence from sexual activity is the best way to avoid AIDS. Their parents will have a chance to have their children excused from the AIDS instruction. And Dr. Kizer's involvement, while important from a medical point of view, will also give the governor considerable in-put in the program.

The issue is too serious for the AIDS education program to be sidetracked or delayed by politics or squeamishness. It must get into the schools as soon as possible.

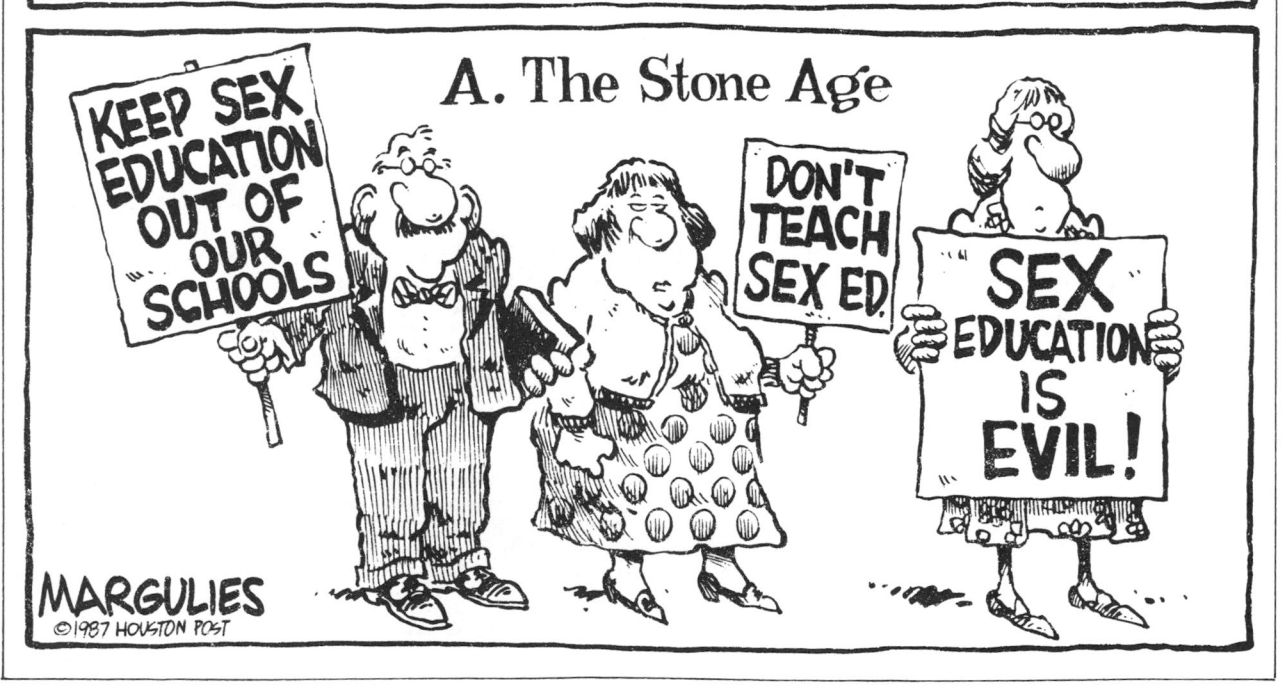

The News and Courier

Charleston, SC, May 15, 1987

The more people know about AIDS, the less the chance of it spreading, and that's why the new, locally produced video on how to protect oneself from contracting the deadly disease should be applauded as being in the best interest of the community.

A few of words of caution, however. No matter how worthy the film is, it should not be mandatory viewing for all public school students. Parental consent should be obtained before children are exposed to the hard facts of life presented in the video. Also, while schools may be convenient locations for educating the public on the problem of AIDS, the film should be shown after school hours and under the auspices of local health authorities, not school teachers or other school officials.

Charleston County's public schools already are saddled with too many extra-curricular activities. The AIDS film should not be added to the "extras" list for the sake of convenience.

If the film is worthy — and we have no reason to believe that it is not — then it should be sufficiently promoted and made available to the community. Children should be allowed to view it if their parents or guardians approve. Adults should be encouraged to see it too. But the airings should not be at the expense of regular studies.

The Des Moines Register

Des Moines, IA
May 20, 1987

If the message is too serious, will people listen to it? If it is too light, will it be taken seriously?

This is the problem facing those who are trying to educate the public about AIDS.

When there must be a balance between the public-health message about safe sexual practices and the public morality that requires discretion in how such a message should be presented, the job becomes even more difficult.

In Iowa, a student group calling itself Award Individuals Deserving Survival has produced a version of "The Wizard of Oz" that is based on the safe-sex message. The troupe has presented its play on the University of Iowa campus to a mixed reaction.

In Illinois, an angry Gov. Jim Thompson in April canceled a performance of a state-sponsored campaign to halt the spread of AIDS when he heard the lyrics of a song written by the Chicago comedy group "Second City."

"The Condom Rag" begins with "You say you want sex that's safe and fun, well jive with us and we'll show you how it's done" and goes on to explain why and how condoms are used. The governor called it "outrageous." "I don't mind targeting the message," he said, "but is that what we should foist on the general public? What about children passing by? . . . People will think we have taken leave of our senses."

One Iowan's reaction to the local "Wizard of Safe Sex" was similar, if milder in tone: "Actually, I think it is pretty good, but I don't think I want my kids to watch."

Are these efforts funny? Offensive? It depends on whom you ask. Humor, like beauty, is in the eye of the beholder; tastefulness is, too.

Still, care should be taken in matching the message to the audience. The message about AIDS is too important to be lost in debate over how it is presented.

Los Angeles Times

Los Angeles, CA, May 10, 1987

It is good news that the White House Domestic Policy Council is considering a national mailing of information about AIDS to every household in America. Good news, too, that Atty. Gen. Edwin Meese III, chairman of the council, is suggesting that President Reagan should speak out on AIDS.

Knowledge that leads to prevention is the only way now known to retard this terrible epidemic.

The memo in which Meese assessed further government action seemed to tilt toward the mass-mailing, though it acknowledged that some citizens may object to getting some "objectionable information."

For the information to be useful, it must be explicit. It will by definition be thought objectionable by some people. But delicacy and reticence can only hinder the efforts that must be made to educate everyone on how AIDS is spread—commonly by semen and blood through anal and vaginal intercourse—and how to guard against it—by the use of condoms with spermicides, by practicing safe sex, by abstinence.

It is literally true that the people cannot know too much about AIDS and ways to prevent it. It is also true, as Dr. Neil R. Schram points out on the page opposite today, that public knowledge about AIDS, about how it is and is not spread, about what each person must do about it, is dreadfully inadequate. It must be addressed in the public schools especially. It must be addressed in the media. It must be addressed by government far more thoroughly and more widely than it has been. An explicit mass-mailing from the White House, with a message from the President, would be most useful.

It was especially encouraging to note that Meese's memo spoke about "the importance of separating public health policies and politics." AIDS is not to be toyed with. It is a specter that haunts us all.

The Wichita Eagle-Beacon

Wichita, KS, April 20, 1987

THE message Lt. Gov. Jack Walker delivered to the first meeting of the Governor's AIDS Task Force was clear: Statewide mandatory sex education in the public schools, including information on the prevention and treatment of AIDS, is the most effective weapon now available to combat this insidious disease. This comprehensive educational program is needed now, Dr. Walker says, not a year from now. Many young lives could be lost in a year's time.

The State Board of Education is considering a proposal mandating sex education statewide. Without question, pushing for a statewide sex education program will present difficult challenges both for the board and for the governor's task force.

A statewide sex education program is needed to assist young people in making the often-difficult choices that are part of growing up. Being prepared to make those choices is vital. Parents often wish to teach their own children about sex, but not all do. Since the AIDS onslaught, the price of not knowing how to avoid contracting the disease could be a human life. Even one young person who doesn't know how the disease is transmitted, then contracts it, unknowingly could transmit it then to many others. That's simply too high a price for living in ignorance.

Kansas' young people need and deserve a comprehensive, statewide sex education program such as the one Dr. Walker — a medical doctor — is suggesting; nothing less will do. Not only do the numbers of AIDS victims continue to rise, but teenage pregnancies still pose a serious threat to the future of young Kansans. The critical need for a mandatory, statewide comprehensive sex education curriculum couldn't be more apparent, or more urgent.

BUFFALO EVENING NEWS
Buffalo, NY, April 13, 1987

SHOULD BUFFALO public schools offer special programs to educate children regarding the dread disease AIDS? The Board of Education has directed Schools Superintendent Eugene T. Reville to form a committee to explore that issue and discuss possible subject matter and the grade levels at which it should be presented.

It is far better that local educators explore than ignore this controversial issue. And controversial or not, some kind of AIDS program is necessary.

Buffalo already has a program of sex education, and AIDS, which is usually transmitted by either sexual contact or intravenous drug use, would become a logical addition to it.

Combatting AIDS, or acquired immune deficiency syndrome, is literally a matter of life and death, since the disease is always fatal. And this disease, once limited mostly to homosexual men and intravenous drug users, is now spreading into the heterosexual population.

President Reagan has called AIDS the nation's "public health enemy No. 1" and endorsed the idea of such educational programs in the schools, while also stressing that they should include both medical and moral considerations. He said details of the local programs should be decided by parents and schools, concerns that will engage the committee the Buffalo board is appropriately setting up.

Medical and educational authorities are stressing the importance of education, since that is, at present, the only way of fighting the disease. The state Education Department is developing a plan to teach about AIDS as early as kindergarten, and U.S. Surgeon General C. Everett Koop has called for frank, open discussion of sexual practices and of how to prevent AIDS.

A recent conference of public health officials in Philadelphia urged a crash educational program beginning in kindergarten but concentrating on junior and senior high schools. Officials stressed that abstinence is the best way of stopping AIDS, but that, since millions of young people are sexually active, information should be made available regarding protective action.

This is, of course, a sensitive area of concern. Vice President Bush recently urged greater efforts to educate the public, including children, but said he would have trouble "teaching very young children that the answer is to use condoms."

That poses the complicated question not only of the content of an AIDS program, but at what grade level certain information is introduced. There is no such thing as "safe sex" outside a completely monogamous relationship. Condoms are an important means of combatting the disease, but they are not completely effective.

Thus, while information about condoms should be part of the public education drive at higher grade levels, any balanced presentation must also emphasize that condoms can be unreliable, especially if used over a long period of time in high-risk situations.

The nation faces a terrible time bomb in the AIDS epidemic, because the development of the disease may come 10 or more years after a person is infected. The number infected may be in the millions, and thus that could also mean millions of deaths.

In one sense, there should be no conflict over how to teach about AIDS, since the religious and medical viewpoints converge. The moralist preaches that "the wages of sin is death," and the medical scientist now asserts that casual sex — even so-called "safe sex" — can mean death. Both recommend fidelity or abstinence as the only sure means of combatting AIDS.

The study committee in Buffalo will be composed of parents, teachers, board members, health experts and possibly students, assuring a useful input of diverse opinion. The panel will face difficult decisions of detail. But a sensitive, informative AIDS educational program can serve everyone's healthiest interests.

ST. LOUIS POST-DISPATCH
St. Louis, MO, July 16, 1987

Public health officials have to join the battle against AIDS — acquired immune deficiency syndrome — on a number of fronts. They must make certain that adequate, humane treatment is available and affordable for those who have the deadly disease. More important, until a cure is found or a vaccine developed, they must launch an all-out educational campaign to stop the spread of AIDS.

But in Missouri, movement on AIDS is slow. As *Post-Dispatch* reporters Peter Hernon and Roger Signor reported in a recent series, little has been done by public officials to prepare for the coming AIDS crisis. Only in the last two weeks has the state agreed to allow Medicaid to pay for the AIDS treatment drug AZT — and even that was only after a class-action suit forced the issue.

Education is the key to stopping the spread of the disease. So far, however, educational programs have engendered controversy, with squeamish parents, including Gov. John Ashcroft, worrying that children will be taught more than they should know about sex. But in coming years, homosexual transmission of AIDS is not going to be nearly so great a problem as infection that occurs through the use of shared needles by intravenous drug users. To reach those who are at greatest risk will entail a campaign that reaches to the very fringes of society. Youngsters — and adults, too — need to know about this every bit as much as they need to know about the perils of unguarded sexual activity.

For the city, county and state, all of which are just now drafting their anti-AIDS strategies, the message is clear: Provide for free, confidential testing, develop humane treatment programs for the afflicted, but above all, spare no expense on educating the vulnerable public.

Chicago Tribune
Chicago, IL, April 24, 1987

One hearing of a state-sponsored rap song called "The Condom Rag" was enough for Gov. Thompson. He wrathfully called it "garbage" and forbade any more performances under his sponsorship. Following that, Mr. Thompson examined a series of skits dealing with AIDS that a Chicago comedy troupe was scheduled to perform at the State of Illinois Center and blue-penciled them all.

Mr. Thompson explained that he "believes very strongly" in sex education for children and AIDS education; this presumably includes the current effort by the Department of Public Health to educate Illinoisans on the causes and prevention of AIDS. But, said the governor, "There's a matter of doing it right."

He did not make clear what is right. Evidently it will be up to someone else to figure out how the state can promote AIDS prevention by the use of condoms without offending Mr. Thompson.

The point is not to ridicule the governor for being prudish (although, as the official who led a televised scrutiny of an alleged rape victim's panties, his sense of propriety does seem flexible). Many people are offended by messages about condoms, even by the word itself, and find it all the more offensive when the subject is treated flippantly or in street language. The rap group's version certainly does that: "Pardon the pun, it's in the bag, all you gotta do is the condom rag."

Yet censoring the message to spare sensitive feelings does absolutely nothing to solve the problem—and the problem, unlike the feelings, is deadly.

AIDS is a rapidly spreading disease transmitted chiefly through sexual intercourse. In most cases, perhaps in all, it is fatal. The most effective ways to guard against it are abstinence, monogamy—staying with one sexual partner—and using condoms.

It is clearly urgent to convey these facts to a wide audience, and there is no delicate or indirect way to do it. Those who want to withhold the warnings until some polite formula is found are setting a very high price on their own sensitivities.

A more serious objection than Mr. Thompson's comes primarily from parents and church groups—those who do not want the state sending youth a double message about sexual activity. "Don't do it, but if you do, use a condom" is hardly a bugle call to morality. To many parents, it is like telling a youngster, "Don't hold up banks, but if you do, use a ski mask."

No one, however, has found a way to keep young people in a wide-open society from hearing about sex or to make sure that what they hear is moral. Today's youth hears not just double messages but multiple ones and must choose among them—the luckier ones with their parents' help. Meantime, warnings that are meant to protect their lives should not be withheld.

The state has its priorities right in trying to alert as many people as possible to the danger of AIDS and the ways to guard against it. Maybe it can be a little more sensitive than it was in the "The Condom Rag," but it should not blush at the effort.

Ryan White Allowed to Return to School

More than a year after being barred from attending Western Middle School in Russianville, Indiana because he had come down with AIDS, 14-year-old Ryan White February 13, 1987 won a county medical ruling that he posed no health threat to his fellow classmates and should be allowed to return to the classroom. White, a hemophiliac who had contracted AIDS from tainted blood products, had gained national attention in 1985, while receiving his schooling by means of a telephone hookup to the school. He returned to school on Friday, Feb. 21, but more than 40% of his schoolmates stayed home. A county judge ruled that afternoon that he could not return the following Monday. The judge said White would be barred from attending school until after a hearing was held to determine whether a 1949 Indiana law dealing with communicable diseases applied to AIDS.

Parents who had tried to keep White out of their children's classes said July 16, 1986 that they would no longer put up opposition. The same day, the Indiana Court of Appeals dismissed their request to overturn a judge's decision that allowed White to return to class. White had been attending Russianville's Western Middle School since April 10. In reaction, the parents of 21 sixth- and seventh-graders set up an alternative school for their children.

The Courier-Journal

Louisville, KY
February 28, 1986

THAT PARENTS should be concerned about the well-being of their children is understandable. But the saga of Ryan White, the Kokomo, Ind., boy who has been barred from school because he has acquired immune deficiency syndrome, is a tragedy in which good intentions have resulted in a less-than-admirable outcome.

The fears of his schoolmates' parents that Ryan, a hemophiliac who acquired the disease from a blood-clotting agent, will infect their children are unwarranted. There is no medical evidence that AIDS, which so far has always proved fatal, is spread through casual contact. Yet, victims are being ostracized — and one drama, which pits doctors against some parents and educators, continues in Kokomo.

After Howard County's chief medical officer certified that he posed no health threat to classmates and teachers, 14-year-old Ryan attended school last Friday for the first time since administrators barred him.

But nearly half of his 360 schoolmates stayed home and it was a short-lived triumph for compassion and reason. By that afternoon a Circuit Court judge had issued a temporary restraining order preventing the AIDS victim from returning to class. Parents of pupils at Western Middle School argued in court that his presence endangered their children's health.

The legal battles are likely to go on for some time. On Tuesday, the judge ruled that parents trying to keep Ryan out of school must post a $12,000 bond within five days to cover possible damages and expenses if their effort fails.

It's possible Ryan may not even live to see his case settled. But the issue must be settled for the good of all the children like him.

The dividing line between reasonable caution and unreasonable fear may often be a thin one; in this case, however, it's clearly discernible. He should be in school.

St. Petersburg Times

St. Petersburg, FL, February 17, 1986

For everyone acquainted with Ryan White — the friends who still play with him, his classmates and their parents, the waitress who refused to wipe the table where he had just eaten, officials of Western Middle School — the subject of AIDS was new, the fear was fresh, and the misconceptions were rampant.

The result was that many people at Kokomo, Ind., unnecessarily have ostracized the young AIDS victim who contracted the dreaded disease when he received contaminated blood during treatment of hemophilia.

RYAN MADE national news last fall when he was barred from school. Officials of the school district said the teen-age boy would not be allowed to attend his seventh-grade classes because he might infect other students.

That happened more than a year ago. Since then, there is new evidence that there is no legitimate reason to ban from the classroom most children with AIDS.

A ruling last Thursday by a county medical officer reflects the facts about AIDS. After examining Ryan, Dr. Alan J. Alder certified him as fit to return to classes and said that he posed no threat to other children or teachers.

AIDS, as many health experts have asserted, is not a very contagious disease. The only known ways of transmission are through sexual relations, contaminated needles and blood transfusions. Recently accumulated information confirms that AIDS cannot be spread by casual contact — a sneeze, handshake or proximity.

The largest and most thorough study of members of families of AIDS victims completed to date adds force to the doctor's decision about Ryan. It provides "conclusive" evidence that the disease does not spread through close, day-to-day personal contact, according to the leader of the research team. The study examined in more detail than ever before the extent to which family members hugged and kissed AIDS patients and shared toothbrushes, drinking glasses, beds, towels and toilets with them. Not one of 100 people who shared homes with AIDS victims showed signs of infection with the deadly virus.

THIS STUDY, along with other evidence, is sufficient to quell the hysteria over the casual transmission of AIDS. Medical professionals, school officials and others in positions to influence public thinking have a responsibility to take a more active role in helping the American people sort out the facts and myths about AIDS.

AIDS is frightening. But as more is learned about the disease, there is less to fear — including allowing children with AIDS to sit in a classroom with other youngsters. Ryan, welcome back to school.

THE INDIANAPOLIS STAR
Indianapolis, IN, April 12, 1986

The debate over the communicability of AIDS may be over as far as Judge Jack R. O'Neill of Clinton Circuit Court is concerned. But some parents of children in the Russiaville school to which AIDS victim Ryan White returned Thursday will not agree.

Ryan, 14, rejoined classes at Western Middle School after O'Neill dismissed a temporary restraining order barring his attendance. Almost immediately three parents met with their attorney to begin planning legal strategies to appeal the decision.

It is questionable whether King Solomon could reach a decision in Ryan White's case that would satisfy both sides. Rights are in collision. No matter which way a judge ruled, one side would consider his decision wrong.

Observers can sympathize with either side and feel certain they are right. They can sympathize with both and accept the dilemma as basically beyond solution.

It seems almost impossible not to sympathize with Ryan White, the accidental center of this long-drawn-out and turbulent nationwide controversy and the innocent victim of AIDS which he acquired through a blood transfusion.

In the midst of this stressful battle he is still able to smile. He inspires admiration. He is a brave young man.

AKRON BEACON JOURNAL
Akron, OH, August 30, 1986

THERE'S something new in the classroom this year: students with AIDS. In Kokomo, Ind., the most famous American teen-ager with AIDS is back in school. For the first time in two years, Ryan White started a new school year with his classmates. There were no protests, no court injunctions to keep him out. Parents didn't keep their kids out, either.

And even though some students were a bit wary, they seemed to accept official assurances that Ryan is not a health threat. Old fears and suspicions have diminished, though not evaporated. But school officials have worked out a system that takes extra precautions to ease the concerns of students and staff. Ryan, a hemophiliac who got AIDS from tainted blood, will use a separate bathroom and eat from disposable dishes. The staff has been trained to deal with emergencies involving the youth.

The situation in Kokomo underscores what can happen when the myths surrounding AIDS are dispelled and reason takes over. For as long as he is able, Ryan can have a semblance of a normal life. A school system, indeed an entire community, has matured enough to solve a crisis.

The same thing is occurring in New York City, where six children with AIDS will be allowed to enroll in school. Parents who organized massive protests last year to keep an AIDS youngster out of class say they will not fight this year. School officials hope that increased awareness about the disease has convinced parents that there is no danger.

In both Kokomo and New York, school credibility is key to community acceptance. Relying on the expertise of doctors, each school system carefully considered the medical condition of each child before making a decision about admission.

Most school districts have yet to confront this dilemma, but there is no reason to wait for a crisis before determining how AID cases will be handled. The Canton Board of Education is considering such a policy now, based upon the recommendation of a 12-member panel made up of parents, educators and community leaders.

The committee's basic conclusion is that each case should be reviewed on an individual basis. The superintendent would consult with a medical team to determine whether the AIDS patient would be a health threat in a school setting. That puts the assessment in the hands of the experts, where it belongs, free of the fear and hysteria that surrounds this disease.

Canton is on the right track, because it also recognizes that community education is crucial if this process is to work. It is laying the groundwork for a policy that may someday head off a potential crisis. The lessons of Kokomo and New York have not been lost on this Ohio school district. Other schools will slowly come to grips with the AIDS age. Until a cure for the disease is found, they simply have no other   ice.

The Idaho STATESMAN
Boise, ID, April 13, 1986

Fourteen-year-old Ryan White finally is back in school in Kokomo, Ind. Let's hope he gets to stay there.

For almost a year, Ryan has been fighting for his right to attend school even though he suffers from acquired immune deficiency syndrome. His battle has been a summary-in-miniature of a national debate: Should children with AIDS be allowed to attend public school?

In Ryan's case, reason and compassion won out over the understandable panic and fear that AIDS provokes.

Ryan contracted AIDS through blood treatments for the hemophilia he suffers from. His efforts to be allowed back in public school have been acted out against a grim deadline. AIDS, which destroys the body's ability to fight off infection, is fatal.

Ryan got to attend only one day of school this year, in February, when a local health officer said he posed no threat to his classmates. But worried parents immediately obtained a temporary injunction kicking him right back out.

On Thursday, a circuit judge ended that injunction, but the controversy goes on. Some parents have taken their children out of class in protest and are pondering further legal action.

Their concerns are understandable – but it's time to let Ryan White be.

All the evidence indicates that AIDS can't be transmitted by casual contact. While small children with AIDS who bite or have runny noses or aren't toilet-trained may pose a health hazard to their classmates, Ryan White doesn't.

Last but not least, the teachers and staff at Ryan's school have been given special health-safety instructions for handling any emergencies.

Ryan White has suffered isolation and ostracism this last year with a dignity and patience that adults would be hard put to emulate. His case has been argued to death. It's time for his community to give him a break, and let him get back to just being a kid.

The Chattanooga Times
Chattanooga, TN, February 26, 1986

In September, 14-year-old Ryan White of Kokomo, Ind., was barred from class because he is a victim of AIDS, a deadly disease involving failure of the body's immunological system. The reason: Parents of his classmates feared their children would become infected. Young Ryan was finally admitted to class last week, after months of legal wrangling and, incidentally, publication of a federal study which showed it was virtually impossible to contract AIDS through casual contact. No matter. The parents persuaded the court to issue another temporary restraining order barring him from school after he had been class for one day, again by arguing that their children's health was endangered. Now, the youth's lawyers has asked the judge to require opponents to post a bond in the case to cover whatever damages Ryan might suffer in the case. Fair enough, we suppose, but it's going to take more than legal tactics to overcome overt ignorance.

AIDS Panic Rocks Florida Town

Arcadia, Florida was the scene of a fire of suspicious origin the night of August 28, 1987 that destroyed the home of a couple whose three sons were hemophiliacs known to have been exposed to the virus that causes AIDS. The fire capped a week of bomb and death threats against Clifford and Louise Ray, their daughter and three sons, and a boycott of the local schools. The boycott had been prompted by the Aug. 24 return to school of the three boys after a year's absence. Arcadia is a DeSoto County community about 50 miles inland from the Gulf Coast cities of Sarasota and Fort Myers.

The boys, who had presumably been exposed to the AIDS virus through the transfusion of blood products administered to ease the effects of hemophilia, had been barred from classes in the fall of 1986, after the local school board had been notified of their condition. The Rays then sued, citing doctors who said the boys posed no threat to other children. Nearly a year later, a federal judge in Tampa ordered the boys—who continued to show symptoms of AIDS itself—readmitted to school.

The Rays were not at home when the fire broke out. A brother of Clifford Ray was asleep in a bedroom at the time but escaped. He was released from a local hospital after treatment for smoke inhalation. On Aug. 29, Louise Ray said that her family would leave DeSoto County. "I never thought it would go this far," she said in a telephone interview from her lawyer's office in Sarasota. On Aug. 30, members of a committee that had been formed to keep the three boys out of DeSoto County classrooms offered the Rays donations of food and clothing. By then the family's plight had attracted national attention, and offers were pouring in from across the country. A family spokesman that day indicated that the Rays wanted any donations from DeSoto County to go toward efforts to educate the community about AIDS.

The Hartford Courant

Hartford, CT, September 6, 1987

The fear of acquired immune deficiency syndrome seems the most irrational, and can be at its ugliest, when it affects schoolchildren.

Consider these recent incidents: When three hemophiliac brothers who tested positive for antibodies to the AIDS virus went back to school in Arcadia, Fla., their presence provoked bomb threats, protests and boycotts. Last week, the boys' home burned in what authorities suspect was arson. The family has fled the county.

In Manatee County, Fla., a school board voted to bar another child who tested positive, and a child with AIDS was kept out of a Belleville, Ill., elementary school after some parents said they would make their children stay home if the afflicted child weren't barred.

After all that has been written about the disease, many parents of school-age children still don't seem to understand that it is virtually impossible for the AIDS virus to be transmitted by the kinds of activities that normally take place at school. Some parents do not seem willing to accept the reassurances of school and health officials who insist that AIDS poses almost no threat of contagion to schoolchildren.

Not a single case of AIDS has been known to have spread from one child to another in a school or day-care facility. AIDS, as everyone should know by now, is believed to be spread only through sexual contact, to a fetus by its mother during pregnancy, by contaminated blood or blood products and by dirty needles shared by infected drug abusers.

Because AIDS is a deadly disease for which no cure is known, it's understandable that parents fear for their children. Educators and local authorities, including school boards, therefore must do as much as they can to inform parents and allay their fears. The sad fact is that in too many school districts little has been done. There are exceptions, of course, including the many towns in Connecticut — perhaps most notably Granby — that have taken prompt, effective steps to devise policies governing the admission of children with AIDS to school.

Having policies about AIDS in schools and providing information about AIDS can't prevent hysteria, of course, but it can erase ignorance. That's more than half the battle.

EVENING EXPRESS
Portland, ME, September 4, 1987

Two American communities recently have taught a compelling lesson in tolerance. From Arcadia, Fla., we have learned how *not* to behave toward persons who carry the AIDS virus. And from Arcadia, Ind., has come instruction in how to make life better for AIDS victims.

All the two communities have in common is their name.

Just ask Louise and Clifford Ray. Their family was mercilessly threatened and their home destroyed by a suspicious fire in the Florida town, all because their three AIDS-exposed sons want to go to public school. Let it be emphasized: None of the three boys, ages 8, 9 and 10, all hemophiliacs, actually *has* the disease.

By contrast, 15-year-old Ryan White does. White, also a hemophiliac, is the quiet young boy with AIDS barred from public school in Indiana two years ago because school officials feared he would spread the disease. A judge disagreed and ordered Ryan reinstated. Local emotions ran so high, however, that reinstatement proved impossible. The White family moved and Ryan this week entered a new high school in Arcadia, Ind.

How was he greeted? "Everybody was real nice and friendly," the boy said. One reason: School officials were among those leading the welcome.

Their behavior stands in sharp contrast to school officials' abject failure to act when the three Ray boys were besieged in Arcadia, Fla. Instead, panic was allowed to engulf the town and drive the Ray children not only out of school but out of town as well. And the Florida town is bewildered by public reaction, which has been heavily critical of the community's actions. "We are not heartless, we are not violent," said a leader of the local boycott.

Maybe not. But they sure couldn't prove it by us.

St. Petersburg Times

St. Petersburg, FL, September 1, 1987

Ricky, Robert and Randy Ray didn't choose to be hemophiliacs, nor did they choose to become exposed to the AIDS virus as a result of the blood transfusions they must endure because of their disease. The boys' parents, Clifford and Louise Ray, certainly didn't choose this fate for their sons. All they hoped for — and that hope has faded in the few days since the new school year began — was a decent education and a better life for their children.

The Ray boys and their family are victims — victims of the cruelest disease that the 20th century has to offer. Yet, just as the victims of leprosy, plague and mental illness were shunned and reviled in the Dark Ages, the Rays have been intimidated and ostracized by a large segment of the community of Arcadia. The Rays now say they plan to move to another town, but their problems will follow them wherever they go.

However, Arcadia's problems will not disappear with the Rays' departure. AIDS continues to spread to communities large and small. In all likelihood, the virus eventually will reappear in Arcadia. It might even turn up in the bloodstream of one of the people who have treated the Ray family so unfairly since the three boys' exposure to the AIDS virus was first made known.

For now, the best that can be hoped is that future victims will receive the kind of support from state officials, starting with Gov. Bob Martinez, that has been so conspicuously lacking in the case of the Ray family. The Ray family looked to the government to protect its rights, and the town of Arcadia looked to the government for assurance that the Ray brothers posed no threat to the public health. In this case, the government failed on both counts.

Rural, isolated DeSoto County does not have the educational and medical resources needed to respond to the crisis that has consumed Arcadia since the start of the school year. Local school officials, who complained that they received no guidance from the state, originally decided to have the Ray brothers attend a separate classroom isolated from regular public schools. They relented only after a court order overruled their decision a couple of weeks before the beginning of the new school year. State and local health officials hastily scheduled meetings to attempt to explain the extremely limited risk to other children, but too many parents were either unwilling or unable to understand the relatively technical medical information.

State Education Commissioner Betty Castor now has proposed that the state establish AIDS guidelines for local officials to use in future cases. The people of DeSoto County might have been spared a great deal of pain if such a plan were already in effect. State experts are in a much better position to revise school admission policies as our knowledge of AIDS increases, and state leadership helps to ease the political pressure now placed on local officials.

However, that leadership must begin at the top. Gov. Martinez has been irresponsibly silent and inactive on this issue. It is his job to do whatever is necessary to protect the rights — and the physical well-being — of families such as the Rays. It is also his job to tell the people of this state that the loud voices of ignorance, superstition and violence will not be allowed to overwhelm the forces of knowledge and reason.

The threat of AIDS is very real, even in DeSoto County, and the parents of Arcadia have good reason to be concerned about the safety of their school children. In the absence of state leadership, those local fears have been exploited, with tragic consequences. The best that can be hoped is that the tragedy of one community will not have to be repeated in the hundreds of others that will eventually be visited by AIDS.

Rocky Mountain News

Denver, CO, September 4, 1987

IN Florida, a family had to flee to another town not long ago when their house was set on fire by angry citizens. The crime: Having three children infected with AIDS virus and wanting to send them to school.

In Jefferson County, a group of parents has been circulating petitions saying any child with AIDS should be kept from school, apparently because the mother of a 4-year-old with AIDS has asked that her son be admitted to pre-school.

No matter how many scientists reassure the public about the limited risk of non-sexual contact with AIDS victims, some people just won't believe it. They react as humans always have to perceived danger: with anger and violence.

Unfortunately, the question whether to send children to school who actually have AIDS (as opposed to carrying the virus) isn't easy to answer. Both sides make good arguments. Opponents point out that people with other fatal, communicable diseases are not usually sent off to work or school as if nothing had happened. Supporters insist the risk is minimal, so why deprive victims of a normal existence?

Until the Florida case, most of the ugliest clashes have occurred over schoolchildren who actually showed symptoms of the disease. Children who merely carry the AIDS virus may appear otherwise perfectly healthy. One of them lives in Aurora.

What exactly are her rights?

We think the answer is much clearer than in a case in which a child suffers symptoms. The only humane, decent response is to permit the virus-infected girl to attend school. Fortunately, that's exactly what the Aurora district proposes. The girl will attend Central High School this fall as soon as school officials are confident that parents, teachers and fellow students have been properly prepared.

To bar the child from classrooms would be cruel. After all, no one knows what portion of infected people ultimately come down with AIDS. Estimates range all the way from 20% to 100%. Nor does anyone know how long the incubation period between infection and the sickness can last. It could be 10 years or more.

To isolate someone who may never be stricken with the disease, or at least not for a decade or more, would be irrational given the remote risk. Aurora has acted responsibly in permitting the girl to attend high school. We only hope parents and students respond with equal maturity and understanding.

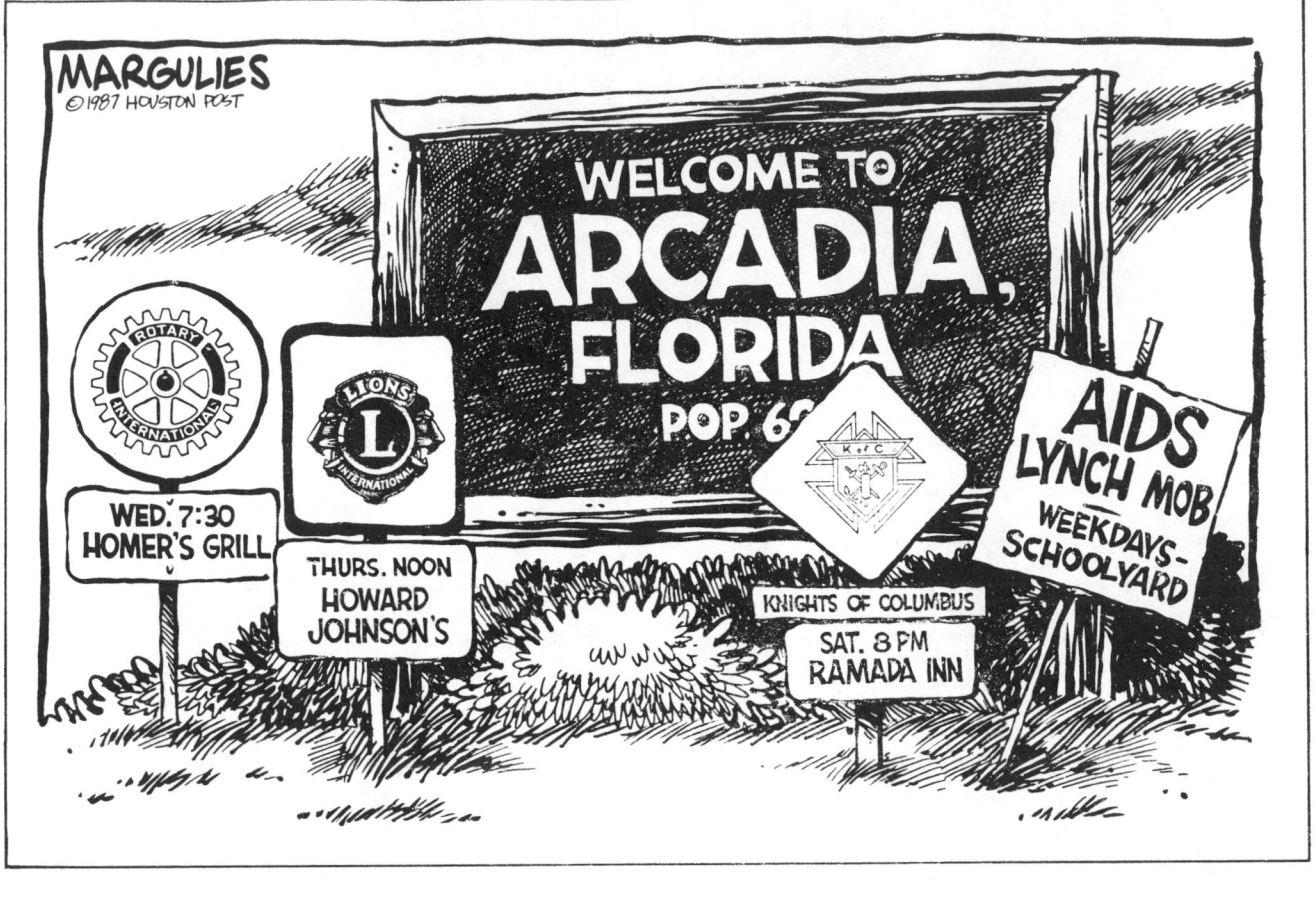

MARGULIES
©1987 HOUSTON POST

WELCOME TO ARCADIA, FLORIDA POP. 6?

ROTARY INTERNATIONAL
WED. 7:30
HOMER'S GRILL

LIONS INTERNATIONAL
THURS. NOON
HOWARD JOHNSON'S

KNIGHTS OF COLUMBUS
SAT. 8 PM
RAMADA INN

AIDS LYNCH MOB
WEEKDAYS-
SCHOOLYARD

Chicago Tribune

Chicago, IL, September 2, 1987

A Florida town called Arcadia has turned its back on a family that has been touched by AIDS. An Indiana town called Arcadia has opened its arms to another. The names and events are a coincidence. But it is a coincidence that highlights how different communities' reactions to the disease can be.

The people of Arcadia, Fla., shunned and harassed the family of Clifford and Louise Ray because their three sons carry AIDS antibodies as a result of treatment for hemophilia. They received threats. Their church shut them out. Residents organized a boycott of the boys' elementary school. The family finally left after its house mysteriously burned.

Hamilton Heights High School in Arcadia, Ind., was as warm and welcoming to AIDS patient Ryan White, 15, another hemophiliac, as its Florida counterpart was cold and heartless to the Rays. Ryan White's family moved to the school district after Ryan's home-

town, Kokomo, Ind., reacted to his condition with a near-panic.

The difference between the two Arcadias is the difference between fear born out of ignorance and compassion supported by public education. A few children were missing from Hamilton High on Ryan's first day at school, but not many. The town was prepared to welcome Ryan because its residents were sufficiently informed of the true dangers of the disease, which are minimal without blood-to-blood contact, such as sexual intercourse or shared use of hypodermic needles. Arcadia, Ind., got the message. Arcadia, Fla., did not.

To fight a plague like AIDS, government must sponsor research. But its responsibilities to public health and welfare do not stop there. It also must show leadership in promoting public education to restore public confidence. Compassion can open the arms of a community, but only after education has opened its minds.

Calgary Herald

Calgary, Alta., September 1, 1987

Nothing justifies the escalating panic linked with growing awareness of Acquired Immune Deficiency Syndrome.

Winnipeg authorities are issuing rubber gloves to teachers to be worn when dealing with students' playground cuts or nosebleeds.

This absurd and pointless precaution looks sensible when compared to the reaction to AIDS in the rural area of Arcadia, Florida.

Arcadia residents Clifford and Louise Ray have three hemophiliac sons infected with the AIDS virus from blood transfusions.

The Rays fought and won a long, bitter court battle to send their boys to school in Arcadia. But, despite their legal victory, the Rays were forced to leave town when their house was destroyed by a mysterious fire.

There is no question that AIDS is a frightening, incurable, deadly phenomenon made that much more frightening because it is spread through sexual intercourse or re-used hypodermic needles or blood transfusions. AIDS may be very widespread because its incubation period is long.

But these facts do not justify taking drastic measures that could isolate and ostracize AIDS victims, creating a version of 20th-century lepers.

Extreme reactions, from absurd precautions to stigmatization of AIDS victims, reinforce social resistance to rational treatment of the AIDS condition.

Fear will drive potential AIDS sufferers underground, making detection, investigation and prevention that much more difficult.

That is the last thing needed to cope with such a perilous menace to public health.

As former United States president Franklin Roosevelt said in a reassuring speech to the American people at the outset of the Second World War: "We have nothing to fear, but fear itself."

The Burlington Free Press

Burlington, VT, September 3, 1987

Is this the age of enlightenment, when man's powers can illuminate the smallest cell and the darkest reaches of the universe?

Or is this the Dark Ages, when the danger of disease can drive us to mindless fear and the burning of witches?

AIDS came recently to a small place called Arcadia, Fla., a kind of Everytown, USA. What happened there should have no place in this century or this country.

Arcadia schools were closed to the three young sons of Clifford and Louise Ray, hemophiliacs who acquired the AIDS virus through blood transfusions. When a court order opened the classroom doors, other parents — including the mayor and his wife — kept their children home. They turned a burning anger on the Ray family. The Rays' church turned its back. The telephone brought them threats.

Then someone burned the family's home down. The Rays say they will not return.

Arcadia has scourged AIDS from its precincts, burned it at the stake.

Whoever held the match, we must all hang our heads at the triumph of ignorance and fear.

Scientists have not yet unraveled every mystery of AIDS, but on one thing they agree. There was virtually no chance the brothers would spread AIDS to their schoolmates.

AIDS is not the Black Death returned. It is transmitted from one person to another in blood or semen, usually during sexual intercourse. Hemophiliacs under a doctor's care don't bleed more than other people. Children in an elementary school classroom don't commonly cut themselves and spread the blood around on the open wounds of their classmates.

Nature doesn't intend parents to react completely rationally when their children are threatened. But we are not mother bears charging mindlessly at any shape between us and our cubs.

What makes us human is the capacity to balance instinct with reason and with knowledge — and with empathy for our fellow humans. Humanity deserted too many residents of Arcadia when AIDS knocked at the door.

In places like Arcadia, Fla. — or Burlington, Vt. — the danger is not that AIDS will descend like the Plague, but that we will allow fear and ignorance to plunge us into a kind of moral Dark Ages.

THE INDIANAPOLIS NEWS

Indianapolis, IN, September 3, 1987

Human beings can be awful cruel to one another.

— Mark Twain

Mark Twain could have written the above sentence today and it still would be true. He might even have cited events in Arcadia, Fla., as proof.

Arcadia was, until recently, the home of the Clifford Ray family. The key word is "was."

The Rays left Arcadia recently because of a tragedy that befell three young boys in their family — a tragedy that was made worse by the needless cruelty of many Arcadia citizens.

Ricky Ray, 10, and his brothers Robert, 9, and Randy, 8, recently tested positive in an AIDS examination. They were exposed to the AIDS virus through a blood transfusion, just as Hoosiers Amy Sloan and Ryan White were.

Testing positive means that they carry the AIDS virus in their blood. But it does not mean that they have the disease.

That probably is no consolation to the Rays. It is likely that at least one boy will contract the deadly disease. It is possible that all three will.

That is quite a burden for three young boys and their family to carry around, even if their friends and neighbors are helpful and supportive. And the neighbors in Arcadia were anything but supportive.

When the news of the Ray boys' misfortune broke, people began picketing the Ray house, trying to keep Ricky, Robert and Randy out of school.

Some who didn't picket phoned or mailed death threats. Others warned that they would bomb the Ray house.

Then, on Friday night, the Rays' house caught fire and burned to the ground.

The Rays were convinced that someone had bombed or otherwise torched their home, and they were understandably distraught. The AIDS crisis and the fire had swallowed the few resources the family had; they didn't know how they would live.

The Rays decided to leave Arcadia. The threats, the harassment and the fire drove them away.

As for Arcadia itself — well, many of that small town's citizens, particularly those who probably set fire to the Rays' house, will have to live knowing that they suffer from something more deadly than AIDS. Something truly worthy of shame.

Brutal inhumanity.

The Record

Hackensack, NJ, September 3, 1987

To the people of Arcadia, Fla., the enemy was AIDS, and it threatened their own children. No matter how many times the authorities assured them that there was no risk in casual contact with AIDS carriers, the parents of Arcadia were unconvinced.

For nearly a year, the three Ray brothers — Ricky, 10; Robert, 9; and Randy, 8 — had been kept out of Arcadia's Memorial Elementary School. Hemophiliacs, they'd contracted the AIDS virus from contaminated blood-clotting products. They were barred from school even though they showed no AIDS symptoms; some people carry the virus for years without developing the disease itself. Last week a federal judge ordered the boys readmitted to school, and the community went crazy. Half the parents kept their children home. The school received three bomb threats. Then, last Friday, a suspicious fire destroyed the Rays' house.

The people who committed these acts of cruelty and hate were behaving in familiar, age-old fashion: They were belling the lepers. They simply did not believe scientists who say that it would be almost impossible for an infected child to transmit the disease. All documented cases of AIDS involve the entry of infected blood or semen into the body of a second person. A hemophiliac child is simply no danger to other children.

In contrast to this ugly, sad story, consider another town with the same name — Arcadia, Ind. On Monday, students and school officials there gave another hemophiliac with AIDS — 15-year-old Ryan White — a warm welcome. Like the Ray children, Ryan had been barred from school in another community two years ago; the family moved and found that the new town accepted the situation without hysteria.

In New Jersey, meanwhile, nine babies with the AIDS virus are languishing in New Jersey hospitals because nobody will give them a home. And, as The Record's Laura Gardner reported on Monday, the number of abandoned AIDS babies is expected to grow.

In order to attract suitable parents, the state Division of Youth and Family Services has announced that it will pay foster parents a premium monthly rate to care for AIDS-infected youngsters. Such parents deserve it, not because of the danger — there is none — but because about half of those babies will develop the disease itself and will die before their sixth birthday. Said the heroic foster mother of one AIDS baby: "You have to have a lot of love, a lot of understanding." You have to accept the child's death.

Communities that have children with AIDS don't face such heartbreak. They need only display common courtesy to the children and their families, teach their own children to do likewise, and resist the unreasoning panic that strips people of their humanity and tears communities apart.

BUFFALO EVENING NEWS
Buffalo, NY, September 1, 1987

THE SUSPICIOUS FIRE that destroyed the modest house of the Clifford Ray family in Arcadia, Fla., the death threats that preceded it and the boycott organized by some parents against the admission of three Ray children to school constitute a shameful episode.

The three boys, aged 10, 9 and 8, carry the AIDS virus, presumably as a result of medical treatment they received for hemophilia, a blood disease. They were admitted to an Arcadia elementary school last week at the order of a federal district judge.

One can understand the concerns of the parents of other Arcadia school children without condoning their actions. And certainly without condoning the frightening train of events that has now led the Rays to withdraw their sons from the school and move to another community.

Arcadia offers a stark example of how the fear of AIDS can find fertile ground among those who are either unaware of the medical facts or refuse to accept them.

Scientists and medical authorities, including Dr. C. Everett Koop, U.S. surgeon general, have emphasized repeatedly that AIDS is not spread through casual contact, in a school yard or the workplace or the home or anywhere else. Dr. Koop says assurances that the Ray children posed no threat to their classmates were "based upon as solid evidence as anything possibly can be in public health." He said he would "have no compunction at all about sending my children or grandchildren to a school where children not only carried the virus, but had frank AIDS."

Given the alternatives of relying upon fears or upon responsible medical opinion, the choice ought to be clear for any parents or for any community or school system.

Americans need to inform themselves about AIDS, and the federal government is about to distribute a new, detailed pamphlet about AIDS prepared under Koop's direction. One way to get copies is through members of Congress. This and other distributions of authoritative information about AIDS, based on facts about the disease rather than fears, can help as much as anything else to prevent repetitions of the Arcadia tragedy.

At bottom, this shocking episode is rooted in too much fear and too little forthright leadership in the small Florida community.

In its aftermath, one of the most rational voices has been that of the boys' mother, Louise Ray. A relief fund has been organized to assist the stricken family. According to their family attorney, Mrs. Ray believes that the "good people over there waited a little too long to help. The crying need over there is for AIDS education."

THE ARIZONA REPUBLIC
Phoenix, AZ, September 1, 1987

WITH their home gutted by a suspicious fire and their three boys shunned like lepers, no one can blame Clifford and Louise Ray for their decision to look elsewhere for a community to call home. The Florida citrus and ranching community of Arcadia effectively has made sure of that by its bigoted behavior rooted in ignorance, not scientific data.

The fear raging through the 6,000 inhabitants of Arcadia is as sinister and disturbing as the fear that keeps alive the white supremacy beliefs of the Ku Klux Klan.

The Rays and their four children — Ricky, 10, Robert, 9, Randy, 8, and Candy, 6 — are innocent yet tragic victims of this communal fear of AIDS, the deadly disease for which there is yet no known cure or vaccine.

The three boys, all of whom are hemophiliacs, presumably were exposed to the AIDS virus through a blood factor they take to make their blood clot. The local school board last fall barred the trio from regular classes. After a yearlong fight, Clifford Ray won a court ruling last month that ordered the boys reinstated.

The ruling did not sit well with parents of other Arcadia children. They kept their children home during a boycott of the first week of classes, a protest that waned in intensity toward the end of last week.

The fire last Friday that virtually destroyed their wood-frame home was the *coup de grace.*

Although there has not been a formal determination of arson, it stretches the imagination that the fire was coincidental. Their home and personal possessions destroyed, the Rays fled into seclusion for their personal safety.

The community resistance encountered by the Rays dramatically points up the need for greater education of the causes, prevention and spread of the virus responsible for acquired immune deficiency syndrome. A concerted nationwide effort could do much to lessen the panic and hysteria such as the embarrassing spectacle in Arcadia ever since the Ray children tested positive for the AIDS virus.

It is understandable that parents unschooled in the ways AIDS is transmitted would be jittery about having their offspring come in contact with carriers of the killer virus. But scientists are convinced that casual contact is not a means of transmittal. Documented cases reveal direct contact of blood to infected blood or semen — usually through sexual intercourse or the sharing of needles and syringes by drug abusers — is how AIDS spreads.

Getting out education materials and information on AIDS should be a top priority. School boards should participate in the dissemination of information instead of, as in Arcadia, responding inhumanely. Community hysteria and ostracizing humans in need of help are ignorant and unwarranted responses in the 20th century.

Bangor Daily News
Bangor, ME, September 3, 1987

In Arcadia, Fla., the Ray family, which includes three hemophiliac, AIDS-infected sons, has been driven out of town by the irrational fears of neighbors who disrupted the school and may have burned their house down. In Arcadia, Ind., meanwhile, Ryan White, another hemophiliac infected with the AIDS virus, met a different reception when he arrived this week at the doors of Hamilton Heights High School. He was enthusiastically greeted by fellow students and school staff. Nobody picketed and only two kids stayed home.

The case of the two Arcadias is a study in contrast. The Rays' persecution and Ryan's reception show the difference that education can make. AIDS can't be spread by casual contact. AIDS-infected blood needs to be handled with care, but hemophiliacs suffer no more tendency to get cuts or to bleed profusely from superficial cuts and scrapes than do other people, say medical experts.

Closer to home, for the past month members of the Bangor Fire Department's ambulance crews have been putting on surgical masks, rubber gloves, and gowns whenever they have administered first aid to bleeding victims at the scene of accidents. This policy should cause concern because seconds can matter when it comes to saving the lives of bleeding victims. It takes precious seconds to don gloves, masks, and gowns.

But it isn't possible to discount the actions of the Bangor firefighters as hysterical or based on ignorance. AIDS can be contracted by handling contaminated blood if one has open cuts or other blemishes leading into the bloodstream. An ambulance attendant not only runs the risk of being spattered by blood, but he also risks being cut at the scene of an accident. Treating an AIDS victim could pose a high risk.

The events in the two Arcadias and in Bangor and in many other places that are slowly adapting to the AIDS epidemic show the need for increased educational efforts to fully inform citizens of what constitutes danger and what does not.

The pathetic circumstances of the Ray family in Arcadia, Fla., could have been averted with the proper leadership. But it is clear that techniques adopted by Bangor firefighters are a realistic reaction to potential problems. Such reactions to AIDS underscore the need for a more intensive research effort so that the disease's spread can be better understood, and its cure realized.

ARGUS-LEADER

Sioux Falls, SD, September 2, 1987

Residents of Arcadia, Fla., ought to feel disgraced.

Death threats and bomb scares weren't enough to chase Louise and Clifford Ray and their three sons out of the community. But a suspicious fire that destroyed the Rays' home sent the family packing with what was left of their belongings. Louise Clifford says her boys, who have all been exposed to AIDS, has **Editorial** been withdrawn from school and the family will leave DeSoto County.

A fire that destroyed their home capped a week of bomb and death threats and a boycott of the elementary school where the Ray boys had returned to classes after being reinstated by a judge.

Unfortunately, the panic in Florida is only a sample of the AIDS overreaction that has infected several communities in the United States.

A child with AIDS was banned from an Illinois elementary school. Parents in Tennessee are threatening a boycott if a young AIDS carrier is admitted. Elsewhere in Florida, a school board has voted to bar another child who tested positive.

In Indiana, a 15-year-old AIDS victim who once faced pickets and lawsuits has moved to a new community and resumed classes without incident. In a highly publicized battle, the boy and his family had to fight for a year for that modest opportunity.

Communities across the nation are failing the AIDS compassion test. All the panic is unwarranted. It's also cruel.

AIDS — acquired immune deficiency syndrome — is a deadly disease. In recent years, it has killed more than 23,000 Americans. But experts have pointed out repeatedly that AIDS is not spread by casual contact. The disease is believed to be spread primarily through the exchange of body fluids in sex or through infected needles used by drug abusers.

There is no record of the disease ever having been spread from one child to another in school or in a day-care setting.

"AIDS is a frightening disease, so it's understandable that parents are afraid, but they don't need to be," Chuck Falles, a spokesman for the federal Centers for Disease Control in Atlanta, said. "It isn't spread by drinking from school water fountains or eating lunch after an infected student."

The Ray boys are hemophiliacs. They show no symptoms of AIDS, but all have tested positive for antibodies to the virus that causes the deadly disease. The boys are believed to have been exposed to AIDS through a blood product they take to make their blood clot in case of injury.

A federal judge had ordered the boys reinstated in school, prompting angry protests from frightened parents and a boycott when classes started.

About the only bright news about the Ray case is that strangers around the nation and the world have offered the family help. The family has received more than enough clothing and has even been offered home.

Strangers' kindness and generosity offset Arcadia's lack of understanding and compassion but certainly does not excuse it.

The Miami Herald

Miami, FL, September 2, 1987

HOW MUCH is one family supposed to take in this good life? The Ray family of Arcadia has three sons with hemophilia. They were exposed to AIDS from a contaminated blood product. That led to community ostracism and now the torching of their home. If there is any luck for the Rays, it is that no one died in that fire.

Fear fed by ignorance turned to hatred. What other result could be expected when community leadership faltered? That anger would stay focused at a distant Federal judge who ordered the boys' admission to school? That the family would slink away although it has few resources?

To be sure, the Ray story touches dark emotions, a dread disease linked to homosexuality, children, and Federal fiats. But this wasn't the first school-admissions case, and the DeSoto County School Board played to community ignorance instead of fulfilling its role in public *education*.

Now the "good folk" of Arcadia are collecting food and clothing for the Rays. Pastors are preaching homilies on open hearts. Where were they before? An open heart requires an open mind, one that listens to reason and facts.

The Ray boys do not have AIDS. They carry antibodies in their blood. There is evidence that hemophiliacs may be less likely to develop symptoms than others. As for exposing others, AIDS is spread by exchanging of body fluids, not school contact. Indeed, the boys' parents and sister do not carry antibodies.

This is why medical specialists recommend what the law insists upon: a case-by-case review of school children with AIDS or AIDS exposure. The school board could have tried hard to ensure that the community understood what was happening, but it threw the problem to the courts and then waited to hold any public workshops.

And what of law enforcement in Arcadia? The family had been threatened. The threats came true. This failure of leadership cries for investigation, for those in authority failed their responsibility to protect this family. Gov. Bob Martinez should order such an inquiry so that the shabby events in Arcadia are never repeated there or elsewhere.

The Washington Post

Washington, DC, September 1, 1987

WHEN A FAMILY member contracts AIDS—particularly when the victim is a young child—it is a terrible tragedy. Imagine then the plight of a single family with three sons, 10, 9 and 8 years old, all infected with the virus. Clifford and Louise Ray of Arcadia, Fla., are the parents in such a family. Their sons Richard, Robert and Randy are hemophiliacs who were presumably infected from blood products they received before the blood supply was made safe. The boys do not yet have symptoms of AIDS, but the odds are overwhelming that they will eventually get the disease.

There are not that many school-age children with AIDS. Most youngsters who have the disease contracted it from afflicted mothers, many of whom are addicts. These children usually do not live long enough to go to school. Older children with the virus, like the Rays, are more likely to have contracted it from contaminated blood transfusions, but that group is limited and no longer expanding. Many of these children want to go to school, and their cases have aroused controversy. The Rays and other parents have had to go to court to force school boards to accept their children—a situation to which other parents have demonstrated resistance.

Last week, many children in Arcadia were kept home because the Ray boys were in school. But attendance was increasing steadily. On Friday night, the Rays' home was destroyed by a suspicious fire that is being investigated by local authorities and the FBI. The community is stunned by this apparent violence, and many who led the school boycott have rushed to condemn the wrongdoer—if there is one—and to help the family. But there is still confusion and differing opinion on the question whether the boys should be at school.

People who are infected with the AIDS virus can transmit it to others—but not casually. Parents have been repeatedly assured by doctors and scientists that children are safe in school; but because the virus is so deadly, fears persist even when the risk is infinitesimal. It is not as easy to overcome this fear—which may be irrational but is understandable—as it is to condemn violence.

The best approach, we believe, is to treat these cases with candor and compassion and to make every effort to treat AIDS children normally. There is no place for either massive resistance or secrecy. Each case should be considered on its merits. Are the children, both the AIDS victim and his classmates, mature enough to understand each other's fears and combat them? Are there responsible adults in the school who can help in emergencies? Are school authorities providing help and reassurance—not just to the family in need, but to all the parents involved?

These steps have been taken in some communities, and with patience and good will this problem—which is temporary—can be worked out elsewhere. No family should have to go through what the Rays are experiencing without the support and sympathy of its community.

the Charleston Gazette

Charleston, WVA, September 2, 1987

ARCADIA, in literature, represents a land of peace and simplicity. In America, it stands for two separate towns and two very different ways of dealing with the disaster of AIDS.

Earlier this week, Ryan White started his freshman year at Hamilton Heights High School in Arcadia, Ind. White, a hemophiliac, contracted AIDS two years ago from a blood transfusion. A junior high school in Kokomo barred him until a court battle allowed his readmission.

However, not until his parents moved to Arcadia and enrolled him in a new school was White able to resume a normal school life. Fellow students have done their best to make the 15-year-old feel welcome. When classes started Monday, several classmates met him in a hall and shook his hand.

Their behavior is remarkable when contrasted to another Arcadia that has been anything but peaceful. Since Aug. 24, Arcadia, Fla., has been in ferment over a court order allowing three brothers to attend elementary school. The little boys, like Ryan White, were born with hemophilia and were exposed to AIDS through contaminated blood transfusions. They show no symptoms other than a positive blood test. Nor have their parents or sister, living with them, tested positive for AIDS.

But many Arcadia residents are in panic. A protest group has been organized. A boycott kept 200 children out of school Friday. Worst of all, the family's home burned Friday night in a blaze police are calling "suspicious."

The ultimate tragedy of Arcadia, Fla., is that its example is likely to be repeated across the country. Parents have every right to worry over the health of their children. But they shouldn't turn savage against unlucky children who are among thousands testing positive to the virus.

The best experts say that AIDS can be contracted only through sexual intercourse or the mixture of body fluids, as occurs when two intravenous drug users share the same needle. Simple precautions will protect schoolchildren.

No less an authority than U.S. Surgeon General C. Everett Koop said of the Florida uproar: "There is absolutely no reason to fear those children being in school." That should be reassurance enough to persuade communities to behave like Arcadia, Ind., not Arcadia, Fla.

Wisconsin State Journal

Madison, WI, September 3, 1987

The Wisconsin State Journal and many other newspapers carried stories the other day that might have caused the average reader to do a double-take.

One story was about the cruel ignorance being displayed in Arcadia, Fla., where three young brothers — Ricky, Robert and Randy Ray — exposed to the AIDS virus had been shunned by church, school and community and their parents essentially run out of town after a mysterious fire gutted their home.

The other news item was about Ryan White, 15, an AIDS victim in Arcadia, Ind., who returned to Hamilton Heights High School and was given a warm welcome.

There are some obvious parallels between these two stories. Both involve young hemophiliacs who were infected with the AIDS virus through contaminated blood products. Both involve small towns named Arcadia (the Florida version has about 6,000 people; Arcadia, Ind., has about 1,800 citizens).

But there the similarities abruptly end. Arcadia, Fla., is an embarrassing example of how AIDS hysteria and lack of education can turn otherwise clear-thinking people into bigots. Arcadia, Ind., is an uplifting case of how a properly informed public can co-exist with a person exposed to AIDS — acquired immune deficiency syndrome.

It is a difference that speaks well for the efforts in Wisconsin to educate adults and children about AIDS, a serious plague but one that nonetheless must be viewed in rational terms.

In the Madison school district, for example, AIDS education is now a requirement in all ninth-grade health classes. Most Madison elementary schools also discuss AIDS during lessons on communicable diseases in fifth-grade growth and development classes. A program for middle-school students is being developed, as well.

The district has also adopted a policy to deal with students who contract AIDS. Basically, it calls for allowing those children (and there hasn't been a reported case yet) in class unless there is a clear danger to other students, teachers or staff.

Most recently, the State Medical Society recommended mandatory AIDS education for Wisconsin schools beginning in the sixth grade. "Mandatory" education seems a lot less intrusive than "mandatory" testing, and it probably would do more in the long run to check the spread of the disease.

The people in Arcadia, Ind., welcomed Ryan White back to school because they knew that the chances of getting AIDS are minimal unless a healthy person (1) has blood-to-blood contact with an infected person, or (2) sexual intercourse with an infected person, or (3) shares a hypodermic needle with an infected person.

No one is so naive to believe that such activities don't take place between some teen-agers, but we should not be panicked into thinking AIDS can be contracted at the water fountain outside the algebra class, either.

The more people know about AIDS, the more they can guard against its spread in fact and in fear.

LOS ANGELES HERALD

Los Angeles, CA, September 1, 1987

As hemophiliac children inadvertently exposed to the AIDS virus in the course of their medical treatments — but as yet showing no signs of the disease itself — it's uncertain how long Richard, Robert and Randy Ray will live. What is certain, however, is that they and their parents will survive a lot longer now that the family has left Arcadia, Fla.

Their legal battle with the public school system has been national headlines for nearly a year. But ironically, it was their recent court victory that signaled the beginning of the end. Demonstrations escalated into death threats, and last week, a probable arson attack injured a relative, destroyed the Rays' home and drove the family out of town.

"We're all level-headed, everyday, normal people," protested the wife of the president of Citizens Against AIDS in School. "The outside world is taking this too seriously," declared a local minister. Explaining that AIDS is treated differently than other communicable diseases, Arcadia's mayor admits that "I know I must sound like a country jerk saying this."

Such ignorance and intolerance, unfortunately, has not been confined to the Arcadias of the world. While few communities, fortunately, have expressed it so bluntly, similar sentiments nationwide have been mounting, along with the number of AIDS casualties. California, where so many AIDS victims reside, is no exception.

Here a second proposed Lyndon LaRouche initiative is now circulating, aimed at mandatory testing and quarantine. Here a new legislative emphasis in Sacramento now focuses on the punitive rather than the preventive. Here the governor has vetoed $22 million in AIDS research funding. Here local officials argue that homosexuals should simply go "straight" and condemn an AIDS information pamphlet as a how-to manual for homosexuality.

Education is clearly the best medicine now available for preventing AIDS. But the educational effort must be expanded to people who aren't in the high-risk groups and to issues beyond avoiding disease. Like tolerance, compassion and common sense. Arcadia reminds us how much elected officials and public policy-makers still have to learn about AIDS.

WINSTON-SALEM JOURNAL

Winston-Salem, NC, September 11, 1987

In ancient Greece, Arcadia was a symbol of rural serenity, a paradise on earth. In modern Florida, Arcadia is less benign. It's the town that banned from school three hemophiliac children of a family named Ray who are infected with the AIDS virus but do not have the disease. Later, when a judge said they must be allowed to attend, their home was burned to the ground. Arson is suspected. It's a reasonable suspicion given some of the attitudes reported among Arcadians.

The mayor has been quoted as believing that the lack of national quarantine measures for AIDS victims is the result of a gay conspiracy. Other townfolk have opined that there's no point in allowing the Ray children in school since they will die long before graduation anyway.

AIDS is certainly frightening enough. And it isn't going to vanish any time soon. Rather, it is destined to spread. And Americans haven't really had to deal with a widespread incurable and infectious disease since the virtual eradication of polio and tuberculosis over a generation ago. So maybe we've forgotten how to cope. But surely attacking what many regard as a plague of medieval proportions with medieval methods isn't the answer.

Through the employment of rational public health and information measures, the AIDS epidemic can be faced and endured. What can't be endured is making scapegoats of its victims, suggesting they be made to wear leper bells, imagining them to be involved in a conspiracy, and torching their homes. Hysteria is a malady more threatening to society than the worst plague ever known.

THE TENNESSEAN

Nashville, TN, September 2, 1987

ARCADIA, Fla. is obviously the home for some hysterical parents. It may also be home of terrorists.

Clifford and Louise Ray and their four children lived in Arcadia. Mr. Ray is an unemployed prison guard who finds seasonal work driving a farm truck. He and his wife have four children — a healthy six-year-old girl and three sons. All three boys are hemophiliacs, and all three carry the AIDS virus, which they contracted from intravenous injections of contaminated blood.

Imagine the pressure of being unemployed, trying to provide for a family of six. Imagine the worry of being the parents of three little boys who have a blood disease that requires close supervision and medical attention.

And imagine the anguish of learning that, in coping with that blood disease, all three boys have contracted the deadly AIDS virus.

Things went from bad to worse. The Rays were told that their sons, who have no symptoms of AIDS, couldn't attend the local public school. The Rays sued and won the boys' admittance.

Then the real trouble started. The lawsuit alerted the entire town of the boys' condition, and an issue that should have been settled in a court of law became an issue in the town. Parents boycotted the school. The Rays received telephone calls — first menacing, then threatening — warning them to keep their children away from school.

Last Friday, the Rays' home and all of their belongings were destroyed by a fire that authorities call "suspicious." The Rays left Arcadia.

The Ray children aren't the only victims of AIDS who have become victims of discrimination. Today in Lake City, Tenn., a 12-year-old hemophiliac who has the AIDS virus but not the disease will find out if he will be able to attend public school. The superintendent will make the decision after consulting with a team of professionals who are familiar with the child's condition.

Some Lake City residents had considered organizing a boycott if the child returns to school, but attendance is now good, and school officials believe a boycott is unlikely. Regardless of the decision about the child, Lake City residents should stay reasonable. A boycott would only harm the children — all the children — by giving them a lesson in discrimination and fear.

A hysteria swept through Arcadia, Fla. when parents found out about the Ray children. Those parents didn't care that neither of the boys' parents nor their sister had contracted the disease. They ignored the medical evidence that indicates that the Ray boys were no more likely to spread AIDS by casual contact than they were to spread hemophilia.

The hysteria in Arcadia was maddening because it was an affront to medical knowledge, and because it was adding tragedy to the already tragic lives of the boys. Society is uncommonly tolerant, however, of the irrational hysterics of parents who are genuinely worried about their children.

The fire that destroyed the Rays' house is another matter. That's not hysteria — that's terrorism, and no amount of concern for the safety of one's children can right that wrong.

The people of Arcadia should be a hundred times more worried about the possibility of terrorists than of the three AIDS carriers. They can't undo the damage done to the Rays, but they should demand that law enforcment officials turn over every leaf to find and prosecute those responsible for destroying the Rays' home so that more victims of AIDS don't become victims of terrorism. ■

Newsday

Long Island, NY, September 3, 1987

The saga of the Ray family in Arcadia, Fla., might well go down as a double milestone in the history of AIDS in America. The apparent torching of their home is a major disgrace, but it could also be a turning point — a tragedy that knocks this nation to its senses.

AIDS (acquired immune deficiency syndrome) is a killer. There's no vaccine or cure, and there may not be for a long time. But that's no reason to succumb to hysteria or ignorance. If either prevails it will as readily eat at the nation's fabric as the AIDS virus corrodes a body's disease defense.

The Ray family's three sons, Richard, Robert and Randy, are guilty of nothing more than being hemophiliacs. But in receiving blood transfusions to treat that condition, they were exposed to the AIDS virus.

That was bad enough. But then they were exposed to an epidemic of ignorance. The Rays went to court to force the school board to accept their children. When the Rays won, many parents had their children boycott classes. And Friday night the Ray home was destroyed by a fire that officials have labeled as of suspicious origin.

Many people in Arcadia — and elsewhere — were shaken by what happened. That the Ray family is now being showered with messages of condolence and unsolicited contributions from all over the world is evidence of widespread sympathy and understanding. Nonetheless the incident should serve to remind all concerned — from the White House on down — that much more must be done in the field of AIDS education. And it must be done quickly.

People must be told again and again that AIDS is transmitted by intimate, not casual, contact; that those who are infected with the virus will not inevitably develop the disease itself, and that those who do become AIDS victims require care and love, not ostracism and isolation.

The lesson of Arcadia, Fla., is that the nation is plagued with not one but two epidemics — the disease itself and the abysmal ignorance surrounding it. While we are awaiting a cure for the former, there's a readily available antidote for the latter: repeated doses of education.

Roanoke Times & World·News

Roanoke, VA, September 2, 1987

IT'S MERE coincidence that two towns named Arcadia have had to deal with a threat of AIDS in their public school systems recently. The similarity between the two localities stops with their name, however.

In Arcadia, Ind., a 15-year-old AIDS victim was welcomed by officials and students on the first day of school Monday. In the Florida town of Arcadia, there were protests all last week and threats against a family with three children who have been exposed to the AIDS virus. When a suspicious fire gutted their home, the family gave up and decided to leave town.

Ryan White's family moved to the Arcadia, Ind., area during the summer to escape lawsuits and protests over his battle to attend school in his old school district, Kokomo. Ryan, a hemophiliac, was diagnosed as having acquired immune deficiency syndrome in December of 1984. It wasn't until last year, however, that Ryan was allowed to start a regular school term.

The protests staged in Arcadia, Fla., when school began last week — and the three sons of Clifford and Louise Ray showed up for classes — have not presented the town in its best light. The Ray brothers — Richard, 10, Robert, 9, and Randy, 8 — are all hemophiliacs who do not have AIDS but who have been infected with the virus.

The fire at the Rays' home last Friday only made Arcadia's public image worse. It's one thing to protest someone's actions; quite another to do him harm.

The cause of the fire that destroyed all of the Rays' belongings hasn't been determined. It's possible — although unlikely — that the blaze had nothing to do with the school protest. Unless mitigating evidence comes to light, it can be assumed that this was an act of hate.

As such, it ought to be a jolt for the protesters. Many of them were stunned by the fire, but no one should be too surprised by this graphic demonstration of just how destructive fear can be.

It's natural for parents to fear for the safety of their children; yet it's important for people to listen to reason. Panic will tear communities apart. Scientists say it's almost impossible for AIDS to be transferred in casual contact among schoolchildren, and there's no reason to doubt them.

School systems all over the country are going to be facing the same problem as this incurable disease spreads. AIDS victims and their families already are suffering greatly. Will their neighbors show them compassion or disdain? Which Arcadia's example will they follow?

The Honolulu Advertiser

Honolulu, HI, September 3, 1987

If you care about Hawaii, you have to hope that what happened in Arcadia, Florida, couldn't happen here. We may have a chance to find out.

Arcadia's the town that cruelly, maybe criminally, drove out the Ray family because their three young sons, victims of hemophilia who need many blood transfusions, tested positive for the AIDS virus.

First, the boys were barred from school. Citing medical opinion that there was no risk for others, their parents got a court order allowing them to enroll.

On the first day of school half the students boycotted classes. Bomb threats followed. When the Ray home was gutted by a suspicious fire that might have been arson, they fled town.

Too many in Arcadia are suffering from a disease. Its symptoms are an excess of ignorance about AIDS (which all evidence shows cannot be transmitted by casual everyday contacts) and a severe shortage of the milk of human kindness.

Hawaii may soon find its understanding and compassion tested. A public/private task force is looking for a home for eight to 12 people at a time — people who have AIDS but do not need to be hospitalized. Sites in Nuuanu, Kalihi and Makiki are being considered. If the AIDS crisis worsens, more homes may be needed.

Hawaii's acceptance of these kinds of care facilities has not been exemplary. As a small community, our NIMBY — Not in My Back Yard — mentality is often strong.

Such worthy causes as a Ronald McDonald House for the families of gravely ill children and homes for patients recovering from mental illness have suffered from the NIMBY attitude.

People have the right and good reason to be concerned about their neighborhoods, to be sure, both for lifestyle and property-value considerations. Areas with lower real estate costs close to town do get more than their fair share of these homes. But the experience of many neighborhoods, once the facilities move in, is that the effects are not as bad as was feared.

With the AIDS epidemic growing, an extra ration of the aloha spirit and human compassion is going to be needed to care for the afflicted. Honolulu shouldn't respond like Arcadia.

Birmingham Post-Herald

Birmingham, AL, September 5, 1987

The AIDS-stricken Ray family of Arcadia, Fla., has been treated abominably, maybe criminally. Instead of compassion, they received harassment, and worse.

The three young sons of Clifford and Louise Ray were infected by the AIDS virus through no fault of their own or of their family. They are hemophiliacs and presumably contracted the virus from blood products needed to control internal bleeding. While they carry the virus, they do not show any symptoms of the disease.

The boys, Randy, Robert and Richard, aged 8, 9 and 10, first were barred from attending public school. When their parents obtained a court order to have them admitted, other parents initiated a boycott of classes and the family began to receive anonymous threats. When the boycott began petering out after a few days, the Ray home mysteriously was gutted by fire; arson is suspected.

Fear of AIDS is understandable, but the reaction against the Rays went beyond reason. There is no evidence that the AIDs virus is transmitted by casual contact, as normally occurs among pupils. And experts in blood disorders say a child with hemophilia and infected with the AIDS virus poses no exceptional risk to others.

A Catholic priest in Arcadia told parishoners that community reaction in the Ray case reminded him of the way people used to treat lepers. "The ultimate tragedy," he said, is to make the Ray children, already with troubles enough, "feel outlawed and unwanted."

In one of the most heartless comments imaginable, an Arcadia resident was quoted as saying: "What's the point of an education for them, huh? They don't need an education because according to statistics I've seen, they only have but five years to live."

That, too, is based on ignorance. Despite a high rate of infection with the AIDS virus among hemophiliacs because of their large need for blood-based products, relatively few have developed active cases of AIDS. At present, the Ray children are among those who have not shown symptoms.

Now that they have been shunned, threatened with death and finally burned out, the Rays have said they are giving up and leaving town. No doubt the people of Arcadia will be relieved — both because the source of their fears will be gone and because they will not have to face the family they have so mistreated.

There are 20,000 hemophiliacs in the United States, of which more than half are believed infected with the AIDS virus. Are they all to be hounded out of town? Or will compassionate Americans find a better way to deal with this problem?

The Orlando Sentinel

Orlando, FL, September 2, 1987

By now everyone in America knows the Ray family has left Arcadia for good. Their DeSoto County home ravaged by a suspicious fire, Clifford and Louise Ray took their three hemophiliac sons exposed to the AIDS virus away from the town that shunned them.

And all because of AIDS hysteria.

Ironically in another Arcadia, students welcomed 15-year-old Ryan White, a hemophiliac who suffers from AIDS, to an Indiana high school this week. There were no class boycotts, no bomb scares, no death threats, no fires.

Why did these two communities react so differently to the AIDS menace? Leadership is the key. Indiana law lays out medical guidelines for accepting students with AIDS. Florida is lacking such guidelines.

Florida ranks second in the nation in cases of children with AIDS. But despite that statistic, state officials have been reluctant to set a policy on AIDS. That has left local officials without guidance. Now state Education Commissioner Betty Castor is proposing developing state guidelines.

But until then, other cases of hysteria are bound to happen. In Pensacola, for example, 150 people persuaded a state agency Monday to abandon its plans to turn a vacant house into Florida's first group home for teen-agers with AIDS antibodies.

Residents complained the sexually active teens were a health threat. State health officials didn't bother to dispel residents' fears. Instead, officials chose to find a new location for a group home.

Who knows, the Beach Haven neighborhood may not have been the right choice for a group home anyway. But by caving in so quickly health officials have ducked their responsibility to set the record straight on AIDS. Irrational fears are left to fester once again. And that could hurt the state's chances of placing a group home anywhere.

In the Ryan White case, Indiana health officials and community leaders moved quickly to quell any hysteria. They met with students, parents and teachers months before White was to go to school. The community had time to get the facts about AIDS.

They learned AIDS cannot be transmitted casually, only by direct blood contact or sexually. They learned that if AIDS were spread casually, then the families of hemophiliacs who have AIDS would have contracted the virus. In fact, none has. Those facts put many fears to rest.

That was not the case in DeSoto County. Parents there got conflicting messages from community leaders and that made it all the worse.

School officials first fought in court to keep the Rays out of school. Then after losing the legal battle, those same officials told parents that the boys, who have AIDS antibodies but not the disease itself, did not pose a health risk to other children. No wonder the Arcadia parents were skeptical.

Other community leaders contributed even more to the hysteria — either by their actions or inaction. Arcadia's mayor took his child out of public school. The Rays' Baptist minister, Carl Fuentes, did nothing. He felt it was better not to discuss the Rays' plight from the pulpit.

There were some leaders who did call for understanding. The priest at St. Paul's Catholic Church asked his congregation to have compassion for the Ray family, to avoid treating them like lepers, to open their hearts and their homes to them. Many of them did.

But for the Rays, it was too little, too late.

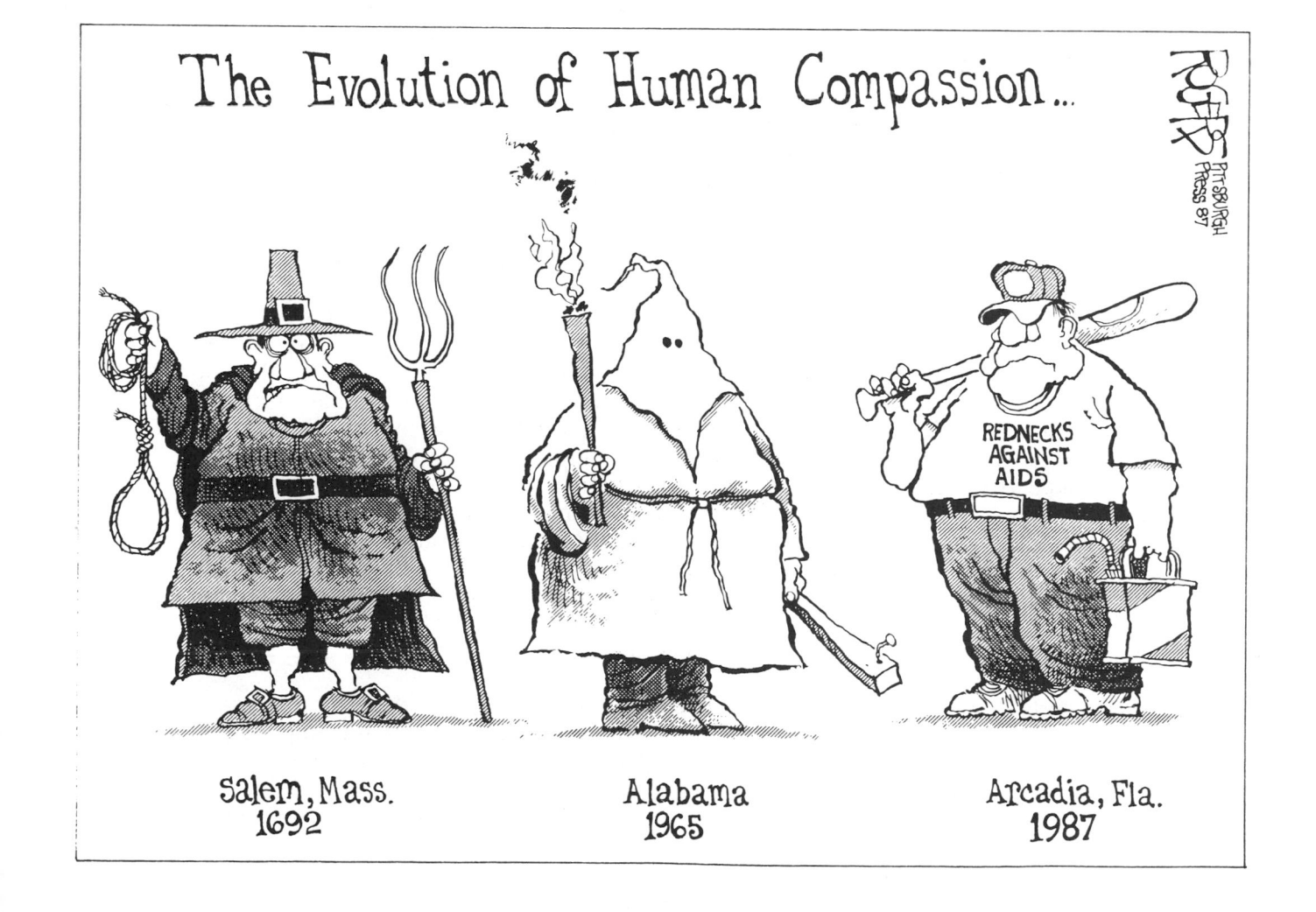

Part IV: AIDS and the Law

The law regulating public health actions is complicated and uncertain. AIDS therefore poses an incomparable challenge for health and policy makers, who must seek methods of reducing its spread and of helping ensure the public safety consistent with the protection of individual dignity and autonomy. The major health cases in which public health policies actions are rooted arose near the turn of the century. However, subsequent advances in medicine and changes in the judicial treatment of individual rights have forced revisions in health law that are not yet complete.

Many of our public health responses to epidemic diseases are decades or even centuries old. The scientific basis and appropriate uses of measures like quarantine have changed considerably as 20th-century medicine has developed a better understanding of the cause and transmission of disease. Concurrently, American society and its judiciary have become more sophisticated about individual liberties: Additional rights have been recognized—ranging from privacy in contraception to attendance at non-segregated schools—and protection of all rights have been enhanced. The AIDS epidemic has presented an invitation to the court system to fully incorporate the legal and medical developments into the health law.

Perhaps the thorniest and most controversial legal issue involving AIDS regards the question of testing, because it is one that crosses the spectrum of social considerations. Prison, military, insurance, immigration and education officials have all expressed a desire for testing but have lacked the proper legal means to implement such measures. At present, there is no readily available test for determining whether a person who has been exposed to the AIDS virus harbors it now, nor is there a test that determines who is infectious. However, a test does exist for determining whether a person has been exposed to the virus. Caution dictates that such persons be presumed to be infectious.

Properly understood, testing is a means, not an end. It provides information whose value depends on the use to which it is put. Testing proposals can be evaluated only in terms of how well they accomplish some desired goal in both the legal and medical arenas. Testing for the AIDS virus can, theoretically, do two things: provide a clearer statistical picture of the prevalence of the virus and identify infected individuals who may benefit from some sort of public health action. On both counts, massive screening is legally problematic. For several reasons, civil libertarians say, a widespread mandatory testing program is an inappropriate and perhaps counterproductive method of doing this, in that a person's antibody status can be a very dangerous piece of information. If their status becomes public knowledge, people who test positively for AIDS may be exposed to discrimination ranging from loss of employment or housing, to denial of insurance, to serious physical abuse. In addition, critics of mandatory testing say, that a negative result may be of little value if the person tested has engaged in high-risk activity within six months before testing, because the antibodies produced do not show up due to the virus' dormancy period. Furthermore, they say, a positive result (even if it is not a false positive) does not reveal whether the victim is actually infectious or will ever develop AIDS or AIDS-Related Complex (ARC). It is precisely for these reasons that confidentiality is regarded as a critical issue in any testing program.

AIDS testing by public health officials has begun to be accepted by the courts as a valid public health measure. The Supreme Court has recognized the importance of maintaining the confidentiality of medical data as well as its faith in the confidentiality protections provided by typical health laws. Current litigation concerning mandatory drug testing by the federal government may foreshadow how the courts will treat challenges to governmental AIDS testing.

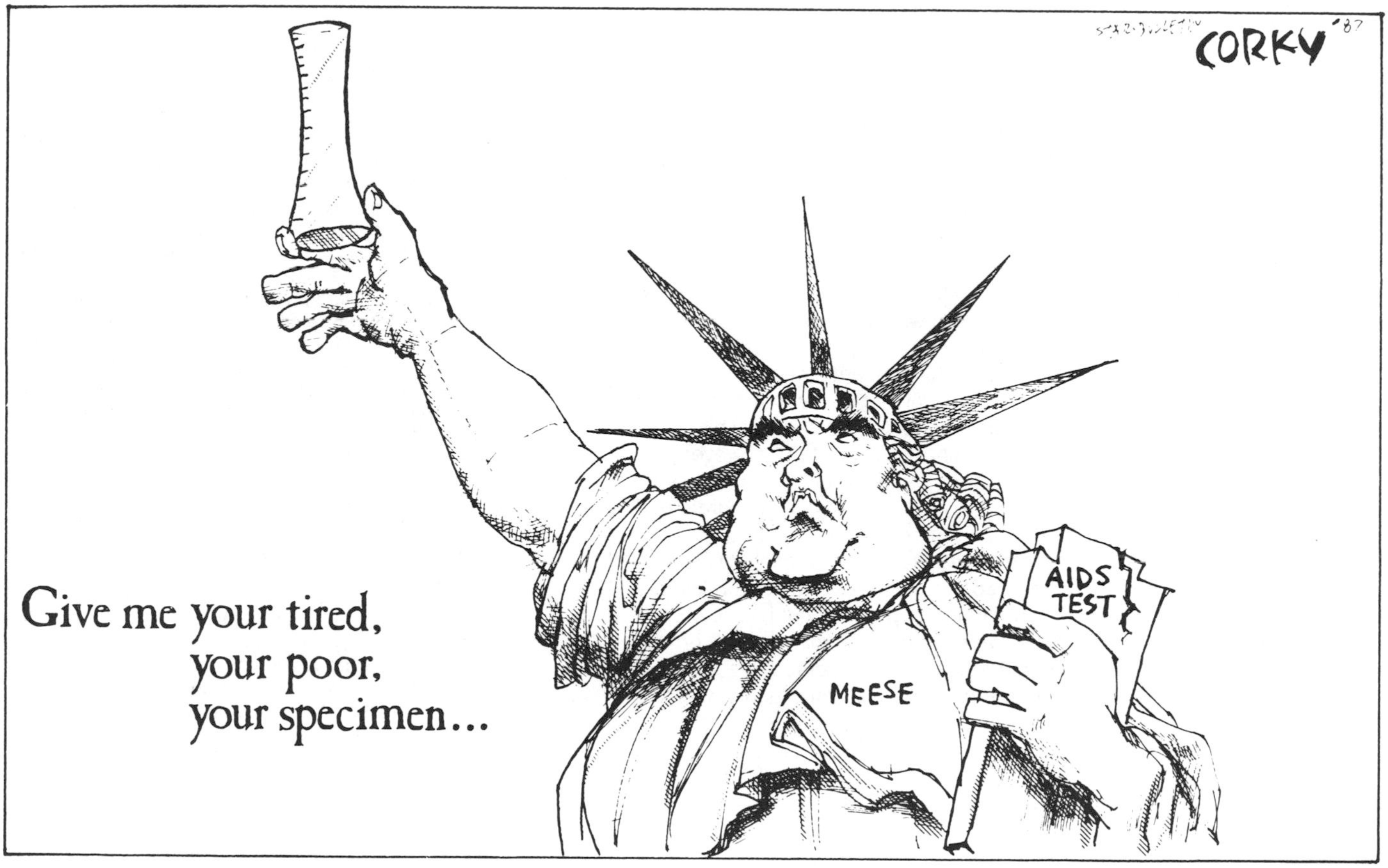

Give me your tired,
your poor,
your specimen...

Meese Details Federal Program to Screen Prisoners

U.S. Attorney General Edwin Meese III June 8, 1987 announced details of a program to test federal prisoners for infection with the virus that causes AIDS. Meese said he had instructed federal prison officials to begin immediate testing for all new inmates. Previously the Bureau of Prisons, which housed more than 43,000 inmates, had tested and isolated only those inmates who had showed symptoms of AIDS. Since 1981, there had been a total of 76 reported cases among federal prisoners. Meese said he had also directed officials to develop a system to test all inmates for the virus 30 days before they were released from prison. Federal probation officers would be notified of positive results. Such information, Meese said, "might affect the probation officer in the type of employment [a parolee] was allowed to have." The attorney general cited "counselor in a day-care center" as the kind of job that "some probation officers" might deem inappropriate for parolees infected with the AIDS virus. Meese also suggested that it might be inappropriate to grant parole to some inmates with AIDS if they posed a danger to the community. Meese said he had ordered the National Institute of Justice, the Justice Department's research arm, to set up an AIDS clearinghouse to assist law enforcement professionals regarding the "ever-increasing risk of unknowingly contracting AIDS through contact with...offenders."

The question of AIDS in prisons had garnered public attention as homosexual activity and intravenous drug use in prisons is an acknowledged and unavoidable reality of prison life.

The American Medical Association (AMA) at its annual meeting in Chicago June 23, 1987 adopted a policy that was more selective as to who should be tested for the virus that causes AIDS than were Reagan administration proposals. The AMA governing board rejected testing of hospital patients or marriage license applicants but recommended that doctors urge people in these two groups to be tested if their family history or lifestyle placed them in a high-risk category. The AMA, however, did endorse mandatory testing of prisoners and would-be immigrants. Mandatory testing of federal prisoners and those seeking to immigrate had already been adopted by the federal government.

The United States had 15 centers for the purchase and resale of blood, it was reported August 23, 1987. The trade in prisoners' blood had died out during the early 1970s because of unfavorable publicity but had revived in part because of the AIDS crisis. Newspaper accounts had reported a drop in blood donations that had accompanied the disease's spread. Deaths from contaminated blood had caused many to associate blood banks with the AIDS virus and to believe that even donating was dangerous.

In a related development, the Los Angeles County district attorney's office June 29, 1987 filed charges against Joseph Edward Markowski, a 29-year-old victim of AIDS for knowingly selling his AIDS-infected blood. The case appeared to be the first in the U.S. in which a commercial blood donor who knew he was infected with the AIDS virus had been charged with attempted murder. Markowski, described by authorities as a prostitute and drifter, was alleged to have sold his blood at least once to a Los Angeles blood company, Plasma Production Associates, and was in the process of doing so again when he was arrested June 25. The charges were, however, dismissed the following December 1 for want of evidence, as required by law, that Markowski had intended to kill anyone. Markowski was acquitted March 2, 1988 of two counts of attempted poisoning for selling his tainted blood

The Washington Post
Times Herald
Washington, DC, June 10, 1987

THESE ARE confusing times for aliens. Many millions of undocumented workers in this country were expected to apply for amnesty under the terms of the immigration law passed last year. So far, the numbers have been disappointing, perhaps because some aliens do not understand the details of the program and others fear the consequences of coming forward. All need to be reassured and encouraged.

Congress understood that some would-be applicants would be reluctant to present themselves to immigration authorities for fear of being rejected and deported. To overcome this apprehension, two important provisions were added to the law. The first authorizes a network of non-government agencies—churches, social welfare groups, ethnic organizations—to accept applications and to do the initial paper work. The second provision forbids the use for any other purpose of information learned through an amnesty application. This protects applicants against criminal charges for using false papers to get a job, for example, and it protects them from deportation based only on this kind of information.

Most recently, aliens hoping to qualify for amnesty have faced new problems. Some have been fired from jobs they have held for a long time because employers believe they will be penalized for hiring illegals. The catch here is that an applicant must show he is self-supporting to qualify for amnesty. Employers are being reminded by the Immigration and Naturalization Service that they need not fire workers hired before the law was passed last November. And fortunately, in tough cases where an applicant can show a steady work history that has been interrupted only because of an employer's misunderstanding of the law, a spokesman for the INS says, the government "will give applicants the benefit of the doubt."

AIDS testing is another worry. This country's immigration laws have traditionally barred admission of those who have contagious diseases, and newly announced regulations make clear that this restriction will be applied to those who carry the AIDS virus. Applicants for amnesty will be tested, and under the law, those who have the AIDS virus will not qualify for the benefit. But the attorney general has given assurances that such people will not be deported because information about their medical condition learned during the amnesty process cannot be used to penalize them.

Much public and private energy has been devoted, in recent months, to helping those aliens who will qualify for amnesty. It is sadly true, however, that there will always be some who prey on the desperation of those who come here illegally and who seek to exploit their vulnerability. This week, in Brooklyn, 21 private security guards and six others who helped them were arrested and arraigned on charges of extortion. They had all, it is alleged, engaged in a scheme to coerce individuals awaiting deportation who had been placed in their custody. It is charged that large money payments and sexual favors were demanded in exchange for arranging an alien's escape and that food was withheld from those who refused to cooperate. Abuse of people who are so desperate and so vulnerable by those in authority is despicable; if the charges are proved, the punishment should be severe.

The Clarion-Ledger
JACKSON
DAILY NEWS

Jackson, MS, July 30, 1987

Sometimes the non-traditional approach to controversial issues is the best.

That's the case now with the decision by the state Corrections Department to begin this weekend selling condoms to the 6,950 state prison inmates.

Currently, at least two inmates at the State Penitentiary at Parchman have AIDS and are in the prison hospital. Another four have been diagnosed as having an AIDS-related virus.

Considering that the incurable disease is already there in the confines of the prison and is likely to be spread, prevention by use of a 25-cent condom is far less expensive than treatment, which can total $50,000 to $150,000 from diagnosis to death. This is not meant to condone sexual activity among inmates. It simply faces the reality that AIDS is real danger and must be controlled.

Nationwide, by 1991, the care for AIDS patients is expected to range from $15 billion to $70 billion.

Money from the sales of condoms at the state prison will be put into a fund to pay for testing of inmates for exposure to the AIDS virus. Again, another need that is being met by clear, reasonable thinking on the part of state Corrections Department officials.

But the sales of condoms to those who are incarcerated in state prisons is not the only facet of the new policy to control AIDS among those confined for crimes. The state also will issue plastic gloves to the 1,279 guards at the state's two prisons and 13 community work centers. The policy also calls for coordinating with state Health Department officials training and education of Corrections Department staff on the disease.

AIDS, by the very nature of the infection, is a subject that most people would care to forget. But the rapid spread of this disease is forcing many people to change the way they think.

The new policy approved by the Corrections Department might seem wrong or silly to many, but in reality it is a practical way of handling AIDS, especially in the confines of a prison.

TULSA WORLD

Tulsa, OK, August 26, 1986

OKLAHOMA corrections officials are right in not overreacting to reports that two state inmates carry AIDS antibodies. (Neither inmate has AIDS, and medical authorities say only 5 to 20 percent of those persons who carry the antibodies eventually contract the disease.)

Inmates, understandably frightened by the thought of AIDS carriers, have requested that the entire prison population be tested.

Corrections officials say there is no reliable test for the disease itself, and testing for AIDS antibodies now is needless. Officials at one facility will hold a seminar to educate inmates about the disease.

Homosexual men and drug users are in the highest risk groups for AIDS. Because homosexuality and drug abuse are common in prisons, a prison might seem to be a likely spot for an AIDS outbreak.

Officials of the U.S. Center for Disease Control in Atlanta, Ga., say there have been some cases of AIDS reported among prisoners in New York, New Jersey and California. Evidence indicates those inmates contracted the disease before entering prison.

According to the CDC, there is no evidence that the incidence of AIDS is higher in prisons.

AIDS is cause for grave concern. Already, it is the second leading killer of men in New York City. But unreasoned, panicked action is not going to help anything.

The Providence Journal

Providence, RI, May 21, 1986

Where AIDS is concerned, Rhode Island correctional officials don't see much difference between the prison community and the larger community outside the walls. They keep inmates' medical records confidential, and are reluctant to isolate prisoners unless they pose a public health threat.

"Civil liberties is a very critical issue here in prison," says Jeff Laurie, deputy assistant director of corrections for rehabilitation, who drew up the department's AIDS policy. "Inmates here are very constitutionally oriented."

Mr. Laurie's approach to this deadly disease largely coincides with one adopted by the state Department of Health — to strike a balance between prisoners' rights and possible risks to prisoners as a group. That seems both sensitive and sensible.

Those who insist that all prisoners be tested for the AIDS virus should confront the pros and cons. To what purpose would mandatory testing be put? Should any inmate found to be carrying the antibodies — indicating that person has been exposed, but does not yet have the disease — be segregated? Should such isolation be promoted for only long-term inmates, or should those serving a year or so be treated equally?

Exposure to AIDS, or contracting the disease, are not crimes, and preventing its spread is a public health issue that calls for the most diligent education program yet mounted, both in the schools and in prisons.

To their credit, corrections officials have emphasized this in their new policy for inmates and staff. Information is really the only public defense against AIDS, and to be forewarned is to be able to avoid the sexual and drug-abuse practices that are responsible for most cases.

ACI inmates also will be screened for AIDS symptoms, counseled if they test positive or are in a high-risk group, and isolated if they actually have the disease, or when the precursor ACR (AIDS-related complex) is present if it is considered medically necessary.

The Corrections Department has taken an intelligent stand on what can become a controversial issue. Prevention, not punishment is the wisest course, inside as well as outside the ACI.

DAILY ◙ NEWS

New York, NY, April 15, 1987

Stephen Joseph, New York City health commissioner, wants to give out condoms to prisoners in city jails. The rules say no sex in jail. The rules are right. But they are hard to enforce—and generally ignored. Homosexuality is rampant behind bars.

Homosexual behavior minus condoms equals AIDS. And Dr. Joseph claims as many as 25,000 people who have been exposed to AIDS enter the city jail system annually.

Why bother with these criminals? First, they're human. But also because AIDS patients can run up over $100,000 in medical bills from diagnosis to death. Cons don't have health insurance. And AIDS doesn't kill overnight.

Which leaves the Department of Correction with three lousy alternatives. It can insist that cons be chaste—and pay the astronomical medical bills of those who fail to comply. It can hire hundreds of extra guards to serve as sex police. Or it can hold its nose, accept the inevitable, and start handing out condoms.

Dr. Joseph favors alternative No. 3. Not because he likes it, but because it makes sense. He's right.

Newsday

Long Island, NY, April 17, 1986

Sex among jail inmates is forbidden. So why give out condoms to gay prisoners as a means of curbing the spread of AIDS? Because common sense tells you that there will always be sexual activity in prisons and homosexual sex is one very major way AIDS is transmitted.

This is why Correction Commissioner Richard Koehler was right to announce a condoms-for-cons pilot program this week. This decision, urged on him by city health chief Stephen Joseph, put aside judgmental moralizing in the interests of saving lives and trying to curb the growth of the AIDS epidemic.

It's too bad, then, that city and state officials can't seem to summon up comparable courage in dealing with intravenous drug addicts. IV drug use accounts for more than one-third of the city's AIDS cases and it's the main conduit for the disease's transmission to heterosexuals. Distributing disposable clean needles to drug addicts might help reduce the sharing of contaminated syringes and perhaps reduce AIDS spread.

Despite the fact that Joseph has won Mayor Edward Koch over to his proposed experimental program, State Health Commissioner David Axelrod has failed to give his approval — even though Joseph informally presented the idea to him more than six months ago. True enough, a clean-needle program makes a lot of people edgy. Critics fear it won't reduce the spread of AIDS but will encourage drug use. Still, studies show that junkies do care about their own health as well as the health of their loved ones. Similar programs in other countries have been remarkably successful, so there is good reason to believe addicts would respond to a clean-needle program. Common sense rather than sermonizing and squeamishness must be used to combat the serious health crisis we're facing.

The Hutchinson News

Hutchinson, KS, January 20, 1986

The first AIDS scare is over at Kansas State Industrial Reformatory, but the concern will certainly not be over.

Tests on the first inmate in Kansas suspected of carrying the disease showed negative results, though, the inmate will continue to be segregated. Obviously there will be continuing concern about his health and that of the other inmates.

State and local law enforcement and health officers responded promptly and effectively to the potential problem this week, once an informant sent word of the possibility. Likewise, state and local officials made no effort to hide the concern from the public.

That is as it should have been.

More than 1,400 inmates at KSIR obviously have more than passing interest in any potential health problem within the facility. Their families obviously have more than a passing interest in a potential health problem. The men and women who work at KSIR have more than a passing interest. And so does everyone else.

This year, 8,000 Americans are expected to die from the disease. At that rate, in a brief period of time, more Americans will have died from AIDS than were killed in the Vietnam War.

Those numbers are tragic, in an epidemic in which the first 10,000 cases alone have run up measurable national costs of $6 billion.

• Neither hand wringing nor panic should be the response to the epidemic. The response should include the precise concern and measured reporting undertaken by Kansas officials this past week. It should include increased national attention to finding a cure, along with increased attention to the details of helping those who need help.

The Washington Post

Washington, DC, July 18, 1987

PRISON OFFICIALS have a tough job. They deal day in and day out with very troubled, frequently violent people, and they often lack the facilities, resources, personnel and community support to do a first-rate job of rehabilitating the inmates in their custody. As a minimum, though, they are responsible for the welfare of their charges and, in particular, for their safety. In this connection, assaults by one prisoner on another are a common problem and a major headache. Fights, homosexual rape and even murder take place within prison walls. Now there is something else, something frighteningly dangerous to worry about: AIDS.

Jerome Baker, who is serving two sentences for armed robbery in an Arlington jail, was notified last week that he carries the AIDS virus. Mr. Baker had requested a test after he was bitten by his cell mate, who is infected. It is possible that the virus entered Mr. Baker's bloodstream when his skin was broken during the attack. He also points out that his cell mate had bleeding mouth sores and had shared his cup and toothbrush. It is also possible that Mr. Baker was infected before he even entered the jail. Because many inmates are intravenous drug users and that is a high-risk group for AIDS, he might also have contracted the infection from an intimate contact with some other inmate.

Prisoners have already filed lawsuits in three states seeking protection from AIDS carriers with whom they are incarcerated. In Arlington, it is the policy of corrections officials not to tell prisoners that another inmate is a carrier, not to segregate carriers unless there has already been dangerous behavior, and not to test inmates routinely, or even on request.

Is this fair to those in custody who have not been infected? We think it is not. Granted, this problem has come up rather suddenly and steps to protect the prison population are still in the planning stages, but those plans must be accelerated. Prisoners are wards of society. They do not have the freedom to decide where to eat and sleep or the right to choose those with whom they must live in close contact. They must be protected and so must the families to whom they will eventually return. "It's truly going to be a headache," says Arlington Sheriff James Gondless of the need to test and perhaps separate inmates. But the inexorable deadliness of the infection makes a swift and effective response by prison officials imperative.

The News and Observer
Raleigh, NC, June 11, 1987

In keeping with President Reagan's call for wider and more routine AIDS testing, Attorney General Edwin Meese has announced details of plans to test federal prisoners and immigration applicants. And while a case can be made for testing these two groups of people, the Meese rules illustrate how easy it is for the country to slide down the slippery slope toward infringing on Americans' rights.

The federal government has well-established legal authority to administer a physical exam to applicants for an immigration visa, and the government has an interest in knowing what sort of health problems it will face within its prisons. But, by ordering a test for inmates due to be released from prison and the submission of results to parole officers, Meese now raises the specter that parole decisions could be influenced by an AIDS test.

The penal system is for confining and punishing people for crimes for which they have been convicted. It should not impose further punishment on people for illnesses they may have contracted. If authorities prolonged a person's punishment as a result of an AIDS test, it would surely violate the Constitution's guarantee of due process and its prohibition against cruel and unusual punishment.

In defense of his rules, Meese says, "It is imperative that the federal government do everything it can to combat this rapidly growing public health problem." In fact, of course, the Reagan administration is not doing everying it can. Testing prisoners and immigration applicants will hardly make a dent in the AIDS epidemic. Meanwhile, the U.S. government as yet to release its $51 million annual contribution to the World Health Organization.

The WHO, an agency of the United Nations, is the organization best equipped to counter the international spread of AIDS. It was the WHO that stifled smallpox as a worldwide scourge. But the Reagan administration often reflects the anti-U.N. bias of its right-wing constituents, and at the moment the United States is the only major nation not to have made its annual payment to the WHO. Fighting AIDS doesn't require violating people's constitutional rights, but it surely means keeping the WHO financially healthy.

AKRON BEACON JOURNAL
Akron, OH, June 10, 1987

ATTORNEY General Edwin Meese has announced plans to implement the first two stages of a program to fight the deadly disease AIDS. The total program was outlined last week by President Reagan and includes some controversial means — not all of them wise — to push widespread, mandatory testing for AIDS.

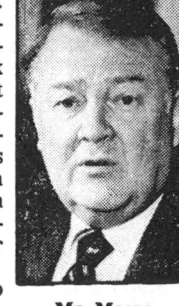

Mr. Meese

The first two steps being discussed by Mr. Meese are probably the easiest to implement, but still are not without problems.

The one that seems to have the fewest number of critics would test immigrants for the AIDS virus and deny entry to those who are infected. That testing will be done under existing laws that require a physical for those seeking immigrant visas, and would include AIDS among the infectious diseases the immigration standards guard against.

The second part of the plan is stirring up more controversy — the testing of the 43,200 inmates of federal prisons. Such testing can work because a prison is a closed population, and can allow better monitoring of sexual contacts. The obvious problem, however, is how to segregate those who test positive for the virus.

As the AIDS epidemic worsens, additional prison facilities will be needed to house and care for the victims, and the additional cost must be figured into any AIDS-treatment program.

Another issue raised by Mr. Meese on the prisoner testing is equally troubling. He suggested that an inmate's infection with AIDS could be a factor in considering whether the prisoner should be released on parole. His reasoning: that a parole board routinely determines whether an inmate would be a danger to the community if released.

That provision, if followed, would be sure to end up in the courts. Withholding or revoking parole for medical reasons seems to violate the Fifth Amendment's guarantee of "due process," and the Eighth Amendment's ban of "cruel and unusual punishment."

Whatever action the government takes, no policy should be considered permanent. Some testing recommended by Mr. Reagan — such as testing couples seeking marriage licenses — seems doomed to waste resources for little real gain. All the testing programs should be constantly evaluated after they are implemented to see if they are worthwhile.

The AIDS epidemic is a growing national crisis with growing costs, both in human loss and in money terms. The nation can't afford to waste resources in ineffective testing programs, any more than it can afford to do nothing to check the spread of this modern plague.

THE DAILY HERALD
Biloxi, MS, July 30, 1987

The state Department of Corrections exercised sound judgment in deciding on specific measures Tuesday to help curb the spread of the deadly AIDS virus in the penitentiary system, including an admittedly controversial plan to sell condoms to inmates.

The decision was not easy. Some department officials wanted to limit condoms to conjugal visits by spouses, fearing their general availability might encourage homosexual rapes. That is what should have been done, although the Health Department recommended making condoms available to all. Such liberal availability is an admission that the prison cannot prevent homosexual activities and rapes among inmates.

Moral issues certainly figure in the debate over acquired immune deficiency syndrome, primarily spread by sexual contact and by intravenous use of drugs. But the fact that there is no known cure for the virus that robs the body of protection against life-sapping ailments is reason enough to give emphasis to ways to minimize its spread.

Mississippi has some 6,900 inmates in prison and in 12 community work centers. Two cases of AIDS-infected inmates, held in isolation, have been reported at the sprawling Parchman penitentiary that has one of the largest conjugal visit programs in the nation. Prison officials have a paramount responsibility to identify carriers of the AIDS-complex virus and to isolate them from the uninfected population.

The problem will be attacked in several ways.

▶ The next 1,000 inmates assigned to prison will be screened with assistance from Health Department officials as a sampling process. A special camp for identified AIDS-virus carriers will be considered if warranted.

▶ An AIDS education program will be launched for the benefit of inmates and Corrections employees.

▶ Inmates identified as carriers of the AIDS virus will not be permitted to engage in food handling, although there are no known ways of AIDS transmission in this activity.

▶ Gloves will be purchased for use by prison staffers who deal with inmates on a daily basis to prevent contact with body fluids in the handling of prisoners who have been injured or wounded.

The use of gloves and other contact prevention apparel is becoming routine for paramedics, surgeons and health service employees whose activities expose them to contact with blood and other body fluids. The federal Center for Disease Control in Atlanta disclosed recently that seven health-care workers have contracted the disease nationally.

The measures adopted by Mississippi's Department of Corrections are a response to a deadly dilemma. They are designed to help protect the general populace as well as prison inmates and to identify and control carriers of the fearsome disease.

DAYTON DAILY NEWS
Dayton, OH, July 6, 1987

AIDS is deadly, and deadly things qualify as weapons.

It didn't take long for a Minnesota jury to make that conclusion. In so doing, the jurors returned a guilty verdict for assault with a dangerous weapon against a federal inmate who bit two prison guards, knowing that he had tested positive for AIDS.

In another case, a California prosecutor is bringing attempted murder charges against a man who allegedly tried to sell his plasma, even though he knows he has the AIDS virus and that his actions could kill. It will be tougher to convict in this case, and again a guilty verdict may not mean much because the man apparently is already very ill.

A very few AIDS victims who, for whatever reason, don't value life can easily create unreasonable fear and hostility toward other AIDS patients. The others don't deserve this backlash, and to prevent it authorities have to react firmly to the crimes of a few.

The Oregonian
Portland, OR, July 2, 1987

The Reagan administration's decision to rule out condom distribution programs for federal prisoners is both premature and unsound.

The government began AIDS testing June 15 of incoming and outgoing inmates — approximately 4,600 per month — at the 47 federal prisons. Initial conclusions will be drawn after two months, with new tests every six months.

Robert Brutsche, medical director of the Federal Bureau of Prisons and head of the testing program, expects tests to show AIDS is no more rampant in prisons than in the general population. He rejected condom distribution as "two-faced" since prison regulations prohibit homosexual sex.

This is unrealistic because uncondoned homosexual activity and intravenous drug use by prisoners are difficult to stop. It is also premature because there is no reliable information yet about the extent and spread of AIDS in prisons.

Condom distribution programs in New York city jails and Vermont prisons began this spring. Until these trial programs yield information, no credible strategy should be excluded.

Brutsche's desire to avoid abetting prohibited behavior is understandable, and pinpoints a major failing of prison system control. Until that is addressed, though, condom distribution should not be ruled out if studies show homosexual sex spreads AIDS in prisons and condom distribution minimizes this.

The public, joined daily by discharged inmates and faced with paying for escalating prison medical expenses, deserves realistic, undivided commitment to cost-effective protection of public health. Brutsche should reconsider. It is not two-faced to oppose the spread of AIDS more than the spread of condoms.

The News and Courier
Charleston, SC, June 22, 1987

President Reagan's call for more testing — voluntary, routine and mandatory — for the Acquired Immune Deficiency Syndrome virus gave experts plenty to think and to talk about recently during the Third International Conference on AIDS held in Washington. And some of the hypothetical questions that have been asked by them are difficult indeed.

What, for instance, do we do about political refugees who test positive for the virus? Should they be sent back to the countries from which they escaped? What will happen to AIDS-infected illegal aliens (those who have been here since 1982) who apply for legal status under the new immigration law? Should they be shipped out even though they probably contracted the virus while living in this country?

Should prisoners who test positive be segregated from the rest of the prison population? If so, where will they be housed and how much would special accommodations cost? Should prisoners who have the virus be granted parole?

The questions are difficult. The response should be tough. Would-be immigrants and prisoners who have the AIDS virus pose a threat to healthy Americans, and the government's first responsibility is obvious.

If a political refugee is found to have the AIDS virus, he should be denied entry into this country. Illegal aliens who have the virus should be sent back from where they came or to another country that would accept them.

Prisoners with AIDS should be isolated from the general population, and, of course, the government would have to pay the bill. If those who have the virus are allowed to remain in the general prison population, they may infect other prisoners and the cost for caring for them would be even more. Prisoners with the virus should not be released on parole because they are clearly a threat to society.

However, there should be room for exceptions, depending on the individual circumstances. If a political refugee, for instance, was infected through a blood transfusion, and if the authorities determine that he is responsible enough to seek out counseling and treatment so as to avoid spreading the disease, an exception could be made.

The overriding truth in all of this, of course, is that few refugees and other immigrants, or even prisoners, would test positive anyway.

THE SUN
Batimore, MD, July 6, 1987

The Justice Department's misguided instincts on controlling the AIDS epidemic rose to new heights recently as it unveiled the specifics of its mandatory AIDS testing plan in the federal prisons. The department rejected entirely the possibility of providing inmates at its 47 federal prisons with condoms — arguing that because homosexual sex was against prison regulations, condom distribution would constitute an implicit sanction of homosexuality.

While Reagan officials are loath to recognize homosexual activity, they are going great guns on the program to identify the infected — a tacit, albeit clear, recognition of homosexuality in its institutions. As of June 15, all prisoners entering and leaving federal penitentiaries were to be tested until Aug. 13, when the results will be made public. Thereafter, the administration says it may discontinue testing new prisoners and instead test prisoners every six months. The admission that sexual activity does occur in prisons and the unwillingness to provide these men with the available protection from disease is shameful. Instead, the administration may use the test results to try to rationalize and muster support for its newest effort — to isolate infected prisoners.

This approach contradicts recommendations from the Centers for Disease Control and the American Medical Association. It makes no sense. An infected prisoner who is sexually active already has infected others. Isolating him is not going to stop the spread of the disease within the institution. Moreover, once infected persons are identified, what will be done with them? Where will the department house them? Will it begin lumping together prisoners on the basis of their medical status rather than the severity of their offenses?

The department's mandatory testing program is off to a misguided start. The Surgeon General repeatedly has stressed the need for wider access to condoms in the general population. Those convicted of crimes deserve no less.

LEXINGTON HERALD-LEADER
Lexington, KY, July 2, 1987

The Reagan administration has turned thumbs down on a proposal to provide condoms to federal prison inmates to curb the spread of AIDS. Instead, the administration may consider separate prisons for victims of the disease.

Why? Because handing out condoms would be inconsistent with regulations forbidding homosexual acts.

This is a ludicrous assertion.

Curbing the spread of AIDS is a cheaper, safer program than grouping together prisoners of different security needs on nothing more than AIDS virus exposure.

Like it or not, homosexuality is a fact of life in prisons. Distributing condoms won't stop the spread of this deadly disease in prisons, but the practice could help slow the spread. That's more important than clinging to regulations that are far from reality.

The Atlanta Journal
THE ATLANTA CONSTITUTION
Atlanta, GA, June 20, 1987

The mandatory testing of prisoners, prospective immigrants and illegal aliens for the AIDS virus, though sound in principle, has not been as well thought out as Attorney General Edwin Meese would us like to believe. His plan leaves several serious questions unanswered.

For example: What would become of illegal aliens, applying for amnesty, who test positive? They could be denied legal status, but they couldn't be deported on the basis of test data; by law, all information obtained in connection with an application for amnesty is confidential.

What of the 87,000 who have already applied for legal status under the new immigration law and had medical examinations before the AIDS blood test was required? Will they now have to be re-examined?

What of political refugees found to be infected with AIDS? Would they be sent back to the countries they left?

Meese also fails to consider the impact of his decision to notify probation officials about AIDS-positive prisoners about to be released. Their medical conditions might be appropriate factors in deciding whether or not to release them and what jobs they could hold, he said. But where would they be cared for, if not in prison? At whose expense?

And if prisoners who have served their time could be detained, what is to prevent the government from moving to quarantine law-abiding citizens?

These are difficult questions, deserving more than the cursory notice they have received so far from the administration, blithely racing to implement its new rules.

Unless special provisions or exceptions are made for those who fall between the cracks of Meese's dragnet, the government would be relegating them to a permanent underclass — carrying a lethal infection but unable to work or obtain health or housing assistance legally. This can't be what the government has in mind.

THE ATLANTA CONSTITUTION
Atlanta, GA, July 2, 1987

The administration has finally decided what to do about the spread of AIDS among federal prisoners: It will look the other way.

It will not provide condoms to inmates, calling the idea "inconsistent" with prison regulations banning homosexual activity. Which is tantamount to removing the bars, because nobody's supposed to escape.

There is talk of separate prisons for AIDS victims, but that would create staffing problems, force the grouping of all classes of prisoners and deprive uninfected inmates in the general prison population of protection against inmates not yet diagnosed.

State prison officials are more realistic and more concerned about checking the spread of AIDS wherever possible. Recognizing there is no way, short of isolating every prisoner for the duration of his incarceration, to prevent homosexual activity altogether, Vermont and New York now provide condoms to inmates who request them. Other states are expected to follow suit.

So should the administration, dangerously wrong in its initial decision to leave the majority of federal prisoners at risk.

Far more susceptible than law-abiding citizens to diseases transmitted primarily through homosexual sex, they must be protected during their incarceration — to keep offender rehabilitation from becoming a death sentence and to protect the rest of the population after their release

THE DAILY OKLAHOMAN
Oklahoma City, OK, September 19, 1987

FEAR of the unknown is adding to the AIDS crisis.

That is pointed up by the corrections officer at the Conner Correctional Center in Hominy refusing to go on duty without knowing which specific inmate under his supervision had tested positively for AIDS antibodies.

In another instance, a prison employee had personal contact with an inmate in an emergency medical situation involving bleeding. The employee got blood from the inmate on his hand and didn't know until afterward that the inmate had tested positively for AIDS antibodies.

Corrections department officials wisely clarified their policy, assuring staff members they will be notified in advance when they are to have contact or might have contact with inmates with AIDS or AIDS antibodies. Some inmates have tested positive for the antibodies but officials said no inmate is known to actually have the syndrome inself.

At least, there is less fear in knowing than in not knowing. More care can be taken to avoid exposure.

Knowledge is an important weapon in the battle against AIDS and in coping with the myriad of problems created by the crisis. With that in mind, the creation of a special AIDS study committee by Oklahoma Senate chief Rodger Randle and House Speaker Jim Barker can be beneficial.

But the scope of the AIDS problem is so complex and far-reaching — encompassing moral and ethical issues as well as the scientific and medical aspects — the state legislative committee will be wise to rely heavily on the resources and findings of President Reagan's AIDS commission now studying the dilemma.

The Des Moines Register
Des Moines, IA, August 24, 1987

Homosexual acts between inmates are a fact of life in prisons, and now that AIDS has become an issue, prison officials must decide how far they must go to protect prisoners from the disease.

Iowa prison officials have decided to stand by their policy of prohibiting sex between prisoners, which means there will be no distribution of condoms, as some groups have urged, and condoms will still be contraband.

The officials are not naive. They concede that, despite their "total abstinence" policy and rigorous security systems, homosexual activities occur. They see the no-condoms policy as a matter of consistency: Saying sex between prisoners is forbidden while handing out condoms is a contradiction that could damage discipline.

This reasoning explains why the prisons don't issue clean hypodermic needles to protect drug-abusing inmates from AIDS. The logic is hard to fault.

To those who may think it heartless to deprive inmates of protection from a deadly disease, Deputy Corrections Director Paul Grossheim says that since both practices are illegal and contrary to policy, prison officials will condone neither by providing equipment.

The AIDS-in-prison question comes down to how far the state must go to protect prisoners from themselves. As a practical matter, there are so few Iowa prison inmates with documented cases of AIDS — only seven incoming inmates have tested positive in nearly two years — that it isn't worth contradicting the policy of not condoning sex between prisoners.

At the same time, corrections officials would be wise to institute a hard-hitting AIDS educational program, so that no prisoner can say he or she didn't know the consequences of engaging in sex.

And it goes without saying that the prison system has a duty to protect every inmate from homosexual rape, especially now that AIDS has entered the equation.

The Hutchinson News

Hutchinson, KS, July 2, 1987

An AIDS victim in Los Angeles has admitted that he was "so hard up for money" that he sold infected blood 23 times.

"I know AIDS can kill," the 29-year-old former male prostitute said as he was being booked on four counts of attempted murder and six other felonies. He is thought to be the first AIDS victim to be charged for knowingly selling or donating infected blood.

If he is convicted, the sentence will be irrelevant.

But that should not lessen the need for the indictment or the judgment that may follow. Victims must be accountable for their actions, just as non-victims must be accountable.

THE INDIANAPOLIS STAR

Indianapolis, IN, July 1, 1987

Somewhere in Los Angeles, a nightmare will become real.

Someone in the City of Angels will receive a blood transfusion, contract AIDS and die because a male prostitute knowingly sold his AIDS-tainted blood.

Joseph Edward Markowski explained to police why he sold blood: "I know that AIDS can kill. But I was so hard up for money I didn't give a damn." Presumably, Markowski offered the same reason for his decision to continue selling sex after he received his AIDS diagnosis.

Los Angeles city officials are attempting to give Markowski an after-the-fact lesson in social responsibility by prosecuting him on 10 criminal counts, including attempted murder. And they are trying to control the damage Markowski has done by tracing his blood donations and tracking down his sex partners.

Most likely, however, officials won't be able to find every pint and person Markowski infected, and tragedy will follow.

That's why it's important that other cities follow Los Angeles' example and vigorously prosecute those who knowingly infect someone else with AIDS. Punishing Joseph Markowski probably won't save the persons he has imperiled, but it might protect many others by discouraging AIDS victims from following Markowski's example.

And that might stop a few more nightmares from becoming real.

Rockford Register Star

Rockford, IL, July 9, 1987

What we don't know about AIDS, including how to kill off its epidemic, is gigantic. But the California legal case now developing tells us what we do know about AIDS, that it kills.

District Attorney Ira Reiner has charged a Los Angeles man believed to be a male prostitute with the following: attempted murder, assault with intent to do great bodily injury and attempted poisoning.

The defendant, Joseph Edward Markowski, 29, is being held under $1 million bond. What he is accused of doing, the act that triggered 10 charges in all, was to sell his blood to a Los Angeles plasma center knowing he had AIDS-contaminated blood.

Reiner said the defendant acknowledged he could be spreading acquired immune deficiency syndrome (the AIDS virus disarms the body's mechanism for resisting disease) but "didn't give a damn" because he needed the money.

The California charge is unprecedented in the annals of AIDS — and may be difficult to prove. For one thing, presence of the virus does not automatically produce the disease. Also, the plasma center involved screens its plasma to detect whether it contains AIDS. The concern, however, that prosecutor Reiner articulates is one heard everywhere: AIDS virus transmission can be the first step toward a resultant death. It will rest with the litigants to prove that murder is attempted when someone admits the virus into the blood market.

THE LINCOLN STAR

Lincoln, NE, August 14, 1987

The charge is ludicrous.

The Douglas County attorney admitted he considered filing an attempted murder charge against a man who tested positive to exposure to the AIDS virus who spat on a crime lab tech in the Omaha jail.

Attempted murder? Was the technician in danger of drowning? It would be as likely that as getting AIDS from spittle.

Law officers incur a range of anti-social behaviors in the course of their work. As disgusting as it is to be spit on, it's a leap of imagination to believe it's analogous to being assaulted with knife or gun.

Educating emergency personnel about AIDS is a more reasonable response than enacting specific laws to deal with so-called AIDS crimes, as Douglas County Attorney Ron Staskiewicz has proposed.

Such cases are red herrings. They'll make bad laws.

Nebraska has laws against assault and even specific laws protecting police that are applicable to situations in which an individual is trying to cause bodily harm to another.

However, Staskiewicz may be on the right track with his call for a task force to create AIDS guidelines for the state's law enforcement agencies. The task force must seek information from reputable health authorities, such as the state Health Department or the Centers for Disease Control, and from the homosexual community, which has been in the forefront in AIDS education.

Much less would merely confirm law enforcement's own phobias, enacting them into policy that would not greatly protect the officers nor do much to improve the general public's awareness of AIDS.

If current projections are correct, AIDS will drastically alter our society and will require special responses. But as a society we are being derailed from the real AIDS issues by fear and ignorance.

A much more important set of questions concern how America, community by community, will address the medical, financial and psychological needs of people with AIDS. Will we provide nursing care? Will livable, affordable housing be available? Will we shun and ostracize our neighbors? Will we force the sick into poverty? Will we allow fear or reason to dictate public policy? Will we extend or withdraw friendship and spiritual support in their times of need?

Answering these questions is crucial to how we survive this disease. We haven't time to spend with our noses buried in law books, or lobbying the Legislature, because we want to prosecute an AIDS patient for spitting. We're so busy chopping down one tree, we don't notice the threat to the forest.

Los Angeles Times

Los Angeles, CA, July 6, 1987

Joseph Markowski is a 29-year-old drifter with AIDS who is so emotionally unstable that the authorities have tried five times in the last five months to have him confined in a mental hospital. But under the laws he could not be held against his will, and each time he was released and left to roam the streets.

Destitute, he twice sold his contaminated blood to private blood banks and engaged in prostitution despite his disease. As a result, he now stands charged with four counts of attempted murder— a charge brought by Dist. Atty. Ira Reiner, who is trying to stretch the law beyond what it was intended to cover.

No one ever got the blood that Markowski sold, and the chances are extremely small that anyone ever would have. All donated blood is routinely screened for the AIDS virus before it is transfused into another person. Nor is there evidence that the man with whom Markowski had sexual relations picked up the AIDS virus in the process.

What's more, attempted murder requires malice. There must have been an intent to kill, which appears to be missing in this case. Markowski has reportedly told investigators that he "didn't give a damn" what happened to anyone else, but that statement falls short of intent to kill, especially given Markowski's history of mental instability.

Markowski's conduct was both dangerous and reprehensible. But there are adequate laws on the books to cover such situations. In this case attempted murder does not appear to be one of them.

Roanoke Times & World-News

Roanoke, VA, July 3, 1987

JOSEPH Edward Markowski is a miserable person by any measure of the human condition. He is a homosexual, and therefore an outcast in the eyes of good portion of the population. He is a male prostitute, which places him in the seamier ranks of the gay population. He has AIDS, which means that, unless a cure is found soon, he won't live much longer.

And now he's charged with attempted murder.

The deadly assault weapon is Markowski's own blood. Los Angeles police brought that charge against him after he sold his blood, knowing that it carried the AIDS virus. District Attorney Ira Reiner quoted Markowski as saying: "I know that AIDS can kill. But I was so hard up for money I didn't give a damn."

So Markowski was willing to spread his misery around — not only among his homosexual sex partners but to any innocent medical patient who might be unfortunate enough to use his contaminated blood.

Reiner said the attempted murder charge can be made to stick if he can prove that Markowski intended to kill someone. The DA thinks the accused's own statements will support the charge.

That raises some interesting points. Reiner can spread his affliction in other ways besides giving blood. He can spread it through sexual relations. He can spread it by injecting drugs into his veins and sharing the needle with someone else.

Anyone who knows he has AIDS and engages in sexual activity is aware that he may be communicating death to his partner. Anyone who knows he has AIDS and shares a needle with someone else knows that he may be passing on something even deadlier than the drug.

Should AIDS victims, then, be subject to murder or attempted murder charges if they engage in any of these activities?

Reiner seems to be stretching the definition of murder somewhat to get his conviction. Yet there should be some legal sanction against anyone's knowingly passing on a deadly disease, whether by selling blood or by other voluntary actions.

In the case of AIDS victims, the courts may have problems finding an appropriate penalty. If a person has AIDS, he is already effectively under a death sentence. Should laws provide that sexually active AIDS carriers be locked up for the rest of their lives to protect the public? Or should we leave it to their potential sex partners to take the necessary precautions?

In the case of blood sellers, the public is particularly at risk. Dr. James Mosley of the University of California School of Medicine heads a federally funded study of transfusion safety. He says the donor system has excellent safeguards for blood, plasma and most products but there's a remote chance the AIDS virus might survive processing of the anti-clotting factor concentrate.

Another expert on blood for transfusions said it is unlikely the virus-infected blood would escape detection.

"It should have been picked up," said Dr. Carl P. Treling, a pathologist at Hollywood Presbyterian Medical Center, which operates a blood bank.

There's a *remote chance* the virus might survive . . . It's *unlikely* that the virus-infected blood would go undetected . . . . It *should* have been picked up . . .

None of these assurances sounds completely reassuring. Until California finds out exactly what happened to Markowski's blood, no one in the LA area can feel completely confident in accepting a transfusion or using blood products for other medical purposes.

We may not have enough jail cells to hold all the AIDS carriers who continue to engage in sex. But at least their sexual partners know the practices that place them at high risk. They have a choice, and they also have measures to protect themselves.

But the recipient of blood may be someone whose illness or injuries leave little choice but to accept a transfusion. Such persons should be protected from those who would pass along death to the unwary just because they're hard up for money.

While medical science is struggling to find a cure for AIDS, it would be nice if it could come up with a safe, synthetic substitute for human blood for transfusions. Great progress has been made in assuring the safety of blood for transfusion, particularly blood collected by the American Red Cross. But accidents do happen. The wrong blood type can be used. Occasional cases of hepatitis are traceable to transfusions. And several people contracted AIDS through transfusions before tighter safeguards were inaugurated.

In many cases, surgery can be performed without blood. Safe blood substitutes are available in other instances. And techniques have been devised for storing the patient's own blood.

We're told that the incidence of AIDS is likely to grow dramatically in the next few years. We need to protect ourselves in every feasible way. So long as human blood is transfused into medical patients, we run a chance — remote or not — that the virus will find its way into an innocent body. Rigorous safeguards at the point of donation and at the place of processing will reduce the risk. But we would be better off if we didn't have to use blood in the first place.

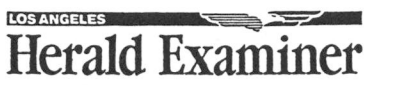

Herald Examiner

Los Angeles, CA, July 1, 1987

The headline's a grabber, but like L.A. District Attorney Ira Reiner's trumpeted "attempted murder" charges against AIDS patient Joseph Markowski, it distorts the issue.

Reiner is right, of course, to take seriously the threat Markowski posed to the community. The 29-year-old drifter, who allegedly sold his contaminated blood and prostituted himself, knew that he had AIDS and that he could be endangering the lives of others. If he's found guilty, he should be locked up.

But if he's so obviously dangerous, how did he manage to go undetected for so long? Why was he prematurely released last week from mental health observation, where he was sent after lunging wildly at a bank guard and screaming "Kill me! Kill me!"?

A successful prosecution will keep Markowski contained. But don't bet that it will do much to stop the spread of AIDS. No amount of punitive actions, like the battery of bills Sen. John Doolittle, R-Roseville, is trying to force through the Legislature, will prevent deranged or simply evil people from wantonly threatening the lives of innocent bystanders.

But that threat has been overblown by the kind of attention the Markowski story generated. In the six years since we've known about this disease, there have been but a handful of reported incidents of AIDS patients who knowingly attempted to pass on the virus — out of 37,870 AIDS cases. That's a remarkably low ratio.

And it suggests that the great majority of people who have AIDS, when educated and counseled properly, won't spread it. Unfortunately, education and counseling continue to be poorly funded, both on the state and federal level.

In the face of such a seemingly overwhelming danger like the AIDS epidemic, citizens might be heartened by the DA's busting the Markowskis of this world. But battling this disease effectively will require more work.

California could reinforce its own efforts by adopting San Francisco Assemblyman Art Agnos' AB87, which would set up an AIDS Commission to coordinate the state fight. It's a less dramatic approach, certainly, but a lot more sensible one.

All in Military to Be Tested

The Defense Department October 25, 1985 issued guidelines for the testing of all 2.1 million military personnel for signs of AIDS. The announcement was the first official acknowledgment of the plan, which would rely on a recently developed blood test. The action was easily the most dramatic taken by any government body to defend against the disease. As reasons, officials listed the need for rapid deployment anywhere, without concern for soldiers' health, the use of vaccinations that could kill an AIDS sufferer, and the need for soldiers to supply blood transfusions. Finally, some officials said the military did not want the costly burden of caring for the victims of the disease.

The first indication of the plan had been the Defense Department's announcement August 30, 1985 that it would screen recruits. Those found to have been exposed to the AIDS virus would be turned down. Under the Oct. 25 guidelines, exposed personnel already in the military would not be discharged. But they would undergo yearly retesting and be barred from overseas deployment. Those actually suffering from the disease would be granted honorable discharges under medical conditions. The Defense Department said Oct. 28 that it would automatically discharge persons who, during screening for AIDS, admitted to drug use or homosexuality. This reversed a statement to the contrary made three days earlier. Personnel would twice undergo a test called the enzyme-linked immunosorbent assay (ELISA). Those who registered signs of AIDS would then be tested by the so-called Western blot method, a more thorough and expensive process.

The Wichita
Eagle-Beacon

Wichita, KS, October 25, 1985

WORD that the Defense Department has decided to test 2.1 million current U.S. military personnel, as well as new recruits, for AIDS is sure to inspire controversy. Not only will that be a task of monumental logistical scope, but some are sure to see the AIDS testing as a violation of privacy rights and a military crusade against homosexuals.

But Defense is right to proceed with the AIDS testing, despite the difficulties it poses. As the principal guarantors of the national security, the armed forces can ill afford epidemics of any nature. Given the variety of ways with which AIDS can be spread and the close quarters in which some military personnel serve, it's directly in the interest of national security that Defense discover potential AIDS victims and remove them from the ranks.

To their credit, Defense medical officials seem determined not to succumb to the atmosphere of hysteria that now surrounds AIDS. For example, the first of two tests Defense reportedly will use in preliminary screening for the AIDS virus, the ELISA blood test, isn't intended as a diagnostic tool, and isn't 100 percent accurate. Defense officials seem to understand that, and plan to have those who repeatedly fail take a second, more reliable, test. Only then, officials say, would medical decisions that could affect the careers of the servicemen and women in question be made.

As Defense's AIDS testing program gets under way, Congress should monitor it closely. It's important that suspected victims aren't arbitrarily deemed homosexuals and hounded out of the service, and that the AIDS stigma doesn't follow suspected victims into civilian life. What seems a legitimate step to protect the men and women charged with defending the nation shouldn't be allowed to degenerate into a witchhunt.

ST. LOUIS POST-DISPATCH

St. Louis, MO, October 31, 1985

The Defense Department wants to test all military personnel for AIDS, offering honorable discharges to those with the disease while restricting the assignments of others who are merely shown to have been exposed to AIDS antibodies. The Pentagon has a good case for needing to be fully informed of the medical condition of the men and women it relies on to protect the nation's security. Those stationed overseas — or who might be sent there in an emergency — must be both healthy and able to give uninfected blood to their wounded comrades.

While noncombatant personnel who are AIDS carriers may be a less immediate threat to the efficient functioning of the armed forces, the separation between fighting men and women and those serving in a support capacity is not neat or simple. Soldiers, sailors and airmen brought back to the U.S. for medical treatment may need blood from those stationed at home, and are routinely in close contact with their comrades in a variety of other circumstances that may facilitate transmission of the disease. Thus, if combat personnel are to be tested, all who serve in uniform should be tested as well.

But there are serious problems with the Pentagon's program. If the military is to learn the maximum amount about the transmission of the disease — not only for its own purposes but for the benefit of medical science as well — it must receive candid information from those tested about how they contracted AIDS antibodies or the disease itself. Such candor may involve the admission by an individual of drug use or homosexuality. Yet the current Pentagon plan is to discharge — honorably or otherwise, depending on the circumstances — all who reveal they have engaged in either practice.

This would defeat the very purpose of learning more about the disease because it would encourage military personnel to lie about their past activities either to protect their careers or, in some instances, to avoid dishonorable discharge, which usually results in the loss of veterans benefits. Secretary Weinberger at first considered confidential interviews but then rejected them. He should reverse his decision and restore them to the program. It is manifestly more important to track accurately the pattern of the transmission of AIDS than to root out all homosexuals from the military.

The other troublesome problem associated with the Pentagon's testing program is the encouragement it may provide to other institutions to begin their own testing programs. These could easily result in firing (or refusing to hire) all AIDS-exposed individuals in the private sector. This would be grossly unfair, considering that of the nearly 1 million people presently identified as carrying AIDS antibodies, only 14,000 have actually come down with the disease. The Pentagon's testing program shouldn't be allowed to determine how the rest of society treats the problem. The nation needs a comprehensive policy on the handling of AIDS-exposed individuals now.

The Courier-Journal
Louisville, KY, October 26, 1985

IF, as one Washington lawyer suggested, the military's motivation for testing personnel for AIDS were merely to "ferret out homosexuals," then defending the decision to proceed with those tests would be difficult. But however one feels about the rights of homosexuals, or the military's policy of expelling personnel who are proven to be homosexuals, one must recognize that there are valid reasons for testing the 2.5 million men and women who serve in the Army, Navy, Marines, Air Force and Coast Guard.

One reason is perceptual. To keep up enlistments, military officials need to assure recruits that barracks life doesn't include exposure to AIDS. Of course AIDS isn't transmitted by simply sharing barracks with a victim of the disease. But as a recent *New York Times*/CBS News poll indicated, Americans are so uninformed about AIDS that 27 percent of them believe it can be spread by toilet seats.

Even if soldiers needn't be protected from toilet seats, they could benefit from other sorts of protection. AIDS is transmitted through blood, and in a combat or terrorist situation all military personnel are viewed as "walking blood banks." If a fallen soldier received contaminated blood from a comrade, then what was meant to be a lifesaving transfusion could turn out to be life-threatening.

Further, before military personnel are sent overseas, they typically receive vaccinations, which contain live virus. Even a small amount of virus can run rampant in the system of a person who has AIDS, since the disease wipes out the body's immune system. For that reason, a person with AIDS exposes himself to still another kind of risk if shipped abroad: Exotic places harbor exotic diseases, and the AIDS victim will be especially vulnerable to them.

The armed services already routinely test personnel for venereal disease. But critics believe AIDS testing is different. The fear in the gay community, of course, is that the military, which has made no secret of its desire to rid itself of homosexuals, will use AIDS test results to further that purpose. But that would be a mistake, as the military knows, because homosexuals are not the only members of the armed services at risk of contracting AIDS.

Last month, a researcher at Harvard told a Senate subcommittee about "accumulating evidence" that prostitutes were spreading AIDS among their customers. That evidence includes Army findings that five percent of a group of soldiers seeking treatment at a venereal disease clinic in Berlin had been exposed to AIDS.

Military officials vow that those found to have the AIDS virus in their blood will not be expelled from the armed forces. Rather, those who have been exposed but show no signs of the disease may have their duties and assignments limited; those who actually have AIDS will be treated. "Nobody," said the official who announced the decision to begin the testing program, "would be forced to leave the service."

Still, curbs on one's duties amount to placing a limit on one's career. And, as gay rights activists observe, this will happen more often to homosexual and bisexual men, since they constitute 72 percent of those who have contracted AIDS so far. That is unfortunate, but it can hardly be called discriminatory. Heterosexuals who are unlucky enough to contract the virus will be treated in the same way.

Pittsburgh Post-Gazette
Pittsburgh, PA, October 23, 1985

With its plans for screening military personnel for AIDS, the U.S. Defense Department appears to be recognizing — and preparing to deal with — the special problems that Acquired Immune Deficiency Syndrome poses for the armed forces.

Obviously, AIDS is no more lethal for soldiers and sailors than for anyone else. Yet the military has a special — and legitimate — concern about the presence and transmission of any communicable disease in its ranks, even in peacetime. (AIDS is not an extreme problem for the military. Only about 100 cases have been reported so far.)

The military is not known for an excess of delicacy where personal privacy is concerned, but the architects of the AIDS screening program seem to recognize the importance of both privacy and accuracy.

Under the plan now being discussed, all military personnel will undergo initial screening — the so-called ELISA test — for antibodies to the virus associated with AIDS. To avoid erroneous conclusions at this early stage, those who test positively twice will be given more refined screening by the so-called Western blot test that determines the presence of the AIDS virus with a high degree of probability. The results of that test will then be used to indicate the need for extensive clinical examination for definitive signs of failure in the person's immunological system.

To their credit, the services intend to follow the guidelines of the Centers for Disease Control in dealing with the spread of AIDS. Those guidelines put emphasis squarely on medical criteria and, in a military context, ought to exclude the possibility of panicky responses.

Unless the soldier being screened chooses to make a public disclosure, the result of all stages of testing for AIDS would not be known by anyone other than the soldier and the medical officials who are conducting the tests. Awareness of an individual's illness may be difficult to confine, however, if the disease obviously manifests itself. In that circumstance, a person would be processed for a medical — and honorable — discharge — to receive needed medical care at a Veterans Administration hospital. In that event, AIDS would not be specified as the reason for the discharge on an individual's service record.

A more delicate issue presents itself when the Western blot test determines a high probability of the presence of AIDS virus in the blood of an individual who does not exhibit other symptoms of the disease. Fortunately, the services appear inclined to recognize that individuals in the military services — like their counterparts in civilian life — are capable of continuing normal activities.

Care must be taken, however, to monitor for signs that the disease has begun to undermine the person's health. And for persons in that gray zone of exposure before AIDS has begun to injure the individual, the military should be especially scrupulous in following the Centers for Disease Control guidelines.

Except in very special circumstances, such as in combat-ready brigades where one soldier might be expected to donate blood for a comrade, there appear to be no sound medical reasons for reassignment. The Secretary of Defense, in his final implementation of this policy, should instruct the services to allow an individual to continue on active duty until AIDS actually has begun to compromise his health.

Mandatory AIDS Testing Opposed By CDC Forum

Federal health officials concerned about halting the spread of AIDS in the U.S. said February 3, 1987 that they were considering expanding use of the AIDS blood test to all patients admitted to hospitals, women seeking prenatal care and couples applying for marriage licenses. The test was currently required only of blood donors, active-duty military personnel and recruits and State Department Foreign Service officers.

The proposal was prompted by the continuing spread of AIDS and the threat it posed to unborn children, according to Dr. Walter Dowdle, deputy director for AIDS programs at the national Centers for Disease Control in Atlanta. "We need to continue to search for any possible way to affect the course of this epidemic," said Dowdle. "We are trying to explore ways to use the test for prevention." According to Dowdle, children would be the intended beneficiary of premarital and prenatal testing to detect exposure to the AIDS virus. He said it would be up to prospective parents to decide whether to bear children and, if a pregnant woman tested positive, it would be up to her to decide whether to have an abortion. He also said the CDC was not proposing that people who showed signs of infection be denied marriage licenses. Dowdle stressed that officials were considering the proposal as a way of sparking wide debate on measures public health officials might take to control the fatal disease. "This is a consensus building and multi-stop process," he said. "It is not our intention to have a federal statute."

Participants in a federally sponsored forum in Atlanta on the control of AIDS reached broad agreement February 25, 1987 on the need for wider use of the blood test to detect exposure to the AIDS virus. However, they came out squarely against a Feb. 3 proposal by the CDC to expand mandatory blood testing for AIDS in the U.S. to a variety of groups. The Atlanta forum had been convened Feb. 24 by the CDC largely to give public health officials and other interested parties an opportunity to debate the proposal. The two-day forum, which had originally been designed to accommodate a small number of participants, was attended by hundreds. Participants included state and local health officials, civil libertarians and gay-rights activists. Mandatory testing for the AIDS antibody was opposed almost unanimously.

The conferees, however, recommended offering voluntary testing to three groups for which mandatory testing had been proposed, namely people being treated for sexually transmitted diseases, those being treated for intravenous drug use or their sexual partners, and, in some circumstances, pregnant women. On the other hand, the conferees came out against expanding even routine use of the AIDS blood test to two other groups, namely hospital patients and applicants for marriage licenses. It was argued that the virus was still not widespread enough to justify the financial cost of routinely testing large groups that were, in essence, drawn almost at random from the general population.

During the conference, it was repeatedly stressed that expanded use of the AIDS antibody test would have to be accompanied by adequate funds for counseling and by tight controls to keep medical records confidential. The absence of federal legislation to prevent discrimination against people found to be infected with the AIDS virus was seen as a major problem. It was pointed out that such discrimination only obstructed efforts to fight the disease by driving infected people underground.

The conference ended on a stormy note as members of a militant New York City-based gay activist group, called the Lavender Hill Mob, shouted "15,000 of us are dead!" and "You've murdered us all!" at panelists. They and other militants charged that federal health officials had not been sufficiently concerned about AIDS before it came to be viewed as a threat to heterosexuals. Representatives of mainstream gay groups, however, applauded the conference's firm rejection of mandatory tests for AIDS and even took credit for creating the climate that led to this verdict.

THE KANSAS CITY STAR
Kansas City, MO
October 22, 1985

Some health officials are now advocating tracing the sexual partners of AIDS victims to do blood testing and counseling. The need to check the spread of the disease is obvious. Public safety, in the absence of an AIDS cure or survival rate, is so threatened it justifies pursuing a course of mandatory tracking.

This time a disease is not just a disease. AIDS has become a symbol and a cause. It frightens and it tests, and depending upon who is speaking, it is America's major public health issue or a dare line for homosexual civil rights. That makes a policy decision controversial. But by doing nothing, officials also make policy. Research indicating the disease is increasing beyond established risk groups intensifies pressure for duplicating steps already followed with venereal diseases. Other facts also make the proposed checks attractive: It is believed people can carry and transmit the AIDS virus without being sick themselves. And there is a long dormant period for the virus.

Civil liberties experts are fearful that such a practice would undermine individual rights. It would be especially bad, they say, because the highest risk populations are homosexual men and intravenous drug users already insecure in civil liberties. People identified as having the virus, symptoms or antibodies, or who could acquire them because of a relationship, could easily become targets of discrimination. The disease could become a cover for deep hostilities. Yet most cases of AIDS, however acquired, seem to be traceable back in a chain to homosexual intercourse. If the disease comes to the general population in epidemic proportions, hostility toward homosexuals could become truly deep.

It's a gloomy outlook, one no decent American wants to see materialize. Along with policy to act should be policy to protect. Certainly there's precedent. The United States has done a balancing act between public welfare and private rights since its founding, stumbling badly on occasion but for the most part combining responsible policy with compassionate behavior. There's no reason it can't happen again.

Even the cynical hope fervently, though perhaps privately, that scientists will discover a cure and prevention quickly. In the meantime, people should have as much protection as possible regardless of their sexual preferences.

The Miami Herald

Miami, FL, September 25, 1985

FEAR OF AIDS (acquired immune-deficiency syndrome) has gotten the better of Metro commissioners. They've tentatively voted to require that all food-service workers in Dade be tested for the disease. Broward commissioners ought to resist pressures on them to do the same.

The commissioners' motivation is not in question. Aware of how the AIDS panic has hurt restaurant patronage in several other cities, they properly want to calm fears and protect food-service jobs.

Inadvertently, though, the Metro commissioners may have sent the wrong signal. Medical experts say that AIDS is *not* spread by the kinds of contact that food handlers have with a restaurant's patrons or with their food. By ignoring this advice, commissioners implicitly seem to be questioning it. This may heighten the public's fears, not calm them.

What's more, commissioners ignored the very practical concerns expressed by Dade's health director, Dr. Richard Morgan. He pointed out, among other things, that the AIDS test is time-consuming and costly. The costs would be borne by Dade County, which has fiscal problems of its own, or by food-service workers, most of them low-paid. Other public-health needs — including the search for an AIDS cure — would represent a much better use of the several million dollars that Metro's AIDS test would cost.

That is especially evident when one notes the test's inability to do what is expected of it. Dr. Morgan says that testing all 80,000 of Dade's food-service workers would take a year. So even if AIDS were spread through food — which it is not — the test would be of dubious value. A food-service worker might test "clean" one day, become infected the next, continue working, and escape detection for months.

Moreover, the high worker turnover in this seasonal business means that large numbers of these costly tests would continue to be given indefinitely. Thus the costs would not necessarily diminish much after all current workers had been tested.

The AIDS-test requirement is part of a broader health-card ordinance that commissioners tentatively approved the other day. When it comes up for final approval, they should toss the proposed AIDS test into the disposal.

Chicago Tribune

Chicago, IL, April 10, 1985

Chicago Health Commissioner Dr. Lonnie Edwards is wrong to protest federal guidelines requiring that blood donors be informed if tests show that their blood contains antibodies to the virus linked to AIDS (acquired immune deficiency syndrome).

The new test for AIDS antibodies is being phased into use in the nation's blood banks, after its approval early in March by the Department of Health and Human Services. Blood found to have AIDS antibodies will be discarded. By late April, all blood banks in the Chicago area will be doing such screening.

But the antibody test is still controversial. It cannot show whether a blood donor currently has AIDS. A positive result only indicates that a person has been exposed at some time and in some way to the virus believed to cause the usually fatal disease—not that he is immune to it or that he will eventually become ill and die of it. Another problem is that the test is not totally accurate; both false negatives and false positives can occur.

Some homosexual groups oppose the use of the AIDS screening test on the grounds it could violate individual privacy or that a third party might obtain test results and use them to discriminate against donors. But the presence of AIDS virus in the nation's blood supply is becoming a serious problem. Dozens of recipients of blood or blood-based products have already died of AIDS presumably acquired from blood donors. In a few instances, these victims have passed the disease on to their spouses and young children.

The safety of the nation's lifesaving blood supply must be protected. Whatever its shortcomings, the AIDS antibody test is currently the only way possible to screen out blood donations that could be hazardous.

Some health officials fear that some persons who are told they have a positive AIDS antibody test will misunderstand the significance of the information and will be unnecessarily confused and frightened. Because there is no cure or effective treatment for AIDS, there is no point in arousing needless anxieties, they argue.

But it's ethically wrong to withhold health information from the individual it most concerns. A positive test result should be reported to the blood donor with a clear statement of its meaning and an offer of counseling or further diagnostic tests if necessary. It is unfair to those with a positive test to let them continue donating blood, unaware that it will be discarded later when the antibodies are detected.

Another argument against disclosure is that homosexuals and others in high-risk groups may sign up to donate blood just to get the results of the AIDS antibody test, thereby increasing the dangers of contaminating the blood supply.

But if people at risk of AIDS are so eager to have an antibody test that they would sign up to donate blood just to get that information, it should be made available to them outside of blood banks. Chicago health officials have considered setting up special clinics where the AIDS test can be given without a blood donation. They should do so as quickly as possible, whether or not federal money is available to help.

Medical concern that AIDS is spreading to the general population is growing. The number of victims is still doubling at least every year and some public health officials predict that new cases could total 200,000 by the end of 1988, at a cost of $10 billion to $20 billion for hospital care alone. No effective treatment or vaccine seems likely soon. But the new screening test should help protect potential victims among blood recipients—even if it means discarding some blood that may be falsely identified as hazardous. And those whose tests show AIDS antibodies have a right to know it—even if it means some needless anxiety.

SYRACUSE
HERALD-JOURNAL
Syracuse, NY
February 20, 1985

Since 1981, when doctors first recognized the deadly Acquired Immune Deficiency Syndrome (AIDS), they also have recognized that it could be spread through transfusions of infected blood or blood products. And yet, federal health officials continue to drag their feet about licensing a test for blood donors.

Last week, even as New York and other states prepared to put such a test to work, Margaret M. Heckler, U.S. secretary of health and human services, said: "Additional weeks will be required for manufacturers to provide the needed data on the operation of the test and for the Food and Drug Administration to review it."

There was no indication of how many weeks the delay would last.

Don McLearn, a spokesman for the FDA, said his agency had requested more data from the manufacturers but he also indicated that should not have resulted in the delay announced by Heckler. He said the FDA knew of certain weaknesses in the test, but added, "The test with its known limitations is better than none at all because we will still get a purer blood supply."

▽   ▽

Officials of the American Red Cross, which supplies the nation with about half its 12 million blood transfusions each year, had said last week they knew the test was not perfect, but that it was a good one.

At least 177 patients — of the 8,314 cases reported to the Centers for Disease Control in Atlanta as of early last week — are known to have come down with AIDS as a result of transfusions of blood or blood products, including 61 people with hemophilia who rely on injections of a blood substance called Factor VIII.

All indications are that as the spread of AIDS continues, the lack of a test makes accepting such transfusions a life-and-death gamble on the part of the patient. Without an approved laboratory test, blood bank officials have no way of detecting AIDS-contaminated blood. Their only alternative — which has proven reasonably effective — is to ask members of groups considered high risks to refrain from donating blood.

▽   ▽

Obviously, however, this kind of voluntary screening cannot be a substitute for clinical testing.

One of the reasons, apparently, the test has been held back is that it is not 100 percent accurate and could, in the minds of some doctors, unfairly stigmatize some people who take it. The groups most at risk for contracting AIDS are male homosexuals, intravenous drug users, recent immigrants from Haiti, hemophiliacs and, now, recipients of blood transfusions.

There is a feeling that a mistakenly positive reading of the blood test could attach a stigma to the donor . . . that he or she is a homosexual or drug user, for instance. When balanced against the lives of prospective recipients, that's a small, if unfortunate, price to pay.

A safe test that will screen out all of the infected blood, but has other deficiencies, has to be better than no test at all.

San Francisco Chronicle

San Francisco, CA, February 26, 1987

FRIGHTENING NEW estimates of the spread of the AIDS virus underscore with dramatic urgency the need for more widespread tests in the battle against the viral disease that has already killed nearly 18,000 people throughout the country.

A total of 1.5 million Americans are now believed infected with the virus that causes acquired immune deficiency syndrome, according to the federal Centers for Disease Control. That's one in every 160 people.

Nationally, it is estimated that one in every 80 males is infected, compared with one in every 1000 females. In states with a high prevalence of AIDS, such as California and New York, one in every 30 men may be infected. Counting only the men between the ages of 30 and 39 in such high-prevalence states, one in nine is believed to be carrying the virus.

THE FIGURES are projections, but officials believe further testing will render the estimates more accurate.

Expanded use of the blood test for infection with the AIDS virus would be a major weapon in the efforts to stem the epidemic. The examination should be routinely offered by such health care providers as physicians, clinics that treat people with sexually transmitted diseases, drug treatment centers and prenatal care clinics.

Not only will the tests help determine the extent of the disease, they will be useful in deterring people from spreading the disease further.

STRONG LEGISLATION is needed to ensure that test information remains confidential, avoiding possible stigmatization that could create discrimination in employment, housing, the right to enter public places, life insurance and medical insurance.

Such protection from the unauthorized use of their names would encourage people who are in risk of infection to seek out the testing for any sign of the virus.

Rocky Mountain News

Denver, CO, March 31, 1987

ONE of the most controversial bills of this legislative session receives another hearing this week, in the Senate. The bill requires doctors to report the names and addresses of people who test positive for exposure to the AIDS virus.

Although we have backed the bill, in recent days we've come to doubt whether the case for reporting names is as strong as its proponents and we have suggested. There *are* good reasons to keep a list of names, but there also are good reasons — and perhaps better ones — for not even asking for names in the first place.

Before senators follow their House colleagues and approve this bill, they should carefully weigh the arguments. Their goal must be to devise a program that results in as many high-risk people as possible seeking testing and counseling. If lawmakers believe name-reporting hobbles that goal, they should strike it from the bill and replace it with the option of anonymity.

Proponents of reporting names argue that Colorado has a respectable record compared with other states in AIDS testing, even though this state has already begun to keep a list of names. They're correct, but it's not clear these comparisons mean much.

For one thing, other Rocky Mountain states have far smaller high-risk groups — gay men, intravenous drug users, etc. — and thus their citizens have far less reason for concern.

Even comparisons with states such as California and New York are distorted by the fact that some gay groups there have opposed *any* testing. Colorado's gay community has never taken a similar stance.

What we do know about the situation here is that gay leaders insist homosexual men are avoiding the test because they don't want to give their names. We also know that a substantial percentage of people who elect to be tested provide false names. Finally, there is the testimony of several doctors that some of their high-risk patients — even a few with AIDS-like symptoms — refuse to submit to the test.

Since many people who test positive for exposure to the AIDS virus change their sexual behavior, the fact that anyone avoids the test out of reluctance to give his name should concern us all.

It's possible, of course, that the advantages of reporting names outweigh the unfortunate side effects. According to the state Health Department, name reporting assists in identifying high-risk groups, permits officials to define factors that increase the risk of contracting AIDS, helps trace former sexual partners of infected individuals, permits followup counseling, and may someday be useful in deciding who receives the first samples of antiviral medication.

As critics point out, however, several of those goals have been achieved elsewhere without recording names. Meanwhile, the department itself has revealed that it only traces sexual partners on a limited basis anyway.

All of which leaves lawmakers facing the following question: Do the remaining reasons the department provides really justify scaring an unknown number of high-risk people from the test and prompting so many others to lie?

Count us among the newly skeptical.

The Union Leader

Manchester, NH, May 17, 1987

We find no fault with mandatory AIDS testing for couples about to marry, such as the requirement in the bill that was defeated last week, so long as the public realizes that this is but a beginning, not an end, for testing and that a low "positive" response shouldn't be read to mean that the AIDS threat is not genuine.

Couples aspiring to matrimony and, presumably, monogamy are not likely to be in prime risk of this disease. Then again, science seems so baffled by the AIDS menace, and has had to revise its opinions and projections so often, who's to say that a widespread pre-marital testing program won't turn things upside down yet again?

What baffles us is both the ferocity with which Gov. Sununu has responded to critics of the testing and some of the reasoning advanced by those critics.

Gov. Sununu claims that his testing idea is just coincidental with that advanced (on the same day) by Vice President Bush, whom the governor backs for President. That claim would be more believable were Sununu's protestations of such a link a bit less vehement and his response to critics — including much of the health community — a lot less vitriolic.

Sununu does neither this cause, nor his own political future, any good with an attitude that comes across as: I'm right and the entire state, national and world health community is wrong.

Still, one wonders at the logic of some of the critics. Since the AIDS test has a high degree of false readings, or so they claim, it's unfair to upset people's lives. Instead, say the critics, let's just test prisoners and drug-users. What are they — dog food?

It is becoming clear that AIDS is a great danger to an awful lot of us. To combat it, AIDS testing will be required of us all. So what's wrong with getting the general public accustomed to that via an easily grouped class?

Omaha World-Herald

Omaha, NE, March 9, 1987

Mandatory testing programs cannot reasonably be ruled out as a means of trying to slow the spread of AIDS. Society has the responsibility to protect itself from the epidemic, which is being compared to the plagues that infested Europe in the Middle Ages, sometimes wiping out the populations of entire cities.

During a recent meeting at the Centers for Disease Control in Atlanta, a number of public health officials spoke out against mandatory screening of people applying for a marriage license, entering a hospital, receiving treatment for another sexually transmitted disease or seeking services from a family planning clinic.

Syndicated columnist Joan Beck was on the mark when she wrote that some officials seem "more concerned about protecting the civil rights of victims than safeguarding the health of those not yet infected."

The principle of the public's right to protect itself against communicable diseases is nothing new in America. It hasn't been too many years since public health officials quarantined people who had measles and mumps. Separate hospitals were maintained for victims of tuberculosis to reduce the chances of their spreading the disease. Even today, children can't go to school unless they submit proof that they have had certain shots.

Part of the reluctance of health officials to face reality on the question of AIDS is due to pressure from homosexual rights organizations that oppose mandatory testing. A coalition of homosexual rights groups, in a statement to the health officials in Atlanta, asserted that mandatory tests are "not an ethically acceptable means for attempting to reduce the transmission of infection."

Mandatory screening is not a new concept, however. Generations of marriage license applicants have been tested for syphilis — without arguing that it would be more ethical to do away with the tests and risk giving birth to a syphilitic child. More than half the states still require blood tests for couples seeking a marriage license.

If society can justify these steps to reduce the risk of venereal diseases or birth defects, surely it can accept screening programs to slow the spread of a disease for which there is no known cure.

In Haiti and parts of Africa, the primary mode of AIDS transmission is sexual relations between men and women. Because the appearance of symptoms is delayed, authorities say, it is possible that hundreds of thousands of men and women in the United States have been infected and, without knowing it, are spreading the virus to their sexual partners. Screening for AIDS carriers might not save people who are already infected, but it would give those people the opportunity to stop imposing a possible death sentence on every sexual partner.

As for homosexual rights groups that consider mandatory screening unethical, a question of hypocrisy exists. They demand more from the public in terms of research, treatment and compassion — and even recognition of their way of life as an "alternative lifestyle" — without being willing to share in society's efforts to protect itself. Such groups would be more consistent if they followed a philosophy of "no mandatory tests, no public-supported treatment."

DAYTON DAILY NEWS

Dayton, OH, June 10, 1987

There probably will come a time when people will look back and wonder why there was so much debate about whom to test for AIDS.

When the thousands who are carrying the virus today actually come down with the syndrome and are dying, the testing issue will look very different.

Even so, it's appropriate that policymakers are thinking and debating hard about mandatory tests. They need to be concerned about confidentiality for victims and the possibility of sending those who are in high-risk groups underground.

After all those things are understood, however, the discussion gets back to one fast principle: In addition to preventive programs that encourage uninfected people to avoid risky behavior, one obvious way to stop the spread of AIDS by those who carry the virus unsuspectingly is to find out who has it and counsel them about how not to pass it on.

The military was the first to implement mandatory testing, and justifiably so. Beyond its desire for healthy troops, the military doesn't want to pay for the tremendously expensive care AIDS patients require. Already the Veterans Administration is responsible for an estimated five percent of the nation's AIDS victims.

Additionally, the military is concerned about a contaminated blood supply. In combat, transfusions often take place in the field. The military needs to try to keep its ranks AIDS-free.

Prisoners are another group that should be tested. They belong to a high-risk population because of the prevalence of drug abuse among criminals. In addition, sodomy — both consensual and forced — frequently occurs in institutions. (AIDS is passed through sexual conduct or by sharing needles or any other exchange of blood or semen.) Inmates need to be told if they have a deadly and communicable affliction, and some segregation has to be practiced.

It's also appropriate for the government to test immigrants for AIDS. The law long has required immigrants to be free of contagious diseases upon entry. Again, the intent is to stop the spread of disease, not punish victims.

The Star-Ledger

Newark, NJ, August 21, 1987

Developing a national strategy to cope with an epidemic, about which really little of any substance is known, admittedly is a highly complex, difficult undertaking. Nevertheless, there is an emerging political consensus for mass testing, an approach favored by President Reagan and a growing number of state officials.

There are problems with testing on this massive scale—the sheer huge numbers involved and the medical uncertainties of test results. The Reagan administration's plan calls for testing of federal prisoners and immigrants. Mayor Edward Koch wants to test foreign visitors arriving in New York City. Other officials have proposed random testing.

Some questions are raised by these calls for tests: Where do we draw realistic parameters? And, even more important, what do they really accomplish? In a practical context, the best that can be hoped for in testing is that the results would be useful for establishing an AIDS medical profile, determining the depth of the problem, and possibly as an empirical basis for projecting its spread.

In a positive context, these would be valid reasons for selective AIDS testing. It makes sense to test newly arrived immigrants; the same is true for prisoners, segregating those who are infected. But it would be impractical to test the millions of foreign visitors arriving each year; nor is it likely they would be a significant source for spreading the dread disease.

Testing would be helpful, too, for tracing the incidence of the deadly virus. But there is no substantive medical evidence presently available that testing would serve any purpose in inhibiting or halting the spread of AIDS. It should be noted, moreover, that the whole population is not at high risk. In the United States, the disease appears to be generally confined to such high-risk groups as homosexuals, drug addicts and their sexual partners.

A more useful national strategy would be a massive educational program—outreach projects that would provide counseling and guidance for high-risk groups. In this structured context, the emphasis would be focused on the source of greatest concern in terms of inhibiting the spread of this terminal disease—counseling and aiding the victims who are carriers.

These are essential intervening official responses, a means of trying, in the best way we can, to contain this devastating medical problem until the day when medical research is finally able to come up with the thus far elusive cure.

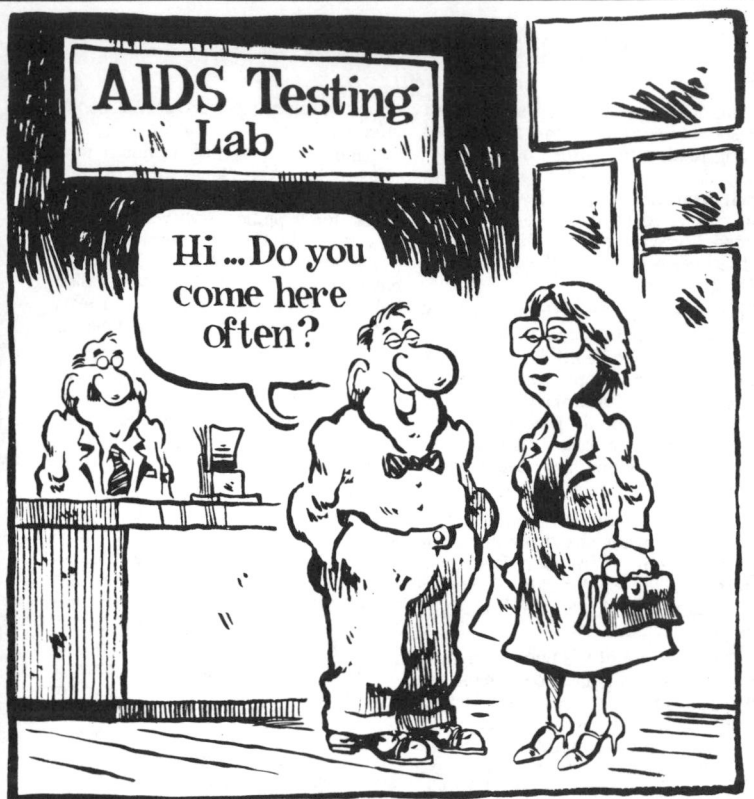

Chicago Tribune

Chicago, IL, January 25, 1987

That controversy about testing anonymous blood samples for AIDS antibodies is silly and could jeopardize an important source of information about the deadly disease and how rapidly it is spreading.

The study involves screening a sampling of blood specimens from a general cross-section of patients who are hospitalized for reasons not connected with AIDS. Normally, such blood specimens are discarded after the prescribed blood tests are completed. All identification except age, sex and race is removed from the blood samples, which are then frozen and stored; a representative group of samples is later turned over to laboratory workers for AIDS testing. Even the several hospitals taking part in the survey are not identified.

What researchers aim to find is an indication of how widespread infection with the AIDS virus has now become. Current estimates range widely from 1 to 2 million people, but both figures could be gross errors. Most data now available come from blood tests given to armed forces recruits, from blood banks and from studies of high-risk groups such as homosexual men and intravenous drug users. But these estimates aren't representative of the general population.

Critics of the new study object that the AIDS testing is being done without permission of the subjects. But they suffer no risks, inconvenience or expense. And limiting the study only to those who agree to participate would distort results and destroy its usefulness.

Another objection is that a patient's identity might be disclosed and his privacy violated. But the study's design seems to make that impossible. Labs, blood banks and venereal disease clinics all manage confidential material without problems and this program goes well beyond all of those in its safeguards.

It also troubles some opponents that when a blood sample does test positive for AIDS antibodies, there is no way to identify and notify the individual who is infected. He could remain ignorant of his AIDS status and could spread the virus to others.

But who should be tested for AIDS under what circumstances and what should be done with the information are other issues that require more public debate and education. Such problems are not involved in this particular survey. Public—and private—decision-making about AIDS requires more data about how far the virus has spread in the general population. That's why this survey needs to be done.

The Seattle Times

Seattle, WA, March 18, 1987

IN JUNE 1985 an editorial in the AMA Journal made headlines across the nation. The editorial was a call to arms against AIDS.

"Not since syphilis among the Spanish," it read, "plague among the French, tuberculosis among the Eskimos, and smallpox among the American Indians has there been a threat of such a scourge. Until a technological method of prevention and treatment can be developed, it will be necessary to contain this virus by changing the lifestyle of many people — by no means all of them homosexual men."

This week the federal government launched a nationwide information blitz to effect those lifestyle changes, with an emphasis upon monogamy and the use of condoms. But that move was overshadowed by news of another federal anti-AIDS effort — an effort that will cause widespread anxiety, but appears to be necessary.

The U.S. Public Health Service, in a bulletin to be released tomorrow, will recommend that tens of thousands of Americans who received blood transfusions — especially those who received multiple transfusions — from 1978 to April 1985 be tested for the AIDS virus.

The first date coincides with early recognition of the disease; the second with the introduction into blood banks of testing for the AIDS antibody. Disease-control officials say the nation's blood supply is "measurably safer" since the beginning of the screening program.

As for the information plan, Health and Human Services Secretary Otis Bowen says this:

"Our best hope today for controlling the AIDS epidemic lies in educating the public about the seriousness of the threat, the ways the AIDS virus is transmitted, and the practical steps each person can take to avoid acquiring it or spreading it."

Education may be the best hope today, but some observers see the recommended voluntary screening of 1978-85 blood-transfusion recipients as the harbinger of a much wider AIDS mass screening program.

Dr. Eugen Berkman, immediate past president of the American Association of Blood Banks, says that if universal screening is what federal health officials "really think we ought to do, they ought to take the bull by the horns and do it."

Testing and counseling facilities are far from adequate for such a program. This is all the more reason why thoughts such as that articulated by Berkman merit a full and prompt official response.

The Dallas Morning News

Dallas, TX, February 28, 1987

Aggressive testing programs would be one way to help control the spread of acquired immune deficiency syndrome throughout the population. But for such an effort to have a chance for success, the testing would have to be voluntary and given with a guarantee that the results would be kept strictly confidential.

Medical authorities gathered in Atlanta this week to discuss the role of testing in curbing the spread of AIDS. The issue is of paramount importance. Up to 1.5 million Americans may be carrying the virus that causes the deadly disease, but many of them probably are not aware that they have been infected.

The idea of widespread mandatory testing was discarded by most of the health officials at the conference — and for good reason. As the medical authorities concluded, any testing requirements that were too broadly applied would discourage people most at risk to the fatal disease from seeking health care.

Far preferable is the suggestion that health officials do whatever they can to encourage individuals to screen themselves by voluntarily taking the test that shows the presence of AIDS antibodies in the blood. Then, presumably, those who are found carrying the virus would act to stop its further transmission.

If voluntary testing were to work, however, there would have to be some reasonable assurance of anonymity or confidentiality. Because of the fear of discrimination, many people probably would not undergo the testing if they thought the results might be released at some point in the future.

In addition, a successful testing effort would have to include comprehensive counseling. Besides providing support to those who have been told they are carrying the germ of a terminal illness, such counseling would stress the importance of their taking steps to prevent others from becoming infected.

With about 70 percent of all AIDS cases having occurred among homosexual or bisexual men, the gay community has worked to educate and protect itself from the disease. As AIDS spreads to the general public, that same emphasis on voluntary testing needs to be adopted by others who think they are at risk.

THE PLAIN DEALER

Cleveland, OH, February 9, 1987

He. Will you marry me?
She. Only if you pass the AIDS test, dearest.

Romance, 1987. Who would have thought just five years ago that courtship would be so tainted? And who would have thought just a year ago that officials at the highest levels of government would be considering whether to require couples to address such a matter as Aquired Immune Deficiency Syndrome.

Such is the march of AIDS, and such is the struggle of science, which so far has been unable to best the bewildering, incurable disease. Last week, officials of the Centers for Disease Control (CDC) in Atlanta said they were considering recommending AIDS tests of all applicants for marriage licenses, and of everyone who is admitted to a hospital. Civil libertarians are upset by the call for mass testing, almost as much as many people are frightened by the disease itself.

Despite much that is known about AIDS, the general populace isn't dealing with the spread of the AIDS virus very well. AIDS is spread only through sexual intercourse or exchanges of blood, as through contaminated needles used by drug users. The disease cannot be spread through casual contact, in home, at school or at the workplace. Its advance can be checked relatively easily by practicing "safe sex" or by the sterilization of needles used by consumers of drugs taken intravenously. Panic and hysteria need not be part of the equation.

Yet, high risk groups—homosexuals and drug users—as well as a growing number of heterosexuals, are playing a dangerous everybody-else-but-me-game. A recently completed study of homosexual men in Cleveland found that 75% ignore "safe sex" practices. The Atlantic magazine reports in its current issue about a couple, both of whom tested positive for AIDS antibodies, who went on to conceive a child, which likely will be born with AIDS, and will die.

Meanwhile, the costs of the disease continue to rise. The average medical cost for treating an AIDS patient is nearly $150,000. Lost earnings because of the early death of the first 10,000 AIDS cases reported in the country are estimated to have totaled $4.69 billion.

With that as background, officials of the CDC have decided to convene a forum later this month to discuss countermeasures, such as the tests of marriage license applicants and hospital patients. Public health officials will be asked to suggest other approaches as well.

There's no guarantee that more widespread testing would be effective in halting the spread of the disease. And the tests are expensive. Last year, 12,427 marriage licenses were issued in Cuyahoga County. At $25 a test, that means a total cost to newlyweds of more than $1.2 million, money that could be better spent elsewhere, given the fact that so few people will test positive. Costs for hospitals also would mount, for tests in the case of hospital admissions often are inconclusive given the fact that patient illness easily can skew results. Then there's the question of discrimination against those found to test positive for the AIDS antibody. The tests are supposed to be confidential. But can officials guarantee that insurance companies, which receive patient records along with the bills, will not pass the word along to employers? At the very least, Congress will need to act by providing anti-discrimination legislation before any mass testing takes place.

But CDC officials all the same are taking the proper approach. They have concluded that it's time for a more thorough public discussion of AIDS countermeasures. Yet, they have expressed caution about acting too quickly. They deny that their goal is a federal requirement for mass testing. The Feb. 24-25 Atlanta forum may not provide many conclusive answers. But it will provide for a badly needed debate.

The Providence Journal

Providence, RI, May 30, 1987

President Reagan and his Domestic Policy Council seem to be edging in the direction of supporting mandatory AIDS tests for immigrants seeking permanent U.S. residence.

It's a sensible idea, and probably about time. The medical profession is talking about it; so are the public health agencies, lawyers and civil libertarians. Even Congress is beginning to consider the proposition.

Last week the Senate rejected such a proposal, which had been attached to a supplementary spending bill, but as Senate Minority Leader Robert Dole of Kansas points out, "We're facing an epidemic, and the president of the United States must provide moral leadership."

The political debate has begun, and is already being conducted within the Reagan administration itself. On the general subject of mandatory testing, Education Secretary William J. Bennett favors it, while Surgeon General C. Everett Koop opposes it. Dr. Koop believes that public education and the use of contraceptives are sufficient lines of defense at this time.

He is correct about their importance, but if AIDS is the potential scourge that Dr. Koop says it is, steps to prevent further introduction of the malady from abroad are hardly out of order. Health tests always were a part of immigrant processing to block contagion. Certainly, all immigrants from all countries should be treated with fairness and equity. But the first responsibility of the government is to the citizens of this country, and the United States has no obligation to admit people who are capable of spreading this dread disease, and endangering the resident population.

For those who test positive, two different tests should be administered in order to eliminate the possibility of false-positive results. The price of such prudence may be considerable — but not when compared to the introduction of the virus from foreign shores, or the potential cost of mass programs of treatment and care.

Education is vital, but testing of immigrants is a legitimate additional method to limit the number of AIDS carriers within the country. Refusing entry to those with a capacity to transmit such a disease is a valid exercise of governmental authority.

Herald Examiner
LOS ANGELES

Los Angeles, CA, May 5, 1987

O fficials at the Centers for Disease Control say their proposal to recommend wider AIDS virus testing is a means to stimulate debate. Indeed, civil libertarians and pragmatic medical authorities are facing off over the idea of testing all applicants for marriage licenses as well as everyone who is hospitalized or treated for pregnancy or venereal disease. There's a way out of this conflict, but it will require the federal government to take charge, which it has so far failed to do.

Those concerned about civil rights have reason to worry about widespread testing. The confidentiality of medical records, particularly in hospitals, is easily violated. Publicly revealing that someone has AIDS could cost that person his or her job, housing, insurance — there are pitifully few protections for those who contract the illness or test positive for it.

Nonetheless, there is a compelling medical need to find out how broad this epidemic is, and to warn those who might have AIDS or who simply show signs of the virus in their bloodstream. Widespread testing could be one tool in the effort to curb the spread of the disease.

Of course, this strategy should only be implemented if its dangers are mitigated. All those tested should be counseled. For those found to have AIDS, the current treatment must be made available. Testing shouldn't replace preventive education, which is still the only proven weapon in the fight against AIDS.

Perhaps most important, there must be a guarantee of confidentiality, similar to the rules currently in place in California. All Americans must feel secure that they won't be persecuted or devastated financially if they test positive. The best way to avoid such a travesty, and to halt the discrimination AIDS patients now face, is to enact a federal law to prohibit such bias.

In short, what's needed is a broad-based approach to the epidemic. Widespread testing could be part of such an effort, but it cannot be a substitute for it.

The Record
Hackensack, NJ, August 16, 1987

Mandatory testing to identify people exposed to the AIDS virus may sound like an efficient way to slow the spread of a terrible disease. But Congress should be wary of proposals to require that large numbers of people be tested and that positive results be passed along to public-health authorities. This pseudo-solution would cause more problems than it would cure.

Rep. William E. Dannemeyer, a Southern California flag-waver for any number of conservative causes, is leading a group of fellow Republicans on a crusade for more testing. States would be encouraged to enact laws requiring AIDS tests for anyone between the age of 15 and 49 who's admitted to a hospital; anyone receiving treatment for a venereal disease; and anyone applying for a marriage license. Labs would be required to send positive results to public-health officials. States that didn't comply would lose a portion of their federal aid.

Opinion polls show that Mr. Dannemeyer is onto a popular idea, and it's easy to see why. Everyone agrees that the spread of AIDS must be stopped. With venereal diseases like syphilis and gonorrhea, it's common public-health practice to follow a chain of sexual contacts, advising the victim's partners to seek treatment. Why not with AIDS?

For many reasons, say health experts. First, testing brides-to-be and their fiancés is simply a waste of effort; very few of these people would have been exposed to the AIDS virus. Even in the case of high-risk groups — homosexuals and intravenous drug users — the existing tests are far from conclusive. A positive reading can be false. Second, the tests are expensive (up to $100 or more) and complicated, and there's no way to administer them on a broad scale without creating a large and costly network of new testing centers. Such centers are so overloaded now that people who come in for voluntary tests at public clinics in New York must wait four weeks for results. In Los Angeles, the wait is seven weeks.

Syphilis and gonorrhea are curable. For someone exposed to the AIDS virus, there is no cure — only a warning that he or she could spread the infection. But you don't need an AIDS test to know that it's dangerous to share drug needles or engage in promiscuous sex.

Finally, there's the problem of confidentiality. AIDS still carries a terrible stigma in this society. No matter how carefully the test-result files are maintained, many AIDS carriers will legitimately worry that the information might leak out — costing them their health insurance, jobs, or even their homes. Mandatory testing would raise the level of distrust between health workers and people at risk for AIDS.

People who think they may have been exposed to the AIDS virus may indeed want to have themselves tested. But broad-scale mandatory testing would be a waste of limited resources and an assault on privacy. Instead, Congress should concentrate on research to develop a cure, on better access to health care and health insurance for AIDS victims, and on public education.

Los Angeles Times
Los Angeles, CA, February 5, 1987

President Reagan's adviser for domestic policy, Gary L. Bauer, has endorsed broader mandatory testing for AIDS and a stripping away of some of the regulations designed to guard confidentiality. He is not alone. Other politicians and officials are responding to the growing peril by proposing other extreme measures. If they have their way, they will do much more harm than good, and will weaken the programs most likely to be effective.

Testing can be useful both to the person being tested and to the epidemiologists tracing the spread of this disease. But the minute that testing is made mandatory, it will become less effective because critical populations will avoid it at all costs.

The principal barrier at this time is the absence of effective federal and state guarantees against discrimination. Once those guarantees were in place, there would be a new readiness from people at risk to cooperate in voluntary testing programs because they would know that their health insurance, their housing, their jobs would not be denied them as a result of the findings. There is a curious contradiction in that many of the people who are most aggressively advocating mandatory testing programs are also opponents of the very anti-discrimination guarantees that would facilitate testing.

One area of mandatory testing favored by Bauer is for those intending marriage. There is no question that people who have had promiscuous sexual activity should have themselves tested for the AIDS antibody before marriage, and without exception before pregnancy. But if that test is made mandatory, those most at risk are most likely simply to avoid it, according to public health experts, and the very people whom one would hope to be warned would be excluded.

That is why the Centers for Disease Control has recommended against mandatory testing. There is a strong a consensus of support for that view among state public health officials as well. A committee of five experts in California recommended making voluntary AIDS testing centers widely available. That makes sense.

AIDS testing cannot be done in isolation from effective counseling, however. Those who test positive to the presence of the virus need immediate and often continuing psychological support. This need for support is becoming clearer with the accumulation of statistics now demonstrating that more than half those who test positive will, over succeeding years, develop either AIDS or the AIDS-related complex, ARC.

Surgeon General C. Everett Koop remains opposed to the extreme measures being talked about within the White House domestic-policy staff. Dr. Koop is supported by the Centers for Disease Control. The President will be wise to heed the professionals.

The Miami Herald

Miami, FL, February 8, 1987

THE TRIAL balloon sent aloft by the Centers for Disease Control (CDC) should be allowed to drift off into the clouds. The CDC's proposal to test for AIDS all those who are admitted to a hospital or who apply for a marriage license would be a waste of resources that should be directed elsewhere.

AIDS (acquired immune-deficiency syndrome) indeed is a major health threat to the nation. But why not focus testing and education funds on those who are in major risk categories, such as homosexuals and drug abusers? It would be a waste of money to test the blood of an elderly woman entering the hospital for cataract surgery or of virginal or sexually discreet couples seeking to wed. In Florida, where more than half of all hospital admissions are paid by Medicare, the wastefulness of such a broad brush is obvious.

There are more-effective ways to achieve the same ends. If the point of the premarital test is to protect potential offspring from being infected by their mother, then widespread public education should urge those who have put themselves at risk to get the test.

If the point of widespread testing is to help forestall the spread of the disease to other adults, then health authorities should face the need to trace the sexual contacts of those known to be infected. Such tracing now is routine for those infected with other venereal diseases, most of which can be treated successfully. Yet, such tracing is considered by some to be a civil-rights violation when applied to AIDS.

The sudden emergence of AIDS five years ago, its deadliness, and its overlay of moral issues has created an atmosphere of fear. Public policy based on fear tends to be sweeping, expensive, and ineffective. AIDS already demands much of the public purse and will continue to do so. Policy to prevent its further spread should be focused carefully to get the most benefit for the dollar.

Richmond Times-Dispatch

Richmond, VA, June 2, 1987

Contrary to the insinuations of those who, with malice aforethought at a Hollywood-glittery AIDS fund-raiser in Washington, booed and hissed President Reagan's calls for more routine AIDS testing, the latest federal recommendations represent no gross encroachment on human liberty and privacy.

The president said immigrants should have to test negative for the presence of AIDS antibodies before being granted entry or permanent resident status. That's hardly draconian: Immigration law already bars those who suffer from "dangerous contagious disease." Surely AIDS, which is expected to claim more American lives by 1991 than the Vietnam and Korean wars combined, qualifies. As for testing federal prisoners, that is a step that can be justified because of the problem of homosexual promiscuity in the close, confined quarters and the danger of further spread into society when the inmates are released.

Mr. Reagan's call for marriage-license AIDS testing was doubly permissive. First, it would leave the decision to the states and localities, where the authority for premarital testing has traditionally been. And second, it would be up to couples to decide if they wanted to take the test. No one would be forced to do so, or be denied a marriage license because one or both partners tested positive. For peace of mind for those planning to have children, however, routine AIDS testing may well be advisable. Better to detect evidence of the virus before pregnancy than after, when the choice might be between an abortion and birth of a child doomed to die of AIDS.

So moderate were Mr. Reagan's recommendations, in fact, that one must wonder if 10 years from now, by which time the AIDS body count may have exceeded the American toll in World War II if no cure is discovered, public opinion will hold that it was a case of too little, too late.

News-Tribune & Herald

Duluth, MN, May 23, 1987

The Reagan administration's second try on AIDS is better — but still a long way from what the government should be doing.

A presidential aide said Thursday Reagan favors mandatory AIDS testing for marriage license applicants and immigrants.

Since many states already test about-to-be-wed folks for syphilis and other diseases, we can't see AIDS tests as a serious problem. And a test for the killer virus would likely be among the least problems facing someone seeking to enter the United States.

But neither use would likely have a real effect on the growth of what is increasingly seen as a world health threat. And the tests would be a mistake if they siphoned limited money away from the real battle.

As columnist Ellen Goodman notes elsewhere on this page, the Reagan administration has done precious little to help its constituents deal with the AIDS virus.

Mandatory testing: It's simple, it's easy to understand, it sounds strong and definitive. It's easy to see why his advisers could sell Reagan on the idea.

And, as we said, it is a step forward from earlier comments by administration officials on the dread disease — which seemed to consider a lack of premarital and extramarital sex as a definitive federal program.

But most public health officials — including Reagan's own surgeon general — agree public education is the only effective tool we have now to combat the spread of AIDS.

And what entity is better able to fill that function than the federal government? The answer, of course, is none. But, as columnist Goodman noted, that huge federal bureaucracy has focused more on the AIDS feud than the AIDS facts.

Birmingham Post-Herald

Birmingham, AL
February 12, 1987

Federal officials had barely mentioned a possible widening of AIDS testing before the American Civil Liberties Union and some spokesmen for homosexual groups jumped all over the idea.

The criticism is premature.

Testing for AIDS is now required of blood donors and military and State Department foreign service personnel. Officials at the Federal Centers for Disease Control are considering recommending routine testing also for hospital patients, applicants for marriage licenses and women seeking prenatal care.

The agency has not made a hard and fast proposal. It is not suggesting a federal law requiring wider testing. If it makes any firm recommendation at all, it would be to health and government officials at the state level.

Alabama health officials are already considering an expansion of AIDS testing and other steps. An AIDS Prevention Council, comprised of medical, church, government and civic leaders, will meet for the first time today to consider ways to slow the spread of the deadly disease.

All CDC officials are seeking is similar talk at the federal level. They have invited about 250 public health officials and representatives of civil liberty groups to discuss the issue at a meeting Feb. 24-25 in Atlanta, where the federal agency is headquartered.

"The time is ripe to discuss these ideas in an open forum and to make certain we do not overlook any possible way" to curb the disease, said Dr. Walter Dowdle, AIDS director for CDC. "This is a consensus building and multi-step process," he said.

The seriousness of the problem is obvious. About 30,000 cases of AIDS have been diagnosed in the United States, and another 2 million persons are believed to be infected. Not everyone carrying the AIDS virus comes down with the disease, but those who do will die, and those who don't might spread it to others. The U.S. surgeon general has compared AIDS to the Black Death that struck Europe in the 14th century.

Homosexual groups fear that widespread mandatory testing will result in the loss of jobs and other discriminatory actions against persons who test positive, even though they may never develop the disease. The ACLU fears an infringement on the privacy rights of individuals.

These are legitimate concerns, but they must be weighed against the need to protect public health. Dr. Dowdle wants to explore these issues at the Atlanta meeting. There's nothing wrong with that.

Chicago Tribune
Chicago, IL, June 2, 1986

In its attempts to deal with the fatal, contagious and frighteningly mysterious disorder of AIDS, government is faced with a troubling set of legal questions. The Illinois Senate has sent to the House a bill that offers a reasonable approach to them. It is designed to encourage members of high-risk groups to be tested and receive counseling, yet protect their privacy.

Sponsored by Sen. William A. Marovitz and based on the preliminary report issued by the Governor's AIDS Interdisciplinary Advisory Council, the bill calls for testing for the antibody to the AIDS virus after the subject of the test has received counseling and signed a release.

The names of those who test "positive" would be reported only to health officials engaged in AIDS-related research or others with a "compelling interest" such as the Centers for Disease Control in Atlanta, the Illinois Department of Public Health, organ or blood donor programs, a funeral director or embalmer, or a legally authorized representative of the subject of the test. Unauthorized disclosure would be a crime.

The bill deals with a number of problems. Health officials and members of the known high-risk groups—particularly homosexuals, hemophiliacs and intravenous needle users—need information. But fear of public disclosure and the shunning that might follow have prevented many from receiving testing and counseling, which includes encouragement to make changes in their lifestyles. The problem is further complicated by the absence of a test for the AIDS virus itself. Apparently, few of those who test "positive" for the antibody actually get AIDS, yet public fears tend to place a social stigma on all antibody carriers, once word gets out.

Unfortunately, the bill, which passed 56-0 in the Senate, may run into trouble in the House, where recent debate over AIDS prevention has turned all too quickly into arguments over homosexuality. The Marovitz bill is a practical approach, and it deserves passage.

The Oregonian
Portland, OR, January 1, 1986

Later this month the Oregon Health Division will ask the Legislature's Emergency Board for permission to continue its free testing program for the AIDS-virus antibody. The major issue will be how to offer the tests, not whether to offer them.

A number of gay organizations want the state to offer the tests anonymously. They fear the names of the people who test positive for the antibody — only a small minority of whom will develop the disease — will fall into the wrong hands and be used by employers and health insurance companies to discriminate against them. Based on a historic presumption of generalized discrimination against homosexuals, the gay community's fears are understandable. But based on actual experience with public health records, the fears are unjustified.

While the Health Division opposes anonymity, it conducts its AIDS-antibody tests with the same confidentiality that protects all public health records. In fact, more. The results of the antibody testing are doubly shielded by a special provision in state law that exempts records for sexually transmitted diseases from search and subpoena. That confidentiality has never been breached, and there is no reason to expect that anyone who would misuse the information could get it now.

Actually, though open to all, the state's antibody test sites were established to serve people who were giving their names anyway in search of a blood test. Last spring, blood banks, all of which require identification, found that worried members of high-risk groups were giving blood solely to find out whether they carried the AIDS virus. To relieve the burden on the blood banks and to prevent possible contamination of the blood supply through false-negative test results, the state opened the alternative test sites.

But the benefit of the free test clinics goes beyond the 100 people a week served by them. The confidential record of names and results gives the Health Division a valuable epidemiological tool to track the spread of the virus and the frequency with which carriers of the virus actually develop the disease. Because high-risk people frequently seek retesting, having names prevents a duplicated count that may artificially inflate the prevalence of the virus and may confuse efforts to monitor the effectiveness of the state's risk-reduction education programs.

The state is on an epidemiological search, not a witch hunt. It still tests, free, samples from patients who preserve their anonymity by going to a private doctor. No matter where they come from, all blood samples go to the testing lab with codes that carry no identifying information.

Even people who go to the public clinics are not required to show proof of identification, and the Health Division is aware but disappointed that some give false names. In rare cases, giving a false name or no name at all can cause unnecessary stress. In California, the only state that mandates anonymous testing, one public clinic told a man he tested positive, only to discover after he left that his test result was negative. Without a name, the clinic had no way to tell him the good news.

The risks of confidentially attaching a name to a test result are imagined. The benefits are real. They should not be sacrificed to calm understandable but unfounded fears.

THE ATLANTA CONSTITUTION
Atlanta, GA, December 20, 1986

Many judges are already ordering convicted prostitutes to be tested for the AIDS virus, but some aren't, and, though judges especially dislike being told how to operate, they cannot afford to ignore the latest recommendations of the Georgia Board of Human Resources: that they require the testing of convicted prostitutes, male and female.

Such proposals sometimes elicit grumbles from advocates for AIDS victims, who fear sufferers might be singled out for discrimination. That's a legitimate concern, but it is not an immediate danger and there are compelling reasons for moving aggressively on testing prostitutes.

Recent studies indicate that AIDS is spreading twice as rapidly among straights as among gays, through intimate sexual contact and the use of infected syringes by drug addicts. Prostitutes appear to be one of the sources of the spread.

Court-ordered testing would help in two ways: First, by identifying those who pose a public-health threat and need assistance; second, by generating more accurate statistics than are being churned up by Atlanta's voluntary testing program.

Only one in 80 prostitutes has tested positive for AIDS in Atlanta, compared with 5 percent and 40 percent respectively in similar programs in Seattle and Miami, but the Centers for Disease Control has warned that the actual rate of infection among prostitutes may be "significantly" higher.

So far, the questions about AIDS outnumber the answers, but the case for court-ordered testing is clear.

☰ The Cincinnati Post

Cincinnati, OH, March 27, 1987

The legal wrangling over court-ordered blood tests for AIDS is likely to continue for a while, until the legislature classifies AIDS as a venereal disease. Yet, such testing in sex-related cases has merit, and the judges who order it should work with public health officials to ensure its success.

Municipal Judge Edward Donnellon was the first to order an AIDS test, mandating one for a convicted prostitute. Judge David Albanese followed by ordering tests as a condition of bond as well as in sentencing, and at least two other judges have said they will follow suit in similar sex crimes.

If for no other reason, court-ordered testing is justified so that public health officials will have more data at their disposal. They can combine that data with information from voluntary tests to paint a more accurate picture of the extent of AIDS in Cincinnati, what groups have it and who is most at risk.

Armed with more data, health officials can do a better job of educating the public about AIDS. That's important because education is the best way to combat this deadly disease for which there is no known cure.

Beyond that, however, tests serve a limited purpose. Results are confidential, so a judge can only hope that a person who tests positive will act responsibly, seek counseling and refrain from conduct that may infect other people. It's a slender hope, since people convicted of sex crimes aren't acting responsibly in the first place.

And here's another caveat: Before judges go overboard, they should consider the burden being placed on the Cincinnati Health Department. The department is one of the few places in the county geared up to handle AIDS testing and the counseling that should follow it. Those tests cost money—$5 to $10 for the antibody screening and $25 to $35 for the follow-up—and the demand for them is growing.

Requests for AIDS tests rose dramatically after the federal Centers for Disease Control recommended them for people who received blood transfusions between 1978 and 1985. This week, U.S. Surgeon General C. Everett Koop recommended testing for people considering marriage or pregnancy.

Albanese and his fellow judges are justified in joining those in the vanguard of the testing movement. They should be committed, also, to working with health officials to ensure that testing is adequately funded and achieves maximum results.

The Miami Herald

Miami, FL, February 28, 1987

THE TENSIONS between public-health officials and civil-rights guardians over AIDS continues unabated. A conference this week served more to define the questions than to answer them. The major point of contention is who should be tested and what should happen to the results.

AIDS (acquired immune-deficiency syndrome) is spreading among the general population. In those states such as Florida where many cases have been reported, one of every 30 men (3.34 percent) and one of every 75 women (1.35 percent) may carry the antibodies that are evidence of exposure. At least one-third of those carriers will develop AIDS within eight years.

Earlier this month, the Federal Centers for Disease Control (CDC) touched off a controversy by suggesting that all persons entering the hospital or applying for a marriage license be tested. The costs of such a program would far outweigh the benefits, and few at the CDC conference in Atlanta supported it.

The watchword, said civil-rights guardians, ought to be voluntary testing, and the experience of the present voluntary program gives this argument some support. Operating at 1,079 sites, the program tests some 50,000 persons a month. Most are in the high-risk categories of homosexuals, drug abusers, and hemophiliacs. Of them, 19 percent have tested positive for exposure to AIDS. But is that program enough? Some employers and Government agencies now are requiring tests, but society has not moved to require them of those convicted of crimes putting them at risk, such as drug abuse and prostitution.

What of the results? One faction is saying that the results must be kept confidential so that those who test positive will not lose their health-insurance benefits or jobs even though AIDS does *not* spread through work-place contacts. Confidentiality is easy to defend, but not if it extends to efforts to block the tracing of contacts. Otherwise, those at greatest risk — the spouses and lovers of the infected — may never know of the risk to their lives without tests. Such tracing of contacts now is routinely done with less-severe sexually transmitted diseases. It makes little sense not to do so with AIDS.

Minneapolis Star and Tribune

Minneapolis, MN, August 22, 1987

In recommending broader testing to detect the spread of AIDS, the U.S. Public Health Service last week set the stage for a serious effort to fight the epidemic on its home turf. The new policy calls for routine but voluntary testing of groups most susceptible to infection, and sidesteps President Reagan's counterproductive plea for widespread compulsory screening. The agency has picked the policy most likely to contain the virus and the devastation it inflicts.

The new guidelines correctly stop short of the strategy urged by the president in June. Declaring that AIDS "is surreptitiously spreading throughout our population," Reagan called for mandatory AIDS-antibody testing of a wide array of groups — including marriage-license applicants and hospital patients. But that approach would have concentrated the costly tests on segments of the population least touched by AIDS.

The Public Health Service favors focusing testing and counseling on more likely targets: drug addicts, people with sexually transmitted diseases, partners of risk-group members, prostitutes and women of childbearing age with identifiable risks for infection. The guidelines also endorse making tests available to individuals at less risk, but stress that all AIDS tests must be voluntary and all test results confidential.

If AIDS were racing through the population, a blanket screening plan might make sense. But mounting evidence suggests that the AIDS virus remains largely confined among gay men and drug users. As the Centers for Disease Control announced last week, AIDS is not spreading at the expected rate among heterosexuals who stay away from drugs. Even in New York, where the virus has already infected half a million people, only a tiny minority appears to have been exposed through heterosexual contact.

That finding should not prompt Americans outside high-risk groups to let down their guard against the disease. But it does underscore the validity of the Public Health Service's testing approach. Since AIDS chiefly afflicts the high-risk groups originally stricken, compassion and logic dictate helping them first and most.

Detroit Free Press

Detroit, MI,
March 23, 1987

AS THE AIDS virus has spread through the population, physicians, policymakers and others have argued about what the government's role should be. Some have suggested that mandatory tests be given to applicants for marriage licenses, pregnant women or those seeking treatment for sexually transmitted diseases. The constitutional hurdles and psychological opposition to mandatory tests, however, are tremendous, and there is a risk that mandatory tests would be counter-productive.

An extensive program of voluntary testing, however, could be a viable alternative. Reports on increased interest in blood tests among heterosexuals in Long Beach, San Francisco, Boston and other centers of the AIDS epidemic strongly indicate that the public would support such a program.

Some people in high-risk groups have argued that the early detection of AIDS only starts a death watch without improving an individual's chances for survival. Others fear discrimination if test results are leaked to employers or insurance companies. Moreover, mandatory tests for AIDS would constitute a gross violation of the individual right to privacy which is intolerable in a free society. The fear of driving AIDS underground is also a strong reason for caution in resorting to mandatory tests.

Voluntary, strictly confidential tests would not raise questions of constitutionality, and, moreover, they may provide a wealth of information needed by epidemiologists to fight the epidemic. Dr. June Osborn, dean of the University of Michigan's School of Public Health, is among those urging the federal government to establish a program that provides anonymous AIDS tests on request. With proper safeguards, she believes people would step forward.

AIDS is often spread by people who do not know that they carry the virus. If a person who believes he or she has come in contact with the virus can be tested without fear of reprisal, the assumption is the person will not spread it unwittingly.

The idea of confidential and voluntary testing may not sound radical enough in the face of the AIDS crisis. It is a proper role for the government to play, though, and the establishment of a voluntary testing program would be well worth the effort.

The Virginian-Pilot

Norfolk, VA, February 6, 1987

Doctors at the federal Centers for Disease Control in Atlanta propose blood testing for acquired immune deficiency syndrome (AIDS) of all patients admitted to hospitals, women seeking prenatal care and couples applying for marriage licenses. Considering the virulence of the AIDS virus — the U.S. surgeon general recently compared the epidemic to the Black Plague, which killed a third of Europe's population in the 14th century — most Americans presumably would support reasonable, if wide-ranging, preventive measures such as the CDC is considering.

But state public-health officials and gay-rights groups promptly expressed skepticism about the proposal. Health officials say the cost of AIDS tests would be as cost-*ineffective* as the premarital blood tests recently discontinued by many states. In Virginia, for example, blood testing of prospective newlyweds was stopped in 1984 because $2.6 million was being spent each year to test 125,000 people to detect barely a dozen cases of venereal disease. Gay-rights activists fear discrimination against and quarantine of homosexuals who test positive for AIDS.

Those objections are rooted in long experience. But it is the future of AIDS that should be the focus of debate. At the rate that the disease is spreading, the U.S. Public Health Service has predicted that AIDS could rank among the nation's top 10 killers by 1991. If current projections come true, AIDS will have come a long way in a short time — from five "unusual" cases of a mysterious disease documented by the Centers for Disease Control in Los Angeles in 1981 to 54,000 deaths a year nationwide a decade later. Currently, no cures or vaccines exist, and the disease is virtually 100 percent fatal. Clearly, the public-health threat posed by AIDS calls for general mobilization.

Is the Centers for Disease Control's blood-testing proposal appropriate? Critics say it is not, because it fails to take aim directly at the high-risk groups of homosexuals and intravenous drug abusers. True, hospital patients, women seeking prenatal care and prospective newlyweds are not high-risk AIDS groups — for now. But what about the future? Why not target the widest reasonable spectrum of Americans? Why not concentrate, as the CDC proposal does, on children, among whom, according to PHS predictions, the disease will spread most rapidly by 1991?

Preventive measures such as blood tests, balanced with civil-liberties protections, are prudent. But the blood-testing proposal is only a trial balloon. Even if the proposal advances to become a recommendation later this month, it will not be a mandate. Acceptance or rejection of such a recommendation will rest with the states, not with the federal government.

The Centers for Disease Control proposal, then, is a timely way to alert states that it's time to start devising prudent health-protective measures against the spread of AIDS — but with this caveat: Privacy and civil-liberties guarantees may need to be strengthened to protect patients who test positive for AIDS from discrimination. Given the fear and hysteria surrounding the disease, the confidentiality that attaches to doctor-patient relationships may not be sufficient to stop leaks of positive AIDS-test results. State lawmakers should consider stiff sanctions to safeguard AIDS victims from social stigmas.

The Register-Guard

Eugene, OR, February 7, 1987

The national Centers for Disease Control announced recently that broader AIDS testing programs would be recommended to the states — programs that could include blood tests for all hospital patients, pregnant women and people applying for marriage licenses. Broader testing has its place in the national effort to stop the spread of AIDS, but health officials should choose better target groups.

AIDS is transmitted almost exclusively through sexual contact or through shared use of intravenous needles. The mechanisms of transmission suggest obvious candidates for a stepped-up program to detect the presence of the AIDS virus. Drug addicts or prostitutes and their patrons, for instance, stand a far better chance of having been exposed to the virus than hospital patients. AIDS tests should be expanded to include those groups before being required of other segments of the population.

Despite rising fear that AIDS is spreading among society at large, the disease remains largely confined to specific groups. Last year there were 1,100 cases of AIDS among heterosexuals who had no history of intravenous drug abuse, compared with fewer than 100 three years earlier. But such cases continue to constitute a low percentage of all AIDS cases, and nearly all of them can be traced back to a sexual encounter with a drug user or male bisexual.

This does not mean that the general public should be unconcerned about the risk of AIDS. The five-year incubation period for the disease allows it to spread undetected through long venereal chains. People who are uncertain of a sexual partner's history need to know more about AIDS and how to prevent the disease. It must also be recognized that such uncertainty is more common than many care to admit.

The general public therefore needs education about AIDS and its means of transmission so that people can take sensible steps to minimize the risk of contracting the disease or avoid it altogether. Testing — particularly mandatory testing — should be reserved for groups that are known to be at risk and are in a position to endanger others. Universal testing of blood donors makes sense from that standpoint; it's needed to protect the nation's blood supply.

The groups listed in the preliminary proposals by the Centers for Disease Control, however, deserve a far lower priority. Hospital patients, pregnant women or people planning to marry cannot automatically be defined as being in greater danger than college students, hockey players or job applicants. Some members of each of those groups may be in danger because they belong to or have been associated with, directly or indirectly, high-risk groups. The high-risk groups themselves, not larger segments of the general population, should be the focus of attention in testing programs.

The Washington Post

Washington, DC, February 7, 1987

A CONFERENCE THAT is sure to be highly charged and controversial is scheduled to be held in Atlanta later this month. The invited participants are serious professionals who take different positions on an issue of national importance, and men and women on both sides believe their positions are not only intellectually correct but also ethically imperative. They will be discussing a recommendation that a broad program of testing for AIDS be put into effect.

Doctors at the federal Centers for Disease Control are concerned about the continuing spread of AIDS, which has already stricken 30,000 Americans. While difficult to transmit, it is invariably fatal. It now affects primarily homosexual men and intravenous drug users and has begun to spread to persons outside these two high-risk groups. Public health experts want wider testing so those who carry the AIDS virus can be notified and advised, specifically so they will not inadvertently spread the disease. Testing is already required of blood donors, people in the military and certain federal employees, for example foreign service officers. The CDC now suggests a discussion on whether applicants for marriage licenses, hospital patients, pregnant women and those treated for venereal disease should be tested too.

Others, primarily civil libertarians and gay groups, oppose widespread testing for a number of reasons. It is certainly an invasion of privacy—although it may be a justified one—but the main concern of opponents is that the tests will be used to discriminate against AIDS victims. Will test results remain confidential? Should they be kept confidential even if it means the disease will be transmitted to others? Will people discovered to be carrying the AIDS virus lose their jobs? Will they be forbidden to marry or pressured to have abortions? Will they be quarantined? These are all legitimate questions, and not one answer is clear, just as it is also legitimate and prudent for public health officials to want to identify carriers, track the disease and take steps to contain it.

Dr. Walter Dowdle, director of AIDS programs at the CDC, emphasizes that the conference is preliminary. No federal statute is in the works, and the CDC intends only to offer advice to state public health officials. Jeffrey Levi, political director of the National Gay and Lesbian Task Force, welcomes a dialogue, suggesting that objections to testing might be overcome if more counseling and education were provided and discrimination problems worked out. The conference is designed to stimulate open debate on the public health and civil liberties aspects of the epidemic and to begin building a consensus on how to proceed. The meeting is a constructive step, and it comes not a moment too soon.

St. Petersburg Times

St. Petersburg, FL, February 9, 1987

There are two aspects to AIDS that seemingly make the case for widespread blood testing, as suggested last week by federal health officials. It is an invariably lethal disease that for now can only be prevented, not cured. Its victims can harbor the virus for years, infecting others, before it makes its presence felt. Shouldn't they be warned? Shouldn't prospective parents, above all, be made aware of the danger?

The issue is complicated, however, by the extraordinary stigmas and fears that AIDS evokes. Straight people are dying of it, too, but the extent to which the public still perceives AIDS as primarily a disease of homosexuals gives all victims reason to not want their identities known. Beyond that, the mere suspicion of AIDS provokes such mindless panic that victims have been fired from their jobs, thrown out of school, evicted from their homes and even rejected after death by some undertakers. Those who suggest mass testing acknowledge that confidentiality is imperative, but they cannot guarantee it.

There might be less resistance to testing had the Reagan administration not gone out of its way to foster discrimination against AIDS victims. The Justice Department has argued to the Supreme Court that it is legal for an employer to fire a diseased worker simply because the employer fears the employee might communicate the disease to others. Under this view, the fear doesn't even have to be well-founded.

AIDS, it bears repeating, is not spread by casual contact, but only by sexual intercourse and contaminated blood.

The Centers for Disease Control has aroused a storm of protest with its suggestion for testing of all hospital patients, pregnant women and marriage license applicants. As some civil libertarians and health experts have pointed out, mass testing could "drive the disease underground," especially considering the Justice Department's medically uninformed attitude toward the civil rights of sick people. Yet the discussion initiated by the Centers' proposal is timely and necessary. Society has a strong interest in finding and alerting potential carriers of the disease. The questions are whether it can be done in ways that respect their privacy and other civil rights. Would they be forced or merely encouraged to identify their sexual partners? Would infected couples be sterilized, or merely advised not to conceive children? Would victims risk quarantine? Bizarre as these questions sound, they are legitimate fears to those who suffer from the disease or have been tested positive for its antibodies.

Yet the disease is serious enough that even some spokespersons for the homosexual community concede the need to discuss the testing question and its ramifications. Jeffrey Levi, political director of the National Gay and Lesbian Task Force in Washington, said that if the government combined testing "with a major counseling program, a general education program, anti-discrimination protections and dealing with the health insurance issue, then I think we could begin to talk."

A society that wants potential AIDS victims to come forward and be tested is manifestly going to have to protect their interests as Levi suggested. It may even be necessary for society to pay for their health and life insurance, in the larger interest of keeping them from going underground. Above all, society must put aside its exaggerated fears of AIDS and stops treating AIDS victims as if they were modern lepers. Without such progress, the case against routine testing will remain very strong.

THE DAILY OKLAHOMAN
Oklahoma City, OK, May 27, 1987

DAY by day, Americans are becoming more aware of AIDS.

Apparently a greater awareness has set in at the White House as well. The Reagan administration appears to be close to getting a handle on the issue, with a meeting of the Domestic Policy Council scheduled to develop recommendations.

Indications are that President Reagan is leaning toward mandatory testing, a position favored by conservatives. Up to now, the administration has been sending mixed signals on what to do about the disease, which has killed more than 20,000 people in the United States.

Ironically, Surgeon General C. Everett Koop opposes testing and advocates expanded sex education, while Education Secretary William Bennett is promoting stern public health measures. A gauge of congressional sentiment was the 63-32 vote in the Senate against an amendment calling for testing of immigrants and marriage license applicants.

The killer epidemic not only threatens human life but has the potential to bankrupt health systems through spiraling costs. In New York City, for example, AIDS cases added $400 million in hospital expenses last year and health officials believe the cost will be more than $1 billion a year by 1991.

Whether President Reagan comes out strong for mandatory testing or other strategies is yet to be decided. The important thing is for the administration to speak with one voice on the AIDS issue.

Meese Orders Testing For Immigrants

U.S. Attorney General Edwin Meese III June 8, 1987 announced details of programs to test would-be immigrants for infection by AIDS. The attorney general was elaborating on a key aspect of the policy introduced May 31, 1987 by President Reagan. Meese announced that he had directed the Immigration and Naturalization Service (INS) to develop a program to test all would-be immigrants for AIDS as well as illegal aliens applying for legal status. Aliens who applied for an immigrant visa overseas, the attorney general said, would be tested overseas if possible and would be informed if they tested positive. Those who tested positive would be denied entry to the U.S. Foreign governments would generally not be told of the test results. Illegal aliens who tested positive would be ineligible for legal status or amnesty, under the new immigration law. However, they could not be deported on the basis of such data because all information obtained in connection with an application for amnesty would, under the law, have to be kept confidential. Immigration officials, however, would be instructed to deny such aliens permanent legal status because of their medical conditions.

THE LOUISVILLE TIMES
Louisville, KY
April 26, 1986

The Reagan administration's proposal to test immigrants for Acquired Immune Deficiency Syndrome (AIDS) and to exclude those who clearly have this incurable diseases is reasonable. Persons who have certain other infectious illnesses have been denied admission to this country.

However, the difficulty is that the screening test now available is not reliable and its widespread use might result in unfair decisions. In addition, it would be costly. Until a better test is available, public funds could be spent more productively on finding cures for the disease.

The fairness issue was raised back in January, when Health and Human Services Secretary Otis R. Bowen proposed the testing. The Public Health Service last week issued regulations that would give consular officials authority to require aliens seeking to visit or settle in the United States to undergo screening for AIDS.

Existing rules now bar from entry persons with infectious leprosy, active tuberculosis and a number of sexually transmitted diseases. Clinically diagnosed cases of AIDS are appropriate additions. But the blood tests — mandatory now at blood donation centers — would provide neither a reliable nor a fair basis for barring aliens from this country.

Many physicians argue that the test isn't a diagnostic tool; rather, it shows whether a person has antibodies to the AIDS virus. The presence of antibodies merely indicates whether someone has been exposed to the disease — not whether he will, in fact, develop AIDS. Nor does it accurately conclude whether someone will be able to transmit the virus.

That's the reason a positive reaction on the screening test should not be sufficient justification for preventing a person from entering the United States. The same would be true, for instance, in the cases of people who have been exposed to TB. While antibodies may show up on a test, only active cases of these diseases should be grounds for exclusion.

AIDS is a major American health problem. The Centers for Disease Control have recorded nearly 20,000 cases — half of which have been fatal.

Federal health investigators have not found a cure, although they say that AIDS can be contracted only in a few ways — sexual contact, contaminated syringes or, in some cases, through transfusions of blood and blood products.

It's baffling. It's disturbing. Preventing persons with active cases to enter this country makes economic and social sense. But let's also focus on the drive to find a cure — the most effective way to spend tax dollars.

THE PLAIN DEALER
Cleveland, OH, February 13, 1986

The usually rational U.S. Department of Health and Human Services has shown that hasty fears and prejudices about AIDS have infected more than the general public. The department recently asked that AIDS be added to the list of seven serious, infectious diseases preventing immigration into the United States. The others are leprosy, tuberculosis and five types of venereal disease.

The idea is creditable and logical. The problem is that, as of the present, there is no good test for AIDS, only for its precursors and clues. The better tests for the clues to AIDS are highly subjective; not easily—or cheaply—used by the contract doctors U.S. consulates abroad are likely to employ. By raising the issue before the technology is able to respond, Health and Human Services is opening a Pandora's Box of tough civil rights and medical ethics concerns about screening for AIDS.

The department's proposal, not yet public and awaiting administration cost review, has already proved controversial among public health specialists who wonder: How will it be implemented?

The current answer is unacceptable. HHS is asking for public comment on the possible use of commercial tests, used to keep the blood supply safe, to screen immigrants for AIDS. But the tests check only for AIDS antibodies. They test to see if someone has been exposed. They are hastily developed blanket tests meant to safeguard the nation's blood supply, not to measure health risks for individuals. No test has yet been developed that can determine whether someone has been infected and is contagious.

Exposure may or may not lead to infection. Although there is growing evidence that the presence of AIDS antibodies means the AIDS virus is also in the body, no one knows for sure how the AIDS virus functions. According to current information, from 20% to 40% of those testing positive for AIDS antibodies—after an incubation period ranging from months to seven years—will contract the fatal disease.

For those reasons, federal agencies charged with public health and welfare, including HHS, unanimously have recommended against using the blood screening tests to weed through the general population, or as part of job, school or other applications.

Part of the danger with the current test—the one proposed for use on immigrants—comes from its two-step process. The first step is an easy, fast and inexpensive test that's a very rough indicator of AIDS antibodies in the blood. The second, used to confirm the first test, is a complex, expensive, time-consuming process requiring skillful interpretation. How many would just use the cheap and easy test, the rough test? How many lives and livelihoods could that destroy? How easy would it be to use the test to discriminate against homosexuals, a group at high risk for exposure?

U.S. Rep. Barney Frank, D-Mass., who serves on the House immigration subcommittee, fears debate on the proposal will discredit a test that's valuable in research, and will "roil the waters unnecessarily" concerning what society should and shouldn't do to protect itself.

Research is now being directed at new and better AIDS tests, including a cheap and easy secondary test for the antibodies, and tests for the presence of the AIDS virus. Until medicine and science provide the tools to avoid the excessive cost and human hardship that seems certain to occur using the current screening process, the administration should shelve the proposed immigration test.

The Boston Globe
Boston, MA, May 2, 1986

Americans can forget about any serious help from the federal government in dealing with AIDS, if the first public health recommendation to carry the weight of law is an example. The recommendation – under terms that are pointless – would ban the admission of anyone with AIDS into the United States.

The ban would apply only to applicants who are so sick with AIDS that their illness could be spotted by a non-medically trained immigration officer. People that sick with any disease are not admissible anyway, so there is no need for a specific AIDS ban.

Furthermore, people with acute and deadly AIDS are the ones least likely to spread the disease to others because by the time AIDS is in its terminal stage, its victims carry little virus. To combat the transmission of AIDS to the United States by foreigners would require the detection of AIDS carriers.

Carriers are the ones most likely to transmit the disease because, though they show no symptoms, they continuously harbor the AIDS virus. To detect AIDS carriers among healthy-appearing immigrants would require a blood test of all.

Yet, the proposed restriction deliberately does not impose an AIDS blood test on emigres, visa seekers, exchange students, temporary workers or tourists. A spokesman for the US Public Health Department said the reason is the risk of inaccurate results.

The larger concern is that foreign countries could impose AIDS blood tests on Americans seeking to travel, study or work abroad. Since AIDS is vastly more widespread in the United States, a blood-test requirement would exclude more Americans from travel than foreigners.

The rationale behind the proposal is to add AIDS to the seven "dangerous" diseases – five venereal diseases, tuberculosis and leprosy – that historically had been grounds for excluding aliens from receiving a permanent immigration permit. Placed on the Immigration and Naturalization Service list in an era when there were no effective treatments, none of these diseases now stands in the way of obtaining entry because all can be controlled or cured with drugs.

Prevention of the spread of AIDS is not the main purpose behind the proposed ban on aliens, said a Centers for Disease Control specialist. Rather, it is to keep out people who would be able to work and who would get sicker – and whose medical care would be a burden to American taxpayers. This exclusion is now applied to aliens who are mentally ill or retarded.

It is not known how many immigrants might pose an AIDS risk, but estimates are very low. An AIDS specialist has noted that the United States, with its huge caseload, has been a far greater exporter than importer.

In the face of a massive AIDS epidemic at home, federal agencies should concentrate on effective ways to combat it. They need not look abroad for a specious AIDS problem to solve.

FORT WORTH STAR-TELEGRAM
Fort Worth, TX, February 7, 1986

Within the next couple of months someone may come forth with some compelling reasons why permanent immigrants to the United States should not be subjected to AIDS screening.

Unless that happens, Health and Human Services Secretary Otis Bowen's order requiring the tests for persons immigrating to this country seems to be sound policy.

Some public health officials within Bowen's department opposed the order, which must be published for 60 days before it becomes final, on the grounds that it might encourage other countries to retaliate against U.S. citizens abroad. They point out that the United States has the largest number of reported cases of acquired immune deficiency syndrome in the world.

That argument does not appear to hold water. Given the relatively high incidence of reported AIDS cases in this country, it would seem only appropriate that other countries would take the same kind of steps to protect themselves from importing AIDS that Bowen is proposing for the United States.

Prospective immigrants to this country can be excluded from establishing residence here if they have one of five sexually transmitted diseases — syphilis, gonorrhea, chancroid, granuloma inguinale and lymphogranuloma venereum.

Since AIDS is worse than all of those curable or controllable diseases combined, it is only reasonable that any country should take steps to avoid allowing infected persons to become part of its permanent population.

Fort Worth, TX, April 29, 1986

The federal government not only has the right to bar immigration into the United States by AIDS victims, as is being proposed, it has the responsibility to do so.

In a proposed regulation published in the Federal Register, the Centers for Disease Control said acquired immune deficiency syndrome should be added to the list of seven "dangerous contagious diseases" that are grounds for refusing entry to the United States.

The seven diseases currently on the list are tuberculosis, leprosy, syphilis, gonorrhea, granuloma inguinale, lymphogranuloma venereum and chancroid. The last five are venereal diseases.

The proposed regulation would give the United States the authority not only to prohibit AIDS victims from entering the country but also to require medical tests for tourists or students seeking entry if AIDS infection is suspected.

It would primarily be aimed at refugees, foreigners seeking permanent immigration to this country and foreigners engaged to marry U.S. citizens. The test also could be applied on a discretionary basis to foreigners seeking a tourist or student visa to the United States.

An official of the National Lesbian and Gay Health Foundation expressed fear that the regulation would be used to discriminate against homosexuals, the principal high-risk group for AIDS. Perhaps it would, but failure to enact the proposed regulation could cause far greater harm to a far larger number of people than random cases of discrimination.

AIDS is a serious health problem and is growing more serious by the day. The government is fully justified in taking whatever reasonable steps it deems necessary to prevent its spread.

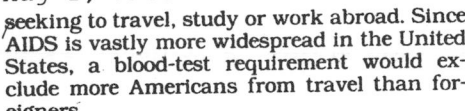

Herald Examiner
Los Angeles, CA
February 5, 1986

AIDS is a contagious and deadly disease. There's no denying that. So when the Secretary of Health and Human Services Otis Bowen recently approved an order to include AIDS on the list of infectious ailments that prevent immigrants from entering the U.S. to become citizens, some applauded. Noticeably absent from that crowd were many of Bowen's own public health officials, who recognize the pitfalls in such an order and advised against it.

The problem lies in determining who has AIDS and who doesn't. Unlike syphilis or gonorrhea, two other diseases on the U.S. Immigration checklist, AIDS testing is still inadequate at best. At worst, it can be terribly misleading. A positive result does not indicate that a person has the disease, merely that he or she has been exposed to the virus that causes it. Experts estimate that only about 10 percent of those who test positive will ever contract AIDS. Moreover, a negative test result doesn't guarantee that a person is free of AIDS or that he or she won't come down with it in the future, because it may take months for antibodies to form after contact with the virus.

Although Bowen's order would be required only for prospective immigrants, some fear that other countries would retaliate by insisting on testing American tourists, whose country has more AIDS victims than any other.

As the issue is debated in Washington, Angelenos can take heart in the way Archbishop Mahoney has reacted to the AIDS crisis. No stranger to controversy, Mahoney announced last weekend that he will ask Mother Theresa of Calcutta to consider opening a hospice for AIDS victims in L.A.

"Even in the midst of this suffering and pain," said Mahoney as he presented the proposal, "we must find a reason to look up." That's good advice for everyone – including the Department of Health and Human Services – as the AIDS tragedy continues.

Insurers Weigh Tests; Gay Bias by Insurers Opposed

Because AIDS primarily affects disfavored minorities, such as gay men and intravenous drug users, and because of the high costs of its medical treatment, decisions regarding AIDS and insurance are politically charged. How society allocates the costs of an expensive disease among different interests with widely varying degrees of political and economic power has been determined, in part, by how insurance companies have responded to the AIDS crisis. The questions lingering between the lines of most insurance issues are who will deal with the financial burdens of AIDS and how will the financial burden be divided?

The nation's state regulators of insurance December 11, 1987 approved model guidelines that would bar insurance applicants from being asked whether they were homosexual. The National Association of Insurance Commissioners, meeting in Orlando, Florida, adopted the rules. The regulations were not binding in themselves, but the individual states were urged to put them into force. Insurers wanted to guard against applicants with AIDS, and gay rights activists feared the insurers might discriminate against homosexuals to do so. Both insurers and gay activists sat on the advisory board that drew up the guidelines, and groups representing the two interests praised the results.

The rules would forbid not only direct questions about sexual orientation, but also the search for clues in an applicant's zip code, marital status or choice of beneficiary. Insurers would be able to ask directly if an applicant suffered from AIDS or AIDS symptoms, but the rules did not say whether or not insurers could require AIDS tests. This was the issue that most divided insurers and homosexual groups. As of January 1987 seven states and Washington, D.C. barred use of the tests for insurance screening.

Previously, Richard Schweicker, the president of the American Council of Life Insurance, November 1, 1985 had said the insurers would insist upon their "historic right to classify according to risks" and test applicants for signs of AIDS. Schweiker said the council did not support questions about lifestyle to discover if applicants belonged to such high-risk groups as homosexuals and drug users. That method was being considered by some companies, although most states barred inquiries about sexual preference.

The Washington Times

Washington, DC, July 23, 1986

Congress is unlikely to overturn D.C. Council's act making those who test positively for AIDS a uniquely privileged group, immune from having insurance actuaries examine this aspect of their medical profiles. It is just as well, say those who oppose the AIDS measure but favor D.C. home rule. Well, what about a referendum?

Two civic activists, Dino Joseph Drudi and the Rev. John Bussey, urged D.C. Council to put the insurance bill to a vote rather than let Congress decide, thereby avoiding an embarrassment to home rule. (Mr. Drudi was a campaigner for the statehood initiative.)

But Council was variously indifferent and hostile, so Messrs. Bussey and Drudi have had to file their referendum proposal with the Board of Elections. This means the inevitable challenge to the wording of the referendum and, once that hurdle is jumped, 13,300 valid signatures by Aug. 6 — in practice, 20,000 or more, since many will be pronounced invalid.

While pacifying home-rule enthusiasts, a referendum also would underscore the problems with home rule, as now constituted. In the 1973 District of Columbia Self-Government and Governmental Reorganization Act, Congress showed that it thought of Washington as a city. Reasonable enough, since it is one. But since it is not part of a state, many of the issues normally faced at the state level inevitably must be faced by city government — by, that is to say, a 13-member council.

This is no argument for statehood, but it may be a reason for a larger and more representative City Council, one able, among other things, to resist special interest pressures and protect ordinary insurance customers.

THE SACRAMENTO BEE

Sacramento, CA, April 1, 1986

Private companies searching for an AIDS vaccine face a daunting problem: The costs developing a vaccine are high and the potential economic rewards of success are uncertain. The market for an AIDS vaccine, which might be administered only to the high-risk part of the population, is likely to be small compared to the potential sales from other biological products. And no company can afford to ignore the recent explosion of damage lawsuits that has driven more than half of U.S. vaccine manufacturers out of the business. Their efforts to develop a vaccine could be slowed without public incentives and liability protection, say Genentech and Chiron, two California biotechnology firms at the forefront of AIDS vaccine research.

To encourage those companies to stay in the hunt for an AIDS vaccine, Assemblyman John Vasconcellos and a bipartisan group of legislators have responded to their pleas with a package of incentives. Their legislation, AB 4250, would provide $6 million to California manufacturers for human trials of an AIDS vaccine and would guarantee state purchase of 1 million doses of an FDA-approved AIDS vaccine from companies here. The bill would also limit the liability of a California AIDS vaccine manufacturer to losses arising from negligence or misconduct; all other losses from adverse reactions to the vaccine would be paid from a state compensation fund.

No one can say for sure that such state incentives will guarantee the development of a successful AIDS vaccine. But given the deadliness of the AIDS virus and the continuing spread of the disease, it's essential that all promising vaccine research go forward as quickly as possible. The incentives Vasconcellos and his colleagues are proposing will make it possible for the companies to push ahead harder. If that extra effort shortens the search for a vaccine by even a few months, hundreds of lives can be saved.

Ideally, those incentives ought to come from Washington. But federal AIDS officials, preoccupied with their own national research program centered at the National Cancer Institute, have been cool to requests for help from the companies, which are their major competitors in AIDS vaccine research. Until Washington is prepared to address problems of liability and compensation for AIDS vaccine manufacturers on a national level, passage of AB 4250 would be a useful way of keeping California's inventive biotechnology companies in the vaccine race.

THE ARIZONA REPUBLIC
Phoenix, AZ, June 3, 1986

POWERFUL gay rights organizations have found another way to make the general public subservient partners in the depravations of an aberrant lifestyle.

By treating the disease AIDS as a civil rights issue instead of a public health threat, efforts to protect the population at large from the spread of the deadly virus have been thwarted.

Now, under legislation passed in California and Wisconsin — six more states are considering similar measures — and, most recently, the District of Columbia, the public will be required, in addition to tax-supported treatment, to bear private insurance costs of AIDS.

Under the new D.C. law, the most sweeping measure passed to date, private insurers are prohibited from denying life or health coverage to people who test positive for exposure to acquired immune deficiency syndrome.

In addition, the law stipulates that insurance companies cannot even charge, during a five-year "grace" period, higher premiums for a person testing positive for AIDS exposure.

No matter that insurance companies routinely evaluate blood pressure, test for indicators of diseases such as diabetes and cancer, and base acceptance and rates upon such risk factors as age, gender, smoking, occupation and general health conditions.

And never mind that insurance companies must honor policies in force — including group plans that require no testing — and are fully prepared to pay all AIDS-related claims under existing and future contracts, just as claims are paid for other medical conditions.

No, under these new restrictions, the "risks" associated with AIDS are to be borne by the general public, who will subsidize the insurance premiums of AIDS sufferers, the majority of whom choose to take part in "high-risk" activities that lead to the spread of the disease.

Health experts estimate that 500,000 to 1 million people in the United States now carry antibodies for the AIDS virus. The Center for Disease Control has projected a doubling of confirmed AIDS cases by early fall of this year and a further doubling by early 1988. If that trend continues, the total number of confirmed AIDS cases could reach 100,000 by late 1989.

With an insurance industry estimate of an average treatment cost of $140,000 per victim, the public will be required to pay a staggering price for an incurable, yet preventable, disease.

It's a tragic irony that in the name of preventing discrimination, a nation is put at risk by the uncontrolled spread of a deadly disease, while at the same time required to pay dearly, both in terms of human lives and personal income, for that grave mistake.

Richmond Times-Dispatch
Richmond, VA, May 24, 1986

When a person applies for life insurance, the insurance company can require that he be tested for heart disease, diabetes or other potentially life-shortening ailments. It can take into account in setting its premiums whether the person is a heavy smoker or a non-smoker. It can refuse to insure a person deemed to be at high risk, or it can set higher premiums for him.

Risk-based insurance may rankle those denied coverage or favorable rates, but it makes sense. Otherwise, healthy persons would have to pay huge premiums to subsidize the infirm and the short-lived.

Yet in the District of Columbia, there will be one exception to risk-based insurance, if a recent preliminary action by City Council should stick. Council decreed AIDS, a lethal contagion, to be off-limits to risk-assessment by health and life insurers. No D.C. resident who tests positive for exposure to the AIDS virus could be denied insurance. Moreover, for at least the next five years, companies could not charge those who test positive for AIDS higher rates than those who don't.

To be sure, AIDS-antibody-testing is controversial. It only indicates that a person is at some increased — not yet precisely defined — risk of eventually coming down with AIDS. Yet a degree of elevated risk is all that, say, detection of a heart murmur signifies. No one, however, suggests declaring persons with congenital heart defects a protected class.

The D.C. legislation goes far beyond opposition to antibody testing, however; it is, in fact, unprecedented. California and Wisconsin also prohibit insurers from using the AIDS antibody test as a screening device, but they permit the use of other tests that show abnormalities in a person's immune system. The D.C. measure does not. Even more ominously, it would not even allow insurers to use any future test that may reliably detect the presence of the AIDS virus itself.

In effect, the D.C. council has treated AIDS, a sexually transmitted disease, like a civil rights issue rather than a major public health problem. It has decreed that people who have been exposed to the AIDS virus have a right, should they come down with the incurable disease, to have their considerable medical expenses subsidized by non-AIDS-suffering payers of insurance premiums. Council members claimed that overzealous lobbying by the insurance industry backfired. But it equally could be said that intensive lobbying by the D.C. homosexual community, the highest-risk AIDS group, paid off in enactment of legislation that is grossly irresponsible.

The Washington Post
Washington, DC, May 9, 1986

AIDS IS NOW the leading cause of death for men between 21 and 44 in New York City. The epidemic is growing, and no cure or vaccine is yet in sight. The disease is particularly terrible because it strikes young people and is invariably fatal. While scientists continue work to conquer the plague, others must deal with different problems, some of them without precedent, that involve the care and treatment of AIDS patients. Public funds must be spent, not only on research, but also on health and social services for those afflicted. And difficult civil liberties questions must be considered in an area where individual rights and the public health are both at stake.

Next week, the D.C. Council will consider legislation concerning insurance for people who have been exposed to the AIDS virus. The bill—a bad one, we believe—would prohibit insurers from using the results of any test that detects the presence of AIDS antibodies. According to the federal Centers for Disease Control, these tests are extremely accurate and while not everyone with antibdies will contract the disease, just as not every three-pack-a-day smoker will die of lung cancer, those who test positively are at great risk. The bill would even forbid a company representative to ask a person applying for insurance whether he has already taken such a test, and if so, what the test revealed. After five years, upon petition to the superintendent of insurance, and under certain conditions, a company might be granted permission to use these tests, but even then it could

not refuse to sell a policy to someone who tests positive. The company could only ask the superintendent to permit a rate differential.

Do present insurance practices—those that would be changed by this bill—violate the civil liberties of those exposed to AIDS? No. Such patients are now treated in exactly the same way as those at risk from other diseases. Heavy smokers, the obese, those with abnormally high blood pressure or a family history of diabetes are all subject to inquiry about these facts and may have to pay higher premiums for health and life insurance. Insurers understandably want to treat AIDS in the same manner. They are not refusing to cover the disease under existing policies, nor do they plan to base an insurance decision on a single test for antibodies. Insurers simply want to be able to assess the risk they are assuming—as they do for every applicant—and set a price based on objective medical facts.

Rates for health and life insurance are now set on the assumption that people under 35 are not often sick and seldom die of illness. AIDS skews these assumptions, and unless information about the disease is allowed to be taken into consideration, cost shifting on a massive scale will occur. The gay community in this city has done a good job educating the public about the disease, helping to care for the victims and assisting them in coping with employment, landlord-tenant and government benefits problems. The pressure for special treatment from the insurance industry, however, is unreasonable and should be defeated.

The Toronto Star

Toronto, Ont., December 30, 1986

Many Canadian insurance companies have added a test for the AIDS antibody to the series of blood tests some would-be buyers of life insurance policies have to undergo. And if the test is positive, the companies won't insure the applicant's life even though the presence of the AIDS antibody doesn't necessarily lead to the disease.

Federal Health Minister Jake Epp, calling the insurance companies' practice "unfair," is having his department investigate whether it's also discriminatory. That's certainly appropriate. But because insurance companies are subject to provincial as well as federal law, Ontario's superintendent of insurance could also do some investigating.

Buying and selling life insurance are market transactions; no one is compelled to have insurance and those who sell it are entitled to use the best scientific and statistical methods possible to determine the longevity of potential policy-holders. From such assessments, insurance risks are determined and premium rates are set. Smokers, people with high blood pressure or diabetes and alcohol abusers, for example, all pay more for life insurance than do healthy people who buy policies when they're young.

Some people with some types of cancer can't get insurance at all. AIDS is a killer, though little else is known about it, and insurance companies can hardly be questioned for refusing to cover a terminally ill applicant. But the disease has only been known for a few years and it is not clear that everyone who has the antibody — meaning he has been exposed to AIDS — ends up with a full-blown case of the disease.

The superintendent of insurance can ask the companies to prove the causal link — and that the incidence statistically justifies denying life insurance to all carriers of the antibody.

DAYTON DAILY NEWS

Dayton, OH, May 11, 1987

Most AIDS strategies ought to be decided by public-health experts as a health issue, not by politicians as a moral crusade. Of course, lawmakers have to decide how much to allocate to what kinds of AIDS programs — care, prevention, research and regulation of businesses (such as insurance) that play a role in the issue. But generally, health officials — more interested in results than moralizing or politicizing — should have the strongest official, guiding role.

Some proposed political solutions to the problems could backfire. For example, it is easy to advocate widespread, mandatory testing for AIDS. But that could cause high-risk people to flee, especially those who fear they might be punished for negative test results. And even a test clearance doesn't guarantee safety if habits don't change. The current system of testing, for the most part voluntary and confidential, seems to be working OK.

For the time being, it seems wiser to try hard to change people's habits. Public agencies have to push for safety measures, even if that includes advocacy of condoms and clean needles. At the same time, abstinence can be promoted as the safest option — but the government can't afford to be so moralistic that it loses its audience or fails to reach those who are going to mess around anyway.

It is silly to advocate quarantines, since AIDS isn't like other epidemics that have been contained that way. Those diseases were communicable through casual contact, had obvious and debilitating signs throughout the infection, and created sickness fast; AIDS has none of these characteristics.

Politicians have to refrain from popping off because they think they are the ones who have to "do something." For example, Rep. William Dannemeyer, R-Calif, wants to make it a felony to spread the disease knowingly. But that has not been a problem, and if this were a problem, how smart would it be put the person in prison where the disease could not be treated well?

The government needs to stay away from threats and focus on the threat itself: AIDS and a careless, uninformed attitude toward it.

The Washington Times

Washington, DC, March 31, 1987

Most of the talk about AIDS has focused on its devastating human toll, as it should. But another AIDS threat has yet to be addressed sufficiently: socialized medicine boomers, with the acquiescence of even some conservatives, are exploiting AIDS in an effort to expand federal funding and control of health care.

Over the past four years, the feds have spent more than $1 billion to fund AIDS research and education programs, and that's only the beginning. According to the Department of Health and Human Services, AIDS will cost the Medicaid program up to $800 million this year and $1 billion next year. Big bucks, to be sure, but less than a quarter of the direct medical cost of AIDS patients, and the drive is on, not surprisingly, to use this gloomy statistic to harangue the Reagan administration into picking up the rest of the tab.

AIDS funding is "grossly inadequate," says the AFL-CIO's Bert Seidman, who wants Washington to bar insurance companies from "discriminating" against people with the AIDS infection (even if they are far more likely than average to contract the disease).

Rep. Henry Waxman, meanwhile, accuses Ronald Reagan of "stubbornly refusing" to support greater appropriations for AIDS. His solution, few who know his record will be thunderstruck to discover, is national health insurance.

A lot of people who should know better are going along. Former HHS Secretary Richard Schweiker, now president of the American Council of Life Insurance, says the only way to solve the AIDS problem "is with federal resources." And Sen. Orrin Hatch, generally a sound thinker, wants to amend the administration's catastrophic health insurance bill — already catastrophic enough for the taxpayers — to allow Medicare coverage for home health care. These are the moderates. One shudders to think what all this will cost once the Teddy Kennedys and Henry Waxmans perform their surgery on it.

None of this is meant to minimize the horrible suffering AIDS patients must endure. The question is not whether to assist the victims, but how. Far from alleviating the problem, guilt trips and new fiscal time bombs can only serve to render it more intractable still.

USA TODAY

Washington, DC, February 26, 1987

The next time you try to buy an insurance policy, you may be in for a surprise: an AIDS test.

Even as health officials flash the caution light on AIDS testing this week in Atlanta, the nation's insurers are stomping on the accelerator. Increasingly, they are giving tests before issuing policies.

If you test positive for the AIDS virus, 91 percent of the nation's insurers won't insure you, even though carrying the virus does not necessarily mean you will get the disease.

Critics call that discrimination and invasion of privacy.

Insurers respond that if they cannot make decisions based on risk, AIDS — which costs $40,000 to $150,000 per patient — will kill them as surely as it kills their clients. Further, they say, if those at high risk aren't penalized, those at low risk will have to make up the difference.

Insurance industry wailing usually evokes no more sympathy than a fat man griping about the loss of his fifth dessert. But in this case, the industry is right.

Barring insurance testing, as California and the District of Columbia have done, creates protection for AIDS victims that is denied to everyone else.

Smokers pay more for insurance than non-smokers. People with histories of diabetes are subjected to tests and can be refused policies. It would be unfair to treat someone carrying the AIDS virus, with far greater risk of death or disease than either a smoker or a diabetic, differently.

Price and availability of insurance should be based on risk, and the only fair way to evaluate risk is by testing — careful, accurate testing done only by consent.

At the same time, those who test positive need an assurance of privacy. Right now, that assurance is sadly lacking.

Insurance companies routinely swap information through a central clearinghouse, which means the records are not very closely guarded. Laws are needed to impose criminal penalties on companies and individuals who disclose test information to anyone but the patient.

Society must then face up to the question of who will pay to treat this epidemic. Eleven states have already arrived at the same, partial answer: insurance pools for people with high-risk illnesses, much like the long-established pools for high-risk drivers.

Here's how the law works in Illinois: People who are denied insurance are covered by a pool of insurance companies and charged 135 percent of the state's average insurance rate. The money goes into a pool to pay claims, and the state picks up the difference if the money runs out.

Congress is considering legislation to provide tax incentives for such pools. It should pass that legislation.

For those who are too poor to pay the pool premiums, we will all pay the cost through Medicaid, as we should.

Meanwhile, being asked to take an AIDS test should act like a sharp jab in the ribs, reminding us that AIDS is no longer only a problem for gays and drug users. It is a problem for us all. That problem is as close as the insurance policy in your desk drawer.

WORCESTER TELEGRAM

Worcester, MA, June 10, 1987

The national debate over AIDS has quite properly focused on questions of prevention, detection and finding a cure. A less exalted — but no less controversial — question is: Who will pay for the billions of dollars in medical care and other costs of the epidemic?

A new study by Rand Corp. indicates the nation's bill for treating patients with acquired immune deficiency syndrome could exceed $37 billion for the five-year period from now to mid-1991. Researchers at the West Coast think tank estimate that AIDS will consume about 1 percent of total national health spending and 3 percent of Medicaid payments during the period.

One aspect of the cost debate is of particular interest in Massachusetts. For the past two years, gay-rights groups have lobbied for legislation that would bar Bay State insurance companies from testing prospective customers to see if they have AIDS.

Senate Bill 1629 — now tied up in study committee and unlikely to be acted upon this year — is a bad idea. It would undermine a bedrock principle of insurance practice. It is the right of insurers to charge higher premiums to customers with medical conditions that increase the chance they will become ill or die young — or to refuse insurance where early death is a high probability.

Such premium surcharges are a vital part of insurance practice. They ensure that customers with average health risks will not pay unfairly high premiums to subsidize clients with pre-existing conditions that put them in a high-risk category. Prospective insurance customers are routinely screened for heart disease and diabetes. Most insurers do not test routinely for AIDS infection, but they properly reserve their right to do so before approving the sale of large policies to people in high-risk groups.

Banning AIDS screening would enable a person infected with the disease to buy large amounts of insurance or make large increases in existing coverage. Insurers say the practice is not uncommon now and might become widespread if AIDS screening were banned.

AIDS is invariably fatal, and insurers now suspect that virtually everyone infected with the virus may eventually die of AIDS-related complications. Consequently, the payout on life insurance policies is a near certainty — not a risk — and the cost will be borne by other policyholders.

The number of payments in AIDS deaths is relatively small now, although it is increasing rapidly. In 1985, State Mutual Life Assurance Co. of America paid on policies of three AIDS victims; the number jumped to 26 last year. With an estimated 1.5 million to 2.5 million people already infected, the spiral is bound to continue.

Although the screening ban proposed in the Senate bill is clearly undesirable, advocacy groups lobbying for it do have legitimate concerns that must be answered, including questions about the accuracy of the current tests. However, improvements in testing in the past year or so are making that a matter of diminishing concern.

Another fear concerns the possibility of public disclosure. The stigma attached to AIDS stems from the fact that it usually is contracted through homosexual acts and the sharing of infected needles by intravenous drug users. Disclosure could have serious consequences, particularly in the victim's place of employment. However, the insurance industry correctly points out that it routinely handles highly sensitive information about its customers and has a good track record for maintaining confidentiality.

Customers who buy insurance policies should not be targeted for an additional financial burden created by one high-risk group. Instead of lobbying for shortsighted plans like the proposed screening ban, advocacy groups should put more effort into developing a long-term national strategy for coping with AIDS and AIDS-related costs.

THE SUN

Baltimore, MD, April 9, 1987

After considerable wrangling, Social Security officials decided in 1983 to classify AIDS as a disability, providing victims with benefits. It was a humane decision, but only half a promise.

While disability payments provide additional income, critical Medicare coverage does not kick in for two years after eligibility. Most AIDS patients don't live that long. During the 24-month waiting period, the majority "spend down" — depleting assets and savings for treatment. That often leaves spouses or family members destitute.

The government has made exceptions for similar medical emergencies. Medicare, for example, routinely pays for dialysis — regardless of the patient's financial status. Now a House bill would do the same for AIDS patients. It would waive the 24-month waiting period. Thus, a person would be eligible for Medicare benefits when he or she qualified for disability income — presumably at the time AIDS is diagnosed.

The bill's underlying intent is on target, but the cost almost certainly will be a political stumbling block. Estimates on the average cost of caring for an AIDS patient vary widely — from $40,000 a year to over $100,000. With 17,000 to 18,000 diagnosed AIDS cases now, and the number expected to soar, passing such a measure without providing the enabling funds would be a superficial response to a complex issue. And entirely irresponsible from a budgetary standpoint.

Debate is ongoing in both the House and Senate about ways to expand the catastrophic health care proposal proffered by Health and Human Services Secretary Dr. Otis Bowen. So far, none of the alternatives includes AIDS in its definition of catastrophic illness.

From both an emotional and financial perspective, that is precisely where it belongs. Federal coverage for AIDS would be far more feasible if the costs were integrated into more expansive health-care coverage. Implementing such a plan should be a legislative health care priority. The only alternative is to sentence victims and their families to impoverishment and to doom some states to intolerable Medicaid burdens. A responsible federal government can do neither.

Supreme Court Upholds Georgia Sodomy Law

The Supreme Court June 30, 1986 refused to extend the right of privacy inherent in the Constitution to homosexual activity and newspaper editorialists around the nation were quick to draw a connection between the ruling and AIDS which is most contracted through sodomy. The court upheld, by a 5-4 vote, a Georgia law that made sodomy a crime, punishable by as long as 20 years in prison. "We are quite unwilling," Justice Byron R. White said in the majority opinion, to assert "a fundamental right to engage in homosexual sodomy." Justice Harry A. Blackmun, in a heated dissent, said the case was not about whether there was a fundamental right to engage in homosexual sodomy but "about 'the most comprehensive of rights, and the right most valued by civilized men,' namely, 'the right to be let alone.' The right of an individual to conduct intimate relationships in the intimacy of his or her home seems to me to be the heart of the Constitution's protection of privacy," Blackmun said. Although the Constitution contained no specific mention of a right to privacy, the Supreme Court had taken a stand since 1965 that it was implicit in the Bill Of Rights. Thus a right of personal privacy had been recognized for married couples in a 1965 ruling. A woman's right to abortion also was based on the right of privacy. But the court ruled out any such right in this case. "Any claim...that any kind of private sexual conduct between consenting adults is constitutionally insulated from state proscription is unsupportable," White said. The privacy right did not "reach so far," he said.

The opinion rested mainly on the established precedent of state laws making sodomy illegal—from the 13 original states in 1791, when the Bill of Rights was ratified, to 1986, when 23 other states had laws similar to Georgia's outlawing sodomy. Blackmun said the long history of antisodomy laws did not mean that the laws were proper or the court should accept them. The court had held in other cases, he said, "that mere public intolerance or animosity cannot constitutionally justify the deprivation of a person's physical liberty." Actually, the Georgia law covered heterosexual sodomy as well as homosexual sodomy, a fact pointed out by Blackmun. The court's opinion did not rule out enforcement of the sodomy laws in Georgia and most other states against heterosexual activity. But this had not been the practice in the past.

The Record

Hackensack, NJ, July 2, 1986

In 1969, police raided a homosexual social club in Greenwich Village called the Stonewall. It was no different from anything they had done scores of times before. They would simply bust in, arrest the proprietor, disperse the patrons, and padlock the door. No rough stuff, nothing dangerous, just a clear message that the authorities would not sit idly by and allow their city to degenerate into a Sodom-on-the-Hudson.

But this time, instead of accepting their fate meekly as they had so many times before, the gays rebelled. After years of being shoved around by cops, sidewalk preachers, and street-corner John Waynes, they shoved back. For two nights running, they threw bottles and stones and chalked "gay power" on the walls. The ferocity of the protest astonished the police and, for that matter, probably astonished the gays as well. In hindsight, Stonewall can be seen as a turning point in American social history. Not only was it the birth of the gay-rights movement; it was an affirmation, since widely accepted throughout society, that the sexual practices of consenting adults are their own business. The job of the police is to prevent crime and guard the public's safety, not to go snooping in bedrooms.

This week we had another turning point — in the opposite direction. By the narrowest of margins, the Supreme Court upheld a Georgia state law forbidding "sodomy" between consenting adult homosexuals. Not merely is it the state's job to "establish justice, insure domestic tranquility, provide for the common defense," in the language of the Constitution; Justices White, Burger, Powell, Rehnquist, and O'Connor have now told the states that they're free to supervise bedroom intimacies. From Atlanta to Boston, Trenton to Sacramento, legislatures may now draw up rules as to who may engage in sex and how they may do it.

What next? State laws on how often and in what position? A statute relegating sex to certain hours of the late evening? Perhaps an official handbook on sexual rules and regulations for Atlanta and portions of adjacent De Kalb County? Of more immediate concern, if gay sex is illegal in Georgia, can the authorities there now go after gay-bar owners for promoting a criminal conspiracy?

Seventeen years after Stonewall, it seems, we can expect more such raids, this time with the approval of the U.S. Supreme Court. You'd think that if the right of privacy means anything, it is the right to engage in consensual sex in the confines of one's home. But now the Supreme Court says no. It is a giant step backward.

THE INDIANAPOLIS NEWS
Indianapolis, IN, July 5, 1986

Indiana once had a sodomy law on its books that was similar to the Georgia law that the U.S. Supreme Court narrowly upheld earlier this week.

In its wisdom, the Indiana General Assembly repealed that law more than a decade ago. One of the incidents that led to the sentiment to repeal the law was the filing of criminal charges by a disgruntled wife against her husband, charging him with committing sodomy on her.

Legislators concluded that the state had no business in bedrooms of private individuals, refereeing their most intimate conduct.

From a strict constructionist point of view, the Supreme Court's 5-4 refusal to strike down archaic sodomy laws in Georgia and 23 other states is understandable.

As noted in the majority opinion, until the 1960s every state had an anti-sodomy law on its books; thus, there can be no claim that such statutes violate a traditional right to privacy. Furthermore, the U.S. Constitution does not expressly grant a right to privacy.

But clearly, a presumption of privacy permeates the Constitution.

As former Justice Louis D. Brandeis wrote many years ago, the right to be left alone is perhaps "the most comprehensive of rights and the right most valued by civilized men."

Another reason why sodomy laws should be stricken from the books has to do with selective enforcement of such laws.

According to various surveys, nearly 80 percent of all adults have at one time or another violated such strictures. Yet, virtually no one is ever prosecuted.

In Georgia, there had not been a prosecution for violation of the law in the last half century. The state even declined to pursue its prosecution of the individual whose arrest instigated the lawsuit challenging the sodomy statute.

And, finally, the Supreme Court would do well to practice a little consistency.

Only a few weeks ago the court struck down another state statute that required physicians to read a fairly innocuous statement about abortion procedures and alternatives to abortions to women seeking to undergo an abortion. The court ruled that such a requirement violated a woman's right to privacy.

How the court can square that decision with the reasoning in the Georgia case is a mystery.

THE SACRAMENTO BEE
Sacramento, CA, July 3, 1986

The Supreme Court's narrow decision to uphold Georgia's sodomy law is hardly surprising. This is not a court prone to assert socially controversial rights, much less open new constitutional territory. Nor, to be fair, was it an easy decision to make. The issue here, after all, was not the wisdom of a law forbidding oral or anal sex between consenting adults, but the question of whether such conduct — conduct offensive to many people — is nonetheless constitutionally protected in the privacy of one's own home.

But that makes the decision no less frustrating — frustrating not only because it's wrong but because it leaves so many other issues unresolved. The court's majority dwelt on the homosexual aspects of the Georgia law: It was a homosexual, Michael Hardwick, who brought the case, and Justice White, in his lead opinion, chose to emphasize again and again that none of its previous privacy decisions — in cases involving contraception and abortion, for example — "bears any resemblance to the claimed constitutional right of homosexuals to engage in acts of sodomy that is asserted in this case."

But the Georgia law does not single out homosexuals, nor, in fairness, could it really do so. It simply defines the act. As Justice Blackmun pointed out in his dissent, "The sex or status of the persons who engage in the act is irrelevant." Its targets, indeed, seem to have included both heterosexual and homosexual conduct. Hardwick's claim that the law involves an unconstitutional intrusion into his privacy, therefore, "does not depend in any way on his sexual orientation."

Which is to say that the law could be applied to anyone, and thus opens what is probably a majority of sexually active adults to the danger of prosecution. The fact that such laws are probably used selectively — against homosexuals in most cases, against other unpopular or vulnerable individuals in others — doesn't mitigate that danger. On the contrary, it makes enforcement of such statutes all the more invidious.

The real issue in this case, therefore, is not homosexual sodomy but, as Justice Blackmun said, about the right to be let alone. The right is essential because it constitutes "a central part of an individual life . . . The fact that individuals define themselves in a significant way through their intimate sexual relationships with others suggests, in a nation as diverse as ours, that there may be many 'right' ways of conducting those relationships, and that much of the rightness of a relationship will come from the freedom an individual has to choose the form and nature of these intensely personal bonds."

The majority in this case argues that if sodomy is constitutionally protected, then incest must be, too. But that analogy is patently false: Incest and the acts prohibited by the Georgia law don't fall into the same moral, political or medical categories. Where intimate sexual relationships are conducted in private and where they carry with them no greater social hazard, as incest surely would, the attempt of the state to interfere creates many more dangers — dangers to individuals, dangers of social controversy — than it prevents. The Hardwick decision ends a generation that enlarged the right of privacy and gave new heart to official tolerance in America. The eye of the state is back in the bedroom.

The Kansas City Times
Kansas City, MO, July 2, 1986

The Supreme Court has made a pronouncement in an area, that of human intimacy, which it has no business regulating. Neither majority behavior, nor the existence of old local laws, nor religious dictates is adequate defense for institutionalizing discrimination.

Now, unless state and municipal leaders are courageous in separating civil rights from sexual behavior through statute and ordinance, the fair treatment of homosexuals — and eventually, perhaps, heterosexuals — is at risk of moving backward.

If the Supreme Court ruling on homosexual conduct is to be applied narrowly and strictly to that minority in this society, such people may well face increased bias on many sides, from employment to housing. This upholding of the Georgia sodomy law can, at the least, lend its flavor to every public dealing with gays.

If the ruling is, however, as dissenting Justice Harry A. Blackmun wrote, not at all about homosexual sodomy but about privacy and people's right to be different, it is a sad Independence Day prelude.

Undoubtedly, justification for the court interpretation will be found on many sides by those who view intimacy between people of the same sex as abhorrent. What is anathema to the court will carry weight in ostracizing AIDS sufferers.

Moreover, thoughtful Americans will find more questions than solutions in this decision. Is similar heterosexual practice protected under constitutional guarantees when homosexual practice is not? Many state laws, including Georgia's, say it isn't. What other areas presumed to be personal might next be raised to the public stage? If intimacy and the home are not private, what is?

In its anxiety to avoid breaking new ground, or "discover new fundamental rights" in the Constitution, the court apparently has made exactly the mighty leap it said it wanted to avoid.

In upholding Georgia's way, the high court found no constitutional protection for this conduct by homosexuals. The law was challenged as an intrusion into individuals' right to privacy.

How are these lawbreakers to be discovered and charged? There is, after all, a Fourth Amendment in the Bill of Rights. It says that "The right of people to be secure in their persons, houses, papers and effects, against unreasonable searches and seizures, shall not be violated. . . ." Surely the Constitution takes precedence over the Georgia Legislature's notion as to what is immoral and therefore a crime.

THE COMMERCIAL APPEAL
Memphis, TN, July 11, 1986

FIVE members of the Supreme Court have ruled that states may punish homosexual conduct in the bedroom as a crime; four say the decision intrudes on privacy.

That division may be fairly close to the general split of public opinion on the issue, even though sex between persons of the same gender was once universally condemned by law throughout the United States. Now, 24 states and the District of Columbia still have laws against homosexual conduct, while 26 states have moved away from them.

IT IS UNCLEAR how the court majority's opinion affects certain sexual practices between consenting heterosexual couples.

The ruling in a Georgia case obviously was intended to apply to homosexual conduct. But the state law that the court upheld prohibits sodomy without reference to whether it is between homosexuals or heterosexuals.

In any event, the decision is unlikely to change sexual practices in the privacy of American bedrooms to any appreciable degree. Police will not be any more inclined now to peep into windows to see what sort of activity is going on than they were before.

In fact, the Georgia case came before the court largely by accident. The homosexual who challenged the law was arrested after a police officer saw him having sexual relations in his bedroom with another man when the officer came to serve a warrant on an unrelated legal matter.

What would be unfortunate is if the Supreme Court's action leads to a round of homosexual bashing and a circumscription of civil rights for a segment of the population whose sexual preferences are different from the norm. To some extent this is already happening because of the AIDS scare.

The majority opinion, written by Justice Byron White, said no judgment was being made on whether state laws against sodomy are wise or desirable. What White said the majority wanted to make clear is that the Constitution does not provide a fundamental right to engage in homosexual sodomy.

WRITING FOR the four dissenting members, Justice Harry Blackmun said that the majority misread what the case was about. He said the case is about "the most comprehensive of rights and the most valued by civilized men" — "the right to be let alone."

Recognizing that people can differ on such an emotional issue, we are inclined to believe that Justice Blackmun is on the better track. Sexual activities between consenting adults in the privacy of the bedroom should not be the government's concern.

The Chattanooga Times

Chattanooga, TN, July 5, 1986

The Supreme Court, in a bitterly divided 5-to-4 vote, has upheld a Georgia law that declares sodomy between consenting adults a crime. But the ruling rests on a shaky, if not fatally narrow, premise: that "the respondent (the original plaintiff in this case) would have us announce . . . a fundamental right to engage in homosexual sodomy." That was not the issue in this case at all. As Justice Harry Blackmun wrote in an eloquent dissent, quoting the late Justice Louis Brandeis from an earlier case, the litigation decided Monday is about "the most comprehensive of rights and the most valued by civilized men," namely "the right to be left alone."

It is easy, but intellectually lazy, to use this decision as a vehicle for condemning the practice of sodomy, which as defined by the Georgia law involved both oral and anal sex. But condemnation of such practices breaks no new ground. Many religions, including Judaism and Christianity, prohibit sexual relations between members of the same sex as violations of divine law. Such prohibitions still stand despite the seemingly increased prevalence of homosexuality.

But as Justice Blackmun pointed out, the Georgia law at issue does not address itself solely to homosexual activity; the language is broad enough to encompass such activity even if it is engaged in by a heterosexual couple. In that regard, therefore, the real issue becomes the extent to which a state can regulate private and intensely personal actions among adults. It is irrelevant that states are unlikely to set up "bedroom patrols" to search for instances of illegal sexual behavior. The point is that the court has dramatically restricted the rights of privacy it has previously enunciated — in cases involving decisions, such as contraception, that only individuals can make, and in cases involving certain places without regard for particular activities engaged in by the occupants.

Georgia argued that its law should be upheld because the actions it prohibits have been condemned as "immoral" for centuries. But the mere fact that a majority of society condemns an essentially *victimless* act, and has done so for years, does not necessarily mean that the majority can impose that view on others, even if the view is rooted in a religious base. Justice Blackmun argues persuasively that"the legitimacy of secular legislation depends instead on whether the state can advance some justification for its law beyond its conformity to religious doctrine." And later: "A state can no more punish private behavior because of religious intolerance than it can punish such behavior because of racial animus."

The state's legitimate right to protect public sensibilities justifies laws barring sexual activities in public places. Similarly, it has the right to protect individuals, particularly minors, from actions committed in privacy, even in the home, such as sexual abuse of children. But there is a difference between those responsibilities, and attempts by the state to enforce laws against persons who happen not to accept the values of a majority of society.

Since 1961, 26 states have repealed laws prohibiting homosexual acts of the sort included in the Georgia law. Does that mean the residents of those states approve of such conduct? Of course not. It simply means they saw no point in retaining unenforceable laws and, more important, that the state has more important things to do than attempt to regulate what consenting adults do in private. The Supreme Court's decision is a regrettable step backward in the protection of privacy.

THE SAGINAW NEWS

Saginaw, MI, July 7, 1986

Nowhere is a right to privacy mentioned in the U.S. Constitution. But a Supreme Court majority still reasons from those grounds in affirming, for instance, a woman's right to abortion.

Within the broad scope of the document, justices can usually find what they choose to find.

Last week Justice Byron White chose to be blind to the implications of his opinion upholding anti-sodomy laws in Georgia, and thus in Michigan and 22 other states.

Most immediately, the 5-4 decision has brought fears that the decision could validate, even encourage, campaigns of repression against homosexuals.

Gays have cause for concern. A Justice Department ruling appears to allow employers to fire homosexuals virtually at will. In California, a LaRouchite ballot initiative would authorize the quarantine of gays. Now, if legislatures can outlaw homosexual behavior, why not homosexuals?

Other adults, though, should not dismiss the ruling as of no concern to them. As an American Bar Association analysis stressed, "This is much more than a homosexual rights case. At stake is the question of how far a state can regulate all private, consensual, adult sexual behavior and whether a bedroom is safer from police intrusion than a bar room or the street."

No, it isn't, replied the court.

Over the past 60 years, the justices had created a "zone of privacy" where government cannot go without compelling cause. The only cause cited by Georgia was that of "traditions and moral values."

But whose morality? What "tradition" can be forced on people who do not share it? Whose business is it, anyway, what adults do in their own homes — or, for that matter, in a private camp?

The argument, as the ABA summed up, comes down to "whether, in a free and pluralistic society, private morality is to be determined by the majority or the individual."

That's why the decision involves more than sodomy laws. Those are hardly ever enforced anyway. Even the Georgia plaintiff was never prosecuted. The bedroom police are not yet at the door. But if this case signals a new court direction, then it means any personal — and private — adult behavior could be banned.

The court majority may not intend such a broad reading of this ruling. But the Georgia law did not distinguish betwen gays and others. Neither do Michigan's related statutes.

The high court's verdict warns once again that restrictions against one group, no matter how despised, can limit the rights of all. And what's at stake here is nothing less fundamental than, as Justice Harry Blackmun said in dissent, "the right to be let alone." If the other justices look hard enough, they'll find that, too, is in the tradition of the Constitution.

ST. LOUIS POST-DISPATCH

St. Louis, MO, July 2, 1986

The U.S. Supreme Court's decision upholding a Georgia sodomy law is appalling for what it does to the right of privacy, which the high court over many years has been expanding. Twenty-three states besides Georgia — including Missouri — have sodomy laws, some of them applying to heterosexual as well as homosexual conduct. But for the most part, they are not enforced, because they are unenforceable without government intrusion into the bedroom. Now the Supreme Court has in effect given government a license to invade homes and police private morals.

As Justice Blackmun said for the dissenters in the 5-4 decision, the ruling is an attack on the most fundamental right of all — the right to be let alone. Besides threatening the right of privacy, the decision will help to legitimize discrimination against homosexuals. As one gay rights spokesman suggested, courts will find it easier to say that a homosexual parent is unfit to gain custody of a child, or employers will say they don't want to hire would-be criminals.

In holding that consenting adults have no right to private homosexual conduct, the Supreme Court was dealing with a case involving conduct between two males. But the sweeping language of the decision indicated that states can also police heterosexual sodomy — a practice that, however it may be condemned morally, simply cannot be controlled by government except in a police state. The upshot of the decision is likely to be that prosecutors and police will use sodomy laws to hunt selectively for unpopular groups, namely homosexuals.

Since 1961, when all 50 states had outlawed homosexual acts, 26 states, by legislation or court decision, have legitimized such conduct between consenting adults. The Supreme Court has turned back the clock on the right of privacy.

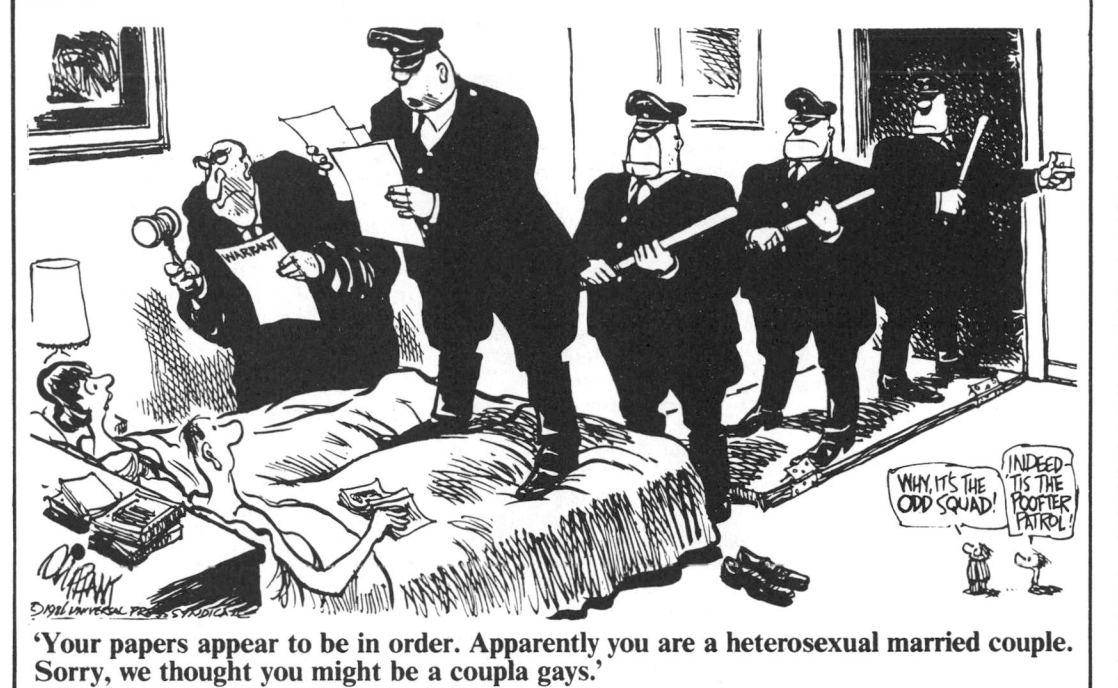

'Your papers appear to be in order. Apparently you are a heterosexual married couple. Sorry, we thought you might be a coupla gays.'

THE PLAIN DEALER

Cleveland, OH, July 3, 1986

Why did Supreme Court Chief Justice Warren Burger vote to reject a homosexual's challenge to the constitutionality of a Georgia state law against sodomy? Because, in part, "Homosexual sodomy was a capital crime under Roman law." That's an interesting fact, and you might think that any reference to "capital crime" is appropriate to a court that upholds the death penalty. But if modern justice is to find literal precedent in ancient Rome, then it will tolerate slavery, incest, the appointment of a horse to the Senate and the use of the White House as a brothel. During the reign of Caligula, the laws of ancient Rome tolerated all of that and worse.

Obviously, the issue of homosexual sodomy requires judicial awareness that is superior to that of demented Roman emperors. So Burger updates his precedents, writing that the 18th century English jurist William Blackstone described homosexual sodomy "as an offense of 'deeper malignity' than rape." That's another interesting fact, although the idea that any sexual act between consenting adults is less tolerable than rape makes you wonder how the English Reformation ever got off the ground.

Burger's point is that 2,000 years of moral teachings cannot be ignored. But it's not the job of modern law to affirm history. And it's not the job of the Supreme Court to rely on fusty, antiquated precedents to establish and defend modern rights. That's especially the case in Georgia, where the law against sodomy (by which is meant either oral or anal intercourse) appears to be selectively enforced only against homosexuals.

In this case, the Georgia law was challenged on the grounds that it violates the constitutional right of privacy. Five Supreme Court justices rejected that argument even though a vast body of recent legal precedent supports it. Like Burger, the majority opinion (his was separate yet consenting) mentioned history: "Proscriptions against (homosexual sodomy) have ancient roots." But more remarkably, the majority ruled that the Georgia

case is not buttressed by other rulings that pertain to privacy and sexual conduct, specifically because even consenting homosexual activity is not connected to "family, marriage or procreation." The lack of such a connection made the court "unwilling" to establish "a fundamental right to engage in homosexual activity."

"Family, marriage and procreation" have nothing to do with private sexual activities between consenting adults. Had the court upheld the challenge, then it might have established a precedent for striking down laws exclusively based on homophobic prejudice. But the Georgia law applies equally to heterosexuals. Married couples can also be prosecuted for "sodomy," although by the Supreme Court's "family" standard, such activity would be constitutionally protected. The double standard is very clear, and so, apparently, is its genesis: the willingness of five Supreme Court justices to accept that homosexuals do not deserve the rights afforded to heterosexuals.

That narrow mindset does indeed justify the invocation of laws enacted by ancient Rome and 18th-century English puritanism. But it is antithetical both to the legal progress that the Constitution symbolizes and to the advancing sophistication of society. It's not likely that this decision will result in the reinstatement of anti-sodomy laws in the 26 states, including Ohio, that have abolished them. But it will slow the decriminalization of private sexual acts between consenting adults.

The court accepts that de-evolution of social standards because it fears getting too far ahead of society. Yet again, it's the court's job to keep the Constitution vibrant. The justices might not want to be made "vulnerable" by decisions that arouse political distress and subsequent efforts to stack the court. That obviously would undercut its credibility. But interpreting Supreme Court decisions is a popular political activity regardless of whether the rulings are viewed as liberal or conservative. To say that vulnerability is a legitimate reason for constitutional restraint is as feckless as citing ancient Rome as an appropriate model of morality.

Wisconsin
State Journal
Madison, WI
July 2, 1986

Five of the nine members of the U.S. Supreme Court, the "conservative majority," have invited themselves into America's bedrooms. That is the bottom line in the court's 5-4 ruling that the Constitution does not protect private homosexual relations between consenting adults, even in their own homes.

The ruling is as spectacularly short-sighted as it is a corruption of the true spirit of conservatism, which in the days before the rise of the "New Right," used to hold sacred the idea that government should not meddle in personal practices that do not adversely affect others.

The court ruled a Georgia antisodomy law could be used to criminally prosecute homosexual conduct between men or women. Besides Georgia, the ruling could affect 24 other states where homosexual sodomy is a crime.

In Wisconsin, sexual acts between consenting adults in private are legal. Former Gov. Lee Dreyfus, a Republican and a conservative in the traditional sense, signed that act into law in 1982 with the following comment:

"As one who believes in the fundamental Republican principle that government should have a very restricted involvement in people's private and personal lives, I feel strongly about governmentally sanctioned inquiries into an individual's thoughts, beliefs and feelings."

Whatever happened to the notion that laws must be enforceable in order to be effective? It seems unlikely even Georgia will initiate "bedroom raids" in search of homosexual conduct, although the case that came before the Supreme Court did begin with just such an arrest.

The court ruling also assumes people choose to be gay or straight, when in fact, medical research indicates people have little or no control over their sexual preferences. It is as fundamental as being born black, blond or left-handed.

Would the nation's highest court rule in favor of a law that criminalizes left-handedness in the privacy of the home? We don't think so.

Those who are concerned about the growing visibility of homosexuality in America should not draw much comfort in the court's decision. It is possible gay people will migrate from states like Georgia to "safe" states or cities, thus swelling the size of gay communities in cities like San Francisco, New York or Madison.

"Georgia does not sound too peachy today," one prominent member of Madison's gay community said.

If there is a positive side to the court's ruling, it is the debate over sodomy laws will be shifted to the legislatures of the various states. Conservatives still believe in states' rights, don't they?

FORT WORTH STAR-TELEGRAM

Fort Worth, TX, July 7, 1986

Proponents of states' rights should be pleased with three decisions handed down last week by the U.S. Supreme Court. In successive rulings, the court held that:

● An Illinois law confining to a state institution a person ruled as being sexually dangerous does not violate the Fifth Amendment guarantee against forced self-incrimination.

● A Puerto Rican law banning advertising of gambling does not violate free speech protections of the Constitution.

● A Georgia law prohibiting sodomy does not violate the constitutional right of privacy.

In each of the three cases, the Supreme Court is returning some of the authority to legislate the safety and well-being of the people where it belongs — at the state level. Too much power has been concentrated in recent years in Washington, and this recent trend by the highest court of the land is a welcome move.

In the Illinois case (about half the states have similar laws), the court held that the Fifth Amendment guarantee does not apply because the state law is aimed at treatment, not punishment. The case involved a man who was declared sexually dangerous after two psychiatrists testified, based on the man's statements to them, that he was mentally ill and had criminal propensities to commit sexual assaults.

In the Puerto Rican case, the court held that states may ban advertisements for products that have "serious harmful effects." The specific case involved a Puerto Rican ban on gambling ads, but some lawyers said the decision appears to clear the way for legislation banning tobacco advertising at the state level.

By upholding a Georgia law making it a crime for anyone, whether heterosexual or homosexual, to participate in sodomy, the Supreme Court probably dashed the hopes of homosexuals in Texas to overturn a similar law in this state. The Texas law was ruled unconstitutional by a federal judge last year, but the U.S. Court of Appeals reversed that judgment, upholding the right of the state to legislate against such practices.

These rulings, we believe, are proper because, under our system, certain governmental functions work better when they are carried out at the local level. There are certain constitutional functions that must be handled at the national level — such as the national defense. But other matters that generally touch on our day-to-day lives can best be regulated at the local level.

Should some states revert to past practices and begin interfering with citizens' basic constitutional rights, the Supreme Court is still there to deal with such matters.

The Des Moines Register

Des Moines, IA, July 3, 1986

The Supreme Court seems to have slipped away from its constitutional moorings and is hopelessly adrift on the question of Americans' right to privacy.

Not three weeks after announcing a sweeping reaffirmation that a woman's right of privacy to choose abortion is constitutionally sacrosanct, the court has ruled that it's proper for a state to outlaw certain sexual acts between consenting adults in the privacy of their own bedrooms.

The court took great pains in earlier decisions to carve out a "private sphere of individual liberty" that is to be kept "largely beyond the reach of government." But now the court is willing to allow that sphere of individual liberty to be breached by the government when it involves sexual acts judged immoral by the state.

The majority — Byron White, Warren Burger, William Rehnquist, Lewis Powell and Sandra Day O'Connor — reached back to everything from Roman law, Judeo-Christian tradition and English common law to statutes in dozens of states to support the contention that sodomy has long been regarded immoral and illegal. The justices forgot only to consult the Constitution.

It is true that certain sex acts, including homosexual sodomy as defined in the Georgia statute, are considered immoral by many if not the majority of Americans. But the Constitution is nothing if not a solid wall against the majority's imposing its moral judgments on the minority.

Provided there are no victims, and the sexual act is performed in the privacy of the home, what possible interest does the government have in the matter?

In his dissenting opinion, Justice Harry Blackmun points out that "what the court really has refused to recognize is the fundamental interest all individuals have in controlling the nature of their intimate associations with others."

The decision is seen by homosexual-rights groups as a setback for their cause, but it also leaves the door open to prosecution of anyone, homosexual or heterosexual, for sexual acts declared illegal by states. It must thus be seen as a disappointing setback for the right of privacy of all Americans.

Detroit Free Press

Detroit, MI, July 2, 1986

In a signal victory for racial justice and the conscience of the nation, the U.S. Supreme Court has solidly endorsed the use of affirmative-action quotas to remedy job discrimination.

The ruling is a powerful setback for President Reagan's five-year assault on the discrimination correctives that became standard in the Sixties and Seventies. Mr. Reagan and his operatives in the Justice Department have argued that numerical hiring goals and timetables discriminate against white job- and promotion-seekers and mustn't be invoked except in behalf of individual minority applicants who can prove they were victims of deliberate discrimination. William Bradford Reynolds, the ultraconservative assistant attorney-general for civil rights, has called hiring quotas "morally wrong."

Writing for the majority, Associate Justice William J. Brennan specifically rejected those views. Upholding court-imposed quotas in cases involving a New York-New Jersey construction union and the Cleveland fire department, he wrote that race-conscious remedies are appropriate where "an employer or labor union has engaged in persistent or egregious discrimination, or where necessary to dissipate the lingering effects of pervasive discrimination." Justice Brennan's point is that such discrimination *can't* be remedied without temporary recourse to reverse discrimination — the tool called affirmative action.

These rulings reverse the drift of the court in recent major decisions. In 1984, the court upheld layoffs of minority workers hired under quota systems. It said, illogically, that the numerical goals could be applied to hiring but not to layoffs. That decision destroyed a minority-hiring plan designed by a federal judge for Newark's virtually all-white police force. The 1984 ruling was broadened in a similar case in May of this year.

While preserving the central goal of minority access to jobs, Justice Brennan tried to answer the legitimate concerns of white workers displaced in the remedial process. He suggested, for example, that numerical hiring goals be reserved for situations in which less disruptive remedies — voluntary compliance, special training courses for minorities, and minority-recruitment campaigns — haven't worked.

The decisions were hailed by rights activists and by Clarence Thomas, chairman of the federal Equal Employment Opportunity Commission. They may lend some comfort to Mr. Thomas, who has been forced by Mr. Reagan to abandon hiring goals in discrimination cases. The decisions may give more direct help to Labor Secretary William Brock, who is resisting presidential directives to drop enforcement of nondiscrimination pledges by federal contractors. Perhaps the high-court ruling will persuade the White House to retreat from this unworthy campaign.

In the midst of victory, however, are the seeds of trouble. Leading the dissents on both decisions was Justice William Rehnquist, who is slated to head the court when Chief Justice Warren Burger retires at the end of this term. Justice Rehnquist insists that Congress intended quotas only to remedy proven discrimination, not as a means to achieve racial balance. The vote margins were narrow. Three justices dissented in the Cleveland case, which reserves half of all fire-department promotions for qualified minorities. Four dissented in the union case, which upheld a 29 percent minority membership goal imposed by a lower court on the Sheet Metal Workers. Analysts have suggested that Mr. Rehnquist will be a much stronger chief justice than Mr. Burger, determined to set a clear course for the court stamped with his own conservative views. That bodes ill for millions of undertrained and underemployed minority citizens.

The Detroit News

Detroit, MI, July 9, 1986

The U.S. Supreme Court infuriated gays, the American Civil Liberties Union, and a host of moral relativists last week when it decided not to overturn a Georgia law that makes oral and anal sex illegal, and refused this week to overturn a Texas statute that forbids such acts among homosexuals. At the same time, fundamentalists like the Rev. Jerry Falwell congratulated the court on helping them keep America morally pure.

The angry gays and the happy Bible-thumpers got the issue all wrong. The court did nothing cataclysmic. It rejected lawyers' attempts to goad it into rewriting state codes, and protected states' rights to regulate certain types of behavior. In the Georgia case, Bowers vs. Hardwick, a police officer was serving a subpoena to Michael Hardwick, who had failed to appear in court to answer charges of public drunkenness. After being admitted to Mr. Hardwick's residence, the officer found Mr. Hardwick and a male friend *in flagrante*. The officer served the subpoena and then arrested the men for violating the state's sodomy statute. Michael Hardwick sued, arguing that the Constitution protected his right to engage in homosexual acts.

The court refused to accept arguments that homosexual behavior is protected by the First Amendment right of free speech, the Eighth Amendment prohibition against cruel and unusual punishment, the Ninth Amendment prohibition against denying or disparaging rights retained by the people, the 14th Amendment's equal protection right, or the court-manufactured right of "privacy," which began as a right to use contraceptives, and later was expanded to protect the "right" to an abortion. A majority of the justices instead noted the Constitution's silence on the matter, and implicitly honored the 10th Amendment, which lets the states regulate matters not enumerated in the Constitution.

In making its decision the court said that people have no "right" to be gay. Significantly, however, it also refused to declare homosexuality a "wrong." It merely noted that the Constitution is mute on the issue. Its ruling thus lets stand the laws of 24 states with no sodomy statutes, as well as the 26 states that outlaw homosexual sodomy, or homosexual and heterosexual sodomy.

The court's decision to let states determine how to treat homosexual behavior implicitly challenges gays, lesbians, and civil libertarians to convince the public that sodomy statutes should be eliminated from the books. Frankly, that's an easy case to make. Most of America's anti-sodomy laws are holdovers from an era in which governments regulated all sexual behavior, homosexual and heterosexual. (Georgia is an exception; its law passed in 1968.) Officials generally ignore these statutes, at least as they concern behavior on private property. Michael Hardwick, for instance, was never tried for sodomy. The prosecutor in Georgia refused to press charges.

The market — in this case, the American legal market — in effect has ruled that anti-homosexuality laws are irrelevant. Although no gay rights or civil liberties group has any national statistics on the number of people prosecuted last year for violating sodomy statutes, it seems clear that the laws seldom are invoked. Michigan offers a good example. The state has such a law, but it hasn't been used by the attorney general's office for years.

That's because state laws already cover the instances in which sodomy statutes might otherwise be invoked. Michigan's law against lewd and lascivious behavior has been used to prosecute the poor wretches who tryst in rest-stops and other public places. A state law that covers the spread of contagious diseases can be applied to individuals who spread Auto-Immune Deficiency Syndrome (AIDS), and assault or rape laws have been used to prosecute homosexual rapists. Similarly, the homosexual seduction or abuse of minors and the use of physical violence during homosexual acts can be punished through existing laws.

The corpus of state laws thus makes a Michigan sodomy statute irrelevant. For that reason, the state should get rid of its sodomy law. Times and mores being what they are, the state cannot expect — nor should it try — to tell people how they should behave privately. Such an action would fall entirely within the boundaries of the Supreme Court's two recent decisions, and would at least eliminate the hypocrisy of having statutes that the state does not and cannot enforce.

Los Angeles Times

Los Angeles, CA, July 2, 1986

That sexual conduct in the bedroom between consenting adults should be beyond the reach of the state and the prying eye of the policeman seems in this enlightened age to be obvious, but not to a narrow majority of the U.S. Supreme Court.

Its 5-4 decision upholding the Georgia law forbidding oral and anal intercourse between homosexuals reflects no doubt a similar division of opinion in the country: 26 states, including California, have repealed their laws forbidding acts called "sodomy" for both heterosexuals and homosexuals, leaving 24 states and the District of Columbia with variations of them still on the books. The Supreme Court ducked the question of heterosexual "sodomy," which includes acts by married couples and which is also prohibited by the Georgia law at issue.

Fortunately the court decision leaves the states on their own; the humane laws of California and the like-minded states are left undisturbed.

The case illustrates nicely how the Supreme Court is called on to apply the general principles of the Constitution to the evolving needs of the nation and its citizens. The case was brought under the relatively new concept of the right of privacy. The right was not explicitly expressed in the Constitution, but it began to emerge in court opinions about 60 years ago, and was declared by the Supreme Court in 1965 to be inherent in the Bill of Rights. The court has applied that right to marriage, child-rearing, conception and abortion.

The right of privacy, said Justice Louis D. Brandeis, the leading early advocate of the concept, is "the right to be let alone—the most comprehensive of rights and the most valued by civilized men." In his eloquent dissent in the Georgia case Justice Harry A. Blackmun argued cogently: "The right of an individual to conduct intimate relationships in the intimacy of his or her own home seems to me to be the heart of the Constitution's protection of privacy."

But Justice Byron R. White, for the majority, citing historical precedent and the reluctance of the court to get into yet another controversy, blandly asserted that homosexual conduct bore no "resemblance" to the other rights of privacy secured by the court.

The rigid and hostile attitude woven through White's opinion will discourage those not inclined to sit in righteous judgment of others, but they can hope, with Blackmun, "that the court soon will reconsider its analysis and conclude that depriving individuals of the right to choose for themselves how to conduct their intimate relationships poses a far greater threat to the values most deeply rooted in our nation's history than tolerance of nonconformity could ever do."

DESERET NEWS

Salt Lake City, UT
July 2/3, 1986

Are Americans really supposed to believe that the police are going to start breaking into bedrooms all over the country?

That's what many homosexuals are trying to insist following this week's controversial but courageous ruling by the U.S. Supreme Court on sodomy.

Since Utah and about half the other states have long had criminal laws against private, consensual homosexual acts without deploying legions of boudoir snoopers, it's absurd to think the new ruling is going to produce much, if any, crackdown.

Even so, it's still an important ruling because of the message it sends to society.

The message is that homosexuality is not just another way of life, that some forms of immorality are much more serious than others, and that government has a right to regulate private conduct when it hurts society — particularly when it hurts as much as homosexuality can hurt the family. Entire civilizations have risen and fallen depending on how stable and wholesome their family life was.

Until 1961, every state had a law making sodomy a criminal offense. Now only 24 states and the District of Columbia have such laws. With this un happy trend has also come more sexual disease. It's about time someone in authority signaled that homosexuality does not have society's approval.

The essence of Monday's Supreme Court decision was simply that homosexuals have no constitutional right to engage in sodomy. It's hard to see how the high court could have ruled otherwise without also ruling that the government has no right to regulate other such deleterious forms of private conduct as incest and drug abuse. Or without saying, in effect, that marriage and the family are merely "alternative lifestyles."

Laws against homosexuality, though never easy to enforce, can still have some deterrent effect — particularly when backed by the nation's highest legal tribunal. With the shocking increase in the incidence of AIDS, the Supreme Court just might be saving some lives as well as striking a blow for simple morality.

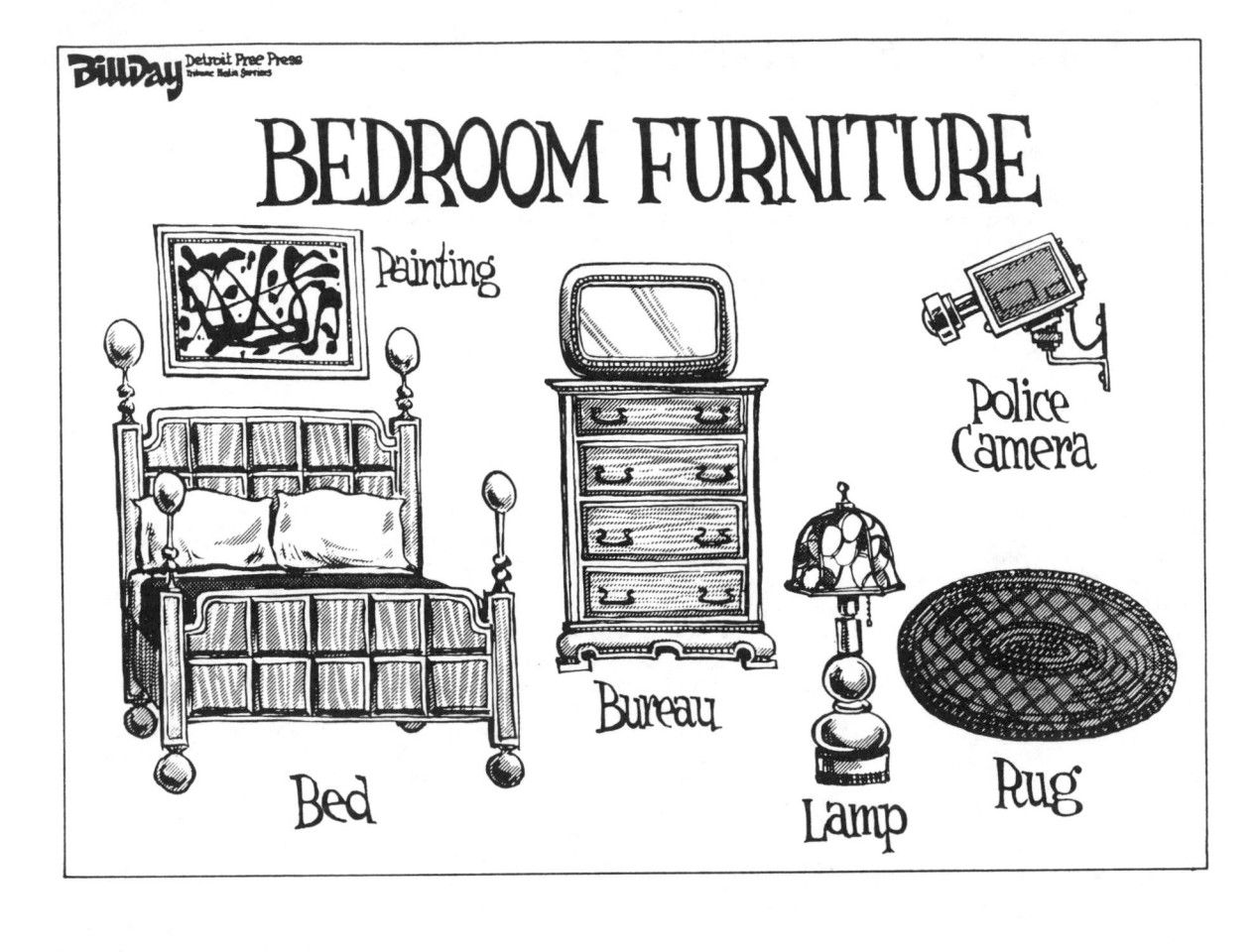

BillDay Detroit Free Press
Tribune Media Services

BEDROOM FURNITURE

Painting

Bureau

Police Camera

Bed

Lamp

Rug

RAPID CITY JOURNAL—

Rapid City, SD, July 3, 1986

Monday, just four days before the annual celebration of Independence Day, five members of the U.S. Supreme Court ruled against freedom.

On a 5-4 vote the Supreme Court upheld a Georgia law which tells consenting adults how they must conduct their sex lives within the privacy of their own homes.

Justice Harry Blackmun, writing for the dissenting minority (Blackmun, William Brennan Jr., Thurgood Marshall and John Paul Stevens), said the decision allows the state to "invade the houses, hearts and minds of citizens who choose to live their lives differently.

"The right of an individual to conduct intimate relationships in the intimacy of his or her own home seems to me to be the heart of the Constitution's protection of privacy."

Blackmun is right.

The court's action upheld a law outlawing sodomy — defined as "any sexual act involving the sex organs of one person and the mouth or anus of another." The majority opinion sidestepped the question of heterosexual sodomy, focusing only on the issue of "consensual homosexual sodomy." The Georgia law also outlaws sodomy between heterosexuals, including married heterosexuals. The court declined to rule on whether the Constitution protects married couples and other heterosexuals from prosecution. But nothing in the decision's language limits the ability of states to enact laws which make heterosexual sodomy a crime.

The majority decision stated that homosexual conduct was not protected by law because homosexuality has a long tradition of being outlawed and is not "deeply rooted in this nation's history or tradition" or "implicit in the concept of ordered liberty."

Following this logic, the justices in the majority (Warren Burger, Lewis Powell, Byron White, William Rehnquist and Sandra Day O'Connor) would approve of slavery because it is "deeply rooted in this nation's history or tradition" and was legal for many years after the Constitution was enacted.

The Supreme Court's most recent ruling sets a dangerous precedent. In 1965 the Supreme Court struck down a Connecticut law which regulated contraception on the grounds the law improperly interfered with privacy. Following the reasoning used Monday by the court majority, such laws might be considered proper.

Simply, the ruling means that states can enact and enforce laws telling people how they may behave in the most intimate moments of their lives.

South Dakotans live in one of the 26 enlightened states that do not make sodomy a crime. This state takes the proper course of outlawing acts which damage others, rather than regulating intimate behavior that some third party might consider offensive.

While lewd public displays or brutality are proper matters for law, private consensual acts are not. The decision will spur shrill efforts by everyone from gay activists to celibate prudes to force their moral opinions on others. Most of society, living somewhere between these positions, should cling to the principle of allowing adults to behave as adults.

Bruised sensibilities sting society. Suppressed liberties maim it.

No level of government — federal, state or local — should tell consenting, mentally competent adults how and under what conditions they may engage in sex in the privacy of their homes.

THE ANN ARBOR NEWS
Ann Arbor, MI, July 2, 1986

The timing of the U.S. Supreme Court's decision on homosexual relations could not have been worse. This year's Fourth of July celebration has been called Liberty Weekend, in honor of the Statue of Liberty's 100th birthday.

But it is our own unique body of liberties which was injured by a 5-4 decision which held that private homosexual acts between consenting adults are not protected by constitutional rights to privacy.

It is a sad day for America when the police are given authority to peek into bedrooms and peer over transoms in an effort to enforce some vague standard of morality on a diverse country.

Is this a preview of the court's expected strict constructionism under its Reagan appointees? Doesn't invasion of privacy mean anything anymore?

How can conservatives, who passionately defend the individual against the power of the state and Big Government, nod in approval of a ruling which does such violence to the concept that a man's home is his castle and that consensual intimacy is absolutely *nobody's* business?

For almost all of us, the last bastion of privacy is one's dwelling. Here a man or woman is allowed to assume a private persona which may be at variance with the one he or she presents publicly. That does not imply it's all right to abuse children in the privacy of the home, or to indulge behavior which threatens the health and safety of others.

But consensual sex among adults in the home is not a fit subject for state regulation or police investigation. And to say that it is highly unlikely the police would go into private homes and arrest adults for engaging in illegal sexual acts is beside the point altogether and seriously begs the issue.

Writing for the majority, Justice Byron R. White used history as a guide. Condemnation of homosexuality, he wrote, has "ancient roots." The original 13 states all outlawed homosexual acts, as did all 50 states until 1961.

White said homosexual activity was not protected by previous decisions involving the 14th Amendment (due process, equal protection) and that it would be "facetious" to suggest that homosexual conduct qualified as a "fundamental right."

Justice Harry A. Blackmun's stirring dissent, however, is worth quoting at some length.

"Our cases long have recognized that the Constitution embodies a promise that a certain private sphere of individual liberty will be kept largely beyond the reach of government."

". . . . The fact that individuals define themselves in a significant way through their intimate sexual relationships with others suggests, in a nation as diverse as ours, that there may be 'many' right ways of conducting those relationships. . . .

"In a variety of circumstances we have recognized that a necessary corollary of giving individuals freedom to choose how to conduct their lives is acceptance of the fact that different individuals will make different choices. . . .

"The assertion that 'traditional Judeo-Christian values proscribe' the conduct involved, cannot provide an adequate justification for section 16-6-2 (the Georgia statute prohibiting sodomy). That certain but by no means all religious groups condemn the behavior at issue gives the State no license to impose their judgments on the entire citizenry. A state can no more punish private behavior because of religious intolerance than it can punish such behavior because of racial animus."

The court in trying to legislate morality has stepped far beyond any notion of ordered liberty. Criminalizing conduct which is engaged in by millions of Americans, married and unmarried, homosexual and heterosexual, is an insult to the rule of law and governing by the consent of the governed.

The issue here, as Blackmun said, is more profound than merely the choice of sexual act. What is at stake is what he called "the fundamental interest all individuals have in controlling the nature of their intimate associations with others."

In other words, human sexuality in its different forms and as practiced among consenting adults belongs in a privacy zone which should be inviolate. It's a tragedy that the court believes something else.

Rockford Register Star
Rockford, IL, July 3, 1986

The government has no business snooping in the bedrooms of private citizens, but that is just what the Supreme Court has legalized in its ruling in the Georgia sodomy case.

We suspect the five justices who voted to reaffirm the Georgia law did so out of personal impulses — out of personal revulsion for certain sexual practices — rather than constitutional logic.

The decision had nothing to do with constitutional rights of individuals — which was the only issue before the court.

The law attempts to curtail certain sexual behavior between consenting adults. That kind of government snooping is insupportable, regardless of moral reservations many people have about this kind of behavior.

Although the Georgia law is aimed at homosexuals, the biggest concern with the Supreme Court ruling is that the law makes illegal various sexual practices researchers claim are routine by many married couples in the United States.

Harvard University Law School professor Laurance Tribe, who argued against the Georgia law before the Supreme Court, said, "For the court to say, even by a 5-4 vote, that Big Brother can enter every bedroom to enforce the morality of the majority on consenting adults in their most intimate decisions I think is a tragic decision."

It is difficult to disagree with that assessment.

Illinois led the nation in 1961 by decriminalizing private sexual conduct between consenting adults. Half the states followed suit. They were 25 years ahead of the Supreme Court in recognizing the rights of the individual in this circumstance.

We hope the court will modify the decision in the future and remove Big Brother from the bedroom.

St. Paul Pioneer Press & Dispatch
St. Paul, MN, July 3, 1986

The Constitution does not confer a fundamental right to engage in private acts of sodomy, even in one's own home, the U.S. Supreme Court has ruled. One hopes the court recognizes the public's right to be fundamentally confused now about what claims to privacy the Constitution *will* protect.

Over the years, the court has ruled that a constitutionally based right of privacy, among other things, prevents states from outlawing mixed race marriage, contraception, private use of pornography in one's home and termination of pregnancy. But that right of privacy does not forbid a state to criminalize sex acts between consenting adults, even in their own homes. So the court now has ruled in upholding Georgia's anti-sodomy law, at least as it applies to homosexuals.

We suspect that most Americans maintain a laissez faire attitude about other adults' private, consensual sexual conduct. Since 1961, when it was illegal in all 50 states, half have decriminalized sodomy between consenting adults. No broad sentiment exists for aggressively enforcing the anti-sodomy laws that survive.

Indeed, the facts of the Georgia case underscore that: The Atlanta district attorney had refused to prosecute the law's challenger, whom a police officer — who had been admitted to the challenger's home and directed to his bedroom by a roommate — had observed in an act of sodomy with another man. (The challenger nonetheless was permitted to continue his lawsuit.) The police were not searching for sodomy law violators. Georgia's state attorney general, who argued the case, said that no one has been prosecuted for violating the challenged statute in the last 40 or 50 years.

The rationale for denying constitutional protection for homosexuals' private consensual behavior was that it was not rooted in the traditions and values of the American people. The court's decision did not call for persecution of homosexuals. Nor did it generally endorse criminal prosecution of consensual adult behavior that the political majority considers sinful.

What the decision *did* do was express anxiety about political backlash against the court's protecting behavior or groups before a national consensus would protect them. To do so makes the court vulnerable as an institution, the majority opinion stated. A case in point is the abortion controversy, which puts immense political pressure on the courts and whose continuing intensity disproves national consensus.

Citizens' expectations of privacy rights may be a bit murky now, but it is clear that the court majority is in no mood to let the Constitution protect bedroom behavior that the legislatures will not.

San Francisco Chronicle

San Francisco, CA, July 3, 1986

THE RIGHTS OF PRIVACY suffered a severe setback when the U.S. Supreme Court ruled that Georgia authorities may arrest consenting adults for what they do behind closed bedroom doors. The decision was a shocking reversal of a long trend toward less government intrusion into private behavior.

Justice Byron White's majority opinion focused on the issue of sodomy between men, but the Georgia law upheld by the court makes no distinction between such sexual activity among homosexual or heterosexual partners. The sodomy laws still on the books of 19 states apply to both sexes, so the decision against oral and anal sex can be used against anyone in those states. married heterosexual couples included.

The 5-4 ruling was, according to the persuading (yet minority) opinion of Justice Harry Blackmun, an assault on the "right to be left alone." The majority, he said, failed to recognize "the fundamental interest all individuals have in controlling the nature of their intimate associations with others."

JUSTICE WHITE'S MAJORITY seemed anxious to use the Georgia case to prove something to court critics and to demonstrate its commitment to strict constitutional construction. The majority went out of its way to declare that it could find no "fundamental right to engage in homosexual sodomy," then added that "the Court is most vulnerable and comes nearest to illegitmacy when it deals with judge-made constitutional law having little or no cognizable roots in the language or design of the Constitution." It's too bad personal privacy had to suffer to make that point.

This case never had to go to the Supreme Court. Prosecutors had decided not to press the sodomy charge against the Atlanta defendant, but he went to federal court in an effort to get the Georgia law declared unconstitutional. It turned out to be the wrong choice, and a classic instance of a bad case producing bad law.

The Register

Santa Ana, CA, July 2, 1986

By upholding a Georgia law against sodomy Monday, the Supreme Court said there is a right way to have sex and a wrong way, and that it is perfectly within the rights of state governments to decide which is which.

It was the court's first major ruling on what is being called a homosexual rights issue, but the idea that governments can use the force of law to impose morality makes the ruling dangerous to everyone, not just homosexuals. Indeed, the Georgia law the court upheld does not mention homosexuals, and seems clearly to apply to heterosexual married couples as well.

Common sense dictates that acts between consenting adults, done in the privacy of their own home, should be beyond the reach of government's policemen. Justice Byron White's majority opinion, however, pointedly disagreed with that approach, saying that "the law is consistently based on notions of morality and if all laws representing essentially moral choices are to be invalidated under the due-process clause, the courts will be very busy indeed."

But that's exactly what the courts should be — busy ruling that moral codes differ from one individual to the next and that people have the right to do what some consider immoral as long as that immorality does not harm others or infringe on their right to act morally.

White noted that, historically, homosexuality has been treated as a criminal offense and never was accorded any specific protection in the Constitution or later interpretations of the 14th Amendment, the chief legal weapon used to attack state restrictions on basic rights.

Unfortunately, while the 14th Amendment of the Constitution precludes the state from depriving any person of "life, liberty or property," it adds the proviso "without due process of law." This enabled the court to deny liberty to the defendant in this case, since there was a law, and due process, however inappro-

priate, was being observed.

Clearly there are crimes — murder, robbery, rape, for example — in which there are victims. There has been force, or fraud. But this time the court was asked to rule on a case in which there was no victim. The Georgia law in question specifically proscribes "any sexual act involving the sex organs of one person and the mouth or anus of another." The justices should have ruled that it was none of the state's business.

Instead, the majority — Chief Justice Warren Burger and Justices White, Lewis Powell, William Rehnquist, and Sandra Day O'Connor — worried that if private homosexual acts between consenting adults were protected by the Constitution, it would be difficult to stop decriminalization of other sexual crimes committed in the home.

They cited incest as an example. But perhaps the court should take on exactly that task and try to define how incest differs, if it does. from any other sexual act between consenting adults. In a case where neither participant feels victimized, it should be impossible to justify state intervention.

According to White, "Victimless crimes, such as the possession and use of illegal drugs, do not escape the law when they are committed at home." But even those who would regulate drug use out of ofttimes misguided concern for the user should be able to see the difference. Whether prohibiting drugs is wise policy or not, there is good evidence that certain drugs can be physically dangerous. The sexual acts in question are not physically dangerous.

The spread of disease and the fear of AIDS are separate issues. The court was asked to judge an act committed in private between consenting adults, fully aware of what they were doing and the possible consequences. The state had no business interfering; the court should have said so.

Chicago Tribune

Chicago, IL, July 2, 1986

The U.S. Supreme Court was at pains to portray its decision upholding a Georgia sodomy law as a refusal to create a fundamental constitutional right to engage in homosexual behavior. But in fact the law that five justices voted to sustain imposes a 20-year prison sentence for any act of sodomy, and so it invites law enforcement attention to the most intimate aspects of the lives of everyone in the state.

By treating this as a homosexual rights case, the court was able to obscure its implications. And it was also able to act as though this were simply a matter of a political majority deciding to set moral standards for a sovereign state. If it had acknowledged the heterosexual aspects of the law, this argument would have sounded pretty hollow. It is hard to believe that a majority of any state, including Georgia, would pass such a law if it believed the law would be enforced as written.

Why? Because most people, even in Georgia, have enough sense to want to keep the police out of their own bedrooms. Maybe they'd be willing to send them into other people's bedrooms, especially if the others are obvi-

ously different. But their own bedrooms? No way. That's the reason Illinois wisely got rid of its sodomy laws years ago.

Imagine what a serious enforcement of the Georgia law would involve. Even married couples would not be spared police interrogation about their sexual habits. If privacy means anything, it must mean that such matters are nobody's business, especially the state's.

The court obviously did not want to extend the reach of the constitutional right to privacy, and it is hard to blame it for being wary. It was the privacy right that caused the court so much trouble in the abortion cases. And in the Georgia case, it was asked to stand against the conviction of a man for engaging in a homosexual act.

But just because five justices of the court have said sodomy laws directed against homosexuals are constitutional, that doesn't mean that Georgia's law is anything but a grand gesture of moralizing that would not last a month if anyone seriously began to enforce it.

THE DENVER POST

Denver, CO, July 2, 1986

THE U.S. Supreme Court, by a 5-4 decision, has upheld a Georgia law threatening homosexuals with 20 years imprisonment for committing acts of sodomy — and theoretically extending the same penalty to married couples who engage in sodomy, including oral sex.

The ruling shocked civil libertarians, who fear homosexuals may face growing discrimination in the wake of the frightening AIDS epidemic. A close reading of the swarm of conflicting opinions in the case, however, suggests that the court may have meant less than either its critics or its supporters believe.

Typical of this divided and meandering tribunal, there is no true majority viewpoint. Harry Blackmun marshalled four votes in his closely reasoned dissent, which attacked the traditional laws against homosexuality. His opinion quotes Oliver Wendell Holmes' maxim that "It is revolting to have no better reason for a rule of law than that so it was laid down in the time of Henry IV."

Byron White countered in an opinion joined by Sandra Day O'Connor and William Rehnquist that there is "no constitutional right of homosexuals to engage in acts of sodomy."

Actually, nobody except White's rhetorical straw men had ever suggested that the Constitution guarantees any specific sexual act. Neither does it specifically authorize you to blow your nose.

What the Constitution does enshrine is the irreversible conviction of a free people that they have a right to live their lives without the government butting into their private business. That right of privacy is at the heart of the landmark 1973 abortion case Roe vs. Wade — a ruling that may well have been the real target of White, Rehnquist and O'Connor. Blackmun, author of the abortion decision, clearly recognized such a threat in his dissent, which underscored the totally inconsistent views toward privacy in Roe and in the sodomy opinion.

But it is notable that White's fourth and fifth votes, Warren Burger and Lewis Powell, issued separate concurring opinions distancing themselves from White's attack on the right to privacy. Burger's opinion is unenlightening and rather uninteresting.

But Powell's opinion seizes on the fact, also emphasized by White, that the Georgia man arrested for committing a homosexual act in his own home was never actually charged with breaking the law in question — because the local grand jury rightly decided it had more important things to do. Thus, he was never tried, much less convicted and imprisoned.

Thus, the court wasn't being asked to right an actual injustice, but rather to issue a kind of term paper saying gay sex is constitutionally protected. The courts are quite properly reluctant to issue such abstract rulings — far preferring to deal with actual rather than theoretical misuses of the police power. Powell's opinion almost shouts that he might vote to free any gay person actually imprisoned by such a law.

Such incarceration isn't really very likely. Even White specifies that his ruling doesn't mean that homosexual acts are illegal, as some cursory news accounts wrongly suggested. It just means that state laws against them aren't unconstitutional in the abstract. States such as Colorado — which has wisely decided not to have police pry into bedroom conduct — are free to continue their sensible restraint. Thus, the chief effect of this ruling may be to underscore the legal maxim that "bad cases make bad law." Gay rights activists made a grave tactical error by choosing to fight this hypothetical case to the Supreme Court.

But the fact remains that, however unnecessarily, the court did rule on a basic test of whether governments are the masters or the servants of the people who elect them — and it botched it.

Only a police-state mentality can rejoice at a ruling which, as Blackmun notes, spurns the eloquent plea of Louis Brandeis that "the most comprehensive of rights, and the most valued by civilized men, is the right to be let alone."

St. Petersburg Times

St. Petersburg, FL, July 3, 1986

The false conservatives on the Supreme Court have chalked up not one, not two but three victories for oppressive government. The Georgia sodomy decision, allowing states to control private sexual behavior, was only the beginning.

The next day, the same five justices subverted the First Amendment by holding that a state can ban truthful advertising for legal products and services as a means of discouraging their use. They also restricted the Fifth Amendment privilege against self-incrimination by ruling that it could not be claimed by an Illinois sex offender who had been imprisoned under a civil mental health statute rather than the criminal law.

It has been a dreadful week for American liberties, an ironic overture to a holiday that celebrates American freedoms.

The advertising case concerned the curious double standard of Puerto Rico, where gambling casinos are legal but are forbidden to advertise to residents of the commonwealth. In earlier cases, such as Virginia's bans on abortion information and retail drug price advertising and the Arizona Bar's prohibition against lawyer advertising, the court ruled that truthful advertisements pertaining to legal activities are protected by the First Amendment. No longer. Writing for the majority, Justice William Rehnquist argued that since Puerto Rico has the "greater power" to prohibit casino gambling, should it so wish, that "necessarily includes the lesser power to ban advertising of casino gambling."

This may be good news to those who would like to prohibit advertising for cigarettes and alcoholic beverages, but where does it stop? States also have the constitutional power to restrict or even prohibit the sale of handguns and other types of firearms. Should they now try to compromise the gun control issue by making it illegal to advertise firearms? And how about the burgeoning industry in radar detectors, which are legal in most states but are sold to further the universally illegal purpose of breaking the speed laws?

The court's position was not only illogical but hypocritical, since only the justices in the minority seemed to acknowledge that the Puerto Rico law permits the casinos to advertise in newspapers outside the commonwealth. Justice John Paul Stevens noted that this "blatantly discriminates" between publications such as the New York Times and the San Juan Star. The greater objection, of course, is that it will encourage state legislators to larger excesses of paternalism and misuse of power. As Justice William Brennan objected, it gives government officials "unprecedented authority to eviscerate constitutionally protected expression."

This newspaper, like all newspapers, has an economic interest in the full freedom of commercial speech. This interest coincides with the national interest in protecting the public from censorship by anyone, whether the person making the attempt is a paternalistic legislator or a paternalistic publisher. If government should undertake to ban tobacco products as a health hazard, fine. But so long as the products are legal, there is no basis for rejecting — or for prohibiting — advertising that describes them truthfully. To invite government to control advertising as a means of indirectly controlling public behavior — which is exactly what the Rehnquist court has now done — is to establish thought control as a legitimate power of the state. It was not a conservative decision. It was extremist.

And so was Rehnquist's other majority opinion of the day, which allowed Illinois to set aside a criminal suspect's constitutional rights in the guise of a "civil proceeding."

Terry B. Allen, an accused rapist, was taken to court under an Illinois civil statute providing for him to be designated a "sexually dangerous person." Upon such a finding, the state would drop criminal charges. But Allen would be held for "care and treatment." In a touch worthy of Kafka, his treatment would take place in a maximum security prison run by the Illinois Department of Corrections. But unlike convicted prisoners serving fixed terms, Allen would be held indefinitely — perhaps forever — until he could prove that he had recovered and was no longer dangerous.

That is what happened. The court, in declaring Allen a "sexually dangerous person," relied on the opinions of psychiatrists in whom he had confided. An appeals court overturned the finding, agreeing with Allen's contention that he should have been warned that his statements to the doctor could be used against him. But the Supreme Court disagreed, saying that the right against self-incrimination is inapplicable to a civil proceeding.

This is a classic distinction without a difference. Allen is being treated like a criminal, and should have been afforded the same constitutional protections that even a criminal enjoys.

The point, as always, is not to protect the criminal. It is to protect the innocent citizen from being abused by the state. If Terry Allen has no rights, neither do you.

There is another society, as it happens, that permits people to be hustled into mental wards with no semblance of constitutional rights. That society is the Soviet Union, which imprisons its dissidents in mental hospitals on the pretext that it, too, is only looking out for their best interests.

Disease Victim Bias Barred in Jobs

The Supreme Court ruled March 3, 1987 that a 1973 Rehabilitation Act law barring discrimination against the handicapped in federally aided programs protected those suffering from contagious diseases. The ruling involved an elementary school teacher with tuberculosis but was construed as applying as well to people suffering from AIDS or other contagious diseases. (See pp. 62-67.)

The 7-2 decision, in *School Board of Nassau County v. Arline*, was specifically targeted by Justice William J. Brennan Jr. in his majority opinion to prevent discrimination based on general "prejudice, stereotype or unfounded fear" that people with contagious diseases were dangerous. The ruling would provide protection for these people against firings or denial of access to the federally aided programs, which included most public schools, federal contractors and agencies and many state and local agencies. Brennan also specifically delimited the ruling. It would not apply to somebody who posed a "significant risk of communicating an infectious disease to others in the workplace," he said.

The 1973 law itself, in barring bias against "handicapped" persons, specified that they must be "otherwise qualified" to do the job or participate in the program at issue. Decisions on these matters would have to be made on a case-by-case basis, the court ruled, under guidelines set down by the American Medical Association in a friend-of-the-court brief. These brought into consideration the nature, duration and severity of the health risk involved, and a finding on the probability of passing the disease on to others.

In the case at hand, that of Gene H. Arline, who was dismissed by Nassau County school officials in Florida, the case was returned to federal district court there to determine if she posed a health threat to others in the system. Chief Justice William H. Rehnquist and Justice Antonin Scalia dissented. They protested that the majority was acting "on its own sense of fairness" instead of on the text of the law. The decision was a rebuff to the Reagan administration, which had taken the school board's side in the case and argued that contagiousness was not a "handicap" as defined by the law.

Detroit Free Press

Detroit, MI, March 5, 1987

THE U.S. Supreme Court's 7-2 ruling that persons who are physically or mentally impaired by contagious diseases may not be discriminated against is an important decision for a civilized nation. The U.S. Justice Department's callous position in the case of a Florida teacher who had tuberculosis and was fired for that reason by a local board of education, was rebuked in the majority opinion by Justice William Brennan.

The Justice Department had argued that an employer who receives federal money could discharge people with such diseases merely because of fear that they might infect others. Undeterred by virtually unanimous expert medical testimony on the issue, Justice Department attorneys persisted in arguing for what amounted to a reinstatement of leper colonies and a requirement that afflicted persons ring bells and cry out, "Unclean, unclean."

People suffering with acquired immune deficiency syndrome (AIDS) have taken heart at Tuesday's high court ruling. Though the court did not specifically mention AIDS victims, the ruling covers them. AIDS victims and even persons who have been exposed to the virus have become, in fact, the lepers of the late 20th Century. Public hysteria breaks out whenever it is revealed, for example, that a child has AIDS or has tested positive for exposure to the AIDS virus. Nothing that doctors can say about the minuscule chance that a person can contract AIDS outside of sexual activity or the use of contaminated hypodermic needles seems to allay the irrational fear. The Supreme Court's ruling in the Florida case will help shore up what doctors are trying to say.

Even though the Justice Department wanted to institute a prejudicial and discriminatory condition where handicapped people are concerned, the Supreme Court in a firm opinion requires that a federal court in Florida now determine if the teacher "is otherwise qualified" for her teaching position. By its ruling the court has advanced the broader cause of handicapped people and given the nation an important lesson in compassion.

The Wichita Eagle-Beacon

Wichita, KS, March 6, 1987

IT'S not OK, after all, for employers to fire workers simply because they have diseases that others fear might be spread. The U.S. Supreme Court rightly said as much Tuesday, plugging a loophole the Reagan administration last year punched in a 1973 anti-discrimination law.

The obvious beneficiaries of the decision, which stems from a Florida case involving a teacher fired because she contracted tuberculosis, are AIDS victims. It was they a Justice Department official had in mind last year in telling employers subject to the Rehabilitation Act of 1973 — any organization receiving federal money in any form — that communicable diseases weren't handicaps, under the definitions of the act. Handicapped workers are protected in the act from job discrimination.

The Justice Department's memo said that fear that a disease might spread — even an unfounded fear — was sufficient reason to fire diseased workers without penalty. That put workers with a whole range of diseases — even non-communicable ones — at risk of losing their jobs. Management needed only to assert a worker's disease caused worry in co-workers, and the act's protections ceased to exist. That's why an official of the Epilepsy Foundation of America said that this week's decision "truly is a victory because epileptics are treated with discrimination based on fear." Epilepsy, of course, isn't communicable.

In bringing people with diseases back under the act's umbrella, the high court didn't say employers can't protect their workers' health. The decision merely requires that a health threat be established before diseased workers are fired. The decision also should encourage employers subject to the act to see if diseased workers might be able to perform other work.

The Justice Department's memo constituted the sort of assault on reason associated with the Middle Ages. In saying ill-founded beliefs about a disease isn't sufficient reason to fire anyone, the high court has brought the debate on this issue back into the 20th Century.

THE KANSAS CITY STAR
Kansas City, MO, March 5, 1987

The Supreme Court set a guide by ruling that the 1973 law protecting handicapped rights covers victims of contagious disease under certain conditions. People who have a contagious disease, the court said, cannot be discriminated against unless they can't do their work because of the condition or there's a real risk they will infect others. The latter clause is crucial and eminently sensible. It's also why the case involving a teacher with tuberculosis is being celebrated by proponents of civil rights for AIDS victims.

Most of the public complaints and flight from workers or students identified as AIDS victims are based on ignorance about how people "catch" the disease. So, unfortunately, is some debate and reaction by officials.

Writing for the majority, Associate Justice William J. Brennan Jr. noted that a point of the federal law being considered, the Rehabilitation Act of 1973, was to replace irrationality with behavior based on sound medical judgment.

"Congress acknowledged that society's accumulated myths and fears about disability and disease are as handicapping as are the physical limitations that flow from actual impairment," Brennan wrote. "Few aspects of a handicap give rise to the same level of public fear and misapprehension as contagiousness . . ."

Although the case the Supreme Court reviewed did not deal directly with AIDS, it's expected the protections will be extended because at issue was the contagious nature of tuberculosis. The ruling specifically applies to recipients of federal funds, which includes most local government units and school districts as well as federal contractors. Private employers are outside the law's jurisdiction.

The court said the law would not bar a federally subsidized employer from dismissing a person who poses a significant risk of spreading a contagious disease. The employer, however, would first have to try to make adjustments so the person could keep working without infecting others. Such an employer would not have to keep infected workers in a job for which they were not qualified to satisfy the affirmative aspects of the statute.

The court has made an appropriate distinction between public safety and the rights of impaired persons.

THE PLAIN DEALER
Cleveland, OH, March 5, 1987

In 1957, when she was 13, Gene Arline was treated for tuberculosis. After treatment, her doctors pronounced her cured, and thereafter she showed no signs of the disease until 1977, when she had a positive reaction to a TB test. It happened again in 1978, and again later that year. Finally, the school board of Nassau County, Fla., where she worked as a teacher, fired her. That decision, based on the contagiousness of tuberculosis, was the first link in an incredible legal chain.

After being fired, Arline contested the decision twice before the local school board. Then she appealed to the state board of education, which ordered her reinstated with back pay. The local board then went to Florida's First District Court of Appeals, which reversed the state board of education. Arline fought back in a U.S. District Court, which rejected her complaint. She then went to the U.S. Court of Appeals (11th Circuit), which overturned the lower-court ruling and sent the case back for review. Meanwhile, the local school board appealed to the U.S. Supreme Court.

Often, the wheels of justice grind too slowly, as proved by the the progress of Arline's case. Tuesday's Supreme Court opinion, however, finally gives purpose to Arline's ordeal. In essence, the court ruled that victims of contagious diseases are handicapped and are therefore protected from discrimination by the Rehabilitation Act of 1973.

What's more, employers may not "distinguish" between the effects of the disease and its contagiousness in order to justify discrimination. Unfortunately, the court avoided the larger issue of whether those who are diagnosed as "carriers," but who have no physical symptoms, also are covered by the Rehabilitation Act.

Often, public apprehensions are not supported by medical opinion. AIDS, for example, is not spread via casual contact, but by contaminated needles or the exchange of bodily fluids such as semen. Obviously, a person who tests positive for AIDS poses no inherent health risk to co-workers. Yet, discrimination against AIDS carriers threatens to become widespread, especially as the trend toward AIDS testing widens.

Congress could not foresee the AIDS epidemic, and so such issues were not explicitly included in the Rehabilitation Act and its subsequent amendments. Yet, the intent of Congress is clear. The act was meant to shield citizens from discrimination based on physical handicap and from discrimination based on the *perception* of a handicap. Obviously, someone suffering from AIDS is handicapped, just as is someone who suffers from TB or the effects of polio. Obviously also, the public fear of AIDS is a handicap for everyone who tests positive, even if they have no symptoms. In that sense, the victims of public alarm deserve as much protection as the victims of the disease itself.

The Charlotte Observer
Charlotte, NC, March 9, 1987

The act would not require a school board to place a teacher with active, contagious tuberculosis in a classroom with elementary school children.
— Justice William Brennan

The case decided by the Supreme Court last Tuesday actually involved a Florida school teacher dismissed from her job because of tuberculosis, not AIDS. But it obviously has particular import for society's handling of the growing number of AIDS victims. On the whole, the decision is good news, for the court said two sensible things:

● People with contagious diseases are covered by federal law protecting the handicapped from discrimination by recipients of federal money, and thus may not be fired or otherwise discriminated against because of irrational fear of contagion.

● But, as the quote above indicates, an employer covered by the law is *not* barred from "dismissing a person who poses a significant risk of communicating an infectious disease to others in the workplace" if the risk cannot be eliminated by "reasonable accommodation." Underscoring that point, the court did not simply order the teacher returned to the classroom; instead, she is to get a lower-court hearing on whether her disease poses enough risk of infecting students to justify her removal from teaching.

Those two points are a solid base of public policy. AIDS is difficult enough to deal with without encouraging public and private measures based on irrational fears. People suffering with serious diseases — whether tuberculosis or cancer or AIDS — do not need to be further victimized by needless loss of employment, education or other social benefits.

At the same time, society has not only a right but a duty to contain serious illnesses. Rational distinctions are not invidious discrimination. If the teacher's illness reasonably threatens her students, then it disqualifies her from the classroom. In weighing the risks in such cases, the greater weight ought to be given to protecting the public health, especially when the disease in question is as deadly as AIDS.

The Washington Post

Washington, DC, March 9, 1987

IN EMPLOYMENT and certain other fields, federal law forbids discrimination against the handicapped. A handicapped person can be not only a person who has an impairment but also a person who is "regarded as having" one. Thus, for example, disfigured or similarly afflicted people who are otherwise able should not suffer discrimination. What, then, about people with diseases that are or are thought in certain circumstances to be contagious? Are they protected or not?

The Supreme Court in a 7-to-2 decision the other day said that they are. This is not as threatening to others as it sounds at first when you suppose that people with all sorts of contagious diseases will have been given the right to remain wherever they want. The most important current implication is for AIDS victims. The administration has argued that "fear of contagion, whether reasonable or not," is grounds for dismissing such people. The court, without specifically addressing all the questions presented by AIDS, said it is not. Otherwise "society's accumulated myths and fears" would rule, which is just the result that the law on the handicapped seeks to avoid.

The decision came in the case of a Florida elementary schoolteacher dismissed because she had recurrent tuberculosis. She appealed on grounds she was covered by the handicapped law. The district court said she wasn't; the appeals court said she was and that the case should go back to the district court for further determination. This is what the justices agreed to.

The decision does *not* say an employer must keep a person with a contagious disease. It does require that steps be taken to make sure the person is not the victim of "prejudice, stereotypes, or unfounded fear." Thus employers and courts in such cases must take into account "reasonable medical judgments" as to the risks involved, as well as whether some "reasonable accommodation" is possible under which the person involved could keep working. Conceivably the teacher here could still be fired, but not summarily.

The dissenters in the case, Chief Justice William Rehnquist and Justice Antonin Scalia, complained that Congress never considered the question of contagious disease and that the majority was stretching the law. But Congress has purposely intervened to alter—rectify—the way the society has traditionally treated people with physical impairments. No particular outcomes are dictated; the goal is merely that their treatment be fair—in the case of disease, that it be balanced and rational. The standard is the right one.

The Cincinnati Post

Cincinnati, OH, March 13, 1987

The U.S. Supreme Court took a major, and justified, step last week toward extending job protection to people with contagious diseases, including AIDS.

The court held that a school teacher suffering from tuberculosis was protected from arbitrary firing by a 1973 law prohibiting discrimination against handicapped persons in programs receiving federal financial aid.

The decision doesn't mean that employers can in all cases be forced to keep a contagious person on the job. What it means is that such a person cannot be fired unless a professional medical judgment is made that the individual clearly poses a health risk to others.

We agree with a spokesman for the American Medical Association who called the ruling a careful balance between two interests: "the right of the victim (of a contagious disease) to be free from irrational prejudice and the right of others to be protected against an unreasonable risk from disease."

The Providence Journal

Providence, RI, March 9, 1987

The Supreme Court created quite a stir on Tuesday with its ruling that a person with a contagious disease can qualify for protection under a federal law aimed at discrimination against the handicapped. But the initial clamor surrounding this case appears to be excessive and premature. This is especially true of those who viewed the decision as likely to have a major impact regarding the topic of AIDS; Justice William Brennan's opinion for the majority explicitly advised that the ruling in this case should not be read to cover "a carrier of a contagious disease such as AIDS."

Section 504 of the Rehabilitation Act of 1973 bars government agencies and recipients of federal funds from discriminating against an otherwise qualified person solely by reason of that person's handicap. The case at hand — involving a Florida elementary school teacher with recurring bouts of tuberculosis — forced the court to enter the maze of definitions created by Congress' 1973 legislation and the subsequent regulatory apparatus of four succeeding administrations. By the time the court emerged, seven of its nine members had agreed that the law was intended to cover people with contagious diseases (the Florida teacher's case was sent back to the lower courts to determine whether her particular medical condition lawfully warranted her dismissal from classroom teaching).

Note well: The court was not establishing a new constitutional right or enunciating a new constitutional principle. It was simply trying to interpret the meaning of a piece of legislation. If the court majority has misconstrued the intention of the 1973 law, as the Reagan administration and Chief Justice William Rehnquist and Justice Antonin Scalia contend, there is a simple and direct solution: An amendment which explicitly states that having a contagious disease is not in itself a handicap within the meaning of the law.

In the absence of such clarifying legislation, where do matters stand now in terms of the important, and potentially momentous, social problem — striking a proper balance between protecting handicapped people from irrational discrimination and protecting the community from dangerous contagious diseases?

The essence of the court's complex argument seems to boil down to this: A person with a contagious disease (like a person with any other kind of handicap) may not be denied a relevant service or benefit solely because of that disease. However, such a denial is proper if the decision is made on the basis of "reasoned and medically sound judgments" concerning the nature, duration and severity of the disease, as well as the probability that the disease will be transmitted to others.

These are reasonable guidelines — provided they are applied in a cautious and sensible fashion. Monitoring this situation will be the continuing task of both Congress, which wrote the law, and the court, which has now interpreted it. Compassion for those who suffer from contagious diseases (including AIDS) is a worthy sentiment, and concern for protecting their rights is a proper goal. But that cannot be used as justification for unnecessarily endangering the health and safety — and rights — of other members of the community.

Roanoke Times & World-News

Roanoke, VA, March 6, 1987

FORTUNATELY, the Supreme Court didn't buy the Justice Department's argument that employers have a legal right to fire AIDS victims because of a "fear of contagion, whether reasonable or not." The high court has ruled that employers, schools and others that receive federal funds may not discriminate against people simply because they have a contagious disease.

The 7-2 decision Tuesday came in the case of a third-grade teacher in Florida who was fired because she had tuberculosis; but its greatest application will be to people with AIDS. The ruling was needed: Too many people are afraid to work, go to school or even live in the same apartment building with AIDS victims.

The Reagan administration has not tried to calm those fears. It intervened in the Florida case on behalf of school officials. A widely circulated Justice Department memorandum last year said employers do not violate the 1973 law barring discrimination of the handicapped by firing employees out of fear that they may spread a disease.

The Supreme Court rejected that interpretation of the law. Justice William J. Brennan wrote in his majority opinion that the intent of Congress was to prevent "discrimination on the basis of mythology."

To allow discrimination based on false fears is to foster those fears. Understanding can't be forced, but recent history has shown that legal intolerance of discrimination for any reason helps bring about a change in public attitudes. The Florida teacher certainly welcomed the Supreme Court's ruling, but its greater value lies in its refusal to condone actions based on a fear of AIDS.

The ruling doesn't mean that people who are sick can never be fired or transferred to other jobs because they have a contagious disease. But the Supreme Court said the law requires that employers base such decisions on sound medical evidence that co-workers are at risk.

That may help calm the fears — based on rumor — that many individuals have of contracting AIDS. Going strictly by *sound* evidence, a worker, student or apartment dweller with AIDS or carrying AIDS antibodies presents no risk to co-workers, fellow students or neighbors with whom he or she has casual contact.

Acquired Immune Deficiency Syndrome is transmitted through sexual contact or through the blood supply. A worker with AIDS won't give it to the person at the next desk by sneezing.

AIDS already carries a stigma because most of its victims in this country have been homosexuals, people who do not have popular acceptance. Rejection of people with the disease at work, at school and at home only reinforces the stigma.

The best hope of stopping the spread of this disease is by identifying all those who have been exposed to it. That will be impossible as long as individuals who make that disclosure must pay too high a price.

The Miami Herald

Miami, FL, March 6, 1987

FEAR is not reasonable grounds for firing an employee. That is the bottom line of a Supreme Court decision that some are hailing as a portent that may protect AIDS victims against discrimination.

The decision doesn't open the doors to people with contagious diseases to stay at work and infect others. What it does is extend the protections given to the handicapped to such persons. If they are employed by agencies receiving Federal funds, this decision gives them the right to have a case-by-case determination of their ability to work and to have reasonable accommodations made for them if necessary.

The case decided by the Supreme Court involved the firing of a Florida teacher because she suffered from recurrent tuberculosis. Gene Arline, 44, was fired by the Nassau County school board in 1978. She had suffered bouts with tuberculosis in 1957, 1977, and 1978. Contagion from tuberculosis is medically controllable, but the board fired her anyway, citing the tender age of her third-grade pupils, and made no effort to place her in another job.

Her attorney, George Rahdert of St. Petersburg, says, "Not for one second would we have suggested that she teach third graders if there were any suggestion of contagion." The school board fired her and stigmatized her by refusing to give her a job reference. Ms. Arline has been free of all symptoms since 1979 but unable to find another job.

Although the majority opinion by Justice William Brennan explicitly noted that the Court was not making a judgment about the employability of AIDS patients, advocates for these patients believe the reasoning will apply to them. AIDS victims — and those whose blood tests merely show exposure — have been fired and denied housing. That's in spite of repeated assurances from medical authorities that AIDS cannot be transmitted through casual contact.

The Reagan Administration opposed Ms. Arline's appeal, arguing that employers have the right to fire employees on irrational grounds, even for having curly hair. With that sort of Neanderthal thinking in the Executive Branch, the judiciary may have its work cut out for it in its pursuit of reason and rationality.

Los Angeles Times

Los Angeles, CA, March 4, 1987

Legislation to implement the AIDS recommendations of the U.S. surgeon general and the National Academy of Science Institute of Medicine is being introduced in Sacramento this week, providing an opportunity for California to move quickly and effectively to meet this increasingly dangerous health problem.

The bill is AB 87, by Assemblyman Art Agnos (D-San Francisco), but in fact it is the product of a remarkable collaboration between Agnos, Dr. C. Everett Koop, the surgeon general, and Dr. David Baltimore, a co-author of the National Academy study, and their staffs.

The presentation of the bill coincides with a visit Thursday to the state Capitol by both Koop and Baltimore. The bill's strong anti-discrimination provisions were reinforced Tuesday by the U.S. Supreme Court decision affirming that persons with contagious disease have the same protections as other handicapped people.

Under terms of the bill, a 21-member commission would be appointed by Gov. George Deukmejian and the Legislature. It would monitor the epidemic, evaluate research and health care and public health needs, make recommendations to all levels of government and propose programs to address particular problems, such as the priority concern about protecting police, fire and first-aid personnel.

The legislation deals at length with testing for the presence of the human immunodeficiency virus (HIV), the probable causative agent of AIDS. The bill affirms the findings of last week's AIDS conference in Atlanta that mandatory testing is not now required and that confidentiality must be assured with the voluntary testing programs. It also emphasizes the importance of voluntary testing, notably for women at risk who are considering pregnancy.

The legislation also sets forth a major program of public education about AIDS, for which the only known defenses are abstinence from sexual intercourse or the use of condoms. Basic instruction about AIDS would be made mandatory for every high-school graduate. The bill calls for the distribution of the surgeon general's report at the junior-high-school level. But it does not provide details of the education program in the public schools. Complementary legislation on AIDS education in the public schools has been introduced by Sen. Gary K. Hart (D-Santa Barbara), and already has passed the California Senate by a vote of 32 to 4.

Agnos won legislative approval last year for more limited legislation that included protections against discrimination, but the measures were vetoed by Deukmejian. Since then the governor's Fair Employment and Housing Commission has ruled that AIDS is a handicap under terms of legislation protecting the handicapped from discrimination. The new bill would make that law. The helpful 7-2 decision of the U.S. Supreme Court on Tuesday, rejecting efforts of the Reagan Administration to deny these protections to those with contagious diseases, would further strengthen the provisions of the proposed legislation barring discrimination—including discrimination in employment, housing and public accommodations.

There is no time to waste. Speedy passage of the Agnos bill could save lives. Using the federal reports, the assemblyman has constructed a compassionate but uncompromising response to the disease, without concessions to hysteria but realistically providing the required resources.

'Catastrophic' Health Care Plan Backed by House

The House of Representatives approved, by a 302-127 vote, July 22, 1987 a bill to expand the Medicare program to protect elderly and disabled persons against "catastrophic" medical costs. The White House had warned July 21 that President Reagan would veto the bill, which contained more funding than an administration proposal put forth by Secretary of Health and Human Services Otis Bowen. The significance of the bill with regards to AIDS was not lost on the nation's editorial writers who pointed out the connections between the bill's passage and the tragedy wrought by the disease.

Before adopting its measure, the House rejected the administration proposal by a vote of 242 to 190. The plan would cost $18.2 billion over five years, according to an estimate by the Congressional Budget Office. Instead, the House adopted the $33 billion, five-year program drafted largely by its Ways and Means Committee. The cost of the program would be met by higher premiums paid by Medicare beneficiaries. The bill was "the most significant and far-reaching expansion of Medicare protection since the program was enacted in 1965," according to Rep. Dan Rostenkowski (D, Ill.), chairman of the Ways and Means Committee.

Not all medical beneficiaries would pay the increased premiums, however. They would be collected only from the 40% of Medicare beneficiaries with enough income to file tax returns. The extra premiums would be collected by the Internal Revenue Service along with individual income taxes. The basic Medicare premiums would continue to be deducted from monthly Social Security checks. Under the bill, out-of-pocket expenses for nondrug Medicare-covered services could be limited to no more than $1,800 a year, and 80% of out-patient prescription drug costs would be reimbursable after a deductible of $500 a year was paid. Coverage for care in a nursing facility would rise to 150 days a year, up from 100 days under the current law. Coverage for hospice care could go beyond the 210-day limit if a physician certified the need. Coverage for home-care visits would be expanded to seven days a week for a maximum of three days generally permitted currently.

THE PLAIN DEALER
Cleveland, OH, July 29, 1987

Medicare rightly has been called the crowning achievement of Lyndon Johnson's "Great Society." In signing legislation that created Medicare 22 years ago, Johnson said, "No longer will older Americans be denied the healing miracle of modern medicine. No longer will illness crush and destroy the savings that they have so carefully put away over a lifetime so that they might enjoy dignity in their later years."

Unfortunately, the cost of providing care has far exceeded the projections of the Johnson administration. Medicare now provides less than half of the cost of health care for the elderly. Even a less-government-is-better president like Ronald Reagan has recognized that Medicare falls short of meeting the needs of older people suffering from catastrophic illness.

More than 18 months ago, Reagan asked for a study. Last November, his Health and Human Services director, Otis R. Bowen, recommended an expansion of Medicare so that no older American would have to pay more than $2,000 in out-of-pocket hospital expenses. The cost would be borne by the elderly themselves, through higher Medicare premiums.

The proposal went to Congress, which to nobody's surprise is taking a more expansive approach. Lawmakers correctly recognized that the administration's proposal was a narrowly focused plan that falls far short of dealing with many aspects of costly, long-term health care. The Senate added some pieces to the Bowen proposal. This week, the House added more, including provisions for physician services and some coverage for care in skilled-nursing homes. The House also included expanded coverage of drug costs.

Now, the president says Congress is doing too much. Reagan, who was less than happy with the Senate version, has promised an outright veto if the House bill survives a House-Senate conference.

Some of the administration concerns are justified. Just as costs outstripped original Medicare projections primarily because of new, expensive medical technology, future costs will continue to escalate. Supporters of the House bill say its self-financing features will place no burden on the federal budget. But there's a risk involved, particularly regarding drug costs. The Health Care Financing Administration and the Congressional Budget Office cannot agree as to the extent of those costs. The Senate wisely was unwilling to act without such information in hand, and chose not to include out-of-hospital drug payments in its bill. The conference committee would do well to take a similar approach.

But other basic elements of the House bill deserve to survive the conference committee. Contrary to what opponents of the bill say, private "medigap" insurance, intended to make up the difference between actual costs and what Medicare provides, is costly, and is not obtained by a substantial number of people. The House bill will provide better coverage at less cost. It will prevent many elderly people from having to exhaust their life savings and live in poverty so a spouse can get nursing-home care. It would expand coverage of home-care visits and hospice care.

The president, in endorsing the Bowen recommendations, said they would "provide that last full measure of security." They will not. Neither would the Senate proposal. Nor will the more extensive bill that came out of the House this week. Even if the House version were to survive the conference committee intact, it would leave many, many Americans unprotected against the devastating economic costs of catastrophic illness. Nonetheless, the legislation is a significant step that deserves a more open reception than it has received from the White House.

LOS ANGELES HERALD
Los Angeles, CA, July 27, 1987

At first glance, there seems little to criticize in the recently approved Medicare expansion bill passed by the House last week. It's necessary for the nation's 31 million elderly and disabled, and it shouldn't cost the Treasury a penny. But there's reason for fiscal caution.

Like its scaled-down counterpart now moving through the Senate, the measure grew out of a Reagan administration proposal to provide catastrophic illness coverage for the nation's elderly and disabled. Both congressional versions significantly expand the White House plan. Should the Senate bill succeed, conference committee members would have to make sure the program had an adequate premium base to support it.

The current bills aim to control Medicare beneficiary costs for out-of-pocket expenses, extend hospital stays and nursing and hospice care. More significantly, the House package would cover outpatient drug prescriptions, which the other two plans would not. And most crucial of all, the congressional plans would be financed not through a flat monthly fee, but by a progressive tax.

Opponents complain that it turns Medicare, an insurance program, into a means-tested welfare program, implying that benefits would then be contingent on need rather than universally available as they are today. But the benefits would remain equally high for everyone. To retain the program's solvency, costs would have to be apportioned by ability to pay, with those in higher-income brackets taxed at a higher rate. But Medicare's payroll-tax component is effectively progressive already.

The legislation's critics raise the specter of AIDS in warning of an uncontrollable cost explosion. That argument points up how much remains to be done for the rest of the nation's population. Congress can read the election returns, in formulating health policy as in everything else. But with problems like infant mortality on the rise, does Congress have any good ideas about how to care for those who may not live long enough to cast their vote?

THE ARIZONA REPUBLIC
Phoenix, AZ, July 22, 1987

WHAT started out as good idea to provide Medicare protection for millions of elderly Americans against the financial calamities of a catastrophic illness seems more like a prescription for disaster now that Congress has got its hands on it.

Originally proposed by the Reagan administration, the catastrophic-care coverage — designed to limit the amount of out-of-pocket expenses a Medicare recipient would have to pay during a long illness — received widespread and bipartisan support when it was introduced earlier this year.

Envisioned by the administration as being supported by a simple, pay-as-you-go increase of less than $5 a month on the optional Medicare premium paid for doctors' fees, the long-overdue proposal now is in danger of turning into a complicated, multibillion-dollar boondoggle thanks to the efforts of well-intentioned, but misguided congressional doctoring.

Adding a dose of this and that designed mainly to stir up political advantage, the congressional versions could price some recipients out of the plan and might very well threaten the financial well-being of the Medicare program itself.

Unlike the administration proposal, the Democratic-supported countermeasures in both the House and the Senate contain provisions requiring higher-income Medicare recipients — who have the financial means to opt out of the plan entirely — to foot most of the bill to pay for the expanded coverage.

With proposed premium payments reaching as high as $50 a month for beneficiaries in the highest tax brackets, neither version takes into account the very real possibility of those higher-income recipients seeking private coverage at lower prices, thereby undermining the financial stability of the whole plan.

On top of that, the House proposal, now nearing passage, includes a provision to pick up most of the cost of prescription drugs for Medicare recipients after a certain annual deductible has been met. Funded by yet another premium added to the cost of optional Medicare coverage — even though there's virtually no data available to measure the potential impact — the prescription benefit adds substantially to the confusion and overall costs of administering the program.

While no one could argue that elderly Americans should have access to needed pharmaceuticals, a hasty adoption of the House plan could do more harm than good. One estimate, by the Health Care Financing Administration, suggests the prescription entitlement program would exceed premium income by $5.5 billion the first year alone, which would then lead to cost-containment measures that would constrain the availability of therapeutic treatment.

On the other hand, the Senate version sensibly suggests that before prescription drug benefits are added, the most appropriate and affordable way to proceed — for the benefit of all — must be determined.

By loading up their catastrophic-care bills with costly add-ons based on unsubstantiated premises, Congress is jeopardizing the financial well-being of the entire Medicare program, which would be an even bigger catastrophe for those the program is intended to help.

The Washington Post
Washington, DC, July 21, 1987

THE HOUSE this week is scheduled to take up a catastrophic health insurance bill that is the most important expansion of Medicare since that program's enactment 22 years ago. The bill owes its existence to the president, who proposed a much more modest plan earlier this year. At the time, he was warned that Congress would take advantage of his offering and expand it. So it has, to the point that the administration is threatening a veto. But this is a good bill which the House should pass and the administration warmly embrace.

Medicare at present helps a person pay the early costs of an illness. Then it tails off, so that a person with a serious illness can face catastrophic costs. The bill would limit these through a cap, after which the government would pick up costs again. The cap in the bill is lower than in the president's proposal, which makes the bill more generous. In addition the bill proposes for the first time to defray high prescription drug costs.

The Congressional Budget Office says the bill would cost $10 billion a year by fiscal 1992, $2 billion of it for the drug provision. The administration fears the drug provision could cost much more, and in any case says the bill now goes too far; its own proposal would have cost only $3.4 billion by 1992. But the bill would not add to the deficit or to the burden on the population as a whole. It carefully includes its own financing mechanism, and the beneficiaries are the ones who would pay—through additions to premiums already charged. The new premiums would also be progressive, rising with income; the president had proposed that everyone pay the same. The states would further be required to pay the premiums and other costs of their poor people through Medicaid. This is in return for the Medicaid money the states would save by the federal government's picking up catastrophic costs that Medicaid now pays.

The drug industry doesn't like the drug provision because it fears the federal funds will be followed by federal regulation, particularly in the form of pressure to buy lower-cost generic drugs. That sounds just fine to us. There may be a skirmish on this issue on the floor; a section of the bill that the industry would like to overturn would require pharmacists to use generic drugs except where doctors prescribe otherwise. But that's a good idea.

Some 33 million people are now enrolled in Medicare, a seventh of the population that almost by definition has extraordinary health-care costs. The bill before the House would mercifully limit these in a fiscally responsible way. There are a lot of areas of unmet need in health care nationally; this is one of the largest. It ought to be an easy aye.

FORT WORTH STAR-TELEGRAM
Fort Worth, TX, July 29, 1987

The overwhelming margin by which the House approved catastrophic illness legislation virtually guarantees that substantial — and welcome — changes are forthcoming in the Medicare program.

But great care must be taken to ensure that those changes make the system more compassionate *and* affordable.

The Senate is expected to begin floor debate on its version of a catastrophic illness bill after the August vacation. The measure that emerged from the Senate Finance Committee, though not perfect, is nearer the desired balance between compassion and affordability than the House bill.

No reasonable voice can question the need for comprehensive catastrophic illness coverage for the elderly. Current Medicare regulations, mandating relatively high deductibles and unrealistic limitations on reimbursement for long hospital stays, offer little hope to patients facing long-term illness. Lengthy hospital stays and expensive medication can wipe out one's savings in a hurry.

Both House and Senate plans would alleviate the situation, but the House bill seems unnecessarily extravagant and calls for entering uncharted territory with little or no advance preparation.

For instance, it calls for 80 percent reimbursement of outpatient prescription drug costs after participants meet a certain deductible. The problem with that is that no one seems to have the remotest idea how much it would cost. Estimates from various supposedly qualified sources range from $1 billion annually to more than $7 billion.

The Senate bill, meanwhile, would put drug reimbursement on hold until a 12-month study could be conducted on pricing and coverage to determine what the actual cost would be.

Both plans would be financed by increasing Medicare premiums and would depart from the present flat-rate system, calling for premiums to be based on a progressive scale. But the Senate version appears to provide virtually the same protection as the House plan at a lower cost, particularly to low-income participants.

The ideal solution would be a bill carefully blending the compassionate aspects of the House plan with the practicality of the Senate's. But if it comes down to an either-or situation, the Senate measure would do the most people the most good for the least amount of money.

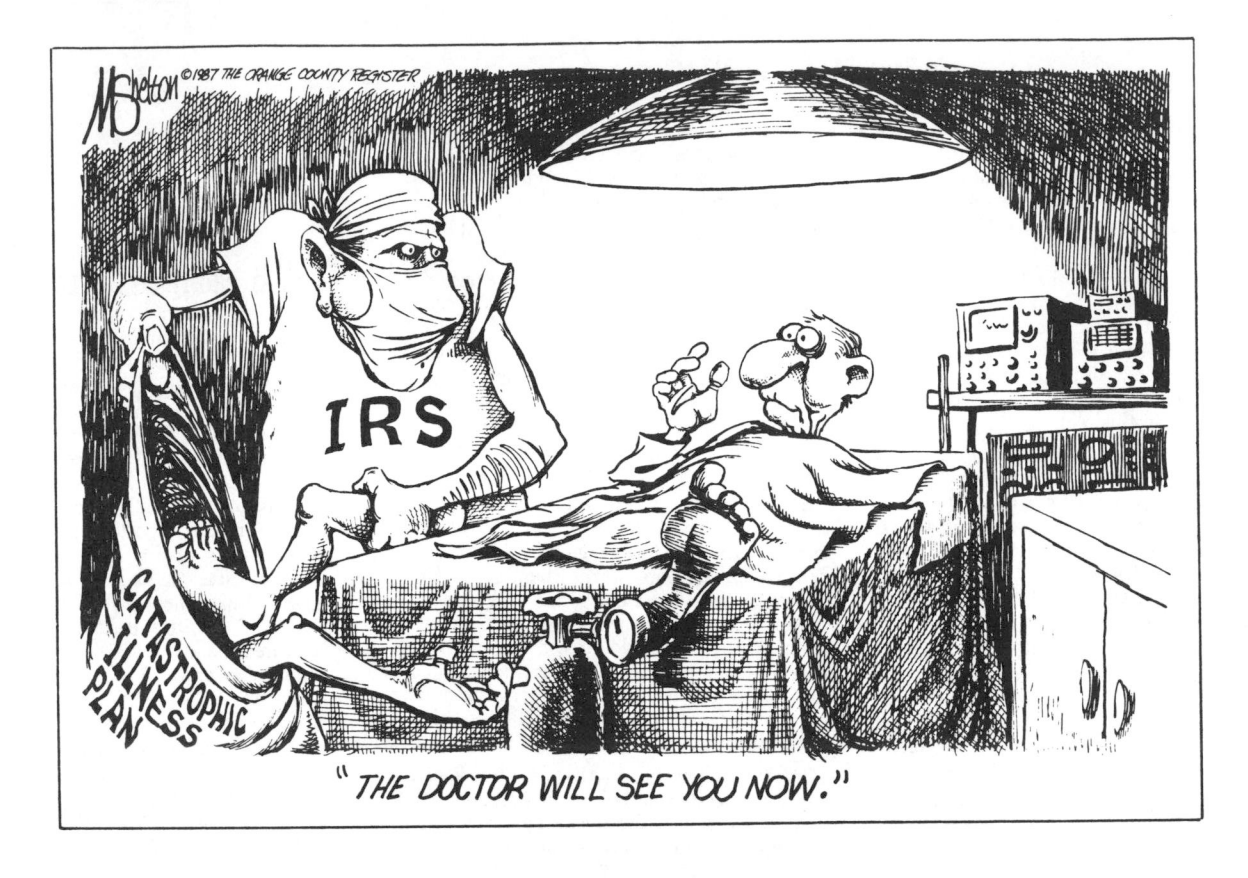

M Shelton ©1987 THE ORANGE COUNTY REGISTER

IRS

CATASTROPHIC ILLNESS PLAN

"THE DOCTOR WILL SEE YOU NOW."

The Morning News

Wilmington, DE, July 27, 1987

FOR ONCE, politicians' hyperbole is right on the mark. "The most significant and far-reaching expansion" of Medicare since its establishment in 1965 is how Congressman Dan Rostenkowski refers to the plan for protection against catastrophic illness. House members passed the plan last week by a resounding 302-127 vote.

Indeed, if the House bill were to become law in its present form — an unlikely event since the Senate is working on a less comprehensive measure — the nation's 31 million Medicare beneficiaries would reap considerable benefits in return for fairly modest premium increases. Also in the bill's way is the fact that President Reagan vows a veto, though he himself last February urged expansion of Medicare coverage for the exorbitant costs of catastrophic illness.

When Medicare was enacted 22 years ago, it was expected to let persons over age 65 get necessary medical care without financial suffering. It hasn't worked out that way.

Medicare coverage for hospital stays, as the seriously ill find out when they start filing claims, now is limited to 150 days, with only the first 60 days fully paid for. Medicare also pays nothing toward medications, except when a person is hospitalized, and the elderly with chronic illness can have horrendous drug bills. Medicare also pays fully only for the first 20 days of skilled nursing-home care and a pittance for the next 80, with no assist afterwards.

Each one of these shortfalls would be corrected under the House measure. There would be unlimited hospitalization coverage. For medications, after a a Medicare subscriber had put out $500 in a year, the insurance would pay for 80 percent of additional medications. Skilled nursing home care would be covered more generously and for 150 days.

The above are just a sampling of the changes the House bill would make. Over five years it is estimated that the cost would be $34 billion over and above the present Medicare cost which runs into the $70 billions. This additional cost, however, according to the bill writers would not come from the Treasury but would be covered by modest premium increases for all subscribers (from the present $17.90 a month to a monthly $26 by 1992). In addition, based on adjusted gross income, there would be an income tax surcharge for those above certain income levels.

There is little doubt that present Medicare coverage can leave folks in the financial hole and that changes are necessary if the intent of the 1965 legislation of ensuring adequate medical care for the elderly is to be fulfilled. But the proposed overhaul may be trying to do too much too quickly.

There is significant doubt that the premiums proposed would adequately pay for the extended benefits. Medicare over the years has cost significantly more than had been anticipated. As a result there have been a mix of premium increases and service decreases. Are we letting ourselves in for another round of raised expectations to be dashed by cost overruns and resulting cutbacks?

Would it not be better to undertake one or two benefit changes at a time rather than the close to a dozen changes in the House bill? For instance, more than 5 million beneficiaries have medicine costs over $500 a year. Many of those folks need help, and in Delaware some get that help thanks to the Nemours Foundation. Adding outpatient medication coverage would help a significant portion of the nation's elderly and should be added to Medicare.

Extended periods of hospitalization, on the other hand, affect thousands rather than millions. Perhaps that benefit should not be added at this point.

Improved coverage of skilled nursing home care, on the other hand, would benefit more persons, especially with the current move to early discharge from hospitals. Similarly, the proposed extension of home-health-care coverage would be a significant plus for a substantial number of people. Both of these items are less costly than hospitalization, so beneficiaries would get more for their premium dollar.

House and Senate conferees should review the Medicare experience of the past 22 years and evaluate where the needs are greatest. They should avoid a Christmas-tree type bill with a politically attractive tidbit for every constituent expected to cast a vote in 1988.

Bangor Daily News

Bangor, ME, July 28, 1987

The U.S. House of Representatives has passed a catastrophic-illness insurance bill aimed at patching one of the gaps in the nation's health-care policy. The Senate has yet to take up action on a different, more conservative version. President Reagan, who has spoken in favor of such a program, has indicated he will veto the House version because it is too costly. But whatever evolves should be a historic contribution to the nation's health-care safety net.

Catastrophic-illness insurance will provide some financial relief for the minority of families of elderly people who end their lives on extraordinary life-support systems. But as Rep. Claude Pepper, D-Miami, has noted: "As a whole (the bill) addresses the issue of health-care costs by the elderly in a very limited manner. In spite of the many benefits of this bill, long-term illness will still remain as the primary cause of financial ruin for millions of Americans."

Pepper is talking about the cost of nursing home and home care that drains the savings of many more people than catastrophic situations. Some observers have suggested that private insurance is the answer, but so far it is not. Many of policies are confusing, inadequate and too expensive for many people who need long-term nursing home or home care. Many people are unaware there are gaps in Medicare.

And almost two-thirds of the insurance policies marketed to senior citizens to fill in the gaps in Medicare coverage pay too little benefits to meet minimum government standards, according to a study by the General Accounting Office. That means they're ripping off the people who are suckered into buying them.

The nation has pieced together a ponderous, expensive and confusing system of health care. It shouldn't cost much more to put together a comprehensive plan that would provide uniformly broad care.

SATURDAY OKLAHOMAN & TIMES

Oklahoma City, OK, July 25, 1987

THE catastrophic health insurance legislation in Congress is a glaring example of a well-meaning effort gone awry.

Last February, President Reagan proposed that the nation's 31 million Medicare beneficiaries be provided protection against financially debilitating illnesses. His plan would extend coverage and limit out-of-pocket expenses. Additional costs would be financed through increased premiums.

Two House committees rewrote the plan, making it more generous and at the same time more burdensome for the elderly. The version passed by the House by a vote of 302 to 127 would produce the largest expansion of Medicare benefits in its 22-year history.

The bill limits liability for costs of hospitalization, physicians' services and even prescription drugs. It provides for care in nursing homes, hospices and at home. Cost of the expanded coverage is estimated at $34 billion over five years, and most of the financial burden would be borne by about 40 percent of the elderly.

Oklahoma's House delegation split evenly on the bill. Joining the state's two Republicans, Rep. Dave McCurdy was one of 14 Democrats on the opposing side. He especially objected to provisions that would force the elderly to pay for costly treatment of AIDS victims. There are currently 4,000 AIDS patients on Social Security disability rolls who will qualify for Medicare coverage after 24 months, McCurdy says. If they live beyond that period, they would have 80 percent of their costs for expensive drugs like AZT paid by Medicare.

Liberals in Congress no doubt would welcome a showdown over enactment of this key item on their agenda of social legislation.

the Charleston Gazette

Charleston, WVA, July 28, 1987

WHILE other industrialized nations provide free medical care for all citizens, America disgracefully can't do as well.

Last week the House of Representatives passed a feeble, inadequate plan to expand Medicare to cover catastrophic health debts of the elderly. It would force Medicare participants to pay all the cost — about $7 billion a year —

through an extra $580 yearly premium, and it wouldn't provide for nursing home care.

Even so, President Reagan fears the plan would incur long-term governmental costs, and he's threatening to veto it.

But you can bet that, if the House voted $7 billion a year for more thermonuclear bombs, Reagan would sign it in record time.

THE SUN

Baltimore, MD, July 27, 1987

From the beginning of the debate on extending Medicare to cover catastrophic health-care costs, it was clear the administration's acute care proposal barely scratched the surface. For the elderly — most of whom live on fixed incomes — any large, unexpected or continuing medical expense can be catastrophic. Costly private insurance policies do not, generally, fill the gap.

While the need was clear, confusion over how to provide affordable benefits was rampant in Congress. Yet the House surprisingly has crafted a feasible bill.

Like the administration's acute care plan, it limits out-of-pocket expenses for hospitalization and physicians' fees. But it goes well beyond the president's proposal, expanding coverage for home care, skilled nursing care, outpatient mental health and hospice care. It also includes a worthy provision ensuring the elderly will not have to impoverish themselves to pay for a spouse in a nursing home.

While the administration's ideological opposition to government expansion is longstanding, it is more irked by a part of the House bill which, for the first time, provides coverage for prescription drugs outside the hospital. After a $500 deductible, Medicare would pay 80 percent of the cost of generic drugs.

We remain skeptical about the accuracy of the

cost estimate, as does the Senate Finance Committee, which has not included a drug provision in its version of the bill. But support for such coverage is strong. An amendment to include prescription drug coverage in the Senate's plan is expected to be introduced on the Senate floor. Clearly, a more precise evaluation of all costs, premiums and deductibles is critical when the bill goes to a House-Senate conference committee. But this provision incorporates the best aspects of two flawed plans and it deserves support and reconsideration.

Equally as significant as the bill's provisions is its financing scheme. The plan approved by the House uses a graduated premium that exempts the poor, while capping the maximum premium for the comprehensive array of new benefits at about $48 a month, collected by the IRS along with income taxes. Under the administration's plan, which uses higher premiums, everyone pays the same — regardless of income. Those who can't afford it don't get coverage.

The House plan needs fine tuning, which we expect in negotiations with the Senate. But overall, representatives have managed to hammer out a bill that offers the prospect of affordably meeting the medical needs of the elderly without taking a penny from the federal treasury. As a result, the nation is closer to the kind of Medicare reform that truly defrays catastrophic health care costs.

Part V: AIDS and American Lifestyles

The decision by movie star Rock Hudson to reveal his diagnosis of AIDS and his homosexuality not only brought information to a wider audience, but also brought sharper focus on the issues of homosexuality and sexual behavior in American society.

Though AIDS has changed sexual practices and brought a reconsideration of lifestyles faster than anyone would have believed possible, persuading individuals to change long-term habits of sexual behavior or drug abuse is extremely difficult. Although recent evidence indicates that carefully designed programs can be effective in the general adult population, many people believe it is equally important to ensure that adolescents, non-English-speaking minorities and drug abusers understand the risk of AIDS. Controversy arises because some people believe that it is inappropriate for government agencies to tell homosexuals or bisexuals how to have "safe sex" or to explain the importance of sterile needles, while others feel that the gravity of the situation warrants such measures.

For many, AIDS poses a severe moral challenge in that promiscuity is a prominent feature of the lifestyles of at least some Americans. The challenge has confronted both those who are not infected with AIDS and those who are. But the issue beyond the commonsense advice that prudence alone requires that the uninfected reconsider the risk of promiscuity, is a *moral* responsibility for the maintenance of good health. The question of moral responsibility for individual health is far from settled because, where the health risks of AIDS and sexual promiscuity are concerned, the health risks are not yet known with enough certainty to permit the judgment that promiscuous people are taking *immoral* risks with their health or the health of their partners. Some in the gay community, for instance, regard calls for more "responsible" sexual behavior as a threat to the community's existence and values, while others argue that it is both prudent and ethical to show restraint in a time of crisis. Happily, at least for homosexual men who are at risk for AIDS, studies have shown beneficial changes in sexual behavior, such as fewer partners and use of condoms.

Researchers are now only beginning to get some hint of the size of the bisexual population because of the growing numbers of bisexuals testing positive for AIDS antibodies. Experts worry that bisexuals' lack of organizational ties and community, along with their fear of losing their spouses and children, may make them the hardest to reach of the potential AIDS-carrying groups.

AIDS poses a major threat to the health of intravenous drug abusers, their sexual partners, and their children. More than two-thirds of AIDS cases resulting from heterosexual intercourse with a member of a recognized high-risk group involve sexual contact with an intravenous drug user. More than half of all children with AIDS have at least one parent who is a drug abuser. Transmission of the AIDS virus among drug abusers results from sharing hypodermic needles and syringes. Proposed options to reduce this practice include: decreasing the amount of illegal drug abuse, providing sterile needles and syringes through public and private agencies, and educating drug users about sterilization procedures and the need to seek out and pay for clean equipment. Though the first option is laudable, neither stricter law enforcement nor the availability of legal alternatives, such as methadone maintenance, has reduced the drug abuse problem in the U.S. The concept of providing sterile equipment, though adopted by some European countries, has aroused considerable controversy, with most arguments focusing on the moral dilemma raised when government organizations provide the materials necessary to carry out an illegal act. Those in favor of the distribution of clean needles and syringes counter that the public health risk presented by AIDS justifies changing the rules. Many public health officials believe that the final option, risk-education and reeducation for intravenous drug abusers, is unrealistic because the target population simply will not listen.

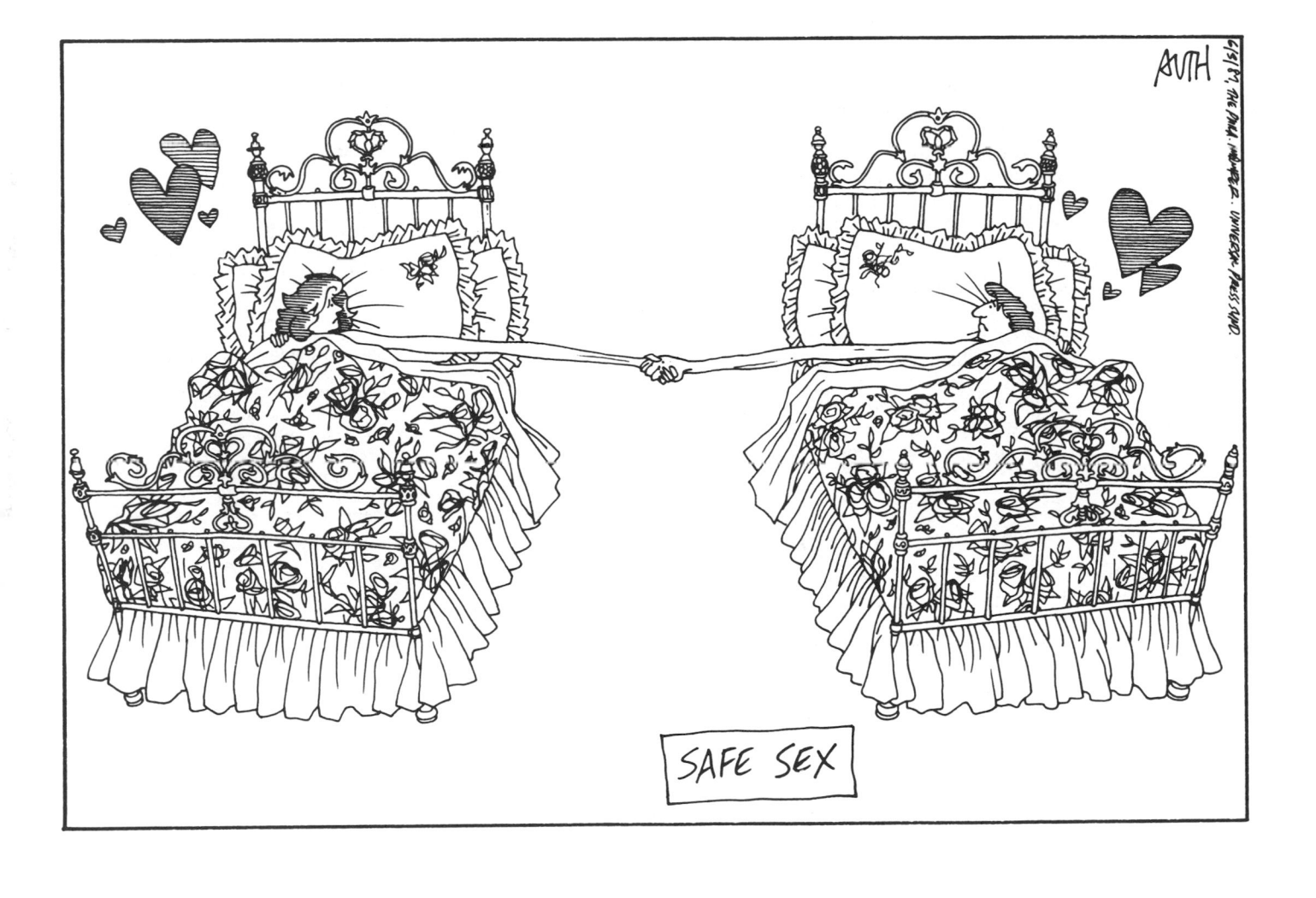

SAFE SEX

AIDS Guidelines Issued; Concern Sweeps Nation

The Public Health Service urged March 3, 1983 that several groups, including homosexual men, drug users and Haitians, refrain from giving blood because it was possible that AIDS might be transmitted through blood transfusions. Most of the AIDS victims observed to date had been homosexual men, but the other groups covered by the warning—drug users and Haitians—were also considered at risk. Recently, a number of hemophiliacs had contracted AIDS, suggesting that the disease could be transmitted through blood transfusions. It was this development that prompted the warning that groups considered at risk should refrain from donating blood.

A group representing hemophiliacs had urged that the government go further, banning blood donations by groups at risk instead of merely recommending that members of such groups refrain. On the other hand, a spokesperson for the National Gay Task Force criticized the Public Health Service action. Blood donation organizations should "screen blood, not people," the homosexual rights advocate said.

Concern had been expressed, however, that the disease was starting to spread into the general population, and there had been cases of health and other workers refusing to have contact with AIDS victims out of fear of contracting the disease. In San Francisco, a city with a large homosexual population and a correspondingly higher-than-average incidence of AIDS, there had been cases of landlords evicting homosexual tenants, presumably in response to concern about the disease, the *New York Times* reported June 14, 1983.

The fact that homosexuals were the largest single group of victims of the disease injected an element of politics and controversy that might have otherwise been absent. AIDS had contributed to a renewal of discrimination against homosexuals in some places, and had furnished a new argument to religious fundamentalists opposed to homosexual lifestyles. Spokespersons for homosexual organizations and political leaders sympathetic to homosexual concerns also contended that the government's response to the disease had been less energetic than it would have been had another group been the victim.

THE PLAIN DEALER
Cleveland, OH, July 6, 1983

In San Francisco and across the nation last week, thousands of homosexuals paraded as part of their annual gay freedom celebration, a celebration overshadowed by the so-called "AIDS crisis."

AIDS (Acquired Immune Deficiency Syndrome) already has killed 644 Americans, most of them homosexuals. The fight against AIDS, as described by Newsweek magazine last week, is the result of an increasing national hysteria ranging from the silly (Beverly Hill women counseling each other to stop kissing their hairdressers) to the serious (Red Cross blood collections are off 16.4% because donors mistakenly fear contracting AIDS).

Much of the blame for the AIDS scare is mistakenly being placed upon the media. Gay leaders contend that irresponsible reporting and editing have contributed to a growing panic. The press has been accused of sensationalizing the AIDS story.

We don't accept that criticism. Sure, as with any story, there have been individual instances of exaggeration or overplay, but the press as a whole is not responsible for the panic. In fact, the gay community has used the press to publicize the disease.

By staging marches, by writing letters, by demonstrations, the gays have turned a little-known disease into a national crisis. Those working at generating public concern have made many scary points comparing the epidemic to the black plague, emphasizing the mystery of the disease and asserting that AIDS is certain to spread among the straight population unless a cure is found.

This is not to question the seriousness of the disease, but to express concern about the "unreasonable fear" cited by the director of the U.S. Public Health Service; a fear that was evident in San Francisco and other cities last week as the gay community marched so soberly and so angrily.

Certainly AIDS is a dreadful disease, an illness for which a cure hopefully can be found. But let us remember that there are many other diseases equally deadly and affecting far more people without the resultant publicity.

Take, by contrast with AIDS, Alzheimer's disease, an illness that affects as many as two million people in this country over 65 years old. It reportedly is the fourth leading cause of death among the elderly and costs for care run into billions of dollars. Yet, until recently, very few people had heard of Alzheimer's disease, very little was known about it.

The gay community deserves respect and recognition, but so, too, do our senior citizens. The former is doing a great PR job; the latter are being ignored.

The Salt Lake Tribune
Salt Lake City, UT
June 28, 1983

By now, most people must know something about acquired immune deficiency syndrome (AIDS) and the growing anxiety over how serious this new health threat might be. Indeed, there is cause for concern but not the hysteria that has reportedly developed in some parts of the country.

The disease destroys, apparently irreversibly, the human body's ability to fight off infection.

Although it has not been determined what causes AIDS, there are reliable indications as to how it is transmitted and what kinds of people are most likely to contract it.

So far, there have been no known cures and the number of deaths, about 600 as of early June, is high. Fewer than 2,000 cases have been confirmed but the rate at which new ones are being reported suggests that the disease could strike 1.5 million people within five years.

Since male homosexuals constitute approximately 70 percent of AIDS' victims, the suspicion is strong that "straights" are unlikely to be afflicted. But the other 30 percent of victims includes hemophiliacs who require frequent blood transfusions, intravenous drug users and, strangely, residents of Haiti.

As publicity is focused on AIDS, instances of babies being born with the malady are being reported and some authorities refuse to accept the present medical judgement that AIDS is not spread by casual personal contact.

Rising public apprehension is being fueled by a mix of ignorance and fear. On the basis of present statistics, homosexual males have genuine cause for anxiety. But as yet there is no cause for alarm for the population as a whole.

Although the number of cases thus far is relatively small, the federal government's health centers have assigned a high priority to finding the agent that causes AIDS and developing a cure. Presumably the same search is on in the private sector, too. Meanwhile, persons who have no reason to believe they are in the high risk segment of the population have minimal cause for concern. Those is the suspect categories are on notice and must judge the distressing odds accordingly.

The Times-Picayune
The States-Item
New Orleans, LA, July 31, 1983

Considering the amount of publicity the new disease called AIDS has gotten and the often panic-tinged nature of it, the conclusion of the state Department of Health advisory board's recent deliberations should be of comfort to the general local population. The judgment is that AIDS is of extreme concern to the medical community and those in the risk group, but not broadly dangerous enough to justify a public health emergency or to directly concern the general public.

AIDS stands for acquired immune deficiency syndrome, and since the causative agent — a yet unidentified blood-borne virus, possibly a new mutant — is not known, the disease is recognized primarily by its effects. What it does is destroy the body's natural immune system so that the victim is vulnerable to common or rare "opportunistic" diseases the normal immune system would have a chance to fend off.

Thus diagnosis can be difficult; an immune system-related illness may or may not be an indication of AIDS. Diagnosis is most certain in unusual and catastrophic cases. Using the conservative definition of the national Centers for Disease Control, there have been eight confirmed cases in Louisiana, including five deaths.

The disease strikes a relatively well defined group: primarily male homosexuals and abusers of needle-injected drugs, and secondarily those who can contract it from blood transfusions. (One cannot contract it by *giving* blood, so while those in the risk group should not give blood, those not in it are encouraged to.) "Haitians" were early placed in the risk group, but fuller investigation has indicated that the Haitian victims were male prostitutes or intravenous drug users.

Public health officials say that since the preponderance of evidence indicates that one can get AIDS only through blood contact, members of the public not in the risk group need not fear contracting AIDS from casual or unwitting association with a victim or a carrier.

Identification and control of the AIDS agent poses a challenge to medical researchers that should be taken up with energy and adequate financing. Those in the risk group can act immediately to reduce their exposure. But the general public, according to the best medical advice, can safely go about their normal lives and leave dealing with AIDS to those directly involved.

The Wichita
Eagle-Beacon
Wichita, KS, August 7, 1983

The seemingly inexorable spread of the disease now identified as Aquired Immune Deficiency Syndrome, and the heavy death toll accompanying it, warrant a serious, concerted response by the nation's health agencies. The fact that AIDS, until recently, had been diagnosed almost exclusively among homosexuals and drug abusers unquestionably has complicated the situation.

Such considerations, of course, should not be the determining factor in whether effective, responsible steps are undertaken. Now, however, in the words of Dr. Anthony Fauci of the National Institute of Allergy and Infectious Diseases, "AIDS is creeping out of well-defined epidemiological confines." The disease has begun showing up in people whose more conventional lifestyles at one point seemed to place them beyond the risk group. Tragically, some of those people are very young children.

Evidence still indicates that intimate sexual contact or exposure through the intermixing of blood are the most likely ways that AIDS is spread. Some research points to some new type of virus as a possible causative factor.

At this point, the only thing known for sure about AIDS is its all-too-often deadly effects. Once contracted, a victim is a likely candidate for a once-rare form of pneumonia or a type of skin cancer that previously was seldom fatal. The AIDS sufferer's body loses its ability to fight off infections and foreign agents, rendering that person susceptible to all manner of such secondary diseases, many of which then can prove mortal.

With mortality rates running as high as 60 percent and doctors having no effective treatment for those whose cases reach the advanced stage, the current "AIDS hysteria" probably was almost inevitable. Some people have refused to provide CPR or other necessary emergency assistance to AIDS victims; there have been cases of blood donations by the public dropping off precipitously, out of the totally unfounded fear of somehow contracting AIDS in the process of giving blood. Emotionalism, however, can't be allowed to rule here.

The central question, of course, must be what can be done. Since AIDS may have a latent stage, those whose lifestyles may already have exposed them to it should refrain from donating blood. They also should consider limiting the number of contacts through which AIDS is known to be passed on — for their own safety, as well as for others'.

And government agencies, such the Centers for Disease Control, can treat AIDS for what it is: a legitimate public health threat that already has claimed more lives than Legionnaire's disease and toxic shock syndrome, combined.

The
Des Moines Register
Des Moines, IA
July 7, 1983

Midwesterners have the reputation of being friendlier and more willing to help a person in need than people from other parts of the country. Though this may be a myth, it would be nice if it were true in the case of the man who has the first confirmed case of AIDS in Iowa.

Iowans' supposed propensity for helping others, and the case of Acquired Immune Deficiency Syndrome, would seem unrelated until one considers what is happening to AIDS patients in other parts of the country. They have been feared and shunned.

In New York, for example, the corrections-officers union has demanded that anyone preparing food in the city prison system be screened for AIDS, and also urged that homosexuals — a high-risk group — be barred from food preparation.

In San Francisco, where there have been many reported cases, horror stories abound. Prospective jurors have refused to sit with AIDS patients, and there have been reports of persons with the disease being evicted from their homes. In one ironic case, a man with AIDS was to appear on a morning television talk show to explain the disease and to tell others there is no risk of contagion from day-to-day contact with a patient. Technicians refused to let the man use a microphone.

Ironically, the man who was willing to talk about the disease had more to fear from the technicians than they did from him. AIDS attacks the body's natural immune systems, leaving the victim defenseless against illness. A summer cold could prove fatal to an AIDS patient.

The disease is most common among homosexuals, intravenous-drug abusers, hemophiliacs and Haitians, but no one knows why. It can be transmitted only through intimate sexual contact, a shared hypodermic needle or, in rare cases, through blood transfusions.

The stigma of the disease as much as the threat of contagion hurts AIDS victims and their families and friends. Despite public-information campaigns and medical reassurances, misinformation still breeds fear where there ought to be compassion.

There is as much a need to cure this fear as there is to find a cure for the disease, for the sake of the patient and those around him.

THE LOUISVILLE TIMES
Louisville, KY, July 19, 1983

Leading medical researchers are baffled by Acquired Immune Deficiency Syndome, but the Moral Majority's Jerry Falwell is not. He believes God's wrath against homosexuality has been unleashed by the mysterious malady that attacks the body's defenses against infection.

Mr. Falwell, who is known for his special brand of hate-mongering in the name of the Good Book, wants President Reagan to round up the nation's homosexuals and isolate them until a cure is found.

Ordinarily, such suggestions would simply be ignored, but Mr. Falwell is not your run-of-the-mill Bible thumper. He is a long-time supporter of Mr. Reagan. From time-to-time he prays with and peddles advice to the President. His radio and television pulpit brings his brand of religiosity into millions of homes every week.

On the subject of AIDS he is both misinformed and misguided. Though AIDS has primarily affected male homosexuals, the disease also strikes hemophiliacs, intravenous users of drugs and Haitian immigrants.

Mr. Falwell offers no clue why God's vengeance has been loosed on those unfortunates, nor does he explain why American male homosexuals have been singled out. Few foreign countries have reported cases of the disease.

Mr. Falwell's quarantine is not designed to protect the non-infected world from AIDS. Rather, he would isolate a particular group in society for ridicule and persecution. Fears about the mysterious illness have already done enough of that. It requires no sympathy for homosexual life-styles to recognize that further inflammatory talk is dangerous to everyone.

THE CHRISTIAN SCIENCE MONITOR
Boston, MA, July 5, 1983

The medical profession still has many questions about what it calls AIDS, an ailment supposed to reduce physical immunity to other diseases. Of at least one thing doctors seem sure: that public fear of infection has become an unnecessary complication in the situation.

The news media are recognizing the problem under headlines such as "The real epidemic: fear and despair." Public and private health officials are trying to ease the alarm with statements such as the one by the chief epidemiologist of a federal task force on the subject: "Suddenly the facts are being misinterpreted to suggest that somehow AIDS is lurking in every swimming pool, the subways, on plates in restaurants, just everywhere. That is simply not the case."

Just this week another federal official noted that the national rate of increase in reported cases appeared to be dropping. (Some 1,640 cases, including about 640 fatalities, have now been reported.) In New York, which accounts for 45 percent of the cases, the increase seems to have leveled off, instead of doubling as predicted earlier, said the health commissioner.

Both media and medical people face the challenge of exposing false fears without contributing to them by manner of presentation.

Possibilities for sensationalism have to be resisted when most of the cases have been linked to homosexual relations or drug addiction. Also to be resisted are the current examples of unreasoning ostracism of members of "high-risk" groups just when realism and compassion are most called for.

Government can foster realism by expediting research on the unanswered questions that tempt fearful leaping to wrong conclusions. Individuals can do the same by recognizing that eliminating fear is an important step in dealing with any human problem — and that all can partake of that love of God which casts out fear.

The Seattle Times
Seattle, WA, September 29, 1983

OFFICIALS of the Seattle-King County Health Department are furious over an unauthorized and unverified list of supposed AIDS victims that has circulated within the Seattle Police Department. The Health Department concerns are fully understandable.

The so-called "AIDS Alert" list was apparently intended to warn police officers against having any contact with the people on the list.

Department officials are investigating the origin of the list and have ordered police to stop circulating it. Whatever the motives of those who drew up and circulated the list, containing 10 names, there are at least three reasons for communitywide condemnation and concern. They are, in ascending order of importance:

First, no identifiable sponsorship. That is symptomatic of a Ku Klux Klan, vigilante-type mind-set that one would like to think does not exist inside the Police Department.

Second, circulation of any such material tends to contribute to hysteria over AIDS (acquired immune deficiency syndrome) inside or outside the department. Specialists on the disease stress there is no evidence that it can spread simply by touching infected persons or their body fluids.

Third, as Dr. Hunter Handsfield, director of the Health Department's Sexually Transmitted Disease Control Program, points out, the list distribution may have done "irreparable damage" to the program, which is dependent on patients' trust that their names will be kept confidential.

That applies not only to AIDS victims, but to anyone in need of the department's help because of a real or suspected infection of any sexually transmitted disease.

It is up to the Police Department's top leadership to insure there will be no recurrence of such disreputable activity within the department.

THE KANSAS CITY STAR
Kansas City, MO, August 5, 1983

When the Department of Health and Human Services officially labels a disease the No. 1 emergency health priority in the nation, it's normal to expect a concentrated attack from several fronts.

Both the unknown and terminal natures of acquired immune deficiency syndrome, or AIDS, are terrifying. Nothing short of finding cause and cure is enough. Given the fact that such investigation cannot be pursued like writing a computer program, that desired solution is going to take time and money.

There have been complaints that the government is dragging its feet. One point that came up in recent hearings was that the $12 million Congress added to federal research efforts on AIDS this year was a congressional initiative. The administration wanted to shift funds from other health programs.

Dr. Edward N. Brandt, the assistant secretary of health in HHS, testified that part of the national strategy to deal with the disease is to continue to redirect money toward research. Setting up a national AIDS hot line and distribution of informational packages to the public are also part of the plan. The strategy, at best, appears modest.

He also testified that if all money being spent on research relevant to AIDS is combined, it amounts to about $166 million this year. That sounds impressive. But health officials and research scientists know even better than citizens upset about the lack of progress that dollars alone don't buy medical breakthroughs. Such elements as leadership, commitment by institutions, pressure from lawmakers and outrage for the suffering of victims help create the atmosphere. And luck helps.

This is no epidemic to put on a corner shelf in the basement. A financial and moral stand must be made, about which there can be no doubt of absolute commitment by private and public institutions. And while we are about such official decisions, it won't hurt to show a decent amount of compassion and concern for the victims. After all, they are the ones suffering and dying.

THE DENVER POST

Denver, CO, August 14, 1983

NO DOUBT, Denver policeman Kevin Boyd by now is thoroughly embarrassed by his hasty retreat from the home of a burglary victim who is suffering from acquired immune deficiency syndrome (AIDS).

The patrolman, interviewing a postal worker who had reported a stolen ring, asked about a box of surgical masks in the man's home. The burglary victim, Henry Pena, told the policeman he sometimes wore the masks to protect himself from infection since his AIDS was diagnosed three weeks ago. In seconds, the policeman was gone.

"From the time I got up off the couch until I got to the door to explain he was in no danger, he was gone. He must've gotten in his police car and burned rubber," Pena told The Post's Marjie Lundstrom.

Patrolman Boyd's reaction is unfortunately typical of the uninformed mythology that shrouds the mysterious disease of AIDS. Although tragically little is known about AIDS, one thing is certain — there is no reason for panic.

The disorder, which robs the body of its ability to fight off disease, so far has been detected in only a minuscule fraction of the population — fewer than 2,000 cases nationwide — and is limited primarily to four specific risk groups: homosexual or bisexual men; intravenous drug abusers, Haitian immigrants and hemophiliacs. Although there's no cure yet and the cause hasn't been pinned down, the best available evidence is that AIDS is transmitted only in extraordinary circumstances: prolonged intimate sex, or invasion of another's bloodstream by the blood of an afflicted person.

Patrolman Boyd obviously wasn't aware of that when he told The Post, "I don't know much about AIDS, but I do know that it's a highly contagious disease and a fatal disease." He may be right about the prognosis; he is wrong about the epidemiology.

In this case, the policeman's ignorance resulted in no permanent damage: He simply made a fool of himself and offended a man who already has been hurt enough. The burglary report eventually was taken by telephone — as are many such complaints — and, in fact, the ring has been recovered at a pawn shop.

But what if Pena had been an accident victim or a shooting victim requiring first aid? It isn't hard to imagine a case in which ignorance and insensitivity could be fatal.

Safety Manager John Simonet's subsequent reaction — to tell the rest of the police force the truth about AIDS — is rational and appropriate, if a bit delayed. Simonet is putting a notice about AIDS in the daily Police Bulletin and says he wants to start a training program to dispel the myths.

That's a good idea, not only for the police, but for others whose job is to help the public in times of emergency. In fact, Simonet did anticipate the problem as it relates to firefighters; they already have been given an informational packet about AIDS.

The new safety manager, who has been in office only since May — tightroping between the old and new city administrations — may not have had time to prevent this particular police-relations problem. But from what Simonet has revealed so far of his management style, Denver citizens have every reason to expect he'll move to thwart the next rumor-fed bogeyman before it jumps out of the dark in similar embarrassment.

BUFFALO EVENING NEWS

Buffalo, NY, July 17, 1983

The recently discovered disease AIDS — Acquired Immune Deficiency Syndrome — has become a serious health problem, and it is stirring fear in many quarters. Some nurses have refused to treat an AIDS patient, and some morticians have been hesitant to embalm AIDS victims.

Obviously any disease that kills a large proportion of its victims and for which there is no known cure is cause for great concern. However, most cases seem to be limited to a few categories in the population.

Almost all those who have contracted AIDS so far have been male homosexuals, intravenous drug abusers, hemophiliacs who may have been infected by blood transfusions and Haitian immigrants. The cause of the disease is unknown, although a virus is suspected. The disease suppresses the body's natural immunity, and the victims often contract rare diseases that are easily resisted by the normal healthy person.

About half the known U.S. cases of AIDS are in the New York City area, and State Health Commissioner David Axelrod has rightly backed measures to fight the mysterious disease. The Legislature has approved state funds to finance studies of the disease in research centers in the state. Federal health officials have announced plans to give top priority to combatting AIDS.

Health officials emphasize that there is no evidence that AIDS can be spread through mere casual contacts. There is no occasion for panic. Nevertheless, uncertainty is bound to remain, since the cause of the disease remains elusive. This makes doubly important the current proposals to launch new research efforts to fight this killer.

The Idaho STATESMAN

Boise, ID, July 9, 1983

In an era of substantial cynicism about society and its institutions, the country's reaction to the terrifying disease called AIDS is in some ways gratifying.

AIDS, which stands for Acquired Immune Deficiency Syndrome, was first diagnosed in 1981. Since then the political system and the medical-scientific establishment appear to have worked remarkably well to address the problem.

From the gay population, which has been hit the worst by AIDS, to the medical community to municipal and federal governments, forces have been marshaled to confine the disease and seek a remedy.

Gay activists have joined with health authorities to warn those who face the greatest risk. Mayors of cities such as New York and San Francisco, prompted both by the political clout of their gay communities and by the obvious health threat, have rallied to support the fight against AIDS.

The federal government this year allocated $14 million for AIDS research and plans to spend at least $17.5 million in the coming year.

Meanwhile, the health-care community has forged one of the most intense medical detective efforts in history.

Predictably, not all the reaction has been positive. Some gays have criticized the federal government for moving too slowly. And some fundamentalist Christians have smugly characterized the outbreak as retribution for the evils of homosexuality.

All in all, though, the national response to a terrible health threat has been admirable. It inspires hope that medical researchers will be able to isolate the cause of AIDS and find a preventative or cure.

In a broader sense, it also gives evidence of our ability, when necessary, to pull together in a humane and rational fashion.

THE ATLANTA CONSTITUTION

Atlanta, GA, June 24, 1983

No threat is quite so frightening as one that defies understanding. The more mysterious the danger, the greater the risk of panic. In the case of AIDS, the strange disease that breaks down the body's immune system, it is important to feed reasonable concern with knowledge rather than fear.

Across the nation, there have been troubling stories. Some AIDS victims have been evicted from their apartments by landlords who fear the disease will spread; studio technicians refused to televise one sufferer; another victim, a prison inmate, was arraigned by officials wearing surgical garb in a criminal courtroom cleared of spectators; embalmers in some areas have balked at handling the bodies of victims.

Some facts to keep in mind:

• There is no cause for fear among the general public that individuals may develop AIDS through casual contact with a patient. That judgment comes from no less an authority than the Centers for Disease Control in Atlanta.

• AIDS is spread "almost entirely" through sexual contact, through the sharing of needles by drug abusers and, less commonly, through blood or blood products.

• The CDC, accordingly, has found that 71.2 percent of the 1,601 AIDS cases reported involve homosexual or bisexual men; 17.2 percent involve intravenous drug users; and .8 percent involve hemophiliacs, persons who suffer from a blood disorder. There is a mystery within this mystery, however: 5.1 percent of the cases involve Haitians, a fact no one can adequately explain. In 5.7 percent of the cases, the victims' lifestyles were unknown or they failed to match the common categories.

• For clinical staffs handling blood samples of AIDS victims, the CDC advises that gloves and clean gowns be worn, that clean instruments be used and that workers take care not to expose open wounds to the specimens. A similar list of precautions is being prepared for embalmers.

Not only does simple justice demand that this disease be fought and treated in an atmosphere of calm rationality. So does common decency.

EVENING EXPRESS

Portland, ME, July 1, 1983

The U.S. Public Health Service has declared AIDS—acquired immune deficiency syndrome—its "No. 1 priority."

And so it should be. A disease exists, its pathology unidentified, yet already it has struck more than 1,640 victims, a number that grows by two new cases a day.

Given the fear that AIDS has generated among homosexual men, drug abusers and hemophiliacs, its primary victims, and among health care personnel and funeral directors worried about potential infection, AIDS is overdue for concerted federal action.

Yet there are those who'd prefer to let the virulent infection run its course unimpeded by the Public Health Service. The Moral Majority, for one, doesn't want government dollars used for AIDS research.

Spokesman Cal Thomas says the group is "opposed to the underwriting of perverted lifestyles by the federal government (except) to keep the disease from spreading to the general populace."

The dismissal is self-serving, and it's uninformed as well. Government response to any disease should not be conditioned by the sexual preferences of its victims.

Homosexual men aren't alone in high risk of contracting AIDS. Despite precautions, the disease has struck hemophiliacs and Haitians.

Fear has convinced some who treat AIDS victims, before and after death, that they can contract it, too. And those fears, too, deserve to be dealt with.

Before any of that can happen, AIDS must be understood.

AKRON BEACON JOURNAL

Akron, OH, July 2, 1983

AS THEY annually do, thousands of gay-rights marchers rallied in major cities across the country last Sunday. But this year one sobering subject preoccupied many participants.

The new factor was Acquired Immune Deficiency Syndrome, a deadly ailment that cripples the body's ability to fight off disease.

AIDS is doing more than killing many victims. It is spreading fear and strengthening old prejudices at the same time it is destroying lives.

People are frightened, because doctors and public health researchers don't know what causes AIDS and no cure is yet in sight.

It is important to keep in mind that even this still-mysterious disease exhibits known basic patterns. More than 70 percent of its victims are male homosexuals, leading scientists to suspect that AIDS is transmitted primarily through sexual contact.

Three other risk groups have been identified: intravenous drug abusers, Haitian immigrants and, to a much smaller extent, hemophiliacs, who require transfusions of blood plasma pooled from thousands of donors.

Since 1979 more than 1,600 cases of AIDS have been recorded. The Akron-Canton area has reported three; one involved a homosexual, one a hemophiliac, one a Haitian visitor.

Scientists first realized two years ago that the disease was more than a random illness. Now they are working feverishly to bring it under control.

We applaud Ohio for joining the fight. Dr. David Jackson, state health director, intends to create an advisory panel and earmark $4 million for community education programs about AIDS. He also wants the Ohio Public Health Council to require doctors to report suspected AID cases.

In time, the disease will be understood. For now, the public hysteria accompanying growing publicity about AIDS is both harmful and totally unwarranted.

Ninety-five percent of AIDS patients fall into one of the four risk groups. There is no evidence that AIDS can be spread easily, by a cough, touch or sneeze. Despite the facts, the behavior displayed by some people has been almost as bizarre as the disease itself.

Landlords have evicted homosexuals; roommates have thrown them out. An AIDS victim resigned from jury duty when fellow jurors in San Franciso objected to his presence. Employees at one company demanded separate phones and toilet facilities from homosexual co-workers.

Of serious public consequence are reports of falling blood donations in major cities. People somehow fear that if they give blood, they may contract AIDS. Those fears have no basis in fact. But blood collection agencies such as the Red Cross in New York and Chicago say fewer donors are showing up.

The hysteria surrounding this new illness can be as deadly as the disease, if it takes hold of otherwise rational people and controls their behavior. Fear based on ignorance won't bring us any closer to unlocking the mystery of AIDS.

THE MILWAUKEE JOURNAL
Milwaukee, WI, August 28, 1983

The Reagan administration has wisely decided to ask for twice the amount originally requested for medical research on AIDS — the mysterious disease that has already killed more than 750 persons. Secretary of Health and Human Services Margaret Heckler announced that she would lobby for congressional approval of $40 million for research instead of $20 million.

That is appropriate, considering that the administration had called investigation of AIDS the nation's No. 1 health priority. The deadly ailment usually strikes homosexuals or intravenous drug users but its ultimate impact could be more widespread.

Heckler herself deserves commendation for recognizing that, as she put it, "The fear of the disease is spreading faster than the disease." To combat undue fear, she went to the bedside of Peter Justice, an AIDS patient in New York. They chatted and shook hands. Heckler said she wanted to demonstrate that public fear of contracting AIDS by such a routine encounter was unjustified. Good for her.

The News and Courier
Charleston, SC, July 14, 1983

Almost everything that is written or said about Acquired Immune Deficiency Syndrome, or AIDS as it is known for short, comes with a thesaurus of nightmare adjectives: horrifying, terrifying, mysterious, dreadful and so on.

Few other diseases in history have aroused so much panic and hysteria. Writers on the subject invariably draw a parallel with the epidemic of plague which raged across Europe in the Middle Ages and was called The Black Death. A better parallel, however, would be with the prevalence of venereal disease in early 19th century Britain and the consequent return to rigid sexual restraints which characterized the Victorian era.

AIDS is certainly not comparable with the plague. Already, enough is known about AIDS to diminish fear, rather than heighten it. Yet misinformation — and subsequent panic — continues to spread. For example, an obviously hastily-prepared news bulletin broadcast recently on a local radio station mistakenly referred to "Hispanics" as being among those who have been afflicted by AIDS. The news bulletin, of course, should have specified Haitians, who make up about 5 percent of the roughly 1,600 cases recorded by the national Centers for Disease Control at Atlanta. Another example of misinformation was a recent edition of the Rev. Jerry Falwell's newspaper, Moral Majority, which showed a "typical" American family — the kind of Mom, Pop and Kids combination hired from a model agency — wearing protective masks. The inference was that AIDS could spread to the population as a whole.

The consequences of sensationalism, carelessness and, even, moral indignation of the kind expressed by Mr. Falwell's followers, are proving to be as dangerous to society as the actual disease itself. We are are not living in the Middle Ages, yet the equivalent of a cry of "Plague!" can produce the most irrational behavior and, with human concern being replaced by blind terror, a great deal of cruelty. Morticians have refused to embalm the bodies of AIDS victims. Nurses have refused to treat patients with AIDS and sufferers can point to a long list of pointless affronts.

Homosexuals, who form the vast majority — some 75 percent — of sufferers are seen as the causes of the disease, not its prime victims. Known homosexuals have become pariahs. Some dentists, policemen and firemen have donned masks and gloves for their encounters with society's new lepers.

The effect of the disease upon homosexuals is devastating enough without society adding to their suffering and anxiety. What is known about AIDS indicates that in the vast majority of cases the disease is transmitted by sexual contact between homosexuals. The other victims have been hard-drug users, who were possibly infected by hypodermic needles, and hemophilics, who likely caught the disease from transfusions of infected blood. The apparently inexplicable five percent incidence among Haitian immigrants may not remain a puzzle much longer. Other Haitians claim homosexuality and drug addiction are also the explanation and that their nationality is irrelevant.

Medical researchers are now fairly certain that AIDS can be traced to a sexual partner, a parent who has the disease, contagion through an infected hypodermic needle, or through a blood transfusion. These hard facts should provide sufficient moral dissuasion against promiscuity, particularly among homosexuals, to make scaremongering and scapegoating unnecessary. The known facts about AIDS are also a further warning to hard drug users of the dangers of addiction and they should also lead to the adoption of measures to protect blood banks from infection.

The panicked reaction to AIDS is bad for society. A good example of this is the sharp reduction in the number of people donating blood. Once again, the way in which blind fear drives out natural human concern, is being illustrated to the detriment of the community as a whole. In order to demonstrate the obvious — that there is no way that any one can contract AIDS by donating blood — Health and Human Services Secretary Margaret M. Heckler gave a pint of her own blood at the Red Cross office in Washington the other day.

Until medical research answers all the questions, we should all try and emulate Mrs. Heckler's action in combating hysteria. The moral lesson to be drawn from AIDS is obvious enough. Fanatical righteousness, allied with medieval fears and superstitions, will not lead to medical or moral enlightenment.

TULSA WORLD
Tulsa, OK, July 11, 1983

THE IMMEDIATE danger to Americans from AIDS — Acquired Immune Deficiency Syndrome — is not the threat of catching the mysterious disease, but secondary hazards produced by public fear.

AIDS is the sometimes disease which destroys the body's ability to fight infection. It is spread by sexual contact, contaminated needles and blood transfusions, according to health officials. Most AIDS victims have been homosexual men.

Since the disease was diagnosed four years ago, it has struck 1,700 people and killed 650. The mystery surrounding the disease has created a public fear totally out of proportion to the statistical odds the average person will contract the disease.

The real threat for the average person is public fear. Because AIDS can be spread through contaminated needles, some people have stopped donating blood. But a person donating blood need have no fear of contracting AIDS. Needles are not reused. Each is a clean sterile instrument. There is no chance of infection from a contaminated needle.

The government needs to reassure citizens that contaminated blood is also not a problem.

The nation's hospitals rely on voluntary blood donations for their patients. Anything which threatens to shut off or curtail that supply is a serious public threat. And that threat is the real public danger of AIDS.

House OK's Bathhouses' Closing; N.Y.C. Targets Bathhouses

The House of Representatives October 2, 1985 approved legislation authorizing the surgeon general to close "any bathhouse or massage parlor" that the official believed to "facilitate the transmission" of AIDS. The measure—an amendment to a bill funding the Labor, Education and Health and Human Services departments—passed by a 417-8 vote, with those opposed arguing that the surgeon general could already close facilities believed to spread an epidemic.

Separately, the New York State Public Health Council Oct. 25 issued regulations against "high-risk sexual activities" in bathhouses and other establishments for homosexual sex. The banned activities were identified as anal intercourse and fellatio, both thought to spread AIDS.

Critics doubted that the rules could be enforced, something the New York plan left to local officials. The chairman of the AIDS Medical Foundation, Dr. Mathilde Krim, said the rules had been adopted on "quick notice" and had "dumped" the issue on New York City, home of almost all the state's gay-sex establishments. The city November 7 forced the first closing under the new regulations, shutting down the Mine Shaft bar.

San Francisco had been the first jurisdiction to try regulating bathhouses. Six establishments had been recently warned by that city of violations, it was reported Oct. 23. Philip S. Ward, a city official in charge of enforcement, said the city's rules met with only limited observance.

Richmond Times-Dispatch

Richmond, VA, October 23, 1985

Say what one will about acquired immune deficiency syndrome being primarily a disease of heterosexuals in Africa, there's no tippytoeing around the fact that in the United States it has been overwhelmingly a homosexual affliction. Nearly three-fourths of AIDS victims are homosexual or bisexual men. More specifically, medical data indicate that this is a disease spread largely by homosexual promiscuity, since a large proportion of victims report having had multiple sex partners.

Given that knowledge and an exponential growth of AIDS cases that could see American hospitals jam-packed with 200,000 dying AIDS patients as early as 1990, the refusal of New York authorities to close homosexual bathhouses that openly promote group sex is absolutely mind-boggling and irresponsible. Gov. Mario Cuomo and Mayor Edward Koch have taken the line that by allowing New York City's 10 bathhouses to remain open under Health Department licensing, officials can educate homosexuals about the kinds of sexual practices that are most likely to spread AIDS. That's like saying firefighters should let a fire rage through a neighborhood so residents can participate in a forum on fire prevention.

News reports suggest that most bathhouses do dispense so-called "safe sex" literature advising against the exchange of body fluids during anal intercourse or oral sex, two practices linked to transmission of AIDS. Some also give out free condoms and copious soap in individual or pump-top dispensers. (Medical authorities say that soap and water are effective in destroying the AIDS virus.) But any benefits of such precautions are surely often erased by these establishments' accommodation of anonymous, multi-partner sex in rented rooms. Consider the following account in an Oct. 14 New York Times news story:

"As a rule, bathhouse patrons can choose between a locker, which costs about $7 for eight hours, or a private room, which costs several dollars more. At the East Side Sauna, which occupies parts of three floors in an office building, there is a steam room and sauna, television and video lounges and what is known as 'the group room.'

"'How do you say this nicely?' said Mr. Schwartz [a minority stockholder in the bathhouse]. 'Basically, it's an orgy room.'"

Quite apart from the morality of publicly tolerated orgies, consider the horrendous monetary cost to society. The average medical tab per AIDS case is $140,000, 60 percent of which comes from tax funds. If the exponential growth of AIDS cases continues, American taxpayers could be forking over tens of billions of dollars in the 1990s to care for victims, however pitiable, of their own irresponsibility. New York officials are being scarcely less irresponsible in tolerating the orgy houses since 6,700 of the nearly 14,000 AIDS cases nationwide come from that bastion of misguided liberalism. And since the AIDS virus is no respecter of state lines, the whole nation has a right to demand that the contagion be squelched at its main sources.

If Mayor Koch and Governor Cuomo will not close these filthy breeding grounds of a disease that now imperils the nation's health, the federal government should do it for them — promptly.

THE ATLANTA CONSTITUTION

Atlanta, GA, December 4, 1985

Continuing attempts to shut down Atlanta's only bathhouse evoke shudders from many of those trying to curb the spread of AIDS — and with good reason.

Let's not kid ourselves. Padlocking the place might persuade some homophobes that officials aren't sitting on their hands while the epidemic rages. But it won't contain the disease, or the kind of homosexual activity associated with it, unless a means can also be found of regulating what goes on in private bedrooms.

An attempt by Fulton County officials to close the club as a public nuisance has been tied up by legal challenges for nearly a year. And as Georgia prosecutors have lately discovered, in a case that went all the way to the Supreme Court and has yet to be adjudicated, they can't even arrest violators of Georgia's controversial, possibly unconstitutional, sodomy law without treading on the rights to privacy.

Which is not to suggest that officials oughtn't to be concerned. Though advertising themselves as facilities where patrons "can relax and exercise in a clean environment," the bathhouses are conducive to anonymous contacts — sex with strangers who may already be carrying the AIDS virus. Club Atlanta, where police claimed to have observed "an orgy" in one large room, also rents private rooms with beds for $12 and requires patrons to sign a statement avowing that they are "not offended by any homosexual activities."

But Fulton County, not the first to wrestle with the special problems posed by bathhouses, seems to have taken a singularly narrow-minded approach in comparison with officials elsewhere. Strategies adopted recently by San Francisco and New York recognize the futility of trying to eliminate gay sex hangouts, concentrating instead on the promotion of "safe sex," not involving the transfer of body fluids. New York has begun random inspections of bathhouses, and three of 14 bathhouses closed by San Francisco in an earlier crackdown are back in business, after agreeing to abide by certain rules.

Controversial as the bathhouses may be, they can be assets in the war on AIDS, centers for the dissemination of condoms and "safe sex" information. To shut them down outright would only further disperse patrons, making them still more anonymous, harder to find and educate — a panic response to a peculiarly resistant problem.

Authorities ought to seek cooperation, not confrontation, with bathhouse owners and patrons; this crisis concerns them all.

DAILY ⏺ NEWS

New York, NY, October 18, 1985

WOULD CLOSING NEW YORK's gay bathhouses stop the spread of AIDS? No. Would it significantly reduce the increase of infection? Arguably, but not certainly. Would it be a proper use of the power of government to close those commercial establishments and to deprive their patrons of the right to use them? *Only* if closing them would yield compelling public health benefits.

Make no mistake about acquired immune deficiency syndrome. It is a horrible disease. It is invariably fatal. Death comes slowly, from another disease against which the victim's immune system can no longer provide a defense.

The suffering, the burden on health care facilities and the costs are dreadful. AIDS is spreading at a potentially catastrophic rate. There is no cure and no preventive vaccine. Medical authorities believe there probably will be none for years, even with relentless research.

AIDS is not a "homosexual disease." It is communicated mainly in three ways: Sexual contact, thus far primarily among male homosexuals; hypodermic needles, passed from one narcotics user to another, and blood transfusions.

WHAT IS THE ARGUMENT *for* closing the bathhouses? That approximately 10 such establishments in New York exist primarily as venues for promiscuous and usually anonymous sexual contacts among gay men. Shut them down, that argument goes, and potentially infectious behavior is stopped or slowed.

But the weakness of that argument is that many of those who patronize these establishments are sexually active to the point of compulsion. They could relatively easily shift to the back rooms of bars, which exist now and would almost certainly proliferate.

What then? Close the gay bars? Police their back rooms? Then much of the activity would shift to back alleys, parks, abandoned piers—or to lofts or apartments devoted to round-the-clock meetings of, say, the Ad Hoc Committee to Study the Aphorisms of Oscar Wilde.

It is further contended that the bathhouses offer an opportunity to educate potential AIDS victims. It's a marginal argument, at best.

The debate raises grave questions about a policy to close the bathhouses. There are other important considerations. All of them must be examined in the context of the gravest of all the threats of the AIDS epidemic.

THAT IS PLAGUE PANIC. It is the danger that, as the disease spreads in total numbers and to broader segments of the population, hysteria is allowed to disrupt, even to destroy, the capacity of government and society to deal rationally with the dangers.

Sensationalism? No. The seeds of panic have been sown—by the nature of the disease itself. Already, they are being nourished by the thoughtless or opportunistic or superficial reactions of people in and out of power.

To what extent is the movement to close the bathhouses, to police bars, and so on, just a coded expression of latent fear and hatred of homosexual behavior and homosexuals?

Homosexuality offends and frightens many people. Does that make a respectable or morally defensible case for punishing or stigmatizing homosexuals? No. Gay men and lesbians constitute a major element of society. The life of the stereotypical gay bathhouse patron is repellant to many New Yorkers—heterosexual *and* homosexual. But to exploit that distaste with political opportunism would be demagogic.

MOST IMPORTANTLY, A DECISION to close the bathhouses and to police their inevitable substitutes could undermine genuinely valuable efforts to deal with the AIDS threat. It would involve considerable official effort, time and expense: policing, litigation, debate and speechmaking.

That would deflect public attention and energy from the difficult and important challenges: Treatment; protection against preventable infection; providing hospital and other prudent medical care; funding the exploding cost of treatment and medical and social support; education, especially of likely victims; basic research toward prevention and cure.

AIDS is a proliferating threat to public health—and public order. Every possible effort must be made to contain, reduce and ultimately eradicate it. To allow coded fagbashing or politically expedient superficial "remedies" to divert energy and funds from effective public health policy would be an act of deadly irresponsibility. It *could* play into the plague panic danger. The zeal for closing a handful of bathhouses reeks of just that.

Close them? *Only* if those who move to do so can demonstrate first that there is a convincing and compelling public health benefit. That has not been done. Yet.

LAS VEGAS REVIEW-JOURNAL

Las Vegas, NV, November 22, 1985

The Nevada attorney general has cleared the way for mandatory testing for exposure to the deadly AIDS virus in the state's 36 legal brothels.

The state's Board of Health has directed the state health division to draw up regulations and seek public comments before a final vote on the regulation by the health board in March.

The health division is planning a program of mandatory testing of the women who work at the legal brothels, and it will be the women or the brothels that pick up the nominal tab for the tests.

As things now stand, a program of voluntary AIDS testing is in place, but only two-thirds of the brothels have agreed to cooperate.

The mandatory tests are needed. As long as prostitution is a legally sanctioned activity in much of rural Nevada, brothels will operate, and they should be kept disease-free. Indeed, one major argument in favor of legalized prostitution is the disease-free environment that is made available when the working women of the bordellos are subjected to regular health check-ups. Surely, AIDS should be added to the list of sexually communicated diseases for which the women are tested.

Not only would the mandatory tests go a long way toward alleviating the anxiety about AIDS of both the women and their customers, the tests could also provide a valuable research tool. There is much dispute about the danger of contracting AIDS through male-female contact. Nevada's legal brothels are unique in the United States and results of the AIDS tests could shed some scientific light on the problem of AIDS.

AIDS is a killing disease that wreaks havoc on the body's immune system. In the United States, more than 14,800 people — 75 percent of them homosexual men — have been diagnosed having AIDS, and more than 7,500 of those have died since 1979. There is fear that the disease is crossing over to the heterosexual population, as it has in Africa, where AIDS is believed to have originated.

A new study out of the University of California at Berkeley indicates that AIDS is more difficult to transmit sexually from men to women than previously believed. The study by the Berkeley researchers, released this week, involved 22 women who engaged in sexual intercourse with men known to be infected with the AIDS virus. Twenty-one of the women showed no evidence of infection.

This may be an indication that AIDS does not easily cross the line to the heterosexual community.

There has been some question, too, about the spread of AIDS to women in Africa, especially Zaire, where AIDS is rampant and has infected many females. Some studies indicate that certain tribal cultural practices in Zaire have aggravated the AIDS problem. One tribal custom involves the use of needles to scratch designs on the skin, and needles, used again and again, may well have contributed to the spread of the disease. One study indicated that many in Zaire accept Western medicine only if it is administered by syringe; the quality of health care is such that needles — often less than clean — are used repeatedly, and this, too, could have helped cause AIDS to spread to the general populace.

Obviously these same conditions do not exist in the United States.

The Berkeley study could be a good sign as far as the Nevada brothels are concerned. But, still, there was that one woman in the Berkeley study who did show signs of being infected. And 22 women is not exactly a definitive sample.

For all these reasons, Nevada health authorities should forge ahead with the testing program in the legal brothels.

Spread of AIDS Continues, Public Fear Mounts

In November 1984 the U.S. Centers for Disease Control (CDC) tallied the cumulative number of U.S. cases of AIDS at 6,993. This represented the total number of cases of the disease since it was first reported in 1981. Of that total, 3,342—or 48%—had been fatal. The CDC reported that as of November 11, 1985 the tally had reached 14,739; of that number, 7,418 had died. The CDC predicted that the total U.S. cases could be expected to double within a year.

These cases were of people who had actually contracted AIDS. Anywhere from 500,000 to more than a million people were thought have been exposed to the virus without actually contracting AIDS. According to news accounts published during the second half of 1985, some 73% of U.S. AIDS victims were homosexuals, and 17% were intravenous drug users. Two percent were hemophiliacs who had contracted the disease through blood or blood-product transfusions. The CDC listed all as high-risk groups. Another 1.4% of the total victims were children, believed to have contracted the disease from their mothers while in the womb or breast-feeding.

The first commercial test to check blood for signs of AIDS was approved by the Department of Health and Human Services in March 1985. The inexpensive process, known as the enzyme-linked immunosorbent assay (ELISA), was designed to be used by blood banks to ward off infected donations. ELISA tested for anitbodies created in response to the virus, known as LAV or HTLV-3. Findings indicated that only 5% to 9% of those who tested positive would actually contract the disease. But it was thought possible that anyone with the antibodies could transmit AIDS.

During 1985, as awareness of the disease spread, so did the public fear of the disease, sometimes exacerbated by misinformation. Medical experts had held that AIDS could not be spread by casual contact; only the sharing of infected blood or semen was thought to be a danger. But skepticism or ignorance of the scientists' claims led to incidents that included the ostracism of AIDS victims. Shortly following the death of screen actor Rock Hudson in October 1985, 15 months after he was diagnosed as suffering from AIDS, the Screen Actors Guild required agents and producers to notify its members if a role required open-mouth kissing.

The News American
Baltimore, MD, August 7, 1985

Fear is the first response to the unknown, and with the mysterious disease called AIDS that fear is heightened because the pariahs of the society — the homosexuals, the drug addicts — are its most talked-about victims. Thus shun those victims, slam the doors on them: We're reminded of the lepers from whom the people of the Middle Ages fled in terror.

But leprosy, hundreds of years before the concept, let alone the term, entered the human mind, was a public health problem. Now AIDS is a public health problem, and the state's health department is forthright in recognizing it as such. The department — which of course would be derelict not to — is ignoring the fear and loathing and has convinced several nursing homes to take in the victims upon whom doors have been slammed. The department will train the nursing home staffs to treat AIDS patients. And it will spend $40,000 in state money to place 20 victims not requiring intensive treatment in foster homes.

AIDS, a condition that breaks down the body's natural immune systems and makes those who contract it vulnerable to killing diseases, got plenty of headlines when the news broke that Rock Hudson is a sufferer. The response of movie people (one former movie person, Ronald Reagan, telephoned the actor to show his concern) has been encouraging in light of the stories of victims being declared unwelcome at school or being denied places to live. Elizabeth Taylor is the prime mover of a Sept. 19 benefit performance that will attempt to raise $1 million for AIDS research. That research is needed, given the disease's mysteries and unknown potential for damage throughout the population. Needed at the same time is the acceptance that AIDS, whose victims are the lepers of the 1980s, has become not a matter of public morality but of public health.

The Hartford Courant
Hartford, CT, August 6, 1985

Diseases whose causes are unknown and for which treatment is ineffectual have always been imbued with special symbolic significance: leprosy, for example, and syphilis, tuberculosis and cancer. When such a disease is fatal, it becomes loaded with even heavier psychic freight and stands as a horrible symbol of humans' dread of capricious death.

Thus, people who fall ill with such maladies often become less the victims of their disease than of the attitudes of those around them. Like those who suffered dread diseases in earlier ages, today's AIDS patients carry a heavy and punitive burden — largely because most AIDS patients have been homosexuals or drug abusers.

The notion of fatal illness as a supernatural punishment for personal sin or community transgression is at least as old as Homer — and as modern as AIDS. But acquired immune deficiency syndrome, although incurable and usually fatal, is not a curse or a punishment; although cruel, it is not more shameful, horrible or gruesome than other fatal diseases. AIDS is a disease, nothing more. It is a malfunction, albeit a drastic one, of the human body that needs to be understood, dealt with and cured.

What has probably retarded research into AIDS is our culture's wrongful contempt for those who, like homosexuals and drug abusers, are regarded as "different" from the rest of society.

But non-drug-abusing heterosexuals, including hemophiliacs and children, have always caught AIDS, too, although their cases received less public attention at first because their numbers were smaller than those of homosexual AIDS patients or those who contracted the viral disease through contaminated hypodermic needles.

Now that AIDS is spreading faster among all groups, the public has become more concerned about AIDS, although funding for research and education and for medical, social and psychological services for AIDS patients is still woefully inadequate.

AIDS will be dreaded and thought of as intractable and malicious until its cause becomes clear and treatment for it found. Medicine, which has discovered cures for leprosy, syphilis and tuberculosis and has made good progress with many cancers, can do the same with AIDS. All that's needed is for the public and the government to begin to think about AIDS, calmly and non-judgmentally, as another disease to be conquered — one of utmost gravity and urgency, certainly, but a disease nonetheless.

As long as AIDS is treated as evil, as an invincible predator, instead of as an illness whose cause and cure might lie within our comprehension and grasp, people with AIDS will continue to be wrongly shunned and the rest of society demoralized by foolish dread and loathing. To conquer AIDS will take far more financial and medical resources than have yet been devoted to the effort. It will be as much a test of our will, and our attitudes, as it is our paramount medical challenge.

ARGUS-LEADER
Sioux Falls, SD, August 27, 1985

Fate has turned in a cruel direction for Rock Hudson: The most dramatic moments of the popular actor's career have come since he acknowledged that he suffers from AIDS — acquired immune deficiency syndrome.

Hudson's jarring disclosure has helped focus attention on a killer disease that

Editorial

federal officials, with good cause, have considered the nation's No. 1 public health priority since 1983.

AIDS, first diagnosed in 1981, attacks humans' immune system, leaving victims more susceptible to deadly infections and cancer. Half of the nation's 12,000 victims are already dead.

Researchers believe that the disease is caused by a virus transmitted through body fluids, mainly blood and semen. Three-fourths of those in the United States known to suffer the disease are gays and bisexual men. But AIDS is not a "gay plague." Misnomers like that wrongly lull people into indifference.

About 20 percent of U.S. victims have been intravenous drug users who contract the disease through contaminated needles, hemophiliacs who receive blood products, and people who receive blood transfusions. In addition, more than 100 children born to infected mothers have picked up the disease.

In central Africa, where AIDS is thought to have originated, hundreds of cases have been reported. An equal number of men and women have been struck. That sug-

gests that heterosexual contact is the dominant means of transmission.

Findings give rise to the fear that AIDS could evolve into a venereal disease, like syphilis or gonorrhea.

"The virus that causes AIDS somehow got introduced into the homosexual population in which the lifestyle tends to spread the disease," Dr. Anthony Fauci, director of the National Institute of Allergy and Infectious Diseases at Bethesda, Md., said. "But it is not and never has been a gay disease. And that has been a problem with public perception for a very long time."

That perception must change. The health of a lot of people may depend on it.

THE SUNDAY STAR
Toronto, Ont., August 4, 1985

Fears, misconceptions and lack of research are all contributing to the public's concern over AIDS. The sexually transmitted disease — acquired immune deficiency syndrome — kills by destroying the body's defences against infections. So far 288 Canadians have contracted it. Of these, 151 men, women and children have died. And thousands more are at risk.

So it's good to see that Ontario is planning to start testing blood samples for the AIDS virus. We're also contributing almost $1 million of the $2.5-million start-up costs of a Canadian Red Cross Society blood screening program that will test blood donations from across the country for exposure to the AIDS virus. And Queen's Park has given $700,000 for AIDS research.

That's part of what's needed. But as experts like Dr. Norbert Gilmore, chairman of the National Advisory Committee on AIDS point out, it's time we did more in two other areas, too: public education and counselling of people with AIDS and their families.

Misconceptions about AIDS abound — not just among the public but among the medical community as well. Experts say that the risk of contracting AIDS is actually very small for most Canadians — those who aren't having sex with someone infected with the virus or who don't receive blood. And now that the Red Cross plans to start testing blood donations, the likelihood of getting the disease through transfused blood should be negligible.

While it's a growing concern — the number of AIDS cases doubles every nine months — AIDS doesn't yet rank as a major killer. Every day 100 Canadians die of tobacco-related diseases. Yet with people like American screen idol Rock Hudson dying of it, AIDS ranks high as a public health worry.

In a recent Gallup Poll, 60 per cent of the people polled said they were afraid of *giving* blood for fear of contracting AIDS. Callers to the Laboratory Centre for Disease Control in Ottawa have worried they might have AIDS because they have met, touched or eaten with homosexuals. Some doctors and nurses have been afraid to conduct autopsies on AIDS victims. These fears are not justified by what we know of the disease.

That's why we need greater efforts by all three levels of government to bolster public understand-

ing of the disease, its risks and the steps individuals and health workers can take to prevent its spread.

For instance, the Ontario government should take a serious look at providing the money for the AIDS Committee of Toronto to meet the heavy demand for public information about the disease and counselling of people with AIDS and their families. The group, which now operates with volunteers on a shoe-string budget and has close links with the homosexual community, has earned praise for its work from Red Cross officials and other health workers in promoting healthy sexual practices designed to stem the disease's spread.

"For a lot of people in Toronto, we're still at a very early stage of learning what 'safe sex' is all about," says Phil Shaw, spokesman for the committee. "If we had more money we could get our message out to people who should be concerned about it — in places like bathhouses, gay bars, health clinics and supermarkets."

Ottawa should show it takes the AIDS threat seriously by setting up a special AIDS unit at the federal disease control centre. The centre needs $500,000 a year to monitor the disease, act as a clearing house for public information, research new testing methods, co-ordinate provincial programs, offer specialized testing that's not available elsewhere, and oversee the screening of blood, sperm and kidney donations.

Canada alone can't hope to do all the research that's needed to combat AIDS. That requires research into prevention, treatment, vaccines, how to bring back the immune system once it has been damaged and how to help people with AIDS deal with the social and psychological impact of the disease. But Ottawa can set out its own research priorities and should be actively soliciting proposals that don't duplicate research being done elsewhere. This might include more research into how the disease is transmitted. Or why some people's bodies are damaged by the virus and others aren't. Or how we can determine who's infectious, since it can take as long as five years for a person who has been exposed to AIDS to show symptoms.

We've had major health scares before. Polio was one in the 1950s. But, with research and a major public commitment to find a solution, we've overcome diseases in the past. There's no reason AIDS should be different.

AKRON BEACON JOURNAL
Akron, OH, October 4, 1985

TWO obituaries are appropriate for actor Rock Hudson, who died Wednesday at age 59.

The first, formal obituary should note the passing of a romantic and comedy star of the 1950s and '60s, a screen idol who gave his audiences the entertainment and escapism that they sought from movies in that era.

It is the other Rock Hudson that many find more compelling, however: A man who kept part of his life hidden and whose death — faced with courage and dignity — focused public attention on a killer disease.

Mr. Hudson died of complications from AIDS — acquired immune deficiency syndrome — a fatal illness that primarily strikes homosexuals and intravenous drug users. In admitting he had the disease, Mr. Hudson helped mobilize the Hollywood community, his many fans and the nation in the fight against AIDS.

This week the House voted to increase funding for AIDS research by 90 percent over the next year, and voted to give health authorities greater powers to enforce preventive measures against the disease. And, because of the attention of recent months, the general public is beginning to understand just how serious the AIDS threat is and that action is needed to halt its spread.

Following his admission that he had AIDS, many people will never feel quite the same about Rock Hudson, the star of those innocent romantic comedies. But, in a message last month to an entertainers' charity, his own words provide perhaps a more enduring legacy:

"I am not happy that I have AIDS. But if that is helping others, I can at least know that my own misfortune has had some positive worth."

DAILY NEWS
New York, NY, August 18, 1985

IN THE WORST CASE, there could be 33,000 victims of AIDS in New York city by 1990. Unless there's a medical breakthrough, they will all die.

That's the highest of the estimates compiled by the Centers for Disease Control in Atlanta. Its lowest estimate for the city is about 8,000 cases. There's not much hope it will be as low as that: There have already been over 4,000 cases here.

People in the Rockaways are up in arms against a plan to put some AIDS patients in the Neponsit Home for the Aged. They fear up to 300 AIDS victims may settle among them.

It's not 300, citywide, but thousands, perhaps over 30,000.

There is a dreadful epidemic, spreading rapidly. Coping with the disaster involves a whole series of painful and difficult decisions by city government and people.

The Atlanta Centers believes that between 500,000 and a million Americans have already been exposed to AIDS virus. Five to 20 per cent, 25,000 to 100,000 people, will contract the disease itself in the next five years.

Exactly one third of all cases in the nation so far have occurred in New York City. So far, all estimates have been underestimates—and the Atlanta figures take no account of people who may now contract the virus. They are talking about thousands of New Yorkers who have *already* been condemned to death.

AIDS is already the leading cause of death among New York males aged between 30 and 40. As the numbers go up, urgent matters of social policy have to be decided.

What happens to an AIDS patient's job? Some firms will summarily sack him, to protect other employes, though the experts say AIDS cannot be contracted in the workplace.

AIDS sufferers have sued to save their jobs. Los Angeles has passed an ordinance prohibiting discrimination against AIDS patients—but that's no more than a gesture.

Court personnel, jurors and cops demand extraordinary protection when AIDS victims appear in court. There have been riots by prisoners jailed with AIDS victims.

The fear of AIDS spreads to a general fear of gays. One gay was sacked when he caught cold, though there was no evidence he had AIDS.

Gays have argued for years that government was not acting forcefully enough to deal with the crisis. Medical research has made rapid progress, though a cure is nowhere in sight. But social policy has lagged far behind.

The city has to provide hospital facilities for sufferers, and that means explaining to communities, like the Rockaways, that the hospital is no danger to them. AIDS is not like smallpox. The educational effort must begin at once: 33,000 patients would need a lot of hospitals.

The Birmingham News
Birmingham, AL, August 23, 1985

The time may be fast approaching when representatives of the health industry, the best legal minds in the state and lawmakers put their heads together to consider options for controlling the spread of the dread AIDS virus and protecting its victims from unnecessary measures.

Investigating options does not suggest a crisis or a present need for heroic measures. But the notion that an epidemic is already ravaging society is firmly established in the minds of many laymen and doctors. Furthermore, Dr. James Alexander, director of the Jefferson County Health Department's Bureau of Communicable Diseases, has characterized AIDS as now in "epidemic" proportions in Alabama.

"Everyone in the U.S. says it is epidemic," says Alexander. "It (the rate) doubles every 11 or 12 months, and it's the same here, too. So if it is epidemic (in the nation), it's epidemic here, too."

In support of his contention, Alexander cites some figures. At this time last year, 10 cases of AIDS were reported in Alabama. Now 26 victims of AIDS have been confirmed in the state.

If no cure or control for the disease is found, and if the rate of increase remains constant, we would have 52 cases next year, 1,664 cases by 1991 and 26,624 cases by 1995.

We are confident that science will eventually find a cure or a control for the disease. Progress toward a cure, however, has been uneven and slow in relation to the need for treatment. The most prevalent cause of infection is regarded to be through sexual contact. Most research indicates that one is relatively safe in other normal contacts with carriers of the virus.

So the prudent person, regardless of his station in society, should find ample cause to avoid promiscuity and any avoidable exposure.

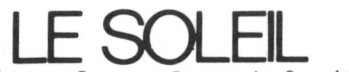
LE SOLEIL
Quebec, Que , August 8, 1985

Le Québec et le Canada ne semblent pas encore gravement atteints par la nouvelle maladie du siècle, le SIDA ou syndrome d'immuno-déficience acquise. Depuis 1981, environ 300 cas ont été répertoriés au pays dont 84 au Québec.

En comparaison et proportionnellement à d'autres Etats, comme l'Australie avec 500,000 cas potentiels, les Etats-Unis avec 12,000 cas signalés et 400,000 personnes touchées par le virus, et certains pays européens, on ne peut parler pour le moment d'une épidémie chez nous.

Mais le SIDA dérange et fait beaucoup parler. Il n'y a pas de journée que les médias d'information ne signalent de nouveaux cas, de nouvelles victimes, de nouvelles statistiques ou de nouveaux modes de transmission. Et il continuera à défrayer les manchettes puisque le nombre de personnes atteintes mortellement double chaque année, que la maladie s'attaque maintenant aux nouveau-nés et se transmet par d'autres voies que sexuelles.

Le virus a été difficile à détecter et à analyser, mais le SIDA a maintenant un visage et on connaît chacune des 9,200 lettres de son code génétique. Il reste à trouver le remède, un médicament qui pourra bloquer son développement, car le SIDA apparaît maintenant comme un mal avec lequel il faut apprendre à vivre.

● ● ●

Il faut surtout arrêter de chercher les coupables et s'attaquer aux causes et aux moyens de combattre et de prévenir la maladie.

Les premiers cas de SIDA ont été connus en 1978 et ce n'est que depuis 1981 qu'il en est question dans l'actualité. Mais au début la maladie semblait conscrite à certains groupes bien identifiés: les Noirs et la communauté homosexuelle.

Cette concentration a nui énormément à la recherche du virus et d'un test fiable pour le dépister. Durant quelques années, on assista plutôt au procès de la communauté homosexuelle. La maladie était considérée comme une vengeance du ciel contre une société aux moeurs dépravées. Les malades devaient être dénoncés, punis et, comme au Moyen-Age pour les lépreux, il aurait fallu les parquer dans quelques coins isolés et les obliger à signaler leur présence au moyen d'une clochette.

Cette mentalité soi-disant bien pensante n'est pas complètement disparue: en Indiana, aux Etats-Unis, un jeune hémophile de 13 ans, contaminé par le virus, vient de se voir interdire l'accès à son école; en Australie, une compagnie aérienne a refusé, il y a quelques jours, de transporter un homme souffrant de la maladie.

Ces préjugés ne font que retarder les recherches pour la mise au point d'un vaccin efficace puisque les sommes d'argent nécessaires n'y sont pas allouées.

La nouvelle faisant état que l'acteur Rock Hudson avait contracté la maladie a eu l'effet d'une bombe aux Etats-Unis. Le SIDA devenait en quelque sorte respectable. Aussitôt le gouvernement américain octroyait $45 millions supplémentaires pour la recherche et la prévention du SIDA. Une fondation était créée en Californie pour ramasser des fonds servant à la recherche sur la maladie. Le Canada, lui, y consacrera $2 millions, cette année.

Mais devant la progression du SIDA et une pression plus forte de l'opinion publique, les gouvernements devront débloquer plus d'argent. Car la maladie s'étend et même la "chasteté et la pureté" ne peuvent plus empêcher le mal de nous atteindre. En même temps que les mentalités, le SIDA a évolué; maintenant il ne fait plus de distinctions de races, d'âges ou de groupes sexuels. Il s'agit bien là d'une maladie de notre époque.

THE SUNDAY OKLAHOMAN

Oklahoma City, OK, August 18, 1985

THE plight of stricken actor Rock Hudson has brought AIDS out of the closet into the glare of national discussion, but the news from the research front is not encouraging.

By now, most informed citizens are aware that the spread of Acquired Immune Deficiency Syndrome constitutes a health threat to the general population, not just to male homosexuals and intravenous drug abusers.

Some reputable scientists are even drawing parallels with the geometric increase in reported cases of AIDS and epidemics of the past, when bubonic plague in the Middle Ages and later cholera, malaria and influenza claimed countless victims.

When the malady first attracted medical attention four or five years ago, it didn't command a very high research priority. Initial data indicated it was confined almost exclusively to homosexual men, drug addicts and heterosexuals who had frequent contact with prostitutes.

This prompted the fundamentalist reaction that AIDS was an angry creator's vengeance upon a wayward people.

What we have learned since is far more frightening. While some 75 percent of all documented cases involve homosexuals and drug abusers, the highly contagious disease is capable of being transmitted to normal heterosexuals and unborn children.

The number of reported U.S. cases, now about 12,000, is doubling every 10 months. Of those, about 9,000 were homosexual or bisexual males and 2,000 were intravenous drug abusers.

But it's spreading even faster in several central African countries, and virtually every country in the world has reported some cases.

At this stage, researchers know quite a bit about the AIDS virus, how it is transmitted and how it systematically destroys the body's natural infection-fighting ability. But there is no cure, nor has there been any breakthrough in developing a preventive vaccine.

Under the circumstances, Oklahoma corrections officials are justified in keeping two inmates who tested positive for AIDS antibodies in medical isolation.

What researchers don't know is how many people may be carriers of the AIDS virus, people who exhibit no symptoms of the disease but are capable of infecting others. While blood and body fluids are the major media of transmission, the virus also has been detected in tears of infected persons.

New York City health statistics reveal that more men between 30 and 39 died from AIDS in 1984 than from homicide, suicide or cancer. At the present rate, AIDS will become the number one killer of NYC males between 15 and 50 by the end of next year.

Research may or may not develop a cure. Meanwhile, there's no reason for circumspect people to panic. For as Dr. James Mason, director of the federal Center for Disease Control in Atlanta, reminds us, "If we could stop drug abusing.. (and) if we could stop the exchange of bodily fluids among members of the homosexual or bisexual community, we could stop this epidemic in its tracks."

The Washington Times

Washington, DC, August 29, 1985

Next month District of Columbia City Council will take up a bill to ban "discrimination" against victims of AIDS. Councilman John Ray says this is necessary so that AIDS victims can "battle prejudice and ignorance."

The bill would also make it illegal to determine whether an insurance applicant has AIDS. Smoking, yes; AIDS, no. D.C. insurance customers will just have to pay the soaring insurance rates that will result. But people already struggling with their monthly bills won't mind, will they, because it's all to "battle prejudice and ignorance."

AIDS research, which deserves unstinting support, is showing the disease to spread in previously unsuspected ways. As ignorance of the virus retreats, the cause for alarm increases. Given this, and given the deadliness of the disease, the inalienable right to protect oneself and one's family from it remains decisive until we have either a vaccine, a cure, or scientific certainty as to how its spread can be avoided.

This right to self-protection is being denied in the case of AIDS only because the affected group is one that is militant, influential, well-to-do on the average (no families to support), and warmly admired by the species of elite that dominates some city councils. Fear of the militant homosexual lobbies' name-calling arsenal and of its electoral clout has paralyzed the normal course of epidemic control.

Many are saddened by the AIDS situation, beyond the obvious fear of catching it, because of a regard for tolerance. Continued tolerance would be easier if healthy citizens were not forced by law to neglect obvious precautions.

THE PLAIN DEALER

Cleveland, OH, August 20, 1985

The actions of Indianapolis law officials after learning a suspect they had arrested was a victim of AIDS is characteristic of much of the paranoia sweeping the nation with regard to the dreaded disease. Rather than prosecute the man, who was accused of stealing a bicycle, or take him to a hospital for treatment, a municipal judge gave the man bus fare for a one-way ticket to Cleveland and ordered him to leave the city.

"Rather than expose court and sheriff's personnel to this hazard," said a Marion County prosecutor, "no charges were filed."

What was exposed was the ignorance of Marion County officials who came into casual contact with the suspect. Deputies wore rubber gloves and gauze masks when booking the man and destroyed pens the man used in signing lockup documents. Excessive? Yes, but not uncommon. Myths and half-truths abound regarding the manner in which the disease can be contracted.

The only proven ways by which the disease can be communicated are by the virus entering the bloodstream, either through blood transfusions or the use of unsterilized needles, or the exchange of body fluids through certain sexual acts. Those most at risk have been homosexuals, hemophiliacs and addicts who take drugs intravenously. Few others need worry about contracting AIDS.

Unfortunately, that doesn't diminish the growing fear among other groups. After all, AIDS first was thought to have been exclusive among homosexuals, which may have contributed to early public apathy for finding a cure. And reports about heterosexual men and women who have contracted the disease, as well as the spread of AIDS in mostly heterosexual African communities, has heightened public alarm. That the disease is often fatal and has no proven cure makes it all the more dreaded.

The question, however, is not that anyone should have fear about contracting AIDS—even those not at risk—but how individuals or a society acts in the face of those fears. The responsible action for Marion County authorities would have been to ensure that the suspect obtained the treatment he was seeking at an Indianapolis hospital. Instead, they dealt with a perceived problem by shipping it elsewhere.

What is most needed nationwide is more public awareness about the dangers posed by the disease and those most at risk. A massive informational campaign would be helpful and could be undertaken without fueling unnecessary alarm. Knowledge should diminish much of the public's irrational fears and allow for more much-needed resources to be directed at finding a cure.

THE SACRAMENTO BEE
Sacramento, CA, September 9, 1985

Catching AIDS is hard; catching AIDS hysteria, unfortunately, is far easier.

In Indiana, 100 parents have successfully sued to keep a 13-year-old AIDS victim, who caught the disease from a blood transfusion, from attending school. In Los Angeles, so many AIDS victims were fired from their jobs, thrown out of their apartments, or denied service in restaurants that the City Council, at the request of health authorities, passed an ordinance banning such discrimination. In Sacramento, the Sheriff's Department issued a bulletin warning deputies of the "potential consequences" of giving mouth-to-mouth resuscitation to homosexuals or intravenous drug users.

The fear of AIDS is understandable. The disease is new and terrifyingly deadly, and too much about it is still unknown. But much of the nervousness about AIDS victims is based on ignorance of the evidence that does exist. Spread by blood or semen, the AIDS virus is not passed through casual contact with victims. There are no known cases of the disease being passed through saliva. The delicate virus cannot be passed, as a cold can, through a sneeze or handshake. Screening studies of health workers conducted by the federal Centers for Disease Control show no evidence that they have been exposed to the virus, even when they have accidentally punctured themselves with needles used by AIDS victims. By all current evidence, only the most intimate forms of contact with AIDS victims — sexual relations or sharing hypodermic syringes — carries a major risk.

Thus, to stigmatize AIDS victims by isolation and shunning is to double their pain for no good reason. "For most infected children, the benefits of an unrestricted (school) setting would outweigh the apparent non-existent risk of transmission," the CDC says. It recommends that children with AIDS be allowed to go to school.

In the case of the sheriff's bulletin, the stigma was placed not only on AIDS sufferers but also on groups — homosexual males and intravenous drug users — known to be at higher risk of contracting the disease. (How a sheriff's deputy, coming upon an unconscious victim in need of resuscitation, is supposed to determine his sexual orientation is a mystery the bulletin left unsolved.) The medical evidence about AIDS suggests that the risk of performing resuscitation is small. For public safety employees, it is far down the list of dangers they face. To imply otherwise only makes more difficult a calm and considered approach to a public health emergency.

Curing the disease has so far proved beyond science's ability. But stopping its spread through common-sense measures and clearing up misconceptions that lead to unnecessary AIDS hysteria are tasks well within the realm of the possible. And the less hysteria there is, the greater the chances of effectively resisting and understanding the disease. What better way to start than having public officials resolve to speak so as to calm fears, not fan them.

THE DENVER POST
Denver, CO, August 25, 1985

THE STATE Board of Health should reconsider its plan to compile a list of Colorado residents who have been exposed to AIDS, the loathsome disease that threatens to become society's new leprosy.

It might be medically desirable to keep track of people who carry the AIDS virus, so researchers can attempt to learn why some develop full-blown cases and others don't. But the side effects of a mandatory reporting rule would be socially unacceptable.

It would be more humane, and probably more effective, to adopt a policy under which the names and addresses of potential AIDS victims would be turned over to public-health authorities only with the individuals' permission.

The underlying issue here, of course, is the stigma attached to the deadly scourge that cripples the body's immune systems. Although the disease has struck down a few women and children, it has been primarily confined to male homosexuals. Thus, a positive reading on the new blood test for the AIDS antibody (an indicator of exposure) means in all likelihood that the subject is gay — and may lose his job, home, friends and health insurance if the results become known.

The Colorado Health Department maintains that it would zealously protect the confidentiality of these records, and nobody doubts it. What people in the gay community fear is that if the nation goes into a panic over AIDS, the state legislature or even Congress might force public-health authorities to release the names of all exposed people so they could be quarantined — even though it is by no means certain that all who carry the virus are infectious, or even that the AIDS blood test is entirely reliable.

The Health Department is right to be seeking all the information it can get on the exposed population. Such data will provide a more accurate and up-to-date picture of the disease than an analysis of those who are actually diagnosed as having AIDS, for it takes three to five years for the symptoms to show up.

But for research purposes, it should be possible to obtain adequate information without taking the names of any except those who do not fear identifying themselves. Moreover, it makes little sense to argue that state authorities should be able to get in touch with potential victims to provide counseling or treatment, in the event that a vaccine or cure is discovered. Anyone who is concerned enough about his health to take the blood test won't be nervous about seeking help.

In short, if anything could increase the health threat posed by AIDS, it would be a rule that would discourage people from taking a test to see if they might have been exposed to the disease.

The Oregonian
Portland, OR, August 8, 1985

The revelation that actor Rock Hudson has been infected with AIDS, the acquired immune deficiency syndrome that leaves the victim exposed to fatal infections, has helped concentrate medical, scientific and political attention on the problem. And about time.

Critics of the current work to combat AIDS are in two categories: Those who believe that a massive national research effort is needed to coordinate diverse studies and those who think political considerations or the mistaken belief that only homosexuals and dope addicts are AIDS victims are hampering the required White House leadership needed to head off a national disaster.

The virus, first seriously noted in 1981, has infected an estimated 1 million Americans, resulting in more than 12,000 active cases, half of whom have died.

In the beginning, the virus, believed to have originated in Africa where it is a heterosexual disease, was seen only among U.S. and European homosexuals and drug addicts and a few individuals who caught it in blood transfusions. It now appears to be spreading into the heterosexual population.

There is good news on the transfusion front. Identification of the virus has permitted development of successful (99.8 percent accurate) screening tests that virtually will end the spread of AIDS through blood transfusions, the National Institutes of Health has announced.

However, research success on treatments and cures will come slowly at the current pace. It usually requires four to eight years of testing to turn a chemical into an approved drug, a process that needs to be speeded up dramatically with this spreading health menace.

Some U.S. scientists argue persuasively that a crash program is needed to coordinate research being conducted at several institutions. What is required is the kind of big push that past presidents gave cancer, heart and other disease programs.

President Reagan, who reportedly has not even mentioned AIDS in a speech, might well consider lending his weight to fighting what his health secretary, Margaret Heckler, recently called the nation's No. 1 health problem.

The Miami Herald

Miami, FL, August 21, 1985

TO CRITICIZE Federal and state health agencies for slowness in recognizing the threat from AIDS (acquired immune deficiency syndrome) is to argue about the past. With a lethal disease spreading geometrically, the future of public policy and public budgets is far more germane to public health.

Last year 346 new AIDS cases were reported, bringing the national total to 12,408. In 1980 the total was *five* cases. Miami, with 393 cases, ranks third among U.S. cities in AIDS incidence. Because AIDS attacks the body's immune system, victims contract a variety of diseases, and incur an estimated $140,000 each in medical bills.

Despite those bills and the crystal-clear need for intensive research, government at all levels has been dilatory in mapping out a comprehensive strategy for coping with AIDS. The Reagan Administration added $40 million to its AIDS budget, for a total of $126 million, but only after first proposing to cut that budget by $10 million. While there have been some rapid and encouraging developments in research, such as identification of its virus and a test for exposure, the Federal Government needs to provide a greater degree of leadership and coordination of research.

Neither the Federal Government nor the state of Florida has addressed the issue of how to pay for patient care and whether to develop specialized hospices for AIDS patients, who frequently die in isolation. Too often, those patients lose their jobs and insurance benefits and do not qualify for Medicaid or Medicare. That means that the costs of their care are passed through to other hospital patients and local taxpayers. Despite these mounting bills, Florida has spent only $576,000 in the past three years on state-funded AIDS counseling, education, and research as compared with $22.7 million in California and $12.5 million in New York.

Government at all levels must strive to formulate public policy that protects both the public and AIDS victims. Medical evidence indicates that AIDS is not spread through casual contact and that AIDS victims, like sufferers from other diseases, should be permitted to work if their physicians concur. The Federal Centers for Disease Control find no reason to exclude young victims from school and will issue guidelines soon. While firing an AIDS victim without proof of his danger to others is discrimination, the issue of refusing to hire one is problematic. After all, that person reasonably can be expected to strain insurance benefits.

The advent of tests for AIDS antibodies has opened the issue of privacy. Florida has a strict confidentiality law for tests at public clinics, but should these tests be used in pre-employment or insurance physicals? They are indications of exposure, not proof of illness.

AIDS first was closely identified only with homosexual sodomy and use of tainted needles by drug addicts. Except for a few unfortunate cases among persons receiving blood transfusions, the public and government considered AIDS as the victims' problem. But AIDS now is spreading through the general population. Of Florida's 781 known AIDS victims, 185 do not fit into a diagnostic category. AIDS is not going away, not getting cheaper, not posing any simpler questions of public policy. Addressing all those issues must be of highest priority in Congress and in the nation's state legislatures — especially Florida's.

THE MILWAUKEE JOURNAL

Milwaukee, WI, August 25, 1985

Many people, including some of those most at risk, have been inadequately aware of the awful dangers posed by AIDS. Others have been panicky, but for the wrong reasons, because of misconceptions. Last week's thoughtful series on the subject by Milwaukee Journal staff members put the dread malady in proper focus.

We want to emphasize some key points, in the hope that clearer understanding of the problem will lead to intelligent, urgently needed action.

First, it must be stressed that the AIDS virus is *not* spread by casual contact, so there is no excuse for depriving its pathetic victims of the care and support they so badly need.

The ailment is transmitted (1) by contaminated needles that intravenous-drug users employ; (2) by transfusion of blood from AIDS carriers, a rare occurrence, given the strict vigilance of blood banks; (3) by sexual contact, primarily from one male homosexual to another but also from bisexual males to their female partners.

Although the risk of heterosexual transmission of AIDS is debated by medical specialists, there's some reason to think the peril to heterosexuals will grow if the epidemic now ravaging high-risk groups is not brought under control.

Even if heterosexuals were entirely free of risk, the problem would still be immense. There are millions of homosexuals and bisexuals, and a decent society cannot be complacent about their fate. After all, there's no scientific basis for the uncharitable belief that homosexuals and bisexuals chose their sexual orientation.

Yet, on a matter in which they do exercise choice, many gays court disaster by deluding themselves about unsafe activities. They must learn to face reality. To indulge in unguarded or half-safe sexual contact is to flirt with a death sentence. Even in Russian roulette, removing most of the cartridges from the revolver will improve the player's statistical odds, but the game still ends in death if played long enough.

Much more must be done by health departments, other public agencies, volunteer groups and gay organizations to make sure that people understand what is safe or relatively safe and what isn't.

Abstinence obviously is the surest preventative, if the least likely to be practiced. Monogamy, growing in popularity, can be the answer for many. Among those who recklessly insist on having multiple partners, the disease-prevention value of condoms (used properly) should not be overlooked.

More widespread testing for the AIDS virus also is necessary, although records must be kept confidential to prevent unfair discrimination.

Yes, the search for vaccines and remedies must be stepped up, too. But control of the deadly contagion is the immediate challenge.

Portland Press Herald

*Portland, ME
August 17, 1985*

A second death in Maine from acquired immune deficiency syndrome this year demonstrates that AIDS is a national health threat, not an offbeat, big-city disease.

The commitment of public money and resources must be stepped up to match it.

So far, Health and Human Services Secretary Margaret Heckler has been more generous with rhetoric than with the dollars required to develop effective medical responses to AIDS.

Granted, Heckler some time ago made AIDS "the No. 1 priority" of the Public Health Service. But what does that mean?

Not enough, the Office of Technology Assessment, a research arm of the Congress, concluded earlier this year. The high public priority accorded AIDS "has not always been supported by financial and personnel resources," the OTA reported.

Public pressure should see that it is.

Total government spending on AIDS, mostly for research, has increased from $5.5 million in 1982 to $97.4 million this year. But the increase can be credited less to HHS and more to members of Congress.

The Reagan administration initially proposed to freeze AIDS spending at present levels for fiscal 1986. Last month, it revised that request to ask for $126.3 million. The money will be spent to monitor donated blood, test vaccines and drugs and conduct AIDS education programs across the country.

Meanwhile AIDS is conducting an education program of its own.

"The diabolical thing about AIDS is that it attacks the very thing that protects you," said Dr. Anthony Fauci, director of the National Institute of Allergy and Infectious Diseases. AIDS is the only known virus that attacks and destroys the human immune system.

First diagnosed in the United States four years ago, the number of AIDS victims is doubling every year. Public health officials anticipate 40,000 new cases over the next two years.

They should be all the priority a strong public commitment needs.

THE ANN ARBOR NEWS

Ann Arbor, MI, August 23, 1985

A sophisticated information society such as ours still has occasion to battle fear and panic. Misinformation and half-truths do a terrible disservice at times.

Nobody in his right mind would downplay the potential public health hazard to this country of AIDS — Acquired Immune Deficiency Syndrome. What we don't know about AIDS is a little frightening in itself, part of which is attributable to its recent identification (1981).

The Rock Hudson disclosure was a great boost to AIDS awareness, much as President Reagan's abdominal surgery focused attention on the need to spot colo-rectal cancers. Unfortunately, the Hudson disclosure also had its dark side.

The homosexual and bisexual male communities, which AIDS has affected heavily, are experiencing a surge of public backlash. In California, for example, a group called the Coalition for Traditional Values is stepping up attacks on the gay community.

AIDS victims deserve help and understanding, not the leper treatment. From the positive diagnosis of the disease to the certainty of death, AIDS victims get one shock after another.

Marc Griffis, director of an AIDS task force in Jacksonville, Fla., put it this way: "They find barriers everywhere they go. They lose their jobs. They lose their money. There's very little government assistance. Even those with insurance have a hard time meeting their deductible. Then they end up in a city hospital where no one wants to touch them."

AIDS has spawned nearly 13,000 cases nationally, a figure that is expected to rise dramatically by the end of the decade. The cost of AIDS to hospitals and taxpayers is enormous. The medical bill of an average AIDS patient runs more than $100,000. AIDS has killed about 6,000 people in the U.S. since it was first identified.

But AIDS is only one of about 25 contagious diseases classified as STD, or sexually transmitted diseases. AIDS is simply the most frightening of the STDs and also the newest. At one time, gonorrhea and syphilis were also accorded epidemic status until major surveillance campaigns in the 1970s reduced their prevalence.

Despite rumors that AIDS can be contracted through casual contact, it actually appears the AIDS virus is very hard to transmit. And despite the fears of hospital workers, there are no documented cases of U.S. health care workers getting infected or sick through clinical contact with AIDS victims.

The "knowns," then, are bad enough. The unknowns of AIDS fuel the worst kind of public hysteria. A clear course of action is to step up AIDS treatment, prevention, education and research programs.

That means more involvement by the government and the pharmaceutical firms than has been seen to date. It means a shift in priorities in national health funding.

Isolation of AIDS victims as though they were lepers and the quarantine mentality are over-reactions. The sense of panic being spread by social institutions which refuse any kind of contact with AIDS victims is based on ignorance and fear. Some of what is being accepted as knowledge of the issue is really misinformation and unsubstantiated material.

Already some people seem to be thinking AIDS will bring this country to its knees and that it is divine retribution for an allegedly deviant life style. Along those same lines, it could be argued that unchecked cigarette smoking and alcohol abuse are sufficient departures from the norm to also be called deviant behavior.

We need to be thinking and working hard on a search for a cure, prevention or treatment of AIDS. Any other approach feeds rather than allays panic.

Edmonton Journal

Edmonton, Alta., August 17, 1985

It's gratifying that the University of Alberta Hospital dental clinic feels a moral obligation to treat victims of Acquired Immune Deficiency Syndrome (AIDS).

Unlike the clinic at University of British Columbia which refuses to work on AIDS patients, the U of A clinic has treated two victims and says it won't turn away others.

True, there are more AIDS patients in Vancouver than Edmonton. But the U of A clinic nevertheless sets an ethical standard to which other clinics should aspire.

The Centre for Disease Control in Atlanta, Ga., advises that special precautions be taken with AIDS victims. And that's reasonable, since AIDS can be transmitted through body fluids.

But AIDS victims should not be denied dental care. They should not be treated as modern-day lepers.

LAS VEGAS REVIEW-JOURNAL

Las Vegas, NV, August 20, 1985

Sexual promiscuity is on the wane in the United States, and while the Moral Majority may not be overjoyed at the reason, folks don't seem to be sleeping around as much as they were.

Morality has little to do with it. As much as anything, fear — fear of AIDS and other venereal disease — seems to be shaping up the personal lives of Americans.

Across the country, health departments are reporting marked declines in communicable social disease. Most officials attribute the trend directly to widespread publicity about herpes and AIDS, particularly the fearful news that no effective treatment has yet been found for AIDS victims.

Nevada figures parallel the national trend. Gonorrhea cases in the state dropped from a peak of 6,776 in 1981 to 4,208 last year. In the same period, syphilis cases decreased from 134 to 104.

From Miami University in Oxford, Ohio, a sociologist reports that virginity is on a rampage among current female college students.

In 1963, he reports, 75 percent of the women he surveyed were virgins. By 1978, the figure had plunged to 38 percent, almost equal that of male students. Last year, a reversed trend was shown when 43 percent of the women surveyed reported themselves virgins.

While no one has analyzed any trends in Nevada's sexual social behavior, the noticeable decline in venereal disease would indicate promiscuous activity is on the wane.

"With the media coverage of herpes and AIDS, people are not having as much casual sex as they were," according to Monte Meador, chief of the Nevada Division of Health's communicable disease section.

Sociologists may soon find that an entire nation's attitude toward premarital and extramarital sex has been reversed because of twin scourges that have frightened people into second thoughts about their personal behavior.

The Seattle Times

Seattle, WA, October 19, 1985

THE Pentagon's decision to test all 2.1 million active-duty military personnel for exposure to the AIDS virus may be open to some points of valid criticism, but simple prudence supports the move.

The decision amounts to an expansion of earlier actions by the military to protect itself from a problem with disastrous potential. Testing for the AIDS antibody has been mandatory for blood donors at military installations since July 1 and has been applied since Oct. 1 to all new recruits.

The decision has been criticized by some groups on the basis that only about 10 percent of persons who test positive for the virus actually contract AIDS. It is difficult to follow such reasoning in view of the fact that anyone with a positive test is considered contagious.

Anyone on active duty found to have the antibody will be placed on limited-service status, officials say. Precisely what this entails has not been worked out, but presumably it would include medical observation and preclude being sent overseas.

No doubt this would be considered an unfair burden on some individuals. That detriment must be measured, however, against the potentially huge protective value of the testing program.

In combat, everyone is a potential blood donor and blood recipient. AIDS can be transmitted by blood transfusions. And military personnel, particularly those going overseas, are required to receive certain vaccinations, some of which can cause an AIDS disease reaction in those carrying the AIDS virus.

AIDS is a relatively new problem for the human race, worldwide, and means of dealing with it are all in the embryonic stage. It is a reasonable conclusion, however, that the Defense Department is ahead of the general population in the steps it is taking at this point.

The Pittsburgh PRESS

Pittsburgh, PA, September 22, 1985

The director of the Allegheny County Health Department, Dr. N. Mark Richards, inadvertently disclosed the other day that a county school teacher was one of 16 persons who had contracted AIDS this year. It touched off a flap that reflects the deep public fears surrounding this disease and the difficulties in dealing with them — here as well as elsewhere in the country.

Edgar J. Holtz, executive director of the Allegheny Intermediate Unit, wanted to know the identity of the teacher. When the Health Department refused to provide it — or even say whether he or she was still teaching, hospitalized, or dead — Dr. Holtz pressed on.

He said he would seek clarification of the rights of school officials to identify students, teachers and others who have been stricken with acquired immune deficiency syndrome.

It's not clear what Dr. Holtz would have done if given the name of the teacher. Or if school higher-ups have any more right to on-demand information about AIDS victims than about those with other medical problems.

Given the relative newness of AIDS — it was first diagnosed only four years ago — there probably aren't any legal guidelines yet in place.

But Dr. Holtz's reaction raises the specter that AIDS victims may be the lepers of the 1980s, not only shunned and isolated by their neighbors but even driven into the most miserable sort of existence.

In other parts of the United States, there have been organized boycotts of schools where children with AIDS are enrolled. Nurses have refused to deal with AIDS patients. Some funeral directors won't handle the bodies of AIDS victims.

The evidence, so far, hardly supports such public fright or hostility.

AIDS, no one disputes, is usually fatal and has no known cure. Yet it's also generally agreed that chances for getting AIDS are remote. AIDS is mostly spread by anal intercourse among homosexual men, by female prostitutes, the sharing of unclean needles by drug addicts, and in transfusions of infected blood. The disease also can be transmitted from mother to child at birth.

But there has been no evidence that AIDS can be spread by casual contact — by youngsters associating with each other in the classroom or playground, by handshakes, by using public bathrooms or even from shared food.

One scientist likened the chances of getting AIDS to getting hit by lightning.

Yet the fears and worries linger, even with such long-odds assurances on AIDS contagion from medical researchers. Especially when much remains unknown about this unusual malady.

Understandably, when parents believe their children's health to be endangered, even slightly, no precaution seems too much. And for others with terrifying fears of even being in the same building as an AIDS victim, no medical data is likely to persuade them otherwise.

In the past, we have seen panic quickly spread over such deadly diseases as polio and diphtheria before vaccines were found for them.

As then, the worries about AIDS are based mostly on deeply imbedded emotions rather than informed judgments. The best knowledge available so far suggests no reason for publicly identifying or isolating AIDS victims as a group.

The county Health Department was right to resist efforts to name any victims and expose them to yet another affliction, one that derives from the fears of others.

The State

Columbia, SC
October 10, 1985

FEAR OF AIDS will increase with the recent death of the well-known actor Rock Hudson, but the fear must be dealt with rationally so there will be no national panic.

One result of the growing worry about AIDS has been a very serious shortage of donors to the essential American Red Cross blood program. The impact is felt here in the Midlands where about half of the normal number of units of blood are presently available because people are not giving.

Lives of patients will be threatened if the shortage grows. A Red Cross spokesman points out that one accident victim alone can use up 60 to 100 units of blood. Surgical patients also depend upon transfusions.

Blood donors should know that there is no risk of their contracting AIDS in giving blood to the Red Cross.

"We don't know all the means of transmission for AIDS at this time," says Dr. Todd A. Kolb, American Red Cross director for the South Carolina region, "but we do know that a person cannot contract AIDS from donating blood.

"All Red Cross blood collections are drawn with a sterile, disposable needle. It is thrown away after a single use," he said.

Furthermore, the Red Cross says patients should not refuse transfusions or forego surgery because of fear of AIDS. Hemophiliac cases, which are being identified now, result from transfusions two to seven years ago.

Blood which is donated today is tested to detect HTLV-III antibodies. The presence of the antibodies does not indicate the donor has AIDS, but that the person was exposed at some time to HTLV-III — and a positive test does not mean that the donor has AIDS or will develop AIDS. The units which test positive are discarded, so those receiving transfusions may be assured there is little chance of contamination.

"There is a very minimal risk from receiving blood transfusions with AIDS, and absolutely no risk from donating blood," Dr. Kolb said.

Former donors and young people who have recently turned 17 should participate when the bloodmobile comes to their communities. I they do not and blood supplies become short, many lives could be endangered.

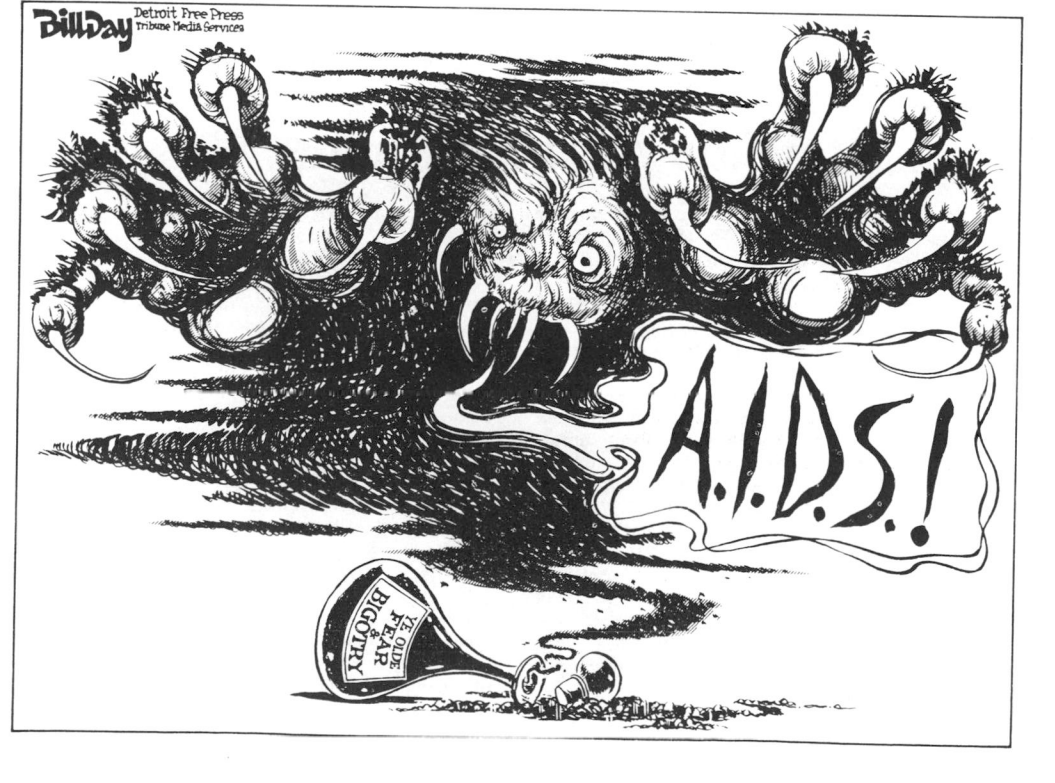

ST. LOUIS POST-DISPATCH

St. Louis, MO, September 20, 1985

In America, 910,000 people will be diagnosed this year as having cancer. One in every three households is affected by mental illness, and 43.5 million people are afflicted with some form of heart disease. Yet none of those diseases is on the lips of most people today. Instead, it is acquired immune deficiency syndrome — AIDS — from which 13,000 Americans are suffering, that has caused a wave of panic that is spreading faster than the disease itself.

One reason for the hysteria is that AIDS is a mystery disease. No one is quite sure of its cause, nor has a cure or vaccine been developed for the deadly illness. What is known is that AIDS is contracted in one of three ways: sexual contact, contaminated needles or blood transfusions. To the best of the knowledge of medical science, AIDS cannot be contracted from toilet seats, doorknobs, by standing next to a person with the disease or by breathing the same air. Although the virus has been discovered in tears of AIDS victims, none of the people with the disease is believed to have contracted it in such a manner. It can't be contracted by donating blood. And no child with AIDS has been known to have contracted the disease through casual contact with other children.

That last point is one that must be driven home to those parents in New York who have refused to let their youngsters attend school because students with AIDS have been allowed to attend. Those parents are wrestling with a situation that has caused many parents across the country these days to consider: What would I do if a child attending my youngster's school had AIDS? The question is a difficult one, and one that has to be grappled with individually. It's only natural for parents to want to protect their children from potential harm.

But one must look at the facts. Studies of hundreds of people living with AIDS victims have failed to indicate any transmission of the disease through daily family contact. No known AIDS cases have ever been transmitted through school or day care. And the Centers for Disease Control in Atlanta has recommended that most children with AIDS be allowed in class and has urged school officials to protect their privacy. "Based on current evidence," the agency said recently, "casual person-to-person contact, as would occur among schoolchildren, appears to pose no risk."

Nonetheless, the questions and concern raised as a result of the lack of knowledge of the disease point toward a definite need for increased AIDS education. Government — federal, state and local — must do all it can to educate the public about the disease. And the public must make a concerted effort to educate itself. No one wants to contract AIDS. But we must not allow ourselves to become hysterical over the disease or lose our common sense about it. Hopefully, increased public awareness, along with potential developments of vaccines or cures, will reduce the hysteria that has captured much of the American public.

St. Petersburg Times

St. Petersburg, FL, September 15, 1985

As the AIDS plague spreads, the hysteria and misconceptions that accompany the deadly new disease grow proportionately. So far, fear has had the upper hand. The cruel result is that victims often are unnecessarily ostracized.

In Virginia, a man with AIDS is told to apply for food stamps through the mail because everyone in the welfare office is afraid to talk to him. In Indiana, a judge drops charges against an alleged thief because he is afraid to have an AIDS victim in his courtroom. In Washington, television crews are afraid to film persons afflicted with AIDS. In New York City, parents are afraid to send their children to school after learning that a second-grader with AIDS is attending classes.

AIDS, or acquired immune deficiency syndrome, is a fearsome disease. It destroys its victims' immune systems, leaving them vulnerable to other serious diseases, such as cancer. The death rate for all AIDS cases to date is 50 percent — 6,376 lives taken. However, the disease takes years to kill its victims. Among those from the early years of reporting, the death rate approaches 100 percent. The number of cases of AIDS relentlessly doubles every year. No one has been cured.

THE TERRIFYING killer presents numerous social problems. One is whether children with AIDS should be allowed to attend public schools. School officials in Florida and across the country are grappling with this emotionally charged and politically sensitive decision.

Some school boards have bowed to public anxiety and have taken the easiest course, banning children with AIDS from regular classes. Others, swayed by the medical evidence rather than uninformed hysteria, have taken a harder but more compassionate and reasonable approach.

New York City school officials, for example, have devised a plan that is both fair to the children and recognizes parents' understandable concerns. The city has set up a panel to review each AIDS case child by child. The panel's decisions have been conservative and cautious, as they should be. Of four children reviewed, one has been given permission to attend regular classes, two are receiving instruction in hospitals and one will be taught at home at public expense.

The panel's decisions reflect the common-sense advice from the federal Centers for Disease Control (CDC), which recommend that many children with AIDS can safely attend public schools because they are not a threat to spread the disease to other youngsters. However, federal epidemiologists advise extra precaution in handling AIDS-afflicted toddlers who drool or wear diapers or exhibit such aggressive behavior as biting.

The only confirmed ways of transmission are through sexual relations, contaminated needles and blood transfusions. There is abundant evidence that AIDS cannot be spread by casual contact — a sneeze, handshake or proximity. Not one of the family members of the 12,000 reported AIDS cases is known to have caught the disease, except for spouses in sexual contact and children born to mothers with AIDS. No doctor or nurse has caught AIDS from a patient. New cases overwhelmingly affect drug abusers and homosexuals.

THE NUMBER of cases of victims who fit none of the high risk groups is growing, but still is only 1 percent of the total. This suggests that AIDS may be transmitted in more ways than originally thought, reason enough for school officials to err on the side of caution but not justification for automatically banning all AIDS children from regular classes.

The vast majority of doctors, including those represented by the Florida Medical Association, concur with the advice offered by CDC. Public panic ought to be calmed by the attitude of thoughtful health experts. Some restrictions on AIDS victims, adults and children, will be necessary to protect the common good and slow the spread of this awful disease. Those decisions need to be based on medical evidence rather than public hysteria.

Dying AIDS victims have been dealt much tragedy; segregating them on the basis of unfounded fear would be compounding the cruelty.

Los Angeles Times

Los Angeles, CA, November 26, 1985

The Los Angeles County Board of Supervisors will meet today to decide what to do about bathhouses frequented by gay men, where AIDS is spread by high-risk sexual activity. The issue is part of the growing problem of public policy and AIDS. Many people, gay and straight, are concerned that as the AIDS epidemic grows, actions will be taken in the name of public health that endanger civil liberties of homosexuals, who have only recently acquired these rights—in fact if not in law—and understandably worry about threats to them. The institution of mandatory blood testing in the military and of insurance screening for the AIDS virus heightens these concerns.

County health officials have recommended that the supervisors adopt a plan to regulate the bathhouses, establish guidelines for safe sex that is to be practiced there and close the places that do not follow the rules. According to the health officials, these steps would be sufficient to p·   the public health, and the supervisors are expected to do at least that much.

But they may choose to go one step further and seek immediate closure of all bathhouses. That would be a mistake. It would signal a policy of blanket action against AIDS that is broader than necessary. It would open the door to more such action in the future and run the risk of making it possible for misplaced public anxiety to trample on individual rights without benefit to public health.

The state of Texas is talking about allowing the authorities there to quarantine some AIDS patients. If quarantine is deemed an appropriate response, who should be quarantined? All AIDS patients? All people whose blood tests positive for the AIDS antibody, indicating exposure to the virus? If the AIDS antibody test is deemed significant to protect the public health, will mandatory national blood testing be instituted?

This is clearly the wrong way to go. If restrictions are going to be imposed to combat the AIDS epidemic, they must be instituted with the utmost care on a case-by-case basis and with scrupulous regard to due process. The decisions must be based on the individual facts and not on politics. That is what should be done now with the bathhouses. Public policy should combat AIDS, not homosexuals.

THE ATLANTA CONSTITUTION
Atlanta, GA, October 7, 1985

It is a tough question that has doctors and civil libertarians understandably nervous. Should public-health officers ask AIDS patients to list recent sex partners, and should they contact the people named? The correct answer is yes. The best defense against this incurable disease is to inhibit its spread. Notification will help with that task.

The risks from this procedure, known as tracking, are obvious. Handled indiscreetly, such lists could devastate many lives. They could abruptly expose private proclivities for marital infidelity or homosexuality. And regardless of how a listee tested for the AIDS virus, the merest association with the disease, if revealed, could result in lost jobs, lost friends and more.

At a time when fear of AIDS sometimes borders on hysteria, such problems cannot be dismissed. Still, the benefits of a well-run tracking program outweigh the perils.

Opponents correctly point out that a person who carries the AIDS virus won't necessarily develop the disease. So they ask: Why should virus carriers be identified when there is no cure if the disease develops — what carriers don't know won't hurt them, will it?

It will — and not only them, but others. One life lived under a burden of terrible knowledge may keep many more lives free of risk. Most people who test positive for the AIDS virus will surely refrain from sexual activity that could spread it.

Those who are at risk should know their status in the event that a cure is discovered. At least seven compounds have been shown to retard the AIDS virus in test tubes, and research continues. A brave confrontation with the truth now might save a life later.

Moreover, such programs can be done discreetly. For years, health departments have tracked the sexual partners of syphilis and gonorrhea patients. Their procedures have created scant fuss.

Yet a successful tracking program for AIDS will require more than candor and discretion. It will demand a thorough public education effort. If those who test positive suddenly become outcasts as a result of flimsy public fears, tracking will surely fail.

Patients will tell less, their partners will deny all and the unintended spread of AIDS will continue unabated. Witch-hunts will only cause more pain. Wisely applied truth is the best medicine.

The Cincinnati Post
Cincinnati, OH, October 28, 1985

The Defense Department's decision to screen all military personnel for AIDS is an appropriate response to a serious health problem.

It is important for the armed forces to isolate victims of acquired immune deficiency syndrome for several reasons:

The Army, Navy, Air Force and Marines are fighting forces, requiring that personnel be in good physical condition.

Eating and sleeping arrangements, as well as other aspects of military life, put individuals in close contact with one another. While it is not believed that AIDS is spread through casual contact, it is better to err on the side of caution when combat readiness may be involved.

In actual combat situations, every member is considered a "walking blood bank" who might be called on to give a transfusion to a wounded comrade. AIDS can be transmitted through blood transfusions.

The proposed testing is not without controversy. Spokesmen for gay rights groups have accused the Defense Department of using the AIDS scare to get rid of homosexuals, who are barred from military service.

The charge is undeserved. The Defense Department would hardly spend the millions of dollars that screening will cost just to harass homosexuals. It is simple fact that most persons who have developed AIDS have been homosexuals.

When the use of illegal drugs became a serious problem in the military, mandatory testing was instituted. Recruits are routinely screened for venereal diseases.

Until more is known about AIDS and ways are found to cure or prevent it, the Pentagon is well within its rights to seek out those who could contribute to an unhealthy environment among the nation's fighting units.

CHARLESTON EVENING POST
The News and Courier
Charleston, SC, October 30, 1985

The mere suggestion by an Indiana insurance company that underwriters try to screen out possible AIDS victims, in part because of the high medical costs incurred in treating them, has evoked cries of discrimination from homosexual groups. Such screening would be unfair not only to homosexuals, the group spokesmen say, but also to young, single heterosexuals, whose lifestyles and ages might cause them to be bracketed in the general classification of insurance applicants who would be subject to special screening. Such objections are predictable, but they lose sight of some realities in the insurance field.

Discrimination is a part of the insurance business — not because of any bias in the popular sense, but because of experience. Coverage and premium rates reflect the risks and probabilities — as determined from experience.

Is it fair that life insurance applicants with a history of heart disease or diabetes are turned down for health reasons? No, it's not. But from the insurers' standpoint it makes economic sense, considering the risks calculated from the morbidity tables.

Is it fair that a 23-year-old man with an unblemished driving record must pay a much higher auto insurance rate than his 46-year-old father, even if both drive the same model car? No, it's not. But the 23-year-old is a victim of insurance experience. The statistics show he is in the age group that is at highest risk on the highways.

There's nothing new in the screening concept suggested in connection with AIDS. It's discriminatory, but no more discriminatory than screenings for other diseases that put applicants at what insurers consider unacceptably high risks.

The Houston Post
Houston, TX, October 22, 1985

In deciding to test all 2.1 million U.S. military personnel for Acquired Immune Deficiency Syndrome, the Defense Department is taking a prudent course without edging over into hysteria.

The reasons for the testing are compelling. After all, the military mission involves combat, which implies emergency blood transfusions among battlefield comrades with no opportunity for screening donors. Also, military personnel are subject to being deployed to almost any part of the world on short notice. If their immune systems are already weakened, this leaves them susceptible to diseases that might not affect the average recruit.

The tests will be administered to *all* personnel, from generals and admirals to privates and sailors. This is as it should be, both for thoroughness and fairness. The procedure will result in the honorable medical discharge of those suffering from AIDS and possible restriction of assignments for those who have the virus but are not ill. This will protect those who do not have the virus and provide valuable medical assistance to those who do.

There is one troubling aspect of the program: Those who test positive will be given medical interviews about, among other things, their sexual behavior. Some commanders are pushing to have those who acknowledge homosexual activity reported to them for discharge proceedings. Even though homosexuality is a cause for dismissal, this is a terrible idea. It violates the fundamental tradition of doctor-patient confidentiality, which exists partly to preserve privacy and partly to encourage disclosure of communicable diseases. If military doctors are compelled to report this, the effectiveness of the whole program will be damaged — and it could become a witch hunt. This must not happen.

That misgiving aside, the program is a good one and should proceed with all due speed.

The Salt Lake Tribune

Salt Lake City, UT, November 29, 1985

For good reason, fear of AIDS has spread throughout the country. To avoid counterproductive hysteria and the unjust treatment that intensifies the victims' suffering, that fright must be tempered with heavy doses of reason.

Hardly a day goes by without more news of the subject. So far, more than half of the 14,125 or so Americans stricken with the incurable, fatal disease have died. Twelve were Utahns. The figures climb inexorably.

Most victims have been homosexual men and intravenous drug abusers, but others have caught the virus through heredity, blood transfusions or sexual contact with infected men and women. Two of Utah's victims were children. Just last week, a Salt Lake County prostitute who could have infected hundreds of men was diagnosed as an AIDS carrier.

Without question, acquired immune deficiency syndrome is an alarming public health problem requiring prompt, effective attention. Finding the cause and cure of the elusive disease has appropriately become the top health priority in the country. Millions of dollars are being and must continue to be spent on medical research in the United States and elsewhere.

While precautions must be taken to control the disease, the public needn't overreact.

The American military, health agencies, schools, prisons and other organizations, both public and private, are developing policies for dealing with victims and carriers. Some of those policies are reasonable responses to what is known about the virus. Unfortunately, though, public misconceptions still are setting off irrational, insensitive reactions to infected friends, family members and acquaintances.

In some states, parents have refused to let their children attend school with AIDS sufferers, even though the U.S. Public Health Service insists the virus is not spread through normal, casual contact.

No Utah schools have confronted an AIDS case yet. But as a precaution, the state's largest school district, Granite, has devised a policy that would treat each case individually. That might work. The fact that Utahns are more inclined than other Americans to worry about contamination in the classroom, however, bodes ill for their first AIDS case.

The Tribune's most recent Bardsley poll shows that 20 percent of parents with children living at home would fight to have an AIDS child removed from school. The national figure is 17 percent. Utahns also are more apt than most to see AIDS as a threat to the general public. And it's at Utah State University that a group of students is using AIDS as one reason to protest the organization of homosexuals on campus.

Special public policies for dealing with AIDS-infected prostitutes and prisoners are in order. When it comes to classrooms, homes and the work place, however, a more relaxed approach applies. Agencies like the Salt Lake City-County and State Health departments and Salt Lake AIDS, meanwhile, have the right idea. They are providing correct, objective information to prevent panic while scientists try to solve AIDS mysteries.

San Francisco Chronicle

San Francisco, CA, November 11, 1985

THE REPORT that some San Francisco homosexual bathhouses and sex clubs continue to allow unsafe sexual contacts which could spread AIDS is no surprise at all. The clubs exist primarily as arenas of promiscuous sexual conduct. As long as their doors are open, they will find customers seeking gratification.

An order by Superior Court Judge Roy Wonder of a year ago allowed the clubs to remain in business as long as "unsafe" sex was prohibited by monitors hired by the establishments. "Unsafe" practices are those which allow the transfer of bodily fluids, and possibly AIDS virus, from one participant to the other.

We questioned the reasoning of that court order when it was first issued. It was, we felt, somewhat like telling someone to go swimming but not to get wet.

THE JUDGE'S ORDER, issued under a law suit brought by bathhouse and sex club owners, overturned a city decision to lock up these places in the belief that there was a clear and present danger. The decision to padlock the baths and sex clubs on medical grounds was a wise one. It still is.

Private behavior between consenting adults can not, and should not, be regulated. But no community should sanction potentially life-threatening activities in places which operate with city business licenses.

Anyone needing confirmation of the seriousness of the situation should consult the latest AIDS statistics. The Center for Disease Control in Atlanta, which began keeping AIDS statistics in 1981, has now counted 14,519 cases, 7,450 of which have ended in death.

SOME HOMOSEXUALS have resisted closure of bathhouses because, they say, the act would represent a denial of hard-won rights and a return of discrimination against gays. We do not believe this view is valid. It is not oppressive or regressive to respond vigorously when a killer is on the loose.

BUFFALO EVENING NEWS

Buffalo, NY, September 9, 1985

AMERICA HAS TO take care of its AIDS patients. It also has to protect its citizens who are not infected. Doing both will take a kind of hard thought and purposeful planning that is only beginning to show itself among public health officials.

Twelve thousand Americans now have acquired immune deficiency syndrome, and the number is doubling every year. This epidemic that seemed to come from nowhere has taken both the public and the medical establishment by surprise, and no cure is in sight. The nation must now figure out how to deal rationally with it.

Testing of potential blood donors and education about the risks facing homosexuals and drug users are important efforts to contain the disease.

But now attention is beginning to focus on the dangers to others from exposure to AIDS patients, and the fine line between unwarranted ostracism of patients and proper protection of the uninfected is not proving easy to draw. There is no evidence that AIDS is spread through casual contact, but the virus has been reported in victims' saliva and even tears.

AIDS is a fatal disease that is only now coming to be understood, as the public is well aware. Research on how it may spread is not yet so far-reaching and definitive that the fears of nurses and health workers, and of parents whose children's classmates have AIDS, can be dismissed as paranoid.

Much of the evidence cited in attempts to reassure the public is based on where and in what groups the disease most frequently occurs, not on biological studies. More basic biochemical research is needed on how the disease can be transmitted.

The New York State Health Department took an important step when it issued official guidelines for hospitals on dealing with AIDS patients. It emphasized the important principle that AIDS victims have the same rights to care as other patients and said hospitals should not refuse patients solely because they have AIDS and should run educational programs for workers.

The guidelines are important in establishing patient rights, but they will not allay all the public's fears or uncertainty about what level of exposure and what kinds of contacts with AIDS victims can be assured to be safe.

School systems face a delicate problem of their own — providing instruction for AIDS children without endangering healthy students. Until the risk of transmittal can be effectively ruled out, home teaching may be necessary, especially for younger students. If school officials do not feel confident they can assure other students' safety, chances should not be taken.

The military took a cautious and reasonable stand in mandating that all new recruits be tested for AIDS and ruling out admission to the services of those found to be carriers of the virus.

As the number of AIDS cases increases and the potential for contacts with infected persons grows, there will be more conflict over where protection of the public ends and ostracism of patients begins. It will be increasingly important for public agencies to step in, as New York has begun to do, with guidelines.

But those guidelines must be based on the latest and best in medical research, so that they inspire real confidence. Research on the spread of the disease, as well as on a cure, must be intensified. And where there is still room for doubt, guidelines must lean toward the side of caution for the safety of the uninfected.

SUNDAY NEWS

Manchester, NH, October 6, 1985

The power of the mega-media, for good or evil, is absolutely amazing.

They can alert and thus prepare a nation for impending natural disaster. For all the hype about Hurricane Gloria, the media still did the public a valuable service.

They can also distort and shape the truth to their liking and on a scale that is breathtaking. Consider AIDS, the Acquired Immune Deficiency Syndrome.

Where has the deadly AIDS virus flourished in America? Most people still know the answer. It has been within the homosexual community, particularly among the most promiscuous of a group that seems prone to multiple partners.

There is little doubt of this fact. From the very first, AIDS was recognized as the "homosexual's disease." It is mainly from within that community that the disease has now been spread, through prostitutes and tainted blood supplies, to the general population.

But while scientists burn the midnight oil to find a cure for the disease, many homosexuals and their apologists scream bloody murder at the very thought that the government would or should shut down their "bath-house" breeding grounds or — heaven forbid — quarantine the carriers.

And it seems to us that the mega-media are now about the business of downplaying, if not deliberately distorting, the homosexuals' role in this impending national disaster.

Oddly, while many in the media take up the alarm for a quick miracle cure for AIDS, they downplay the potential risk and still unanswered medical questions of how carriers — be they defiant, sexual deviants or unfortunate school children — may be affecting the general populace.

The tragic death of the actor Rock Hudson brought forth reams of copy and TV news stories of his inspiring a fight to find a cure for AIDS. But few in the media bothered to point out, in specific terms, the unpleasant facts of how the homosexual actor contracted the disease.

Indeed, when Publisher Nackey Loeb made mention of this in a nonetheless compassionate editorial last week, at least one wire service considered her remarks newsworthy — presumably because they were out of the ordinary.

AIDS is a national tragedy. So too is the misguided and immoral philosophy that holds that homosexuality is but an "alternative lifestyle." It is fast becoming a death sentence and it is endangering us all.

Boston Sunday Globe

Boston, MA, October 6, 1985

As the number of AIDS cases inexorably grows, there is an increasing danger of senseless retaliation against people with AIDS and those who are at high risk for the disease – even though they pose no known hazard to casual contacts.

Some measures being initiated – and some that are being called for – encroach in varying degrees on individuals' civil rights.

Great care must be taken to separate actions that may have some validity as preventive health measures from those that are basically punitive toward the vulnerable groups at high risk for AIDS – homosexuals, drug addicts and prostitutes.

The Defense Department has called for AIDS blood tests for all recruits. Those showing signs they have been exposed to the AIDS virus will be kept out of military service. Although that may be precautionary, it also is illogical, because no comparable tests are being ordered for those already in the service. Diane McGrath, the Republican candidate for mayor of New York City, wants anyone who comes in close contact with the public – doctors, dentists, nurses, teachers, food handlers, barbers, beauticians and prostitutes – to be similarly tested. Those found antibody-positive for AIDS would not be allowed to continue to work. She also wants to close bathhouses, bars, theaters and shops that cater to homosexuals, even though public health authorities know that would not eliminate the contact, but only drive those who frequent such places underground.

The plight of children with AIDS is particularly poignant. Several communities around the country are refusing to allow these children to attend school. Massachusetts, commendably, is following federal guidelines and the advice of the state health commissioner, Bailus Walker, and the communicable disease director, Dr. George Grady, in permitting school attendance by AIDS-stricken children under the appropriate conditions.

Yet, in Washington D.C., separate classes are being set up for children exposed to AIDS, and in New York, district school boards have ousted three children who, though free of AIDS themselves, had mothers with boyfriends in a high-risk group.

Although three states, Florida, California and Wisconsin, have passed laws to prohibit insurance companies from requiring AIDS blood tests, nationally both health and life insurers are weighing the prospects for requiring applicants to undergo AIDS blood-test screening as a prerequisite for coverage.

On the horizon, too, are bills that will confront Congress and the Reagan administration with the issue of protecting the confidentiality of AIDS victims and the estimated 1 million people who have been infected with the virus, but who are symptom-free.

Fear that blood-donor records could be obtained by outsiders is spreading through laboratories and blood banks. The federal Department of Health and Human Services has indicated it will recommend that laboratories inform blood donors who show signs of AIDS exposure that their names may be released to outsiders – such as health departments and, possibly, employers and insurers.

One state, Colorado, has made it mandatory that not only AIDS cases, but also cases of persons with a positive AIDS blood test, be reported to the state health department. By next year Colorado will begin seeking the names of all sex contacts of such persons.

Colorado health officials say they want to follow up on AIDS as they do with other sexually transmitted diseases such as syphilis. While all such reporting is being sought on a confidential basis, the Florida Supreme Court is considering a suit that could open up such records to public inspection.

Historically, the law permits the quarantining of patients with highly contagious diseases that could be spread by coughing or sneezing, or by germs on doorknobs or dishes. But it is enormously premature to restrict the lives and behavior of people who carry a virus that appears to be transmissible only by sexual contact or the exchange of blood.

Experience has long taught that the best way to prevent hysteria and its consequence, unwarranted intrusion on civil liberties, is to keep the public fully and accurately informed.

The Dallas Morning News

*Dallas, TX
October 28, 1985*

What a pity it would be if gay-rights activists or civil libertarians tried to make a civil-rights issue out of a proposal that AIDS victims be subject to quarantine. The proposal comes from the state health commissioner, Dr. Robert Bernstein; the State Board of Health takes it up next month.

The state — any state — has inherent power to protect the public by quarantining the victims of contagious diseases like tuberculosis and cholera.

To say that the victim of a particular disease *may* be quarantined isn't the same as saying he *will* be. The decision to quarantine turns on the likelihood of the victim's passing on the disease to others.

Bernstein explains: "We don't have many diseases, if any, that are worse than (AIDS) in terms of mortality. And if an individual for some reason is spreading the disease knowingly, (the quarantine power) would give us one means of controlling it."

The controversial point, from the gay-rights standpoint, is that quarantined AIDS victims would be prohibited from homosexual relations, lest they spread the disease. But when was there ever a "right" to spread a disease? AIDS isn't a civil-rights issue; it's a medical issue. Let the doctors act accordingly.

Film Star Rock Hudson Dies of AIDS

Rock Hudson, the American actor whose rugged good looks helped him become one of the superstars created by the Hollywood studio system, died October 2, 1985 in Beverly Hills, California, some 15 months after he was diagnosed as suffering from AIDS. The public disclosure of his AIDS illness in July 1985—the first such disclosure by a celebrity of his stature—gained worldwide attention and galvanized public support to fight the disease.

Hudson was hospitalized July 21, 1985 in Paris, France after collapsing at the Ritz Hotel. Early reports had indicated he was being treated for inoperable liver cancer, but the possibility that he had AIDS had also surfaced. A spokeswoman for the actor announced July 25 that Hudson was suffering from AIDS which had been diagnosed a year earlier in the U.S. She added that Hudson himself had decided to make public the nature of his illness. According to the office of Hudson's Beverly Hills doctor, Rexford Kennamer, Hudson had gone to Paris for a second visit to the Institut Pasteur, a medical research institute that had been using the experimental drug HPA-23, then unavailable in the U.S., to treat AIDS patients. Hudson had reportedly received the drug on his first visit to Paris in 1984.

In a film career that began in 1948 and peaked in the 1950s and early 1960s, he twice was voted the top box-office draw in the U.S., in 1957 and 1959; among his best-known films were *Giant* (1956), for which he won an Academy Award nomination for best actor, and *Pillow Talk* (1959), the first of three romantic comedies in which he costarred with Doris Day; after his popularity at the box office dipped in the late 1960s, he became one of the first movie stars to successfully switch to television. His detective series *McMillan and Wife* premiered in 1971 and ran for six seasons. Before he was diagnosed as having AIDS, he had appeared in six episodes of *Dynasty*.

The Boston Herald
Boston, MA
October 4, 1985

ON THE same day that Rock Hudson died, a victim of the dread disease AIDS, so did 20 other AIDS victims. And another 40 people in this country got the news that they too have Acquired Immune Deficiency Syndrome, a diagnosis that at this moment is tantamount to a death sentence.

The difference, of course, is that none of those other people will ever make Page One. Their courage and their suffering will never inspire people to hold glamorous fundraising parties. Many will not even die among the comfort of friends and family as Rock Hudson was able to do, for many are the victims not only of their illness, but of the ignorance, fear and intolerance that has trailed in its wake.

Rock Hudson could have tried to hide the cause of his illness and ultimately of his death. Oh, there would have been the inevitable rumors, but without his own admission, there would be no benefits, no outpouring of time and money from his Hollywood colleagues.

Hudson played out his final role with the kind of dignity and courage he rarely had the chance to display in his screen life. His disclosure became a catalyst for public sympathy and public understanding. The memory of his rugged handsomeness contrasted with his sadly withered appearance in his last public appearance gave his fans a heart-wrenching look at how this disease wends its course.

Hudson in a message read during the most recent fundraiser held by his colleagues said, "I am not happy that I have AIDS. But if that is helping others, I can at least know that my own misfortune has had some positive worth."

It has; and it must continue to do so.

The News and Courier
Charleston, SC, August 19, 1985

When it became know that the movie actor Rock Hudson had been taken seriously ill in Paris, his agent announced that he had cancer. Later, a decision was made to tell the truth about his illness. He has AIDS and he had gone to France for treatment that was not available in this country.

There is much food for thought in the fact that Mr. Hudson's agent decided initially that it would be better for the actor's fans to think that he had cancer, rather than AIDS. Cancer used to be unmentionable. It is a sign of progress — as well as an indication of the advances made by medical science in curing the disease — that it has become a respectable disease for movie actors to have.

It is also a sign of progress that someone, probably Mr. Hudson himself, decided to make AIDS mentionable, although, of course, besides admitting that he had AIDS, the actor was intimating something else. So far, the vast majority of people who are known to have contracted AIDS have been male homosexuals. It is of nobody's concern whether Mr. Hudson is, or is not, a homosexual. It will be a good thing if the publicity that he is giving to AIDS by revealing that he is a victim will help battle the disease and help research to find a cure. But some thought should be given to prevention of the spread of the disease. Mr. Hudson will not be helping to prevent the spread of AIDS if he is used by unscrupulous people to defend promiscuous lifestyles. Mr. Hudson's fame, in other words, should not be used for base motives and his privacy should be respected.

Celebrities are often misused by people with causes. Mr. Hudson has also found himself, quite unwittingly, the champion of people who oppose government regulation simply because he traveled to Paris for treatment that has not been approved by the Food and Drug Administration in this country. Critics of regulation saw Mr. Hudson's encounter with AIDS as a way of dramatizing their opposition to regulation. The drug that he took there — and apparently made him so ill that he was urgently transferred to the American Hospital and then flown back to the United States — was not available in this country simply because it has not passed the stringent regulations demanded by the FDA.

Another pundit, the newspaper editor and columnist Paul Greenberg, whose credentials are as conservative as most critics of government regulation, recently gave a one-word answer to those who oppose watchdogs for the people, like the FDA. That word is Bhopal. We could add many more, like Thalidomide.

There may be a moral to be drawn from Rock Hudson's illness; but it is dangerous to jump to any conclusions on the basis of what we are told about any celebrity.

THE ARIZONA REPUBLIC
Phoenix, AZ, August 1, 1985

THE revelation of Rock Hudson's battle with the killer ailment AIDS, which is associated mainly with homosexuals, should give everybody pause.

Acquired Immune Deficiency Syndrome, a disease that guts an individual's immune system and inexorably leads to death, has leaped out of the closet with the nation's attention riveted on the reclusive Hudson, a Hollywood celebrity and one-time matinee idol.

Hudson's battle to live took him to Paris for treatment with HPA-23, an experimental anti-viral drug developed at the Pasteur Institute. He is now hospitalized in Los Angeles.

The drug has toxic side-effects, and while experiments have shown it to inhibit replication of the AIDS virus, doctors on both sides of the Atlantic emphatically say it is not the panacea cure-all victims are so desperately hoping for.

Still, AIDS victims will grasp at anything to defy death, hoping to hold on long enough until a cure is found, while researchers try to develop a disease-preventing vaccine.

The statistics are staggering for the disease that is spread through sexual contact, blood transfusions and contaminated needles most often used by drug users.

The federal Centers For Disease Control in Atlanta says it has received reports of 11,871 confirmed cases of AIDS. Of those, nearly 50 percent, or 5,917 AIDS sufferers, have died.

That national trend is reflective in Arizona as well.

Of the 55 cases that have been diagnosed since 1981, 26 have been fatal.

The state Department of Health Service reports a doubling of cases every 10 to 12 months.

How many AIDS cases there are isn't precisely known because many are not reported, nor is there a registry to keep track of interstate movements.

Not all AIDS victims are homosexuals, nor is the disease confined to the United States.

Countries in Europe and South America are also reporting cases of AIDS.

The longer the time delay in finding a cure, the more it will inevitably spread, striking not just the "risk" groups of homosexuals, intravenous drug abusers and hemophiliacs, but the general population as well in what epidemiologists call a pandemic.

The U.S. Food and Drug Administration, besieged by pleas to permit usage of HPA-23 in this country, is planning to permit limited "compassionate use" on terminally ill patients perhaps as soon as September.

That, in conjunction with other anti-viral drugs now being tested, is a solid beginning on the road to halting AIDS in individuals whose immune systems aren't already damaged.

Hudson's case has elevated AIDS to new heights of public consciousness, spurring inquiries and interest in what once was known only as the gay plague.

Public health services must continue providing educational materials to AIDS victims. Those homosexual and bisexual males, who account for 75 percent of the victims, have a moral duty to think of the health of the general populace in their societal behavior.

But just that is not enough.

Infusions of money to finance research are needed to find a preventable vaccine, a priority undertaking in the months and years ahead.

The Washington Post
Washington, DC, August 14, 1985

EVEN BEFORE people began responding to the stories about Rock Hudson, attitudes toward AIDS were beginning to change. At first the deadly virus, discovered in 1981, had been thought to be confined to discrete groups, primarily male homosexuals and drug addicts, for whom there was limited sympathy in the society at large. Some uncharitable persons even suggested that there was no public responsibility to search for a cure, since the afflicted had voluntarily chosen to engage in the conduct that leads to the disease. There are other afflictions—alcoholism, drug addiction, venereal disease and even cigarette-induced illness—that have caused people to react this way in the past. But all these have long since come to be regarded as ailments for which it is not just proper but essential that society use its resources to contain and cure. The same, increasingly, is true of AIDS.

There are reasons for this. For one thing, the epidemic has continued to spread at a geometric rate. On Jan. 7 of this year, there were 7,788 reported cases in the United States; today there are more than 12,000, and the figure is expected to double within a year. Since the virus was discovered, 73 percent of its victims have been male homosexuals and 17 percent intravenous-drug users. But there have been others: hemophiliacs, people who have received blood transfusions and the children of AIDS victims. The fact that the malady hit patients who received blood transfusions, a category anyone could be in at a moment's notice, also contributed to alarm in the general population.

Scientists have now solved the blood transfusion problem by developing a test that allows them to screen blood donations for AIDS antibodies. Hemophiliacs and hospital patients receiving transfusions in the future are no longer in a special risk category. They were never more than a small fraction of the victims, but it is right to capitalize on the interest and concern generated by their vulnerability. Research efforts—the federal government will spend $126.3 million next year—have been consistent and productive. The scientific community was well ahead of the general public in addressing this problem.

But laymen must make a contribution too. Preventive efforts, particularly among homosexuals, should be increased. And education must be a priority. Some key facts need to be made widely known: blood *donors* do not contract AIDS; victims do not contaminate clothing, furniture or other objects; and children most certainly do not acquire the disease by being in the same classroom with a youngster who is a victim.

Very few of us will lose our eyesight or need a kidney transplant, yet we do not hesitate to mobilize public sympathy and national resources in aid of those who do, just as we mobilize them to assault diseases associated with social and sexual conduct the majority disapproves. It is good that these things are understood. AIDS is being fought and its victims cared for not because we all have an equal risk of contracting it or because a movie star we admire is a victim or for any reason other than that thousands of our fellow citizens, most of them young, are dying slowly, painfully and in profound despair—and we can do something to help.

DESERET NEWS
Salt Lake City, UT
October 3-4, 1985

Though Rock Hudson's death had long been expected, his passing this week still leaves a particularly painful sense of regret and loss.

How sad that he will be remembered not just for his acting and for the rugged image he portrayed, but also for the fact that he became the first celebrity known to contract AIDS. How disillusioning it was for many fans to learn what this disease indicated about the disparity between Hudson's screen image and his private life.

But keep in mind that Rock Hudson could have spent his last days with his privacy still largely intact and with the nature of his illness known only to his doctors. Instead, he chose to disclose his ailment as a means of focusing national attention on AIDS and of helping to raise funds for research on this fatal affliction. That took courage for a man who valued privacy as much as Hudson did.

Until his case came to light, many Americans were only dimly aware of acquired immune deficiency syndrome or AIDS, an incurable disease whose victims are mostly homosexual men. AIDS can also be acquired by intravenous drug users and recipients of blood transfusions.

As of now, there are 13,611 reported cases of AIDS in the United States, and 6,944 of the victims have died. Those figures don't mean that the disease is only about 50% fatal. Instead, it means that the victims who are still living have been diagnosed recently and have not yet had time to succumb.

The case rate is doubling about every nine months. AIDS is not confined to the U.S., but is also turning up in Western Europe, Africa, Asia, and Australia.

The disease is challenging policymakers as well as scientists. Because of their high rate of vulnerability to AIDS, should homosexuals be identified as such to employers and others? Should children with AIDS be allowed to attend school? If so, should their classmates be notified?

Science, which has conquered many other diseases, may eventually triumph over AIDS, too. Meantime, information and education are essential parts of the defense. As Americans look back on Rock Hudson's career, let them remember with compassion that he helped raise the public's awareness and understanding of a deadly disease.

THE 🏔 SUN

Baltimore, MD, July 31, 1985

There isn't much chance that actor Rock Hudson, who acknowledges he has AIDS, was any better off being treated for the condition in Paris than he would have been at home. One report said Parisian médicos gave him a French drug, HPA-23, which has a slight chance of being effective against AIDS but which has severe side effects. U.S doctors have tried similar drugs, including one called suramin, which is safer because its side effects at various doses are better known. But neither suramin nor dozens of other drugs U.S. and foreign doctors have tested against AIDS have been particularly effective.

Critics say the search for chemicals to treat AIDS is spotty and uncoordinated in both countries. Even though French researchers were the first to discover the virus that causes AIDS, "What we get from France now is the crummiest kind of anecdotal stories," said a Harvard researcher. Other scientists charge that U.S. research is uncoordinated, too. What is needed, says Dr. Martin S. Hirsch of Massachusetts General Hospital, is a "crash program" of carefully controlled tests of several drugs at several medical centers. "It is highly unlikely that the current patchwork of preliminary trials in different institutions will provide definitive answers," Dr. Hirsch said.

There is good reason for a sense of urgency. Besides AIDS victims, there are symptom-free AIDS carriers. Both probably can pass on the disease as long as they live. Not just male homosexuals, Haitians, drug abusers and people who receive AIDS-contaminated blood get AIDS, as was once thought. Some promiscuous *heterosexuals* have gotten AIDS. Mothers can pass the disease to their babies. Scientists fear tens of millions of people may get AIDS in coming years. Even with well-coordinated, amply-financed efforts, it may take years to find effective treatments or preventives.

Rock Hudson returned to Los Angeles after being carried aboard a plane in Paris on a stretcher. We hope the treatment he received in Paris will help. At least his case brings AIDS into the limelight again. Maybe the federal bureaucracy will be moved that much further in the direction of launching the needed crash program.

LOS ANGELES Herald Examiner

Los Angeles, CA
August 7, 1985

Last Monday, actress Elizabeth Taylor visited her hospitalized friend Rock Hudson, who suffers from AIDS. Taylor is the honorary co-chair of an AIDS fundraiser to be held next month. But she is one of many in the L.A. area who give time, energy and money to assist those with AIDS. Notice we say "those with AIDS," not AIDS "victims." For, in dealing with this epidemic, it is as important to avoid hysteria as it is to enforce public-health laws in bathhouses and the like or to step up the research aimed at finding a cure for this mysterious disease. The volunteers we mentioned are playing a crucial role on the anti-hysteria front.

Concerned with the physical, emotional and financial repercussions of AIDS, the volunteers provide a vital social-support system. AIDS Project L.A., for example, helps patients with the difficulties of their day-to-day routines, including getting to and from appointments with doctors. The organization also offers legal services and assists with applications for government benefits. Meanwhile, the Shanti Foundation gives counseling to patients, friends and relatives as well as to survivors of those who die from AIDS. And, finally, there is Aid for AIDS, which raises money to help patients pay their rent and, when necessary, to pay for medication. None of the organizations charges for the services it provides. All rely heavily on volunteers who hold full-time jobs elsewhere and who donate their free time to help.

The entire community, not just patients, owes these volunteers a debt of gratitude.

The San Diego Union

San Diego, CA, July 31, 1985

There are few forces in America more effective than celebrity in focusing national attention on a subject. Rock Hudson's contracting AIDS (acquired immune deficiency syndrome) has given new urgency to this alarming disease.

Spread through sexual contact, contaminated needles, and blood transfusions, the AIDS virus destroys cells that protect the body from disease. Hence, victims usually die from infections, most commonly from pneumonia, and a skin cancer called Kaposi's sarcoma.

In addition to its physical suffering, AIDS carries a social stigma. It has long been viewed as an affliction, somehow deserved, of the homosexual community and its unorthodox lifestyle. Yet, there is an increasing incidence of the AIDS virus in the general population.

Experts predict that as many as 1 million Americans have the virus although they show no signs of the disease as yet. A significant percentage of these persons will develop AIDS and die during the next five years.

So far, the human cost has been significant. The federal Centers for Disease Control (CDC) in Atlanta report 11,871 AIDS cases to date, of which 5,917 have been fatal. AIDS fatalities continuing at this rate will total more than 47,000 by 1987. The AIDS situation in San Diego County is graphically portrayed opposite this page in the commentary by Barbara Peabody.

The medical costs are already enormous. CDC officials estimate the health care bills of the nation's first 9,000 AIDS victims amounted to $1.25 billion and that lost wages and indirect costs amounted to $4.5 billion. These figures are expected to double during the next 12 months as the number of AIDS cases multiply.

AIDS is a relatively new disease to America inasmuch as the virus was not identified in San Francisco until 1976. Medical scientists believe the AIDS virus migrated to the United States through the Caribbean after a disease similar to AIDS was discovered earlier in green monkeys in central Africa. This hypothesis is bolstered by the high incidence of AIDS reported in Zaire and among Haitian refugees in the United States.

As Mr. Hudson discovered in Paris, there is no cure for AIDS. He was treated with an experimental French drug, HPA-23, which stops reproduction of the virus cells. However, the drug also causes liver damage, bleeding disorders, and though halting the disease, does not reverse it.

Researchers have been more successful in killing the AIDS virus in blood-clotting concentrates given hemophiliacs. And, scientists in Boston have produced a protein from the AIDS virus that could serve as a diagnostic test, and later, perhaps as a vaccine.

Recognizing the increasing severity of AIDS, the Reagan administration is seeking a 48 percent increase in funds for AIDS research, with a 1986 fiscal year appropriation of $126.3 million.

A half century ago, a president felled by polio helped stimulate collective national action that helped to bring a cure for that crippling disease. A decade ago, Betty Ford spoke openly about the formerly unmentionable subject of breast cancer. Last month, President Reagan's operation for intestinal cancer brought renewed national attention to that affliction.

Now, Rock Hudson, in acknowledging that he has contracted AIDS, has paradoxically breathed new life into a subject that many Americans have been recoiling from. Already we can perceive a more constructive national consciousness that can mobilize the monetary and medical resources required to combat AIDS effectively.

The Detroit News

Detroit, MI, July 28, 1985

The sight of Rock Hudson wasting away from Aquired Immune Deficiency Syndrome (AIDS) is a sad and moving one. AIDS is aquired through sexual contact or intravenous transfusion of diseased blood; it cripples the body's immune system, leaving it vulnerable to any germ that comes along. There is no cure for the disease; it almost always proves fatal.

Another 12,000 Americans — mostly homosexual men — have been diagnosed as having AIDS so far. Half have already died. For the past several years the number of AIDS victims has doubled every 8 or 9 months.

Though Rock Hudson can easily afford to go to Paris for a cure, it is nonsensical that he had to. The Louis Pasteur Clinic there has done much of the pioneering work in the field. It's been running experiments that seem to indicate that a drug called HPA-23 has some effect inhibiting the potency of the virus in the bloodstream. The evidence is inconclusive, and the Department of Health and Human Services in Washington has repeatedly noted that research on cures is taking a somewhat different path here — drugs other than those at the Louis Pasteur Institute are being tested. None have yet proved effective.

Still, those who are dying and desperate should be able to buy anything that holds out any hope at all, without having to travel to Europe to get it. It is no small irony that transactions likely to net the buyer AIDS — among other things — are for sale on the streets of every city in this country, while possible cures are not. There is no need to repeat the Laetrile debacle. It is possible for the Food and Drug Administration, along with the market — which purveys information with remarkable accuracy — to ensure that dangerous chemicals stay out of the market, while people are allowed to buy whatever placebos they desire.

This incident is likely to spark a renewed round of blaming the federal government for not doing all it could, along with demands for more money. In fact, government scientists, working at the Centers for Disease Control, played a crucial role in the original diagnosis. They have been joined by private hospitals and universities in continued research.

The best research indicates that the AIDS virus is transmitted in bodily secretions — mostly through semen or blood. While some people contract the disease through few contacts, the majority of those with it have had vast numbers of sexual contacts, a trend not uncommon in the gay community. Close study by the National Institute of Health traced the migration of AIDS in the United States to the heterosexual population via bisexual men and prostitutes.

The homosexual lobby is afraid that other Americans are losing patience, and eventually tolerance, as AIDS spreads and becomes a threat to people who don't play Russian Roulette with their sexual practices.

We are afraid that is true. The difference between AIDS and most other fatal diseases is that AIDS is contracted through voluntary, high-risk activity. There is a difference between saying that AIDS is some sort of supernatural punishment — which we do not think — and pointing out that it is the direct result of willful, conscious actions on the part of those who contract it.

It is hard to resist the pathos of men, who once proclaimed their sexuality with glee and now are wasting away in hospitals. Sincere compassion is the proper response to suffering individuals. But it is not an adequate response for society to make.

The most significant real progress — other than to find a cure — can be achieved through changing sexual behavior and attaching enough of a stigma to the promiscuous behavior that leads to AIDS to steer some potential victims clear of it. The best way to reduce the risk of contracting AIDS is: No more sleeping with bisexuals, prostitutes, or gays. People who practice monogamy will not die of AIDS.

Roanoke Times & World-News

Roanoke, VA, July 27, 1985

CONTEMPORARY America has created a cult of celebrity. In a curious way, a person who becomes a celebrity can confer that quality upon other individuals and ideas, even illnesses. Celebrity by association may be the other side of guilt by association. Some people are saying that the revelations about Rock Hudson's health may give the disease AIDS celebrity status.

Doubtless, they are right, at least to a degree. But other, more important changes may result from his condition, too. To begin with, perhaps the sensationalism that has surrounded the disease, because of its initial connection with homosexuality and drug abuse, will abate. Rock Hudson's sexual preference has nothing to do with the larger issue. To speculate or focus on it misses the real point. The AIDS virus has killed more than 5,000 people in this country. Almost 12,000 are reported as having the disease now and the Centers for Disease Control estimate that the number of cases of AIDS in America will double next year.

Though the research is not complete yet, there is every indication that the disease is not transmitted easily. It takes more than a handshake or casual contact to spread AIDS. It requires intimate contact, either sexually intimate or medically intimate through fluid transfusions. Tests have been devised to test donated blood for the AIDS virus, but that will only slow the spread of the disease; it won't stop it. So far, even though there have been few victims, in statistical terms, no one has recovered from the disease and no effective treatment has been found. Every day that passes without a cure puts more people at risk. This is a small, but growing epidemic.

It is not limited to any one group. Even children have been infected through blood transfusions. In Australia, four women were infected through artificial insemination. To attach any social stigma to the disease now is terribly cruel. It is a viral infection, not divine retribution or punishment.

That kind of emotionalism, combined with hysterical fear and misinformation, is counterproductive. If Rock Hudson does give the disease celebrity status, perhaps it will be perceived more rationally. Public health officials claim that everything possible is being done by medical research to find a cure. Other groups say more money is needed. Whichever is true, it's time to examine the problems connected with AIDS without embarrassment or prejudice. Health and Human Services Secretary Margaret Heckler is right when she refers to AIDS as "perhaps the most mysterious disease of our time." Let's solve the mystery and ignore the speculation.

The State

Columbia, SC, August 2, 1985

IT IS HARD to believe that the gaunt, aging face in the news pictures on television and in the newspapers is the handsome, strapping movie-television star, Rock Hudson.

As shocking as his appearance was the disclosure of his affliction — acquired immune deficiency syndrome (AIDS), for which there is no known cure. Its victims are homosexuals, abusers of injectable drugs and hemophiliacs, the disease being spread by sexual contact, contaminated needles and blood transfusions.

The 59-year-old actor is the most prominent public figure to admit he suffers from AIDS, and his efforts to find treatment in Paris have focused widespread attention on the disease. Treatment with various drugs is still experimental, and none so far has rid the body of the virus, although some patients are in remission.

The French are further along in their research than we are in this country, and desperate Americans — more than 100 so far — are arriving in Paris in increasing numbers for treatment. Later this year, some of the same drugs will be used experimentally in the United States.

It is not enough to scoff at the lifestyle of the 11,871 Americans who have been stricken with AIDS — many of them are innocent victims because of blood transfusions which have nothing to do with drug abuse or sexual proclivities.

Nevertheless, it is a dreadful disease, as Rock Hudson's pictures dramatically show, and we hope for a medical breakthrough very soon.

The Miami Herald
Miami, FL, July 29, 1985

ROCK HUDSON is a kind, generous, and talented man who is ill with a vicious, usually fatal disease. He is not playing the role of an AIDS victim; he *is* an AIDS victim. He deserves the compassion that his condition warrants.

The ghoulish quality of the varied public reactions to Mr. Hudson's diagnosis reflects the fear that AIDS — acquired immune deficiency syndrome — generates. It also reflects deep emotional conflicts over sexuality. AIDS victims in the United States have been predominantly, though not exclusively, male homosexuals.

Some heterosexuals seek confirmation of this celebrated patient's rumored homosexuality; perhaps they hope that it would prove their own invulnerability to AIDS. In fact, AIDS strikes children, men, and women alike. Some gay activists demand from the star an intimate sickbed confession; they think that it would enhance their own status.

It is not necessary to know exactly how Mr. Hudson contracted AIDS to know that he is seriously ill. Blood transfusions certainly can spread it, and Mr. Hudson received blood during heart-bypass surgery in 1981. Sexual intercourse, whether heterosexual or homosexual, also can spread AIDS. Some researchers believe that in the Third World it spreads through communal bathing in ponds and through blood-to-blood contact within families. Those communities, however, rarely offer sophisticated medical diagnosis or treatment. The stricken simply die of some secondary infection.

Though there is considerable dispute about the origin of AIDS, there is no doubt about its seriousness. Active cases typically are fatal. More than 11,000 such cases have been reported so far in the United States. The Pasteur Institute in Paris, where Mr. Hudson is being treated, has pioneered research on AIDS but offers no cure. The disease's initial appearance in this country among male homosexuals fostered a lag in public commitment to fund AIDS research.

Perhaps Rock Hudson's suffering will help break that American reluctance to recognize this major threat to public health. As a film giant and a friend of President Reagan, Mr. Hudson commands attention in a way that no previous AIDS victim can. That attention should not seek to invade the privacy that Mr. Hudson judiciously maintained throughout his career. Rather, it should be channeled toward combatting the awful disease that has wasted him to a caricature of the robustness that once was his hallmark.

Pittsburgh Post-Gazette
Pittsburgh, PA, October 4, 1985

It was perhaps more than a coincidence: The movie star Rock Hudson died of Acquired Immune Deficiency Syndrome on the same day that the U.S. House of Representatives approved $189.7 million to study and counter the dread disease — an increase of $90 million over fiscal 1985.

Rock Hudson personified the tragedy of AIDS as no other person has done. Because of his fame, he gave suffering a human face, making the disease real to vast numbers of people untouched by and perhaps indifferent to it. Although he never publicly admitted that he was a homosexual, the group most at risk in the current epidemic, he had to weather the inevitable gossip and speculation.

This he managed to do with a dignity that surely increased public sympathy. His last statement was a model of quiet courage: "I am not happy that I am sick. I am not happy that I have AIDS, but if that is helping others, I can, at least, know that my own misfortune has had some positive worth."

There is a heartening postscript to Rock Hudson's death, one that goes beyond the new resolve by Congress to do more in the fight against AIDS. It came in a characteristically graceful message from President Reagan:

"Nancy and I are saddened by the news of Rock Hudson's death. He will always be remembered for his dynamic impact on the film industry, and fans all over the world will certainly mourn his loss. He will be remembered for his humanity, his sympathetic spirit and well-deserved reputation for kindness. May God rest his soul."

This tribute is all the more admirable when it is remembered that some of Mr. Reagan's closest supporters are of a mind that sees homosexuality as an abomination. To his credit, Mr. Reagan's own humanity on this occasion was not stinted by any ideology or prejudice.

The Dispatch
Columbus, OH, October 4, 1985

Now, at least, we won't have to look at the drawn face, the sunken eyes, or the haunting stare. For a while we needn't think about how he died, but how he lived.

We can remember Rock Hudson the way he was in his glory days of Hollywood stardom, when men were men and the difference between right and wrong was as clear as the nose on your face and the world made a heck of a lot more sense than it does today.

We can remember how he made us laugh and cry, dream and swoon. We can remember his stunning good looks and his powerful presence.

What we saw in the last few weeks wasn't really Rock Hudson. That was an imposter. The real Rock Hudson was 6-foot-4, big, strong, virile, the star of 62 films and many television shows. The kind of guy you'd be glad to invite into your home and be honored if he accepted the invitation.

It's tough to realize how fragile our heroes really are. It's hard to accept that Hudson is dead at all, let alone that he died of AIDS, a disease common to homosexuals and intravenous drug users. He never admitted to being a homosexual, and we may never know if he had a drug habit. We are left to wonder . . .

. . . left to wonder about Hudson, his transformation, and this world we live in. Left to wonder why we idolize — and why we are stunned when our heroes turn out to be human. Left to wonder about things like AIDS. Most of all, though, we are left to wonder about ourselves.

We'll miss Rock Hudson, but we'll miss the simple world he starred in even more.

ST. LOUIS POST-DISPATCH
St. Louis, MO, October 4, 1985

Had Rock Hudson died six months ago, he would have been chiefly remembered as another handsome box-office attraction who successfully made the transition from ruggedly masculine, heroic roles to leading man parts in frothy drawing-room farces and then, finally, to stardom again in television. For years, he was Hollywood's top male star and, through the '60s, he was the town's third ranked money-maker, behind Cary Grant and Elizabeth Taylor.

But last July, the world saw another side of Rock Hudson, for he revealed then that he was suffering from AIDS — the acquired immunity deficiency syndrome that is invariably fatal. When Mr. Hudson chose to make his illness public, he was in Paris for treatment, and to the millions of moviegoers and television viewers who knew him as the prototypical all-American hero figure, the transformation was shocking. Frail, gaunt, ravaged — so Rock Hudson appeared as those who spoke for him acknowledged that he was dying of AIDS.

To have revealed the nature of his illness required no small piece of courage on Mr. Hudson's part. Because AIDS has a strong — but not exclusive — correlation with male homosexuality, a considerable social stigma has been attached to the disease. That stigma, in turn, has both retarded research into this newly discovered and mysterious ailment and perpetuated the veil of ignorance that has been spread over it. Like no act before it, Mr. Hudson's brave admission focused public attention on the facts of AIDS — an essential precondition for any informed response to the disease.

Mr. Hudson's last weeks gave dignity and meaning not only to his life but to those of thousands of others similarly afflicted. That role will outlast all his others.

The Morning News

Wilmington, DE, July 29, 1985

ROCK HUDSON has AIDS, the acquired immune deficiency syndrome. That's sad, you say, but why talk more about him than about the more than 10,000 Americans afflicted with AIDS since 1981, half of whom have died?

Mr. Hudson's case is significant because he is well-known for his roles in film and television. He is a hero to thousands of fans. His being stricken by AIDS puts this always fatal disease into the limelight.

Though AIDS has been written about extensively in the last couple of years, no public idol has previously been identified with the disease. For most Americans, AIDS victims have been nameless, faceless.

Rock Hudson's willingness to have his disease acknowledged publicly changes all that, just as Betty Ford's mastectomy brought breast cancer out of the closet in the 1970s and President Reagan's surgery has done for colon cancer. These folks did not get ill for publicity's sake, but once their diseases were diagnosed, their misfortunes were turned to public benefit.

Mrs. Ford, as far as is known, has had no recurrence of cancer — a good lesson for early diagnosis and prompt treatment. Similar good luck, it is hoped, is in store for the president.

Early diagnosis of AIDS does not halt the fatal course of the disease. So the publicity surrounding Mr. Hudson's illness does not help in that respect. But knowledge of his affliction and recent photographs showing his gauntness should encourage many to use caution in sexual relationships, insist on proper testing of blood supplies, and avoid contamination by drug paraphernalia. The Delaware Division of Public Health, in conjunction with Delaware Lesbian and Gay Health Advocates, has issued a fact sheet on AIDS — its symptoms and advice on how to avoid contracting the disease.

AIDS threatens to assume epidemic proportions — the case rate in the United States is doubling every nine months — unless preventive measures are taken. With no cure in sight (the French treatment Rock Hudson was seeking holds promise of alleviation but not cure), prevention is of prime importance.

At the same time, the scientific search for effective treatment as well as vaccines against AIDS must be sought. The Department of Health and Human Services has ordered significant increases in funding for AIDS research. That may not help Rock Hudson but it could save the lives of many others.

The Birmingham News

Birmingham, AL, October 5, 1985

Rock Hudson died at age 59 from the pernicious disease called AIDS. He leaves behind a mixed bag of achievements — some boring movies, some unimportant but highly entertaining ones and a few of lasting value.

But for one fact, the chances are he would be ranked with scores of film actors who had their moments on stage and then quietly faded from view: He is the first notable victim of AIDS to provide the devastating disease with a human dimension.

Undoubtedly his suffering, attempts to find a cure and his death from AIDS have brought home to Americans the pernicious character of the disease as well as the personal dimension: Money, fame and access to the best treatment are no defense.

If the notoriety of Hudson's last months speeds us toward a cure and a better understanding of the personal costs of the disease, his suffering will not have been without value.

The Seattle Times

Seattle, WA, October 3, 1985

WHEN actor Rock Hudson first publicly acknowledged that he was a victim of acquired immune deficiency syndrome, tens of millions of people around the world abruptly became aware of the fact that the killer AIDS can strike anyone . . . even the rich and famous.

Even though news reporters had the information at the time, Hudson could have "stonewalled" the fact that he had the disease and that it was apparently related to homosexual activity.

Instead, Hudson went public. He appealed for understanding of the disease. He focused attention on the need for funding a major research effort to find a cure. No doubt he helped stimulate a big increase in federal funding for AIDS research.

Hudson inspired a Hollywood gala in his honor that raised more than $1 million and set in motion a private foundation that no doubt will raise millions more for research. A few days ago he personally contributed $250,000 to that cause.

In his recent message to Hollywood friends, Hudson, his body ravaged by disease, said: "I can at least know that my own misfortune has had some positive worth." When he died yesterday at 59, Hudson had that assurance. During his final weeks, Rock Hudson's performance was an award-winner.

Portland Press Herald

Portland, ME, July 27, 1985

Actor Rock Hudson personifies the struggle endured by thousands of Americans who are among the growing number of victims of Acquired Immune Deficiency Syndrome.

Perhaps AIDS needed a well-known face to raise it into full public consciousness. The American public has been curiously unmoved by the numbers: As of this week, AIDS had struck 11,871 Americans and killed half of them. Overall, the number of persons who contract AIDS, an ailment new to this part of the world, is expected to double in 1986.

As a rapidly growing ailment carried across a broad spectrum of homosexual, bisexual and heterosexual persons, AIDS merits not only the highest priority from the U.S. Public Health Service but the money to match it. The spreading scope of the disease belies a public health spokeswoman's suggestion that, even with a new request for funds, "we're doing everything we can."

From the beginning, AIDS has suffered from a kind of public disinterest, related perhaps to its initial occurence among homosexual men with numerous sexual contacts. That disinterest has been costly.

AIDS is a vicious, deadly illness; its victims now include men, women and children. While no one can mandate the discovery of drugs to cure or control it, the American government can intensify research by increasing the money to fund it.

Maine has a dozen reasons to support it. Twelve AIDS cases have now been identified in this state; half diagnosed here and the other half out of state. Of the 12 AIDS victims, five have died.

That's a death rate neither Maine nor the United States should be willing to live with.

AIDS Spreads Through Drug-Addicted Population and Minorities

New York City Mayor Edward I. Koch October 3, 1985 rejected a recommendation by city health officials that hypodermic needles be sold without a prescription. The officials had hoped that making clean needles easily available would check the spread of AIDS among drug users. According to an April 16, 1985 news account, one study found that some 60% of New York City's intravenous drug users had been exposed to the AIDS virus.

According to evidence presented June 3, 1987 at the Third International Conference on AIDS by Dr. Don C. Des Jarlais of the New York State Division of Substance Abuse Services, the spread of the AIDS virus was continuing unabated among intravenous drug users in the U.S. Des Jarlais said that an estimated 750,000 Americans were at direct risk of AIDS infection through exposure to the virus in intravenous drug use. He estimated that about 200,000 drug users, mainly in New York City and New Jersey, were already infected. Des Jarlais said the number of AIDS-related deaths recorded for intravenous drug users would be twice as high if official statistics included those who developed tuberculosis and other diseases not included in the U.S. government's current definition of AIDS.

Blacks accounted for 25% and Hispanics for 15% of U.S. AIDS cases, the federal Centers for Disease Control reported October 23, 1986. Just 12% of the general population was black and 6% Hispanic. The CDC report said intravenous drug use could explain much of the higher risk of infection the minority groups suffered. About 70% of the U.S. women who had contracted AIDS were black or Hispanic. Of U.S. AIDS victims under 15, 58% were black and 22% Hispanic.

The Register

Santa Ana, CA, April 8, 1986

Dr. James Curran, head of the AIDS branch of the federal Centers for Disease Control in Atlanta, has warned that cases of AIDS linked to intravenous drug use, once concentrated in New York and northern New Jersey, are rapidly spreading throughout the nation. Cases among such users have now been reported in 44 states.

This news highlights the importance of a simple reform we first suggested last fall. Why shouldn't present restrictions on the purchase of intravenous needles be lifted?

Intravenous needles are not expensive, but they are difficult to obtain legally. Pharmacies will sell them only with a prescription or under certain other conditions under which they are satisfied that the prospective buyer is a diabetic or otherwise legally authorized to purchase needles. Each sale is carefully recorded.

The result, of course, has not been to eliminate the use of restricted drugs that are commonly injected intravenously, but to make it more likely that drug users will share needles. Thus the dangers already inherent in using such drugs are expanded by the possibility that they will be injected with contaminated needles.

Restrictions on the purchase of IV needles were not intended to increase the spread of infectious diseases like hepatitis or AIDS, but that has been one byproduct of restrictions. With new evidence linking AIDS cases to intravenous drug use, it is becoming apparent that the price of restrictions is too high.

It would be preferable, of course, if people simply stopped using illicit drugs that require needles. No realist believes that is likely to happen, however. The least we can do, then, considering the apparently epidemic character of AIDS, is to make it possible for people to acquire sterile needles legally.

The Record

Hackensack, NJ, August 7, 1986

John H. Rutledge, New Jersey's deputy commissioner of health, is proposing to combat the spread of AIDS by providing addicts with clean, uninfected needles. It's a sound idea; the only thing wrong with it is that it doesn't go far enough.

Dr. Rutledge calls his pioneering idea a "needle-exchange program" and says its purpose is to undercut the "shooting galleries" where dirty needles are passed from user to user and the danger of infection by the AIDS virus is high. Under his plan, a user could walk into a drug treatment center and hand over a used hypodermic needle in exchange for a sterile one. He would also receive drug counseling, along with a stiff lecture stressing the overriding importance of never sharing his needle with anyone. Then, when the new needle goes dull, he could bring it back and turn it in for another.

The proposal is controversial, but its advantages are obvious. Roughly half the intravenous drug users in this state have been exposed to the AIDS virus. If two drug users share a needle, the chances are 50-50 that the needle will be contaminated. If three people share it, the chances are 75 percent. If a dozen people use it, the odds approach 100 percent.

Some people abhor drugs so thoroughly that they are only too glad to see users pay the ulti-mate penalty for their weakness. But the spread of AIDS poses a threat not just to addicts but to society at large. Of the 1,400 people suffering from AIDS in New Jersey, more than 100 contracted it from sexual encounters with drug users — or they are children who had the terrible misfortune to have been conceived by an addict or ex-addict. Surely these people shouldn't be punished for the sins of the users.

The limitation in Dr. Rutledge's program is that it would benefit only those users who have needles of their own — and are willing to come to a treatment center for help. An illegal hypodermic can be expensive, which is why so many users go to shooting galleries where they can be rented for a few dollars. A needle-exchange program would do nothing to protect these people (and their sexual partners and children).

The answer is to allow over-the-counter sale of needles. Opponents of this idea worry that it would encourage the epidemic of drugs. Yet 39 states allow the sale of hypodermics without prescription, and in none of them is drug use markedly greater than in New Jersey and the other 10 states that ban them. In any event, remember what we are fighting here. Intravenous drugs are dangerous, but they pale in comparison with the HTLV-3 virus that carries AIDS.

WORCESTER TELEGRAM

Worcester, MA, January 25, 1986

Should the government supply drug addicts with their needles? The idea, as outrageous as it sounds, has reportedly been discussed by a state Task Force on AIDS. It ought to be discarded.

The concern is well placed — dirty needles can help spread the deadly AIDS virus. Nationally, about 17 percent of AIDS victims are intravenous drug users.

Most addicts would rather risk infection than look for a sterile needle with which to shoot up. Chemical dependency overrides any fears about infection and even the chance of death.

Just the same, the government will appear to legitimize drug use if it starts passing out needles to addicts. As a practical matter, such a program might not work; addicts won't want to make contact with authorities even if they are promised confidentiality.

The inoculation program against hepatitis-B in Worcester shows how difficult it is to get the addicts to cooperate in something for their own good.

Society needs more effective ways of curbing the drug menace and the diseases it spreads. Giving out needles isn't one of them.

Newsday

Long Island, NY, August 5, 1986

The idea of letting drug addicts legally swap dirty needles for clean ones is unsettling in the extreme. Yet just such an unorthodox program may be needed if New York State hopes to halt — or even slow — the spread of AIDS among intravenous drug users, their spouses and their children.

Heroin users who share hypodermic needles constitute the major conduit through which AIDS — acquired immune deficiency syndrome — is transmitted to the heterosexual population. And the incidence of AIDS is increasing at a frightening pace: By 1991, medical authorities predict, 40,000 people will have contracted the lethal disease in New York City alone, and 30,000 will have died.

A needle exchange program should prevent some of those deaths. When the city's former health commissioner, David Sencer, proposed giving addicts clean needles a year ago, he said he thought it might slow the outbreak of AIDS among drug users.

Helping addicts kick their habit would be far better, of course. But that approach won't work in the short term; New York's treatment centers are already overflowing.

New Jersey health officials are planning a carefully monitored, experimental needle exchange plan as soon as they receive legislative approval. And the federal Centers for Disease Control in Atlanta have endorsed such needle swaps in principle — although New York's Mayor Edward Koch and his current health commissioner, Stephen Joseph, are reluctant to institute such a program in the city.

Needle exchange programs for confirmed drug addicts already exist in Amsterdam and in Australia. An experimental plan in New York should exclude casual drug users, be carefully supervised by health professionals and be abandoned promptly if it failed to draw a significant number of addicts. Even if the program failed to reduce the incidence of AIDS, it would at least have exposed some hardened addicts to counseling, treatment and perhaps testing for the disease.

The existing legal prohibition against the sale of hypodermic needles without a prescription might have to be modified to permit a needle-swapping program.

Understandably, many people feel squeamish about establishing a legal source of the paraphernalia drug users need to feed their addiction. But an experimental exchange program doesn't signal approval of drug use. Instead, it's a realistic attempt to deal with the growing menace of AIDS. It may be the only way to prevent confirmed addicts and their families from contracting the disease and thereby widening its range of contagion.

THE ATLANTA CONSTITUTION

Atlanta, GA, June 6, 1986

AIDS is deadly enough to demand a swift retreat from useless public policy. For years, a fashion in the battle against narcotics has been to restrict the sale of needles. For a time, those restrictions made sense. But now that researchers know AIDS strikes through dirty needles, such restrictions are not just passe — they are dangerous.

Several leading AIDS researchers have asked public officials to let go of their reluctance to approve lenient sales of syringes and needles *and* to go a big step further: Doctors have asked that public agencies distribute syringes and needles to junkies. It seems a drastic step, but AIDS is a grave challenge. Since scientists concede that a cure, if there is one, is years away, policy must concentrate on prevention.

Studies show that those who take illegal drugs intravenously get AIDS in frightening numbers. Because junkies have a hard time getting clean needles, they pass used needles on. And they steal dirty ones. The AIDS virus is spread through such blood-borne contamination. Many junkies are also prostitutes, so the virus is passed on to johns, broadening the circle of carriers.

Georgia's AIDS task force never seriously considered the idea of passing out syringes and needles, according to the task force's chairman, Dr. Doug Skelton, who opposes the idea. (Though some states do, Georgia does not ban the sale of syringes and needles without prescription. Many pharmacists, however, do ask for diabetic cards before selling them.) Skelton said his experience with drug-abuse programs indicates that easy access to needles would increase use of narcotics such as heroin.

Skelton may be right. It's possible handing out needles could encourage a few to try shooting up; that would be a tragedy. But most drug addicts survive and many are cured. Not so AIDS victims. The higher priority must be to stop the spread of AIDS.

Chicago Tribune

Chicago, IL, November 12, 1986

If the nation is supposed to be going all out in a war against drug abuse, why is New York City's health department planning to give free disposable needles and syringes to heroin addicts?

The excuse, of course, is AIDS. Intravenous drug users are the second largest group at risk for acquired immune deficiency syndrome because they often share contaminated needles. So some health officials have talked themselves into the idea that giving addicts supplies of disposable needles can reduce the spread of the fatal disease.

The plan, to begin in the next few months, calls for providing the free needles to several hundred heroin addicts waiting for admission to New York City's methadone treatment program. If there is no evidence after several months that the program reduces the spread of AIDS, it is to be discontinued.

But AIDS isn't the only devastating health problem about which the nation must be concerned. The necessary and urgent battle against AIDS must not be fought with tactics and at costs that weaken the fights against other terrible diseases and dangers.

However good their intentions, health officials are wrong to take actions that give government support to heroin addicts. Instead of reducing AIDS, there is risk the plan may increase intravenous drug use by making it easier and by eliminating the fear of AIDS from sharing needles. This ill-advised program should be discontinued before it starts.

Fear of AIDS Puts Condom Ads on TV

San Francisco television station KRON said January 16, 1987 that it agreed to accept commercials for condoms, making it the first major-market station to lift the long-held ban on advertising such prophylactics on U.S. broadcast television. The station's decision to air such ads came at a time when nationwide concern about the spread of AIDS was growing rapidly. Sexual transmission of the fatal disorder had been shown to be curbed by condom use. Great Britain and other Western European nations had already begun airing condom campaigns in an attempt to halt the spread of AIDS. Condom advertising had also already been carried by some cable systems. A spokesman for KRON-TV, an NBC affiliate, said the station had reached an agreement with Carter-Wallace, Inc. to run ads for that company's Trojan line of condoms, the most popular U.S. brand. The station would contribute revenues from the ads to AIDS research and would require that condom advertisers make an equal contribution. It would accept the ads on a six-month trial basis and would not air them "in or around programming targeted to children."

Two affiliated television stations, WXYZ in Detroit and WRTV in Indianapolis, had agreed to broadcast advertisements for Ansell-America's LifeStyles condoms, it was reported Jan. 26. The ads for Ansell-America—whose parent company was Australia's Pacific Dunlop Ltd.—would be somewhat more explicit than the Trojan spots, in which AIDS would not be mentioned directly. But, in common with the ads for Trojans, condoms would not be promoted as birth-control devices. While indicating that they had no problem with the affiliate stations carrying condom advertising, the three major U.S. television networks, CBS, NBC and ABC, continued to resist doing so themselves. They claimed that they could best serve the public interest by continuing to provide information about AIDS through news and special affairs broadcasting. Critics of the ads charged that such commercials only encouraged promiscuity in an age when casual sex is regularly portrayed by network television.

THE TENNESSEAN

Nashville, TN, February 15, 1987

AN old, but once seldom spoken, word is now the topic of discussions from Capitol Hill to church congregations. The word is condom.

In case anyone has missed it, the renewed interest in condoms is not so much because of their use as birth control devices but because they can help prevent the spread of the deadly acquired immune deficiency syndrome — or AIDS. Specifically, the current condom discussions — or more accurately, heated debates — focus on whether or not condoms should be advertised on television.

U.S. Surgeon General Everett Koop thinks they should be. He told the House Health and Environment Subcommittee last week that the threat of AIDS is so great that it "overwhelms other considerations" and that advertisements for condoms would have a "positive health value."

Mr. Koop also quite accurately pointed out that since "television networks do indeed peddle all the attractive parts of sex then they should be willing to also peddle something that might prevent the transmission of sexually acquired disease."

Unfortunately, most television network officials disagree with Mr. Koop. Local network affiliates are free to broadcast the advertisements if they wish, and Nashville's WNGE-Channel 2 is commended for its decision to run them. But representatives of all three commercial television networks told the subcommittee that their networks would not use condom ads because the ads would offend their viewers.

Now what is more offensive — a 30-second television commercial, or a fatal virus with no known cure?

Anyone who believes that the answer to AIDS is abstinence is living in Pollyanna-land. Condoms won't cure AIDS, and they aren't 100% effective in preventing its spread. But they are currently the best protection against this world's worst killer.

Condoms can prevent conception — they can also prevent death. And that message needs to get to everyone it can every way it can. ■

THE PLAIN DEALER

Cleveland, OH, February 6, 1987

Condom. There, we said it. And so have a lot of other people lately. Since it first became the subject of public debate last fall, more than 70 television stations have indicated their willingness to broadcast commercials for contraceptives. Condoms and other forms of birth control recently have begun making cameo appearances in the scripts of prime-time television series as well: in "Cagney and Lacey," "St. Elsewhere," "Kate and Allie" and, this Sunday, on "Valerie." That's a welcome trend. Unfortunately, the trend's characteristics sometimes are unwelcomely trendy.

There are many solid reasons why television stations and networks should lift the ban against such commercials. To begin with, the ban is slightly hypocritical. Ads touting contraceptives are no more offensive than ones selling feminine hygiene products, tampons or remedies for such diverse afflictions as hemorrhoids, gas, diarrhea or constipation. Further, ads for birth-control products offer an important social benefit. By whittling at the stigmas and taboos associated with contraception, they can encourage sexual responsibility. No study has yet been able to associate heightened contraceptive awareness with increased promiscuity. To the contrary, the use of contraceptives encourages people to think about what they are doing in advance. The result doubtless will be fewer unwanted pregnancies and a diminished threat of spreading venereal diseases. Tangentially, ads for condoms also might encourage a better understanding of the role both partners should play in the practice of birth control.

Unfortunately, some of the new commercials sell fear instead of maturity. "I'll do a lot for love," says a woman in one commercial. "But I'm not ready to die for it." Such a message only fuels AIDS hysteria. To be sure, AIDS is a legitimate concern. But to inflate that concern with grim ads of doom for the sake of increased sales is opportunistic. Panic is good for business, or so one condom manufacturer seems to believe. Yet, panic is not good for a nation trying to come to grips with the very real social, moral and medical crises surrounding AIDS, promiscuity and teen sexuality.

Like it or not, AIDS has played an important part in the new acceptability of ads touting birth-control measures. Many station managers say as much. Yet, making that admission doesn't justify commercials that exaggerate popular anxieties. The nation should applaud anything that promises to elevate popular awareness of the need for sexual responsibility. It cannot applaud egregious commercials that are, themselves, irresponsible.

THE BLADE
Toledo, OH, February 15, 1987

AMERICA'S three major commercial television networks are engaged in hypocrisy of the most odious sort by refusing to accept advertisements for condoms.

As U.S. Surgeon General C. Everett Koop said in testimony before Congress, condoms offer the third best form of protection against acquired immune deficiency syndrome, or AIDS, an incurable and uniformly fatal disease that is transmitted mainly by sexual contact.

The two best forms of protection against AIDS are abstinence and sexual activity within a monogamous relationship, Dr. Koop said. But he quickly added that since both of these options seem to be unacceptable for large numbers of people, condoms have assumed a position of central importance in preventing further spread of this modern plague.

Yet representatives of Capital Cities/ABC, NBC, and the CBS Broadcast Group insist that the networks will continue to ban condom commercials even though they are running extensive news coverage of the development. Amazingly, the networks contend that such advertisements might promote sexual permissiveness or cause moral or religious offense to viewers. And, of course, heaven forbid that the networks have anything to do with nasty stuff of that sort.

Those claims are so patently outrageous that the networks are making a national laughingstock of themselves. No single institution in American life has done more to promote sexual permissiveness or more routinely offend those with strong religious feelings about sex than network television.

Daytime soap operas glamorize indiscriminate sex with multiple partners and portray innumerable sexual acts in explicit scenes. Talk shows deal in the most casual fashion with various kinds of orgasms, variations in homosexual and heterosexual behavior, menstrual problems, the penis, clitoris, and other parts of human sexual anatomy.

Situation comedies and dramas are literally crammed with sexual messages. Of course, nobody could take the least offense at those commercials about menstrual products and douches and minipads that supposedly will make every woman more sexually attractive.

America is in the midst of an epidemic of a deadly disease spread by the kinds of behavior portrayed on TV — so frequently, so casually, without regard to the health consequences. The networks should abandon their hypocritical, self-righteous protests and accept advertisements that could be lifesaving for people who adopt the TV ideal and have sex outside of marriage with multiple partners.

Many newspapers and other popular publications already have moved in this direction. The Blade counts itself among those which recognize the importance and have adopted a policy of accepting advertisements presented in responsible format and in good taste.

WORCESTER TELEGRAM
Wocester, MA, February 4, 1987

A few harsh facts of life:

AIDS is a sexually transmitted disease and, at this time, a terminal illness. People who get it face certain death. The disease is spreading — and not just among homosexuals. Intravenous drug users can infect others; mothers may even pass it on to their unborn babies. Medical science has yet to find a pharmacological antidote to the growing menace.

One sure way to avoid the disease is to avoid casual sex. Reliable and caring home and school education about sex and responsibility could do more in the long run to control the disease than any artificial device. For sexually active individuals, however, use of condoms is widely recommended.

It is understandable why there should be so such vehement opposition to television commercials advocating their use. Those opposed to birth control point out that besides preventing disease, they also can prevent pregnancies. These people are concerned about the messages being sent to impressionable youngsters.

But given the awesome threat AIDS poses to society, it is hard to dismiss out of hand commercials for a product to prevent sexually transmitted terminal diseases, as long as they are tasteful and avoid exploitation. Such products, after all, are displayed openly at most drug stores.

If condoms can curtail the spread of a deadly disease, calling attention to their existence is a legitimate function. Those whose moral sensitivities are offended need to consider the lives that may be saved.

The Boston Globe
Boston, MA, February 13, 1987

The surgeon general of the United States, Dr. C. Everett Koop, the newly found AIDS voice of the Reagan administration, is calling for broad preventive measures to try to limit the spread of this modern plague. It is a welcome stance, even though he privately confides that the Cabinet isn't buying it. Koop's forthright guidelines on AIDS bring into even sharper contrast the stark silence on the subject from the White House.

Last October, Koop's report on AIDS urged a bold program of public education to combat the spread of AIDS, including public school instruction that would involve sex-education material.

Since then, he has chosen to defend his report in such unlikely places as the Libertyville University campus of fundamentalist preacher Jerry Falwell and a national convention of religious broadcasters.

As soon as Koop's report became public, he was assailed by conservative columnists and preachers because, "as a health official," he had concluded that America's schools must teach children about AIDS and, indirectly therefore, about sex.

Some see courage in Koop's confrontation with the big guns of fundamentalism on a national AIDS policy. But there is also an aspect of political pandering. Never before has a surgeon general of the United States been expected to placate religious groups to gain acceptance of urgent public health strategies.

Koop now has taken another bold step. He has put the authority of his office on the line, urging television networks to carry commercials saying that condoms provide protection against AIDS. This, too, is a useful maneuver – as far as it goes.

The problem is that the threat posed by AIDS, an impending catastrophe in the view of the National Academy of Sciences, is already so large that Koop's recommendations, six years into the outbreak, seem paltry.

Koop seeks no federal funds for the school or public-education programs that he says are essential. He softened his original call for straightforward teaching about the sexual transmission of AIDS, after a degrading encounter with Education Secretary Edward Bennett, who insists that school material on AIDS stress his own version of moral values.

Koop asks commercial TV to do what he, as the nation's highest health official, does not do – tell the people about condoms, or go further, and make them widely and freely available. Koop wants others to wage massive informational campaigns about AIDS, but he does not commandeer prime television time to warn the nation's people of their peril.

Koop presented his "agenda for action" against AIDS to a Harvard forum this week. Again, it was more talk about action than a schedule for attacking AIDS. For Koop, as for the nation, the major impediment to AIDS action is a White House with blinders on.

THE ☼ SUN

Baltimore, MD, February 15, 1987

Surgeon General C. Everett Koop has done the politically unthinkable. He has gone before a House subcommittee on health and called for condom advertising on television to prevent the spread of AIDS among those people "who will not practice abstinence or monogamy."

Condoms? Abstinence or monogamy? Those are fighting words in this country. But Dr. Koop is saddled with the burden of trying to rein in a disease that, unfortunately, is transmitted through sexual contact. The very nature of AIDS requires the surgeon general to verbalize what few want to hear.

Not surprisingly, Dr. Koop's recommendation fired up the ire of a number of conservative committee members who argued that advertisements for condoms would be offensive to some viewers, that they would encourage promiscuity and that they would not serve desired moral goals.

The opposition is understandable. Promiscuity is not desirable. Further, for people who are opposed to the public discussion of sex on moral or religious grounds, advertisements for condoms may evoke discomfort, even anger. But equally as disquieting should be the more than 20,000 sexual innuendos and encounters aired every year on television, and the countless ads for everything from toothpaste to cars that blatantly sanction carefree sex.

Planned Parenthood recently launched a campaign to point out the error of airing messages that indicate such encounters are desirable, and that they occur without planning and without consequences. If teen-age pregnancy is unconvincing testimony, surely the threat of AIDS should have an impact. Dr. Koop argues that given the potential spread of the deadly disease, advertisements for condoms — the only protection outside of abstinence or monogamy — are unequivocally "necessary" as a matter of public health.

The surgeon general has volunteered to work with the major condom manufacturers to develop ads that point up the public health aspects of condom use and do not encourage sexual activity. Television stations nationwide air public health messages about the dangers of smoking without making the habit appear desirable. The same should be possible in the fight against AIDS.

Clearly, jumping into such a campaign without fuller participation with manufacturers and broader legislative consent would be high-handed. But Dr. Koop's basic commitment to make public health information more accessible to a vulnerable public deserves high praise.

AKRON BEACON JOURNAL

Akron, OH, February 5, 1987

AMERICANS are a contorted mess when it comes to sex.

On the one hand, signs of sex are everywhere in our lives. Television is probably the most useful example. We watch Abby Ewing, her brother-in-law, J.R., and Alexis use sex as a tool of pleasure and power. Stations were bombarded with calls from viewers when *L.A. Law* first introduced the "venus butterfly." For a long time, Frank and Joyce closed out almost every *Hill Street Blues* just before the foreplay began.

Then, of course, there's Dr. Ruth, the ads for jeans and Van Heusen shirts, not to mention those for maxi pads, minipads and douches. Americans have a steady diet of sex imagery and products, and of course, television is just the most prominent carrier of the message.

But there's another side. Suggest that ads for condoms run on TV and a furor erupts. Indeed, that's what has happened of late, and it makes little sense, especially in the context of the spread of AIDS. TV stations have banned cigarette ads from the airwaves because Marlboros and the rest can damage your health, but when confronted with the possibility of saving lives by running ads for condoms, stations balked.

The problem is not just with television — newspapers and magazines have said no to ads for condoms. Part of the issue is that parents simply fear their children discovering sex and want to limit their exposure to it wherever they can. Still, is it unreasonable for these ads to be barred? Contraceptives are hardly a rarity in American life.

When the secretary of Health and Human Services says that AIDS could exceed the proportions of the Black Plague, it is best to spread the word about safe sex. No question Trojan and others stand to profit from access to TV, and some people will be upset, but an awareness of condoms is a part of educating ourselves about a deadly disease.

THE SACRAMENTO BEE

Sacramento, CA, February 15, 1987

Given all that we know about AIDS, it's a simple fact of life, as the surgeon general has repeatedly pointed out, that next to sexual abstinence, the best defense against the spread of the infection is a condom. Admitting this basic truth and doing everything possible to get the message out doesn't entail an endorsement of promiscuity. It's a fundamental issue of medical necessity which, as the surgeon general told Congress the other day, should "overwhelm all other considerations."

But from the very beginning, the clinical battle against this health crisis has been undercut by moral and social attitudes that should be irrelevant to the practical task of saving lives. The conflict several years ago over closing the gay bathhouses in San Francisco, for example, was fought on questions that had more to do with political power than human health. Similarly, the focus on what should be the central issue — how best to prevent the disease from spreading — seems to be getting lost in the current squabble over the refusal of all three television networks, most local broadcasters, and a number of national magazines to allow any advertising of condoms.

For the most part, media executives explain their reluctance on the basis of an untested intuition that such advertising might offend their audience. That's completely irresponsible. Human lives are involved here, after all. It's perfectly possible to devise a tasteful commercial for prophylactics, and almost anyone could name a dozen products these same executives already advertise that are even more offensive and don't do anyone nearly as much good.

In an effort to deflect criticism, KRON-TV in San Francisco has recently announced that it will carry commercials for condoms, but it's turning over the revenues from its advertising fees to AIDS research and will require the condom manufacturers to contribute the same amount. It's nice to support AIDS research, of course, but there's no reason to penalize the manufacturers with what amounts to double-billing for the sake of a public relations ploy. If the station owners are really squeamish about taking money for this kind of advertising, then they should run public service commercials that don't recommend any particular brand. In fact, funding for the preparation of public service ads of this kind should be a part of the budget for the surgeon general, California's AIDS education program, Planned Parenthood and the Advertising Council.

Conservative moralists in the Reagan administration such as the Department of Education's Undersecretary Gary Bauer have expressed their concern that any effort to promote the use of condoms will just reinforce the arguments raised by their adversaries in the gay community that AIDS is not susceptible to moral solutions. But what does that debate have to do with the undeniable scientific evidence on which the surgeon general's recommendations are based? And who's responsible for setting national health policy anyway? The truth is that both condoms and abstinence will work in preventing the spread of AIDS. It's madness to deny one for the sake of the other.

The Oregonian

Portland, OR, February 13, 1987

AIDS has an enormous capacity to cause discomfort even in those who are not afflicted with its deadly virus. The latest victims of AIDS discomfort are television, newspaper and magazine executives throughout the country wrestling with the issue of whether to accept advertising for condoms — the one known physical prophylactic against AIDS short of total abstinence.

More compelling than the delicate question of whether such ads may be offensive to some viewers or readers should be the brutal fact that AIDS is offensive to life, all life, regardless of its religious or moral persuasion.

Particularly uncompelling is the three major television networks' sudden, sanctimonious concern for their viewers' sensibilities. We couldn't have said it better than Rep. Henry A. Waxman, D-Calif., the chairman of a House health subcommittee before which the three networks, on behalf of their viewers, primly demurred from the U.S. surgeon general's request that they carry advertising for condoms:

"The routine promotion of condoms through advertising has been stopped by networks who are so hypocritically priggish that they refuse to describe disease control as they promote disease transmission. While portraying thousands of sexual encounters each year in programming and while marketing thousands of products using sex appeal, television is unwilling to give the life-saving information about safe sex and condoms."

It is not unreasonable to expect from those who have promoted, through their programming, the kind of freewheeling sexual activity that puts its practitioners at higher risk of AIDS a higher obligation to promote prevention through their advertising.

The Honolulu Advertiser

Honolulu, HI, February 12, 1987

When the conservative surgeon general of a conservative administration says it's time for condom ads on television to help slow the spread of AIDS, then it is time.

Surgeon General C. Everett Koop took that message to Congress, but the three major networks say they are keeping their self-imposed ban on condom ads for now, leaving the decision to local stations, except those the networks own.

In Hawaii, the major television stations and daily newspapers, including this one, say tasteful, health-oriented condom ads will be accepted.

Though they can't offer perfect protection, condoms are the only known barrier against the spread of an epidemic which health officials say soon may be more devastating than the Black Plague.

Any medium going into the home where it may be seen by children must be concerned about standards of taste and decency. As a birth control device, condoms do offend the religious beliefs of many people.

But the network claims of modesty over condoms rings hollow. Masses of sexual material (some useful, some exploitive) are used daily to raise ratings and sell products. Discussion of every imaginable infirmity, from backache to bed-wetting, seems appropriate for broadcast, especially if something to alleviate it is for sale.

AIDS is a life and death matter. Not just advertising, but instruction on how properly to use condoms and stern reminders to do so would be a valuable public service, especially on television where so many young people and non-readers get their information.

Abstinence or monogamous fidelity (plus non-use of intravenous drugs) are the only absolute defense against AIDS. But the reality is that many people cannot or will not adhere to these safeguards. Information about condoms is essential to public health in this situation, and the media have a responsibility to help distribute it.

"TV ADS FOR CONDOMS? BUT THAT WOULD BE IN BAD TASTE !!! "

RAPID CITY JOURNAL—

Rapid City, SD, February 15, 1987

Curious. When it comes to increasing ratings, television networks just love controversy. When it comes to saving lives, they hate it.

The American Broadcasting Company has been holding staunch against criticism of its miniseries "Amerika" which begins Sunday evening. The television show portrays an America of the future which has been taken over by the Soviet Union. The concept offends some people and some national advertisers have bailed out rather than risk being connected with the show.

ABC's position to broadcast anyway is correct. The outrage over the series is as silly as the series itself probably is — network miniseries rarely provide much intellectual nutrition. "Amerika" may be of the same ilk as several boneheaded theater presentations of recent years. "Red Dawn," "Rocky IV" and "Rambo" were all cardboard anti-communist diatribes. Those movies made one wonder: If communists are really that stupid, one-dimensional and incompetent, why are we so troubled by them? That's precisely the danger with such portrayals. They lead to unwarranted contempt and underestimation.

However "Amerika" portrays the Russkies and the Yanks, the series is fictional, like a romance novel or "1984." The show may even be a boring dud as are so many heavily promoted television extravaganzas. But just because the concept is offensive to some people's sensibilities is no reason not to screen it. Everything — from "Soap" to "L.A. Law" to "The 700 Club" — is offensive for some reason to some people. The point is that in our society a multiplicity of views are available — and should always be available.

Censorship is more dangerous than exposure to an insipid television series.

Which makes it even more curious that ABC has joined with CBS and NBC in refusing to air commercials for condoms and other birth control devices. Certainly such commercials could be no more offensive than the ads featuring mother and daughter enthusiastically discussing the joys of vinegar douche, or the commercial featuring a leotard-clad female gymnast singing the praises of a sanitary napkin after working out on the parallel bars. Although those are more logical than Mrs. Olson always carrying a three-pound can of coffee around with her.

Bad taste and potential objections aside, promoting responsible sex makes a lot of sense — particularly on a medium where entertainment programs abound with couples diving into bed with nary a question about AIDs or protection against pregnancy. With the growing fear of AIDs and the ill-consequences of unintended teen-age pregnancy, condom commercials have the potential of preventing disaster and death. That's more than can be said for miniseries.

So why does ABC hang tough on commies and whimper over accepting birth control ads? There's one major difference. Birth-control ads will offend viewers who will protest to the networks. The controversy over "Amerika" will cause more people to tune in. It is not a coincidence that the program airs during sweeps week, when networks fight for the highest ratings. Much of the controversy doubtless has been hyped by the network to increase interest.

People offended by "Amerika" have the same choice people offended by birth control commercials have — ignore it. It may be a good week to put Bruce Springsteen on the stereo and curl up with a mystery novel.

The Boston Herald

Boston, MA, February 18, 1987

YOU'VE probably seens the ad: a freckle-faced girl in pig tails proudly declaims into the camera: "Today I learned to have safe sex." She is followed by a whole host of her cohorts making similar declarations about other aspects of sex education.

If you watched the ad with same kind of open-mouthed surprise that we did, you're not alone. The ad for a WCVB-TV series was pulled the other day after the Rev. E.W. Jackson Sr. and several others protested to Channel 5 management that the ads conveyed the impression that it's all right to have sex "as long as it's safe."

The ad was made to promote a series by reporter Jay Schadler on the danger AIDS represents to heterosexuals, certainly a serious topic worthy of exploring. But the guy who did the ad apparently never saw the series.

Granted, news organizations sometimes make mistakes, just like everyone else. But the question must be asked: on such a sensitive topic, isn't anyone talking to anyone else over there at Channel 5?

This promises to be one of the most important issues of the next few years. It deserves more serious treatment and we are glad Channel 5 has recognized that fact.

The Des Moines Register

Des Moines, IA, February 12, 1987

There is a hopeful sign that a long taboo is being broken for the public good. That taboo is against the advertising of contraceptives, condoms in particular.

In the not-too-distant past, it was illegal in many places to carry contraceptive advertising. For the most part, such laws are no longer on the books.

But the concern over giving offense to readers and viewers has continued to stop many segments of the media from accepting such advertising.

But now that is beginning to change. The reason is concern over the spread of the deadly AIDS virus. Medical research indicates that proper use of condoms can slow or possibly stop transmission of acquired immune deficiency syndrome, which is costing society hundreds of millions of dollars as it kills its victims.

Several independent television stations have begun to air carefully scripted commercials that deal with the issue of safe sex without necessarily mentioning either AIDS or birth control. Even muted by rules that strive to balance community standards of good taste with an essential message, these ads serve an important purpose.

Many general-interest magazines have been carrying various types of contraceptive advertising for quite some time, but Time Inc. has just announced that its publications now will accept AIDS-related condom advertising.

Some major newspapers have also reviewed their advertising policies and have begun to accept such advertising. The Register's policy is to accept advertising for all legal services and products — provided such ads meet our standards of taste and truthfulness. The Register will accept condom ads that meet those standards.

This week, U.S. Surgeon General C. Everett Koop told a congressional panel that he favors advertising condoms on network television because of the national health threat posed by AIDS.

•

Still, there is concern that society is not completely ready to accept these decisions, and many parts of the media — including the three major networks and many major news publications — continue to steer clear of these ads. This is a difficult decision to make, but it should be weighed according to the seriousness of the problems.

The cost to society for the treatment of AIDS victims is $40,000 to $150,000 a year for each patient. Although the birth-control aspect is the most controversial issue, the cost to society from unwanted, illegitimate pregnancies, especially among teen-agers, also is great — an estimated $5,378 per child in Medicaid and Aid to Dependent Children in the first year alone.

In both cases, lives are at stake: There is no cure for AIDS and its victims die painful deaths. In the case of an unwanted pregnancy, there often is no escape from the cycle of poverty that limits both parent and child.

Both are subjects that cry out for greater public-education efforts, of which ads for condoms would be one part.

Permitting advertising of contraceptives does not promote irresponsible actions; rather it offers a more responsible alternative than sexual roulette to those who already have made a decision about engaging in sex.

The Philadelphia Inquirer

Philadelphia, PA, February 8, 1987

The Journal of the American Medical Association reported last week that a study it commissioned found that condoms can significantly reduce the chance of AIDS being passed between heterosexual partners. (Homosexuals were not included in the study.) This report, supported by other research, confirmed the obvious — an impermeable barrier prevents the spread of sexually transmitted diseases.

For sexually active people in this perilous age, this is important information to have. It can be found in the news columns of this newspaper, but not in its advertising. Nor can it be found in commercials on Philadelphia's network television stations. With few exceptions, the condom is still not considered an acceptable subject for advertising. (The policy at Philadelphia Newspapers Inc., which publishes The Inquirer, is under review.)

Questions of viewer (or reader) taste are not the real impediment. A tasteful condom ad could be no more offensive than those for feminine hygiene deodorants or hemorrhoid remedies. The problem is that condoms are a form of birth control, and there are powerful forces at large in the land that object to anything that promotes birth control.

Until now, the anti-birth-control lobby held sway with little serious opposition. But AIDS changes the equation. It is a terrifying threat to this nation's health, and yet, if people behave prudently, its spread can be curtailed. Condoms help curtail it, and this should be made known in every way possible. While the government, the schools and the medical community have a large role to play in AIDS education, the condom manufacturers should not be prevented from adding to this informational effort through advertising.

Lincoln Journal

Lincoln, NE, February 12, 1987

As of Jan. 9, according to federal record keepers, 29,137 Americans had been confirmed as AIDS cases. Of those, 16,481 already had died. As of Feb. 5, not quite a month later, the updated figures were 30,632 and 17,542. That means 1,495 additional new cases and 1,061 more deaths.

Between 1 million and 1.5 million Americans are now carrying the AIDS virus. Dr. Neil R. Schram, a Los Angeles internist specializing in AIDS, says. "Even if the spread of the virus stopped today, it is believed that 250,000 to 750,000 would come down with the full-blown disease within 10 years," he adds.

Dr. C. Everett Koop, surgeon-general of the United States and an evangelical Presbyterian — not an irrelevant fact in the boiling national controversy — told an audience at Jerry Falwell's Liberty University recently that nearly 100 million people worldwide could die from AIDS by the end of this century if neither a cure nor vaccine is found.

Dr. Koop found himself the surprised target of sharp criticism from his natural allies within the Christian right when last October he implored Americans to halt promiscuous sex — a view with which there is universal lip-service agreement — and also begin sex education in schools as early as third grade, especially warning youngsters about the peril of AIDS. It was that educational call which aroused the fundamentalists.

The same constituency also is offended by the surgeon general's more current appeal to the television networks: Drop your curb on condom advertising. "The threat of AIDS is so great," Dr. Koop pleads, "it overwhelms other considerations."

There are Americans who regard Dr. Koop as an alarmist, inasmuch as the largest percentage of current AIDS victims are homosexuals or careless drug users, both shunned groups erroneously being being regarded as discrete and confined. Some of these also would be people who might nod agreement with evangelist Falwell's cruel determination that "AIDS could be God's judgment against a nation that chooses to live immorally."

Such assessments are objectionable. The anticipated increase in AIDS incidence among just heterosexuals is on the order of being 20-fold. Unacceptable, too, is a belief that the central defense upon which the nation must rely to halt the spread of AIDS is lifetime abstinence from sexual activity.

That is simply unrealistic.

Abstinence always should be the core recommendation of all sex education programs for young people. But humans are extremely sexual beings, and it is pure folly to prattle otherwise. Pragmatism requires us to help people — juvenile and adult — better understand how they can minimize risks to their own health, if they are sexually active.

Condoms are not a guaranteed 100 percent protection against AIDS (or veneral disease, or against becoming pregnant, if employed for contraceptive purposes). But they are the best current defense short of duplicating the behavior of the Roman Catholic clergy.

A University of Miami School of Medicine study of 45 AIDS patients and their families showed condoms "dramatically decreased" the incidence of AIDS, even with the device's shortcomings. A comparable University of California study of more than 100 heterosexual couples in which one partner had AIDS found condoms, properly and consistently used, protected against further AIDS infection.

These are but two research studies, with relatively small sample groups. Nonetheless, they — and other laboratory studies — justify Dr. Koop's appeal to the dominant culture-molding force in the nation, the television networks. Allowing condom advertising on television "would have a positive public health benefit."

The networks are rethinking their bans on such advertising. If executives could grasp the potential severity of the public health problem, that cerebrating would take very little time indeed.

San Francisco Chronicle

San Francisco, CA, February 12, 1987

THE TELEVISION NETWORKS, so quick to fill the nation's airwaves with violence and sex, are bulwarks of Victorian priggishness when it comes to carrying advertising for condoms to slow down the spread of AIDS.

Network representatives who told Congress this week that they are afraid condom ads will offend portions of their viewing audiences seem to have no such moral misgivings about presenting programs heavy with sexual encounters (mostly outside of wedlock), rape, incest, child abuse, criminal behavior and violence in ever-increasing quantities. Sex on television is no longer limited to off-screen heavy breathing, as anyone who watches soap operas can testify.

The networks ought to pay careful attention to the testimony of U.S. Surgeon General C. Everett Koop. In calling for the networks to lift their ban on condom ads, Dr. Koop said the threat of AIDS to the public health is so great "it overwhelms other considerations."

THE NATION'S TOP public health official said that condoms offer the best protection from the AIDS virus for those who will not practice abstinence or monogamy. Dr. Koop, who has urged candor in discussing safe sex practices in the schools, also expressed particular concern about the rise in AIDS cases in the black and Hispanic communities.

If, as medical authorities agree, condoms can slow down the spread of the deadly AIDS virus, then public health considerations must outweigh the possibility that some viewers may take offense if condoms are advertised on television. To a television audience already accustomed to a daily diet of ads dealing with diarrhea, menstrual cramps, genital odors, hemorrhoids and jock itch, a condom ad is not going to be any big deal.

The Kansas City Times

Kansas City, MO, February 13, 1987

Network executives have been busily explaining that condom ads are not suitable for television because innocent families might be looking. Thursday morning families at breakfast might have been looking at CBS when a man in a red T-shirt gave a similar garment to Mariette Hartley, saying that she would look better in it than he would ("What does he mean, Daddy?") and explaining what was a "T" personality. He gave her a quiz and asked viewers to answer along. He wanted to know whether she ever thought of doing unusual sex things. "You mean with my husband?" she asked saucily, and answered, "Well, yes."

Over on ABC David Hartman was interviewing an actress and two actors about their imminent soap opera denouement. It seems the female character had had a baby by one of the two men, no one knew which. ("Why doesn't she know, Mommy?") The script could not be revealed, of course, but each was asked which man it should be. Broad smiles, giggles and preferences were stated.

We don't know what Willard Scott and Gene Shalit were doing on NBC news. Maybe plugging "L.A. Law" which was said to concern, among other things, Stu trying to persuade Ann to move in with him.

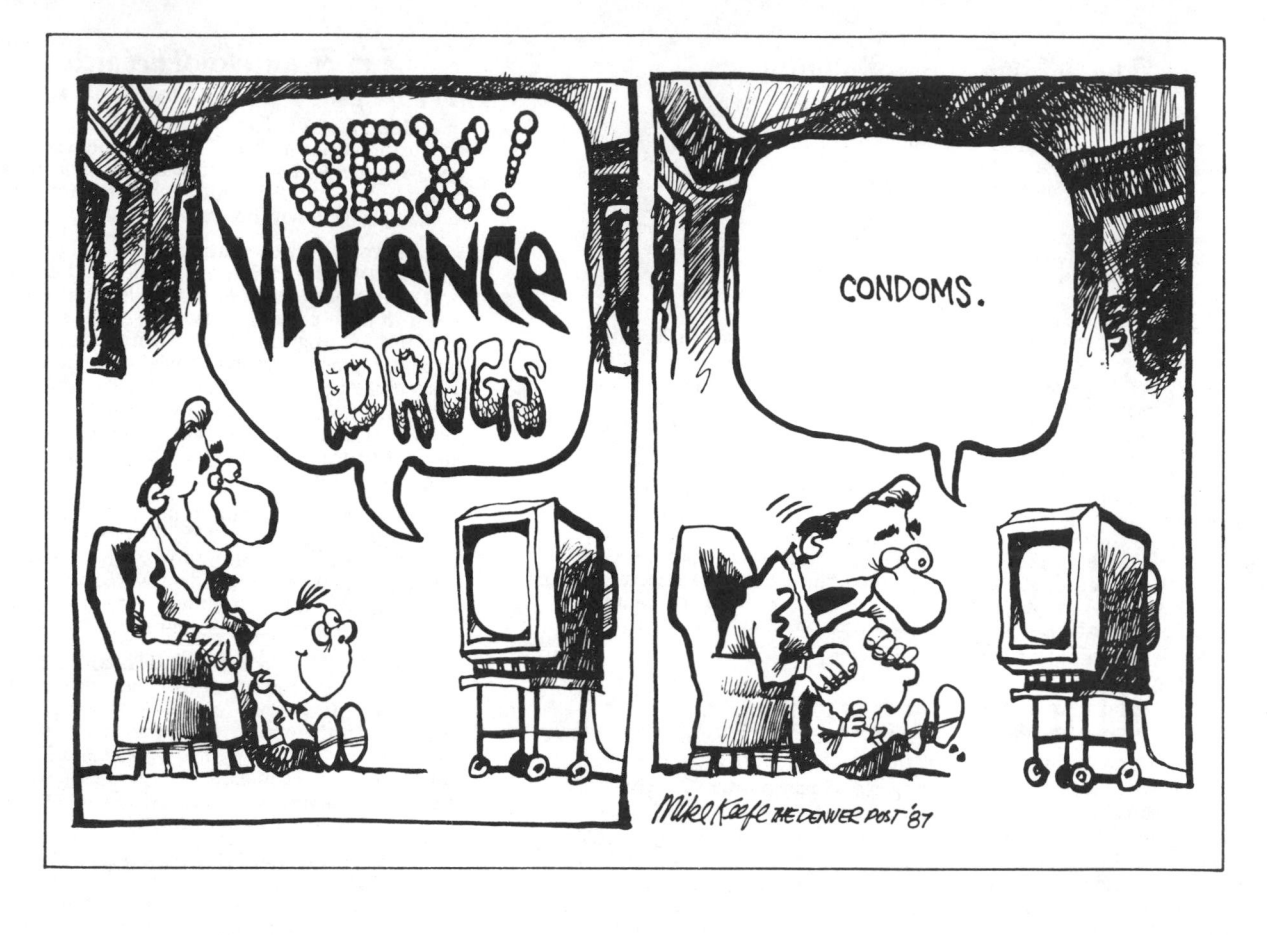

Chicago Tribune

Chicago, IL, February 25, 1987

The search for ways to curb the spread of the deadly disease AIDS has led television stations to question their longstanding ban against advertisements for condoms. CBS, the largest broadcasting operation to change its policy, has made a decision that puts the controversy back at the local level where it belongs. It has decided to allow the local radio and television stations it owns to decide for themselves, while continuing its ban against condom advertising on its network.

The old caveat "sold for the prevention of disease only" on condom packages and vending machines is not as laughable as it used to be. The spread of AIDS, acquired immune deficiency syndrome, has provided a serious, life-saving reason to encourage condom use for those who refuse to practice abstinence or monogamy. Some local television stations, particularly in cities where the AIDS epidemic is most evident, relaxed their policies earlier. Surgeon Gen. C. Everett Koop has encouraged such advertising because condoms do offer effective protection, if used properly by those who insist on taking the risk.

But others, including Joseph Cardinal Bernardin, archbishop of Chicago, fear that condom advertising is an invitation to promiscuity. This position contrasts sharply with the clergy who have made news recently by preaching the virtues of condoms from their pulpits. Some broadcasters have taken the middle-of-the-road position of approving only free public service announcements for condoms. At least, that way no one can accuse the stations of profiting from the controversy.

Concerns for public morality are real, but so is the threat of AIDS. The acceptability of condom advertising to help stop its spread should be left up to the judgment of individual stations, because it is they who know best how to accommodate the needs and moral standards of their communities. Condom advertising can be presented in a manner that is no more suggestive than conventional programming. It should be restricted to hours when children are least likely to be viewing. And it should not exaggerate the effectiveness of condoms at preventing disease, especially when compared with good, old-fashioned moral behavior.

The Union Leader

Manchester, NH, February 22, 1987

The following guest editorial is from the Feb. 13 issue of The Pilot, official newspaper of the Archdiocese of Boston. It expresses very well the opinion held by the Loeb newspapers on this issue.

As a matter of fact, Publisher Nackey S. Loeb announced last week that the New Hampshire Sunday News and The Union Leader will not knowingly accept any advertisements for condom sales.

The Surgeon General says that condoms may help prevent the spread of AIDS. Elsewhere in this issue, Michael Pakoluk raises serious questions about that advice. But for the sake of the argument, let's assume condoms are at least partially effective — that they do provide some protection against AIDS. Should we then encourage the use of condoms? Should family newspapers and television stations carry advertisements for condom sales?

Unless human nature has suddenly changed, the primary market for condoms is not among happily married couples. The proposed advertisements do not appeal to someone whose spouse somehow contracted AIDS. No; anyone who has seen the ads knows that they have a different audience in mind.

The purpose of condoms, as explained in the proposed advertisements, is to make it possible to have sexual intercourse without knowing very much about one's partner. Let's be blunt. Condoms (according to the advertisers' claim) make it safer to have sexual relations with strangers.

Now if the AIDS epidemic has taught us anything it is this: sexual promiscuity — that is, having sexual relations with strangers — is mortally dangerous. So condom advertisers are catering to precisely the sort of behavior that transmits AIDS. And, of course, making a profit on the deal.

We know two things about automobile safety: 1) drunk drivers run a much higher risk of having an accident, and 2) when accidents happen, seat belts save lives. Does anyone seriously recommend an advertising campaign that would urge drunk drivers to buckle up? Of course not; anyone who seemed to condone drunk driving would be labelled, quite accurately, as irresponsible.

By the same logic, if the media want to help stop the spread of AIDS, the only responsible approach is to campaign against sexual promiscuity.

The Record

Hackensack, NJ, February 16, 1987

It was about a decade ago that television discovered the string bikini and the skin-tight T-shirt. Suddenly, breasts, hips, and bellybuttons were everywhere. So were double entendres. But television is never more hypocritical than when it is being salacious. Beneath that leering exterior is a timid and prudish medium with a near-Victorian horror of sex.

In testimony last week before a House subcommittee, Surgeon-General C. Everett Koop called on the big three television networks to lift their ban on commercials for condoms — which, short of monogamy and abstinence, remain the most effective way to block the spread of AIDS. Dr. Koop urged that the ads be aimed especially at minority audiences, since blacks and Hispanics suffer disproportionately the incurable, invariably fatal disease.

Other countries are way ahead of the United States in this area. Adweek magazine reports that the Swedish Sex Education Association runs a television spot in which a woman blows up a prophylactic to the size of a balloon while explaining that condoms are the only reliable way to avoid transmitting sexual disease. "And if he won't put it on," she then says, "tell him it's all off." With that, she lets the air out of the condom, which shrinks to nothing.

But as far as the U.S. television networks are concerned, the spread of AIDS is somebody else's problem. When the television executives testified before the House subcommittee, they wheedled and made excuses. Ralph Daniels, vice-president for broadcasting standards at NBC, worried that some viewers would object to condom advertising "on moral or religious grounds" because, they believe, it "inherently delivers a message about sexual permissiveness which they find objectionable." Vice-presidents of CBS and Capital Cities/ABC voiced similar concerns.

What is really offensive here is the cowardice of the three networks. Condom ads literally save lives. But for fear of an irate letter from a pressure group, ABC, NBC, and CBS refuse to run them. Their behavior is both irresponsible and maddeningly hypocritical. "Sexual permissiveness" is common coin on the networks. If the pressure groups can handle Joan Rivers and J.R. Ewing, they can handle this.

Richmond Times-Dispatch

Richmond, VA, February 16, 1987

The condomization of America proceeds apace. The surgeon general of the United States continues to press television networks to carry condom advertisements as an AIDS-fighting measure. Newsweek features "Kids and Contraceptives" on its cover. In Amherst, N.Y., a Unitarian Universalist Church minister dispenses condoms to his Sunday congregation.

"Too much delicacy about contraception and disease can be harmful," writes George Will in Newsweek. "But a certain delicacy about intimate things does not need to be defended; it is inherently good."

Right. And at Greenfield (Mass.) Community College, condoms evidently are considered a delicacy: Officials there were handing them out to students in the main lobby the other day in a large glass bowl mixed with butterscotch and peppermint candies. Handing them out like candy will not make students more likely to satisfy their sexual appetites, but will prevent pregnancy and disease, officials declared. Uh huh.

America may be gaining condom sense, but that's not necessarily the same thing as common sense.

DENVER POST

Denver, CO, February 22, 1987

NOW THAT some Denver television stations have decided to accept commercials for condoms, it's time to ask whether such ads will really do much to stem the AIDS epidemic. At this point, the answer has to be: maybe, but only indirectly.

This is because the key to controlling the disease isn't simply to persuade people to *buy* "safe sex" products, but to induce sexually active Americans to *use* them.

Public health officials report that the use of prophylactics has ballooned in the homosexual community. But heterosexuals, who still don't perceive AIDS as a serious threat, may not embrace condoms as readily — for several reasons.

Let's face it. These funny-looking gimmicks aren't the easiest instruments of self-protection to deploy. They're annoying to handle, inconvenient to install and tricky to remove — as well as occasionally defective.

Worse, condoms can raise embarrassing questions. Merely by opening the package, a man may indicate misgivings about his bed partner — or that he himself is contagious. And needless to say, a woman who offers a condom to her suitor may convey the same messages. Such troubling connotations can wipe out all the excitement of the encounter.

This would suggest that condoms may sometimes serve as sexual safeguards even when they are left unused. But it's more likely that the prospect of an awkward disruption to the proceedings may lead the parties involved to abandon all precautions — as simply too great a threat to the mutual trust that led to the intimate moment in the first place. Never mind that casual sex without protection might prove suicidal; when the bedroom is only a few steps away, the graveyard can look mighty distant.

Still, advertising the latex sheaths on TV — and thereby making them more socially acceptable — may be the only way to overcome people's natural reluctance.

It certainly wouldn't make sense to require the use of condoms as a matter of law, any more than it makes sense to outlaw "unnatural" acts among consenting adults. And trying to scare people into using condoms won't work either, any more than years of cancer warnings have succeeded in getting people to quit smoking.

Minneapolis Star and Tribune

Minneapolis, MN, February 20, 1987

For fear of offending viewers, the three major television networks refuse to run condom commercials. The networks also fear antagonizing their local affiliates, and believe that one way to avoid that is to observe the longstanding broadcasting policy against advertising birth-control products. Never mind that condoms, abstinence and monogamy protect against the spread of the deadly AIDS virus. Never mind that more people understand the need to combat unwanted teen pregnancies as well as AIDS.

Selective sensitivity to local sensibilities earns the networks a lot of richly deserved criticism. But it also creates a chink in the networks' armor that local stations and viewers can exploit to force more enlightened policies. To its credit, KSTP in the Twin Cities has become one of the grass-roots forces for change.

In its recently launched campaign against the spread of AIDS, KSTP changed its policy and decided to accept condom ads. The station becomes one of a handful in the country to do so. As more stations accept such advertising, the networks are likely to outgrow their phobia against accepting such ads. Because public complaints at the local level might undo that progress, the content and presentation of the ads are critical. Commercials should stress health issues without dwelling on the mechanical aspects of condom use.

Critics point out that KSTP continues to run network fare that portrays casual sexual encounters, a seeming contradiction to its public-service campaign for abstinence and its decision to run health-related condom ads. But KSTP is using a powerful tool for influencing future television treatment of sex and health questions. By running the ads, it is showing the networks that local stations and viewers are ready for such information.

The Idaho STATESMAN

Boise, ID, February 14, 1987

We live in an age of frankness, where prime-time television deals with situations as diverse as euthanasia and teen-age pregnancy. We live in a time of television, whose all-pervasive eye educates as well as entertains. We live, unfortunately, in the age of AIDS.

Television networks could help stem the AIDS epidemic by allowing their powerful medium to advertise condoms as one means of controlling the spread of this always fatal disease. The U.S. Surgeon General, Dr. C. Everett Koop, said as much this week while testifying before a House subcommittee:

"The threat of AIDS is so great that it overwhelms other considerations. And advertising, I think therefore, is necessary in reference to condoms and would have a positive public health value."

We would go a step further. Magazines and newspapers also could advertise the use of condoms as one means of protection against contracting or spreading AIDS.

We do not advocate the advertising of condoms as a means of birth control. This is a public health issue, not a birth control issue.

Although local stations in 11 major cities do allow condom advertisements, the three commercial networks do not, citing the potential for offending their viewers.

Dr. Koop properly urged abstinence as the first line of defense against contracting acquired immune deficiency syndrome, and monogamy as the second. But recognizing that many will not follow that advice, Dr. Koop said the American public must realize that the third and only other protection is to use condoms.

Advertisements for condoms must be done tastefully, under strict network advertising guidelines, stressing the public health message. As Dr. Koop noted, such ads would provide health education at no cost to the government.

Some argue that advertisng condoms will promote sexual promiscuity; but sex, like condoms, is no secret to the young or anyone else. We can't turn our heads from the fact that AIDS has been diagnosed in more than 20,000 Americans since 1979, half of whom have died. There is no cure and no one, so far, has survived.

Understanding that condoms do not provide 100 percent protection, Dr. Koop told the subcommittee that they're better than no protection. By allowing tasteful ads for condoms, television, newspapers and magazines could meet their challenge to inform, educate and, in this case, protect.

Edmonton Journal

Edmonton, Alta., February 23, 1987

CBC's conditional acceptance of public-health advertisements that promote condoms as an effective way to avoid contracting AIDS is a positive step toward heightening public awareness of a terrifying disease that is deadly efficient 100 per cent of the time.

Initially, the CBC balked at changing its policy on condom advertising, fearing it would signal the network's approval of casual sex. But with the disease spreading and with no cure in sight, a compromise was reached: the ads will be balanced with the admonition that "self-restraint" is another way to reduce the risk of contracting AIDS. The ads will not be specific commercial advertisements for condoms. Strictly speaking, they will be public health messages, part of a five-year, $3.7-million campaign by the Canadian Public Health Association.

However effective the ads are in slowing the spread of AIDS, they should be seen only as the start of a broad public-education campaign. While the CBC and such private networks as CTV and Global will soon carry advertisements for condoms, all three major U.S. networks — ABC, NBC, and CBS — still refuse to carry condom ads. Only in the last month has Time Inc. of New York announced that its magazines would accept condom ads and in the last couple of years, few Canadian publications have been asked to accept them.

Since 1981, 898 cases of AIDS have been reported in Canada; 471 of those people have died. In the U.S., more than 30,000 cases have been reported and another 1.5 million people are thought to be carriers.

Various objections can be raised to ads for condoms — that they indicate a tacit approval of casual sex, that they may offend some members of the community. But all of these objections pale in the face of numbers such as these.

The Birmingham News

Birmingham, AL, February 26, 1987

The current debate over the refusal of the major television networks to air condom advertisements, which U.S. Surgeon General C. Everett Koop says are necessary since condoms can help prevent the transmission of AIDS, is obscuring a basic moral issue that the disease raises.

We support all efforts to stem the AIDS epidemic in this nation, but there is a better weapon against this sexually transmitted disease — a return to morality. Only a moral society can stop an illness that owes its persistence to drug abusers and those involved in casual and plural sexual relationships.

AIDS, of course, is not limited to the immoral. The innocent babies of mothers infected with the disease may also suffer from it, so may people with other serious illnesses who, through no fault of their own, have received a transfusion of tainted blood.

But we now know that the exchange of bodily fluids necessary for the transmission of acquired immune deficiency syndrome most often occurs between people who have lifestyles that involve multiple sexual partners, including prostitutes, or sharing hypodermics with fellow drug abusers.

By any traditional moral standards, such lifestyles are wrong.

We agree with the Rev. Edward E. Jones of Shreveport, La., president of the National Baptist Convention of America, who at that organization's convention in Mobile this week declared that fighting AIDS is a "job of education, a job of stern religious teachings and principles."

So long as we tolerate widespread immorality, we cannot effectively stop the spread of AIDS. Condoms may be part of the solution to slowing the spread of this particular disease, but condoms are not the answer to our real problem.

Stopping AIDS — or the disease that eventually will take its place, as AIDS took the place of herpes in our national consciousness — requires us to change our way of thinking. The emphasis must be on morality.

Wisconsin ▲ State Journal
Madison, WI, February 25, 1987

Like the other catch phrase of 1987 — "safe sex" — the rubric of "restoring American competitiveness" can mean different things to different people.

Nowhere does the definition seem broader than on Capitol Hill. Few in Congress have extolled the virtues of "trade protectionism" since former Speaker Thomas "Tip" O'Neill took up golfing, but a lot of formerly protectionist-minded lawmakers are standing tall for "restoring American competitiveness."

Were all of the protectionists converted en masse, or are some of the legislative proposals to improve U.S. competitiveness in the world economy just old-fashioned protectionism in a new wrapper?

This year, Democratic legislators seem to be defining protectionism as any narrowly focused bill to protect a specific industry. Broadly based measures against countries that export more to the United States than the United States exports to them fall under the heading of "restoring American competitiveness."

Neither the House nor Senate trade bills contain language protecting specific industries, for example, but both share broader provisions considered protectionist by the Reagan administration.

One amendment written by U.S. Rep. Richard Gephardt, a Missouri Democrat who announced his presidential campaign this week, would require the president to retaliate against countries that have large trade surpluses with the United States by imposing tariffs and other import restrictions.

Maybe that's "restoring American competitiveness" in Gephardt's book, but in any pre-1987 dictionary, it would fit nicely under the definition of protectionism.

ARGUS-LEADER
Sioux Falls, SD, February 21, 1987

It was almost funny hearing network television representatives explain why NBC, CBS and ABC do not carry condom advertisements.

They told a U.S. House panel last week that such ads would be offensive to viewers of many affiliate stations.

That assessment came from **Editorial** networks that promote promiscuity daily in daytime soap operas and evening dramas. That's an odd assessment because there's probably less gratuitous sexual titillation in an hour of condom ads than in a typical episode of *Dynasty*.

Maybe network executives are starting to recognize the irony. Encouragingly, their resistance to condom ads is breaking down.

Three CBS-owned television stations and NBC's New York station announced Thursday that they would start accepting such ads.

In addition, ABC announced it would begin running a 30-second public service message with C. Everett Koop, U.S. surgeon general, saying the best protection against sexual transmission of AIDS, except for abstinence, is a condom.

Network resistance to such ads would have been comical if AIDS were not such a serious health threat in the United States.

AIDS is a disease that impairs the body's ability to fight infection and cancer. Researchers think it is caused by a virus transmitted through body fluids, mainly blood and semen.

The U.S. Centers for Disease Control in Atlanta predicts that 270,000 Americans will come down with the disease within five years, and 179,000 will die.

AIDS was first diagnosed in 1981. By mid-1985, half of the nation's 12,000 victims were dead. More than 29,000 Americans are known to suffer from the disease now, and the number is growing.

AIDS has been diagnosed most commonly in homosexuals, but it also can be spread heterosexually.

Koop deserves credit for helping break down network resistance.

Koop told members of the U.S. panel that he favors advertising condoms on network television because the national health threat posed by AIDS overwhelms other considerations.

Local stations already are free to carry condom ads on their own. Ads are carried in 11 markets. We haven't heard any public outcry. The only outcry we heard came from network officials.

Network officials apparently misjudged public sensitivity and common sense.

Such ads might provide a valuable health service if, as encouraged by Koop, the ads promote disease prevention rather than sexual activity. The ads also might help reduce the problem of teen-age pregnancy.

We welcome the networks' change of heart.

Winnipeg Free Press
Winnipeg, Man., February 22, 1987

The shyness which the television networks in Canada and the United States have exhibited in the matter of advertisements promoting the use of condoms in sexual activities might be comical if it were not so blatantly hypocritical. The issue arises because of the concern of governments and health agencies in both countries about the spread of AIDS and how best to control it. The use of condoms, it is said, will help prevent the spread of AIDS through "safe sex".

There is legitimate reason to doubt the wisdom of such a campaign. Condoms are not one hundred per cent effective in preventing either pregnancy or infection by other, more familiar, sexually transmitted diseases. They do help, but there is a danger that some infected people may believe that their use will enable them to have safe sex with healthy partners, or that healthy people may believe that their use will eliminate the dangers of a promiscuous life-style.

Neither this nor any other legitimate reason is advanced by the networks in refusing to allow the advertisements. Rather, they cite the question of good taste and a reluctance to be seen to be condoning sexual promiscuity or casual sex. This comes from the same networks that routinely use sex and sexism as advertising gimmicks to promote both their own and others' products in commercials, and which, in their programming, whether it be comedy, drama or movies, depict people fornicating at a furious pace, usually without any of the serious consequences that can result from sexual relationships in real life.

Real life, of course, has as little to do with television advertising and programming as does good taste, which has long been a stranger in network boardrooms. It seems likely now that most networks will permit the advertising of condoms in the interests of the public and their own profits — in Canada CTV and Global networks have indicated they will approve it, and the CBC has amended its policy. This may or may not help to limit the spread of AIDS, but now that the networks have discovered the issues of good taste and sexual responsibility, they could do all of society a favor if they were to consider them in all of their advertising and programming instead of only matters of the public health.

St. Paul Pioneer Press & Dispatch
St. Paul, MN, February 23, 1987

How often events seem to repeat themselves. That's what history has taught over and over again. And now the current issue of Discover magazine adds a new twist to the old aphorism.

In a truncated tracing of condoms, which itself was taken from a new book ("Johnny Come Lately") on the history of condoms, Discover draws a rarely made connection. It is between today's enlistment of the protective sheaths for men in the growing fight against AIDS, and the fact that condoms were used in similar efforts to combat outbreaks of syphilis in medieval times.

Truth be known, the use of condoms began two thousand years ago when the Chinese made them from oiled silk paper, the magazine reports.

We're not sure what to make of this. Except that seeing such an article in a popular family magazine devoted to science and technology adds to a belief that the debate over condom advertising is becoming increasingly irrelevant. Whether the product is promoted in advertising or not, it is receiving plenty of attention in the news columns of print media and on the talk and news shows of the electronics.

INDEX

A

ABC--*see AMERICAN Broadcasting Company*
ACQUIRED Immune Deficiency (AIDS)--
  see individual topics
AFRICA--*see also individual countries*
  New AIDS findings reported--4-5
  WHO gives alert on AIDS in Africa--22-23
AFRICAN Swine Fever
  New AIDS findings reported--4-5
AFSV--*see AFRICAN Swine Fever*
AIDS--*see individual topics*
AIDS Medical Foundation
  House ok's closing bathhouses--180-181
AIDS Testing--*see HUMAN & Civil Rights*
AIDS-Related Complex (ARC)
  Large AIDS toll projected in US--32-33
  FDA approves US AZT sales--36-39
ALBERT Einstein Medical Center
  Reagan names AIDS advisory panel--84-87
AMA--*see AMERICAN Medical Association*
AMERICAN Broadcasting Company
  Fear of AIDS puts condom ads on tv--202-211
AMERICAN Council of Life Insurance
  Insurers weigh tests--150-153
AMERICAN Foundation for AIDS Research (AmFAR)
  Reagan seeks wider AIDS testing--72-83
AMERICAN Medical Association (AMA)
  Meese details prison screening program--126-133
  Supreme Court bars victim
    disease bias in jobs--164-167
AMERICAN Red Cross
  AIDS linked to blood transfusions--6-17
ANSELL America's Lifestyles
  Fear of AIDS puts condom ads on tv--202-211
ARC--*see AIDS-Related Complex*
ARCADIA, Florida
  AIDS panic rocks town--114-123
ARLINE, Gene
  Supreme Court bars victims
    disease bias in jobs--164-167
AZIDOTHYMIDINE (AZT)
  Anti-AIDS drug found successful--28-31
  FDA approves US sales--36-39
AZT--*see AZIDOTHYMIDINE*

B

BATHHOUSES--*see SEX*
BENNETT, Education Secretary William
  Reagan speaks out on AIDS--68-71
BILL of Rights, U.S.
  Supreme Court upholds Georgia sodomy law--154-163
BIRTH Issues
  Mandatory testing opposed by CDC forum--136-147
  Spread of AIDS continues, public fear mounts--182-193

BLACKMUN, Supreme Court Justice Harry A.
  Court uphold Georgia sodomy law--154-163
BLACKS--*see MINORITIES*
BLOOD Transfusions--*see SCIENCE & Technology*
BOWEN, Secretary of Health & Human Services Otis
  House backs catastrophic health care plan--168-171
BRANDT, Edward N.
  AIDS called top priority--46-49
BRENNAN, Supreme Court Justice William J.
  Supreme Court bars victim
    disease bias in jobs--164-167
BROADCASTING
  Fear of AIDS puts condom ads on tv--202-211
BUREAU of Prisons
  Meese details prison screening program--126-133
BURROUGHS Wellcome Co.
  Anti-AIDS drug, AZT, found successful--28-31
  FDA approves US AZT sales--36-39
BUSH, Vice President George
  3rd annual AIDS parley held--72-83
BUSINESS & Industry
  AIDS linked to blood transfusions--6-17
  WHO gives alert on AIDS in Africa--22-23
  Anti-AIDS drug, AZT, found successful--28-31
  FDA approves US AZT sales--36-39
  Fear of AIDS puts condom ads on tv--202-211

C

CANCER--*see SCIENCE & Technology*
CARTER-Wallace, Inc.
  Fear of AIDS puts condom ads on tv--202-211
CBS--*see COLUMBIA Broadcasting Company*
CENTERS for Disease Control, U.S. (CDC)
  AIDS linked to blood transfusions--6-17
  Researchers report finding probable AIDS virus--18-19
  AIDS virus evidence mounts--20-21
  WHO gives alert on AIDS in Africa--22-23
  Large AIDS toll projected for US--32-33
  Hospital infections spread alarm--40-43
  AIDS fears effect school attendance--96-103
  Mandatory testing opposed by CDC forum--136-147
  Spread of AIDS continues--182-193
  AIDS spread through addicted population--200-201
CHERMANN, Jean Claude
  FDA approves French AIDS drug--24-27
CIVIL Rights--*see HUMAN & Civil Rights*
COCKRILL, Dr. Franklin 3rd
  Leaders quit AIDS panel--88-93
COLUMBIA Broadcasting Company
  Fear of AIDS puts condom ads on tv--202-211
CONDOMS--*see PROPHYLACTICS*
CONGRESS
  Heckler defends administration effort--46-49
  Justice Dept says AIDS victims can be fired--62-67
  House backs catastrophic health care plan--168-171
  House ok's closing bathhouses--180-181

CONSTITUTION, U.S.
    Supreme Court upholds Georgia sodomy law--154-163
    Supreme Court bars victim
        disease bias in jobs--164-167
CONWAY-Welch, Colleen
    Reagan names AIDS advisory panel--84-87
COOPER, Assistant Attorney General Charles
    Justice Dept says AIDS victims can be fired--62-67
CRIME
    AIDS panic rocks Florida town--114-123
    Supreme Court upholds Georgia sodomy law--154-163
CURRAN, Dr. James
    AIDS virus evidence mounts;
        exposures feared wider--20-21
    WHO gives alert on AIDS in Africa--22-23
    Large AIDS toll projected in US--32-33

D

DAVIS, Dr. Richard
    Reagan names AIDS advisory panel--84-87
DE VOS, Richard
    Reagan names AIDS advisory panel--84-87
DEFENSE & Military
    All in military to be tested--134-135
    Mandatory testing opposed by CDC forum--136-147
DES Jarlais, Dr. Don C.
    AIDS spreads through addicted population--200-201
DETROIT
    Fear of AIDS puts condom ads on tv--202-211
DOWDLE, Dr. Walter
    Mandatory testing opposed by CDC forum--136-147

E

EDUCATION
    WHO gives alert on AIDS in Africa--22-23
    AIDS called top priority--46-49
    Koop wants AIDS classes--50-61
    Reagan speaks out on AIDS--68-71
    Reagan names AIDS advisory panel--84-87
    AIDS fears effect school attendance--96-103
    Public education stressed
        as prevention measure--104-111
    Ryan White allowed to return to school--112-113
    AIDS panic rocks Florida town--114-123
    Supreme Court bars victim
        disease bias in jobs--164-167
EDUCATION, U.S. Dept. of
    House ok's closing bathhouses--180-181
ELISA--see ENZYME-Linked Immunosorbent Assay
ENZYME-Linked Immunosorbent Assay (ELISA)
    All in military to be tested--134-135
    Spread of AIDS continues, public fear mounts--182-193

F

FAUCI, Anthony
    FDA approves French AIDS drug--24-27
FDA--see FOOD & Drug Administration
FILMS
    Rock Hudson dies of AIDS--194-199
FLORIDA
    Supreme Court bars victim
        disease bias in jobs--164-167
FOOD & Drug Administration (FDA)
    AIDS linked to blood transfusions--6-17

    Approves French AIDS drug--24-27
    Anti-AIDS drug, AZT, found successful--28-31
    Approves US AZT sales--36-39
FOREIGN Aid
    WHO gives alert on AIDS in Africa--22-23
FRANCE
    Researchers report finding probable AIDS virus--18-1
    AIDS virus evidence mounts;
        exposures feared wider--20-21
    FDA approves French AIDS drug--24-27
    Rock Hudson dies of AIDS--194-199
FRIEDLAND, Dr. Gerald
    AIDS through casual contact ruled out--34-35

G

GALLO, Dr. Robert
    AIDS virus evidence mounts--20-21
GAY Men's Health Crisis
    Reagan names AIDS advisory panel--84-87
GAY Rights--see HUMAN & Civil Rights
GEORGIA
    Supreme Court upholds sodomy law--154-163
GREAT Britain
    FDA approves US AZT sales--36-39
    Fear of AIDS puts condom ads on tv--202-211

H

HAITI
    New AIDS findings reported--4-5
    AIDS guidelines issued--174-179
HARVARD University
    New AIDS findings reported--4-5
HEALTH--see MEDICINE & Health
HEALTH & Human Services, U.S. Dept. of (HHS)
    AIDS linked to blood transfusions--6-17
    Researchers report finding probable AIDS virus--18-19
    Anti-AIDS drug, AZT, found successful--28-31
    Large AIDS toll projected in US--32-33
    Heckler defends administration effort--46-49
    Justice Dept says AIDS victims can be fired--62-67
    House backs catastrophic health care plan--168-171
    House ok's closing bathhouses--180-181
    Spread of AIDS continues, public fear mounts--182-193
HECKLER, Margaret
    Researchers report finding probable AIDS virus--18-19
    Defends administration effort--46-49
HISPANICS--see MINORITIES
HOMOSEXUALS
    Researchers report finding probable AIDS virus--18-19
    Large AIDS toll projected in US--32-33
    Koop wants AIDS classes--50-61
    Reagan seeks widers AIDS testing;
        3rd annual parley held--72-83
    Reagan names advisory panel--84-87
    Public education stressed
        as prevention measure--104-111
    Meese detals prison screening program--126-133
    All in military to be tested--134-135
    Mandatory testing opposed by CDC forum--136-147
    Insurers weigh tests--150-153
    Supreme Court upholds Georgia sodomy law--154-163
    AIDS guidelines issued--174-179
    House ok's closing bathhouses--180-181
    Spread of AIDS continues, public fear mounts--182-19:
    Rock Hudson dies of AIDS--194-199

HOUSE of Representatives--see CONGRESS
HOUSE Ways & Means Committee
    House backs catastrophic health care plan--168 171
HPA-23
    FDA approves French AIDS drug--24-27
HTLV-3
    Leukemia virus linked to AIDS--4-5
    AIDS virus evidence mounts--20-21
HUDSON, Rock (1926-1985)
    Spread of AIDS continues, public fear mounts--182-193
    Film star dies of AIDS--194-199
HUGHES, Dr. James
    Hospital infections spread alarm--40-43
HUMAN & Civil Rights
    Koop wants AIDS classes--50-61
    Justice Dept says AIDS victims can be fired--62-67
    Reagan seeks widers AIDS testing--72-83
    Reagan names AIDS advisory panel--84-87
    AIDS fears effect school attendance--96-103
    Public education stressed
        as prevention measure--104-111
    Ryan White allowed to return to school--112-113
    AIDS panic rocks Florida town--114-123
    Meese details prison screening program--126-133
    All in military to be tested--134-135
    Mandatory testing opposed by CDC forum--136-147
    Meese orders testing for immigrants--148-149
    Supreme Court upholds Georgia sodomy law--154-163
    Supreme Court bars victim bias in jobs--164-167
    AIDS guidelines issued--174-179
    House ok's closing bathhouses--180-181

I

ILLEGAL Aliens--see IMMIGRATION
IMMIGRATION
    Reagan seeks wider AIDS testing--72-83
    Meese orders testing for immigrants--148-149
IMMIGRATION and Naturalization Service
    Meese testing for immigrants--148-149
INDIANA
    Ryan White allowed to return to school--112-113
INDIANAPOLIS
    Fear of AIDS puts condom ads on tv--202-211
INS--see IMMIGRATION and Naturalization Service
INSTITUT Pasteur
    FDA approves French AIDS drug--24-27
    Rock Hudson dies of AIDS--194-199
INSURANCE Issues
    Insurers weigh tests--150-153
    House backs catastrophic health care plan--168-171
INTRAVENOUS Drug Use--see NARCOTICS

J

JUSTICE, U.S. Dept of
    Says AIDS victims can be fired--62-67
    Meese details prison screening program--126-133
    Meese orders testing for immigrants--148-149
    Supreme Court bars victim
        disease bias in jobs--164-167

K

KAPOSI's Sarcoma
    Leukemia virus linked to AIDS--4-5

KENNAMER, Dr. Rexford
    Rock Hudson dies of AIDS--194-199
KENYA
    WHO gives alert on AIDS in Africa--22-23
KOCH, New York City Mayor Edward I.
    AIDS spreads through addicted population--200-201
KOOP, Surgeon General C. Everett
    Wants AIDS classes--50-61
    Reagan speaks out on AIDS--68-71
    Public education stressed
        as prevention measure--104-111
KRIM, Dr. Mathilde
    House ok's closing bathhouses--180-181
KRON-TV
    Fear of AIDS puts condom ads on tv--202-211

L

LABOR & Employment
    Supreme Court bars victim
        disease bias in jobs--164-167
    House ok's closing bathhouses--180-181
LABOR, U.S. Dept. of
    House ok's closing bathhouses--180-181
LANCET (magazine)
    New AIDS findings reported--4-5
LAV--see SCIENCE & Technology
LAW & Legal System
    Justice Dept says AIDS victims can be fired--62-67
    Ryan White allowed to return to school--112-113
    Meese details prison screening program--126-133
    Meese orders testing for immigrants--148-149
    Supreme Court upholds Georgia sodomy law--154-163
LAW Enforcement
    3rd annual AIDS parley held--72-83
    Meese orders testing for immigrants--148-149
LEE, Dr. Burton 3rd
    Reagan names AIDS advisory panel--84-87
LILLY, Dr. Frank
    Reagan names AIDS advisory panel--84-87
LOS Angeles
    AIDS linked to blood transfusions--6-17

M

MACDONALD, Dr. Donald Ian
    Large AIDS toll projected in US--32-33
MANN, Dr. Jonathan
    WHO gives alert on AIDS in Africa--22-23
MARKOWSKI, Joseph Edward
    Charged with attempted murder--126-133
MASSACHUSETTS
    AIDS fears effect school attendance--96-103
MAYBERRY, Dr. W. Eugene
    Reagan names AIDS advisory panel--84-87
    Leaders quit AIDS panel--88-93
MEDICAID
    FDA approves US AZT sales--36-39
MEDICARE
    House backs catastrophic health care plan--168-171
MEDICINE & Health
    AIDS linked to blood transfusions--6-17
    Researchers report finding probable AIDS virus--18-19
    AIDS virus evidence mounts;
        exposures feared wider--20-21
    WHO gives alert on AIDS in Africa--22-23
    FDA approves French AIDS drug--24-27

Large AIDS toll projected in US--32-33
AIDS through casual contact ruled out--34-35
FDA approves US sales--36-39
Hospital infections spread alarm--40-43
AIDS called top priority--46-49
Justice Dept says AIDS victims can be fired--62-67
Reagan speaks out on AIDS--68-71
Reagan seeks wider AIDS testing;
   3rd annual AIDS parley held--72-83
Reagan names AIDS advisory panel--84-87
AIDS fears effect school attendance--96-103
Ryan White allowed to return to school--112-113
AIDS panic rocks Florida town--114-123
Meese details prison screening program--126-133
All in military to be tested--134-135
Meese orders testing for immigrants--148-149
Insurers weigh tests--150-153
House backs catastrophic health care plan--168-171
AIDS guidelines issued--174-179
House ok's closing bathhouses--180-181
Spread of AIDS continues, public fear mounts--182-193
AIDS spreads through addicted population--200-201
Fear of AIDS puts condom ads on tv--202-211
MEESE, Attorney General Edwin 3rd
Justice Dept says AIDS victims can be fired--62-67
Details prison screening program--126-133
Meese orders testing for immigrants--148-149
MILITARY--*see DEFENSE & Military*
MINORITIES
Insurers weight tests--150-153
AIDS spreads through population--200-201
MONTAGNIER, Dr. Luc
AIDS virus evidence mounts--20-21
MONTIFIORE Medical Center
AIDS through casual contact ruled out--34-35
MYERS, Dr. Woodrow Jr.
Reagan names AIDS advisory panel--84-87
Leaders quit AIDS panel--88-93

N

NARCOTICS
Large AIDS toll projected in US--32-33
Koop wants AIDS classes--50-61
Meese details prison screening program--126-133
Insurers weight tests--150-153
AIDS guidelines issued--174-179
Spread of AIDS continues, public fear mounts--182-193
AIDS spreads through addicted population--200-201
NATIONAL Academy of Sciences
Public education stressed
   as prevention measure--104-111
NATIONAL Association of Insurance Commissioners
Insurers weigh tests--150-153
NATIONAL Broadcasting Company (NBC)
Public education stressed
   as prevention measure--104-111
Fear of AIDS puts condom ads on tv--202-211
NATIONAL Cancer Institute
Researchers report finding probable AIDS virus--18-19
AIDS virus evidence mounts--20-21
NATIONAL Gay Task Force
AIDS guidelines issued--174-179
NATIONAL Institute of Justice
Meese details prison screening program--126-133
NATIONAL Institutes of Health (NIH)
AIDS linked to blood transfusions--6-17
Anti-AIDS drug, AZT, found successful--28-31

NATIONAL Institute of Mental Health (NIMH)
AIDS linked to blood transfusions--6-17
NBC--*see NATIONAL Broadcasting Company*
NEW Jersey
AIDS linked to blood transfusions--6-17
AIDS spreads through addicted population--200-201
NEW York City
AIDS linked to blood transfusions--6-17
AIDS fears effect school attendance--96-103
House ok's closing bathhouses--180-181
AIDS spreads through addicted population--200-201
NEW York State
AIDS linked to blood transfusions--6-17
NEW York State Division of Substance Abuse Services
AIDS spreads through addicted population--200-201
NEW York Times (newspaper)
WHO gives alert on AIDS in Africa--22-23
Justice Dept says AIDS victims can be fired--62-67
AIDS guidelines issued--174-179
NEW England Journal of Medicine (magazine)
New AIDS findings reported--4-5
AIDS linked to blood transfusions--6-17
WHO gives alert on AIDS in Africa--22-23
FDA approves French AIDS drug--24-27
AIDS through casual contact ruled out--34-35
NIH--*see NATIONAL Institutes of Health*
NIMH--*see NATIONAL Institute of Mental Health*

O

O'CONNOR, Archbishop John J.
Reagan names AIDS advisory panel--84-87

P

PACIFIC Dunlop Ltd.
Fear of AIDS puts condom ads on tv--202-211
PLASMA Production Associates
Markowski charged with attempted murder--126-133
POLITICS
Reagan names AIDS advisory panel--84-87
Leaders quit AIDS panel--88-93
PRESIDENTIAL Commission on AIDS
Reagan names advisory panel--84-87
Leaders quit panel--88-93
PRISONS
Meese details screening program--126-133
PROPHYLACTICS
Koop wants AIDS classes--50-61
Fear of AIDS puts condom ads on tv--202-211
PUBLIC Health Service, U.S. (PHS)
Researchers report finding probable AIDS virus--18-19
Large AIDS toll projected in US--32-33
AIDS called top priority--46-49
AIDS guidelines issued--174-179
PULLEN, Rep. Penny (R, Ill.)
Reagan names AIDS advisory panel--84-87

R

RAY, Clifford and Louise
AIDS panic rocks Florida town--114-123
REAGAN Administration
AIDS called top priority--46-49
Koop wants AIDS classes--50-61
Justice Dept says AIDS victims can be fired--62-67
Reagan speaks out on AIDS--68-71

3rd annual AIDS parley held--72-83
Leaders quit AIDS panel--88-93
Public education stressed
  as prevention measure--104-111
Meese details prison screening program--126-133
Meese order testing for immigrants--148-149
House backs catastrophic health care plan--168-171
REAGAN, First Lady Nancy
  Reagan names AIDS advisory panel--84-87
REAGAN, President Ronald
  Speaks out on AIDS--68-71
  Seeks wider AIDS testing--72-83
  Names AIDS advisory panel--84-87
  Leaders quit AIDS panel--88-93
  House backs catastrophic health care plan--168-171
REHABILITATION Act (1973)
  Justice Dept says AIDS victims can be fired--62-67
  Supreme Court bars victim
    disease bias in jobs--164-167
REHNQUIST, Chief Supreme Court Justice William H.
  Supreme court bars vicitm
    disease bias in jobs--164-167
RETROVIR--see AZIDOTHYMIDINE
ROSTENKOWSKI, Rep. Dan (D, Ill.)
  House backs catastrophic health care plan--168-171
RUTHERFORD, George
  Reagan names AIDS advisory panel--84-87
RWANDA
  WHO gives alert on AIDS in Africa--22-23

S

SAN Francisco, Ca.
  AIDS guidelines issued--174-179
  House ok's closing bathhouses--180-181
  Fear of AIDS puts condom ads on tv--202-211
SATURDAY Evening Post (magazine)
  Reagan names AIDS advisory panel--84-87
SCHOOLS
  Koop wants AIDS classes--50-61
  AIDS fears effect attendance--96-103
  Ryan White allowed to return to school--112-113
  AIDS panic rocks Florida town--114-123
  Supreme Court bars victim
    disease bias in jobs--164-167
SCHOOL Board of Nassau County v. Arline
  Supreme Court bars victim
    disease bias in jobs--164-167
SCHWEIKER, Richard
  Insurers weigh tests--150-153
SCIENCE & Technology
  Leukemia virus linked to AIDS--4-5
  AIDS linked to blood transfusions--6-17
  Researchers report finding probable AIDS virus--18-19
  AIDS virus evidence mounts;
    exposures feared wider--20-21
  FDA approves French AIDS drug--24-27
  Anti-AIDS drug, AZT, found successful--28-31
  AIDS through casual contact ruled out--34-35
  FDA approves US AZT sales--36-39
  Reagan seeks wider AIDS testing;
    3rd annual AIDS parley held--72-83
  Reagan names AIDS advisory panel--84-87
  Public education stressed as
    prevention measure--104-111
  All in military to be tested--134-135
  Mandatory testing opposed by CDC forum--136-147
  AIDS guidelines issued--174-179

Spread of AIDS continues,
  public fear mounts--182-193
Rock Hudson dies of AIDS--194-199
SCIENCE (magazine)
  Leukemia virus linked to AIDS--4-5
  AIDS virus virus evidence mounts--20-21
SCREEN Actors Guild
  Spread of AIDS continues, public fear mounts--182-193
SERVASS, Dr. Cory
  Reagan names AIDS advisory panel--84-87
SEX
  Researchers report finding probable AIDS virus--18-19
  Large AIDS toll projected for US--32-33
  AIDS through casual contact ruled out--34-35
  Koop wants AIDS classes--50-61
  Reagan speaks out on AIDS--68-71
  Reagan seeks wider AIDS testing;
    3rd annual AIDS parley held--72-83
  Public education stressed
    as prevention measure--104-111
  Meese detals prison screening program--126-133
  All in military to be tested--134-135
  Mandatory testing opposed by CDC forum--136-147
  Insurers weigh tests--150-153
  Supreme Court upholds Georgia sodomy law--154-163
  AIDS guidelines issued--174-179
  House ok's closing bathhouses--180-181
  Rock Hudson dies of AIDS--194-199
  Fear of AIDS puts condom ads on tv--202-211
SEX Education--see EDUCATION
SHEAFFER, Linda
  Reagan names AIDS advisory panel--84-87
  Leaders quit AIDS panel--88-93
SOCIAL Security
  House backs catastrophic health care plan--168-171
SODOMY
  Supreme Court upholds Georgia law--154-163
STATE, U.S. Department of
  Mandatory testing opposed by CDC forum--136-147
SUBSTANCE Abuse
  AIDS spreads through addicted population--200-201
SUPREME Court
  Upholds Georgia sodomy law--154-163
  Bars victim disease bias in jobs--164-167
SURAMIN
  FDA approves French AIDS drug--24-27

T

TANZANIA
  WHO gives alert on AIDS in Africa--22-23
TAYLOR, Elizabeth
  Reagan seeks wider AIDS testing--72-83
TEAS, Jane
  New AIDS findings reported--4-5
TECHNOLOGY Assessment, Office of
  Heckler defends administration effort--46-49
TELEVISION
  Rock Hudson dies of AIDS--194-199
  Fear of AIDS puts condom ads on tv--202-211
THIRD International Conference on AIDS
  3rd annual parley held--72-83
THIRD International Conference on AIDS
  AIDS spreads through addicted population--200-201

U

U.N.--see UNITED Nations

U.S. Court of Appeals for the 11th Circuit
   Justice Dept says AIDS victims can be fired--62-67
UGANDA
   WHO gives alert on AIDS in Africa--22-23
UNITED Nations (U.N.)
   WHO gives alert on AIDS in Africa--22-23

W

WALSH, Dr. William
   Reagan names AIDS advisory panel--84-87
WARD, Phillip S.
   House ok's closing bathhouses--180-181
WATKINS, Adm. James (ret.)
   Leaders quit AIDS panel--88-93
WELFARE
   FDA approves US AZT sales--36-39
WHITE, Ryan
   AIDS fears effect school attendance--96-103
   Allowed to return to school--112-113

WHITE, Suprme Court Justice Byron R.
   Court upholds Georgia sodomy law--154-163
WHO--*see WORLD Health Organization*
WINDOM, Dr. Robert E.
   Anti-AIDS drug, AZT, found successful--28-31
WOMEN'S Issues
   Mandatory testing opposed by CDC forum--136-147
   AIDS spreads through population--200-201
WORLD Health Organization (WHO)
   Gives alert on AIDS in Africa--22-23
WRTV-TV
   Fear of AIDS puts condom ads on tv--202-211
WXYZ-TV
   Fear of AIDS puts condom ads on tv--202-211

Z

ZAIRE
   WHO gives alert on AIDS in Africa--22-23
ZAMBIA
   WHO gives alert on AIDS in Africa--22-23